DICTIONARY OF AMERICAN MEDICAL BIOGRAPHY

An institution is the lengthened shadow of one man.
Emerson, *Self-Reliance*

DICTIONARY OF AMERICAN MEDICAL BIOGRAPHY

Martin Kaufman, Stuart Galishoff,
Todd L. Savitt, Editors

Joseph Carvalho III, Editorial Associate

Volume II

M-Z

GREENWOOD PRESS
Westport, Connecticut • London, England

Library of Congress Cataloging in Publication Data
Main entry under title:

Dictionary of American medical biography.

 Bibliography: p.
 Includes index.
 1. Medicine—United States—Biography. 2. Public
health personnel—United States—Biography. 3. Healers
—United States—Biography. I. Kaufman, Martin,
1940-   . II. Galishoff, Stuart, 1940-   . III. Savitt,
Todd L., 1943-   . [DNLM: 1. Physicians—United
States—Biography. 2. History of medicine, modern—
United States. WZ 140 AA1 D5]
R153.D53   1984   610'.92'2 [B]   82-21110
ISBN 0-313-21378-X (lib. bdg.) set
ISBN 0-313-24333-6 (vol. 1)
ISBN 0-313-24334-4 (vol. 2)

Library of Congress Catalog Card Number: 82-21110
ISBN: 0-313-21378-X

First published in 1984

Greenwood Press
A division of Congressional Information Service, Inc.
88 Post Road West
Westport, Connecticut 06881

Printed in the United States of America

10 9 8 7 6 5 4 3 2 1

Contents

DICTIONARY OF
AMERICAN
MEDICAL
BIOGRAPHY

M

McBURNEY, CHARLES (February 17, 1845, Roxbury, Mass.-November 7, 1913, Brookline, Mass). *Physician; Abdominal surgery.* Son of Charles, businessman, and Rosine (Horton) McBurney. Married Margaret Willoughby Weston, 1874; three children. EDUCATION: Harvard University: 1866, B.A.; and 1869, M.A.; 1870, M.D., College of Physicians and Surgeons (Columbia); 1870-71, intern, Bellevue Hospital; 1871-72, studied medicine and surgery, Vienna, Paris, and London. CAREER: 1872-1907, practiced medicine, New York City; at College of Physicians and Surgeons: 1873-80, anatomy faculty; and 1880-1907, surgery faculty; visiting surgeon: 1875-88, St. Luke's Hospital; and 1888-1900, Bellevue Hospital; 1889-1901, sole visiting surgeon, Roosevelt Hospital; consulting surgeon: New York, Presbyterian, St. Luke's, and Orthopedic hospitals and Hospital for Ruptured and Crippled. CONTRIBUTIONS: Foremost authority on the diagnosis and treatment of appendicitis. Demonstrated that a diseased appendix could readily be detected by applying pressure on a tender point, known thereafter as "McBurney's point" (1889). Originated "McBurney's incision" to expose the appendix without cutting the muscle fibres (1894). An early advocate of operating for appendicitis before rupture had occurred. With the aid of a private donation, built an elaborate private operating pavilion in Roosevelt Hospital which became nationally prominent as a center for surgical research and teaching. Required his assistants to wear rubber gloves shortly after William S. Halsted (q.v.) had advised it, insisting that they be worn by all members of the operating team.

WRITINGS: "Experience with Early Operative Interference in Cases of Disease of the Vermiform Appendix," *N.Y. Med. J.* 50 (1889): 676-84; "The Incision Made in the Abdominal Wall in Cases of Appendicitis, with a Description of a New Method of Operating," *Annals of Surg.* 20 (Jul. 1894): 38-43; "The Use of Rubber Gloves in Operative Surgery," ibid., 28 (1898): 108-19. REFERENCES: *BHM* (1970-74), 168; (1975-79), 114; *DAB*, 11: 555-56; Kelly and Burrage (1928), 768; *NCAB* 26: 48-49;

John H. Talbott, *Biographical Hist. of Med.* (1970), 1018-19; *Who Was Who in Am.*, 1:797.

S. Galishoff

MacCALLUM, WILLIAM GEORGE (April 18, 1874, Dunnville, Ontario, Canada-February 3, 1944, Baltimore, Md.). *Physician; Pathology; Endocrinology.* Son of George Alexander, physician, and Florence Octavia (Eakins) MacCallum. Never married. EDUCATION: 1894, A.B., University of Toronto; 1897, M.D., Johns Hopkins Medical School; 1897-98, intern, Johns Hopkins Hospital; 1900, studied in Leipzig. CAREER: Pathology faculty: 1899-1908, 1917-43, Johns Hopkins Medical School; and 1909-17, College of Physicians and Surgeons (Columbia); pathology staff: 1909-17, Presbyterian Hospital; and 1917-43, Johns Hopkins Hospital. CONTRIBUTIONS: Studied and described the flagellation of the malaria parasite of the crow and identified this phenomenon as part of the sexual cycle of the parasite; predicted and observed the same process in human malaria (1896-97). With Carl Voegtlin (q.v.), distinguished the independent functions of the thyroid and parathyroid glands; showed that calcium metabolism is controlled by the parathyroid gland and demonstrated that tetany could be prevented by the injection of calcium salts (1905). Demonstrated in surgical experiments on animals that the acinar tissue of the pancreas could be destroyed without causing diabetes so long as the islets of Langerhans were left intact (1909). Wrote an innovative *Textbook of Pathology* (1916) that went through seven editions in his lifetime and was widely used in medical schools; approached the subject by examining the etiology of various diseases and their effects on the entire body instead of the usual practice of cataloging all of the morbid processes that can effect each separate organ. Persuaded New York City to establish a medical examiner's office headed by a trained pathologist to replace the city coroner, a political post. Made major studies of the microscopic anatomy of the lymphatic system (1903) and of epidemic pneumonia among soldiers during World War I. Worked also on hypophysis, vaccinia, and correlation of the organs of internal secretion. Promoted the study of medical history at Johns Hopkins and wrote a biography of *William Stewart Halsted, Surgeon* (1930).

WRITINGS: "On the Flagellated Form of the Malarial Parasite," *Lancet* 2 (Nov. 13, 1897): 1240-41; "On the Haematozoan Infections of Birds," *J. of Experimental Med.* 3 (1898): 117; "On the Relation of the Parathyroid to Calcium Metabolism and the Nature of Tetany," *Johns Hopkins Hosp. Bull.* 19 (1908): 91-92, with C. Voegtlin; "On the Relation of the Islands of Langerhans to Glycosuria," *ibid.*, 20 (1909): 265-68. A bibliography is in *BMNAS*. REFERENCES: *BMNAS* 23 (1945): 339-64; *DAB*, Supplement 3: 482-83; A. McGehee Harvey, *Adventures in Med. Research* (1976), 22-31; Miller, *BHM* p. 66; *NCAB*, 32: 499; *Trans. Assoc. of Am. Physicians* 58 (1944): 28-30; *Who Was Who in Am.*, 2: 335-36.

S. Galishoff

McCAW, JAMES BROWN (July 12, 1823, Richmond, Va.-August 13, 1906, Richmond). *Physician; Administrator.* Son of Dr. William Reid, physician, and Ann Ludwell (Brown) McCaw. Married Delia Patteson, 1845; nine children.

EDUCATION: Premedical education, Richmond Academy; 1844, M.D., University of the City of New York. CAREER: 1843-1901, private physician, Richmond, Va.; 1853-55, editor, *Virginia Medical and Surgical Journal*; 1856-59, co-editor, *Virginia Medical Journal*; 1858-60, 1865-68, professor of chemistry, Medical College of Virginia; 1862-65, surgeon-in-charge of Chimborazo Hospital, Richmond; 1864-65, editor, *Confederate States Medical Journal*; 1868-83, professor of the practice of medicine, Medical College of Virginia; and dean of the medical school for many years; 1871-73, editor, *Virginia Clinical Record*; former president, Richmond Academy of Medicine. CONTRIBUTIONS: Renowned for leadership of the medical profession. Founder, Medical Society of Virginia, and editor of a number of medical journals. During the Civil War, helped establish and directed the Confederate Army's Chimborazo Hospital, the largest military hospital in existence at that time; 76,000 patients were treated during the war, and the hospital was considered a model of efficiency. Postwar career was a combination of private practice and teaching.

WRITINGS: "Remarks on the Uses and Effects of Sulphate of Quinine," *Stethoscope* 2 (1852): 665-80; "Sick Headache," *Virginia Med. J.* 8 (1857): 34-39. REFERENCES: Wyndham Blanton, *Medicine in Virginia in the Nineteenth Century* (1933); *DAB*, 6, pt. 1: 575-76; F. H. Garrison, "Dr. James Brown McCaw," *Old Dominion J. of Med. and Surg.* 5 (1906): 65-66; John R. Gildersleeve, "History of Chimborazo Hospital, Richmond, Va., and Its Medical Officers During 1861-1865," *Virginia Med. Semi-Monthly* 9 (1906): 148-54; Howard A. Kelly, *Cyclopedia of Med. Biog.* (1912).

P. Addis

McCAW, WALTER DREW (February 10, 1863, Richmond, Va.-July 8, 1939, New York, N.Y.). *Physician; Military surgeon.* Son of James B. (q.v.), physician, and Delia (Patteson) McCaw. Never married. EDUCATION: Premedical education, Richmond private schools; 1882, M.D., Medical College of Virginia; 1884, M.D., College of Physicians and Surgeons, N.Y. (Columbia University). CAREER: 1884-98, assistant surgeon, U.S. Army; 1898-1901, major and surgeon, Spanish-American War; 1902-13, librarian, Surgeon General's office, Washington, D.C.; in charge of museum and library division; and professor of military hygiene and later professor of military and tropical medicine, Army Medical School; 1914-15, army chief surgeon, Philippines, in charge of division hospital at Manila; 1916-17, department surgeon, southern department, Fort Sam Houston; 1918-19, chief surgeon, American Expeditionary Force, World War I; 1919-27, assistant surgeon-general and brigadier general. CONTRIBUTIONS: Outstanding military surgeon, administrator, and professor. An expert on tropical and military medicine.

WRITINGS: Contributed chapters on "tropical surgery" to *Keen's Surgery* 4 (1908): 1075-1138. REFERENCES: Wyndham Blanton, *Medicine in Virginia in the Nineteenth Century* (1933); *NCAB*, A: 89.

P. Addis

McCLELLAN, GEORGE (December 23, 1796, Woodstock, Conn.-May 9, 1847, Philadelphia, Pa.). *Physician; Surgeon; Medical educator.* Son of James, principal, Woodstock Academy and Eunice (Eldredge) McClellan. Married Elizabeth Brinton, 1820; five children, including Gen. George B. McClellan. ED-UCATION: Woodstock Academy; 1816, A.B., Yale University; medical student of Dr. Thomas Hubbard and John Syng Dorsey (q.v.); 1819, M.D., University of Pennsylvania; resident student, hospital of the Philadelphia Almshouse. CA-REER: 1821-25, founded and taught at Institution for Diseases of Eye and Ear; taught anatomy and surgery at home; at Jefferson College (Jefferson Medical College): 1825, founded medical department; and 1826-38, professor of surgery; 1839, founded medical department, Pennsylvania (Gettysburg) College. CON-TRIBUTIONS: Was a highly regarded surgeon and a promoter of medical education.

WRITINGS: *Principles and Practice of Surgery* (1848, published posthumously). REF-ERENCES: *Autobiography of S. D. Gross* (1887); *BHM* (1970-74), 114; *DAB*, 6: 579-81; S. D. Gross, ed., *Lives of Eminent American Physicians and Surgeons of the Nine-teenth Century* (1861); *NCAB*, 4: 139; *Trans., Coll. of Physicians of Phila.* (1846-49).

D. I. Lansing

McCLENNAN, ALONZO CLIFTON (May 1, 1855, Columbia, S.C.-October 4, 1912, Charleston, S.C.). *Physician; Surgeon.* Son of Harriet (Kennedy) McClennan. Married Ida Veronica Ridley, 1883; three children. EDUCATION: Wilbraham Academy (Mass.); University of South Carolina; 1879, appointed to U.S. Naval Academy; 1880, M.D. and pharmacy degree, Howard University. CAREER: Medical practice: 1880, Columbia; 1880-84, Augusta, Ga.; and 1884-1912, Charleston. CONTRIBUTIONS: Leading black physician in late nineteenth- and early twentieth-century Charleston. Established first black-owned drugstore in Charleston (c. 1892). Founded the Hospital and Training School for Nurses (1897) and served as its medical director and surgeon-in-chief (1897-1912). Founded and edited one of the earliest black medical publications, *Hospital Herald*, a monthly journal (1899-1901). Co-founded the Palmetto Medical, Dental, and Pharmaceutical Association, a black organization (1896).

WRITINGS: Brief articles in *Hospital Herald*. REFERENCES: Information obtained from Waring Historical Library, Medical University of South Carolina (Anne K. Donato, curator), Charleston; and Dr. McClennan's granddaughter, Mrs. Maude T. Jenkins, New York City.

T. L. Savitt

McCLURG, JAMES (c. 1746, Elizabeth City County, Va.-July 9, 1823, Richmond, Va.). *Physician.* Son of Dr. Walter McClurg, superintendent, Hampton Small Pox Hospital. Married Elizabeth Seldon, 1779; two children. EDUCATION: 1762, graduated from College of William and Mary; 1770, M.D., University of Edinburgh; 1770-73, postgraduate medical studies, Paris and London. CAREER: c. 1773-1823, private practice, Richmond; during the American Revolution, surgeon, Va. militia, and directed the military hospitals in the state; 1779-83, professor of anatomy and medicine, College of William and Mary; 1787, Va. delegate to the Constitutional Convention; 1786-87, member, Va. Executive

Council; 1797, 1800, 1803, mayor, Richmond; 1820, 1821, first president, Virginia Medical Society. CONTRIBUTIONS: One of the most renowned physicians in Va. during his lifetime. Served as a consulting physician. Essay "De Calore" (1770) is said to anticipate the work of French experimentalists. A second essay on human bile also had great influence on the profession. It developed a new theory in an age when medical theories were very popular.

WRITINGS: "De Calore" (1770); *Experiment upon the Human Bile and Reflections on the Biliary Secretion, with an Introductory Essay* (1772). REFERENCES: Wyndham Blanton, *Medicine in Virginia in the Eighteenth Century* (1931); *DAB*, 6, pt. 1: 596-7; Howard A. Kelly, *Cyclopedia of Am. Med. Biog.* (1912); J. B. McCaw, *A Memoir of James McClurg, M.D.* (1834); *NCAB*, 3: 413; James Thacher, *Am. Med. Biog.* (1828).

P. Addis

McCOLLUM, ELMER VERNER (March 3, 1879, near Fort Scott, Kan.-November 15, 1967, Baltimore, Md.). *Biochemist*. Son of Cornelius Armstrong and Martha (Kidwell) McCollum, farmers. Married Constance Carruth, 1907; five children. EDUCATION: University of Kansas: 1903, A.B.; and 1904, M.A.; Yale University: 1906, Ph.D.; and 1907, postgraduate study. CAREER: 1907-17, agricultural chemistry faculty, University of Wisconsin; chemist, Wisconsin Agricultural Experiment Station; 1917-44, biochemistry faculty, Johns Hopkins University, School of Hygiene and Public Health; 1928-37, nutritional consultant, U.S. Department of Agriculture. CONTRIBUTIONS: Played a prominent role in the discovery of vitamins A, B, and O. One of the first American scientists to employ rats for controlled *in vivo* biochemical experiments. Using these rat colonies, demonstrated that certain fat-soluble and water-soluble substances were necessary for normal health, which he later termed fat soluble A and water soluble B. Artificially producing rickets in animals, proved that vitamin D was the antirachitic factor found in butterfat and codliver oil. Developed the methodology for biochemically analyzing foodstuffs showing that there were nutrients other than carbohydrates, fats, and proteins. Studying the properties and functions of vitamins A, B, C, D, and E, later discovered the significance of many of the minerals necessary for a healthful diet.

WRITINGS: "The Essential Factors in the Diet During Growth," *J. Biol. Chem.* 23 (1915): 231 (with M. Davis); "The Dietary Factors Operating in the Production of Polyneuritus," ibid., 24 (1916): 491 (with C. Kennedy); *The Newer Knowledge of Nutrition*, various ed., (1918-39); "A Study of the Dietary Essential, Water-Soluble B, in Relation to Its Solubility and Stability Toward Reagents," *J. Biol. Chem.* 33 (1918): 55 (with N. Simmonds); "Studies On Experimental Rickets: The Production of Rickets by Diets Low in Phosphorus and Fat-Soluble A," ibid., 47 (1921): 507 (with N. Simmonds, P. G. Shipley, and E. A. Park). Writings listed in *BMFRS* and *BMNAS*. REFERENCES: *BMFRS*, 15: 159-71; *BMNAS*, 45: 263-335; *DSB*, 8: 590-91; Elmer Verner McCollum, *From Kansas Farm Boy to Scientist* (1964); *NCAB* C: 477-78; Eleanor McKnight Synder, "Elmer Verner McCollum," *J. Am. Diet. Assoc.* 52 (1968): 49.

C. Borst

McCORMACK, ARTHUR THOMAS (August 21, 1872, near Howard's Mill, Nelson County, Ky.-August 7, 1943, Louisville, Ky.). *Physician; Public health* *officer*. Son of Joseph Nathaniel (q.v.), physician and sanitarian, and Corinne (Crenshaw) McCormack. Married Mary Moore Tyler, December 15, 1897, four children, divorced; Mrs. Jane Teare Dahlman, October 16, 1924. EDUCATION: 1892, B.A., Ogden College, Bowling Green, Ky.; 1892-93, University of Virginia, Charlottesville, Va.; 1896, M.D., Columbia University, College of Physicians and Surgeons; 1896-97, internship, Paterson General Hospital, Paterson, N.J. CAREER: 1897, began the practice of medicine and surgery, Bowling Green; in Warren County, Ky: 1897-1908, health officer; and 1898-1912, assistant state health officer; 1901-43, founder and editor, *Journal of the Kentucky Medical Association*; 1908-12, established and operated St. Joseph's Hospital (42 bed), Bowling Green, with his father, J. N. McCormack, and their associate, Lillian H. South (q.v.); 1900-1908, surgeon-general, Kentucky National Guard; 1907-43, secretary, Kentucky Medical Association; 1917, at beginning of World War I, commissioned major and organized Base Hospital No. 59; 1917, appointed by General Gorgas to succeed him as chief health officer, Canal Zone (with rank of lt. colonel), where he completed the construction of Ancon (now Gorgas) Hospital; 1922-36, secretary, Kentucky State Board of Health; 1936-43, commissioner of health, Ky.; 1920-c.1930, founder and dean, School of Public Health, University of Louisville; president: 1924, Conference of State and Provincial Health Authorities of North America; 1937, American Public Health Association; and 1940, Southern Medical Association. CONTRIBUTIONS: As a public health officer (1877-1943), made some of his greatest professional contributions. Simultaneously served as secretary, Kentucky Medical Association, and editor, *Journal of the Kentucky Medical Association*, which he helped launch (1901). Through his official offices in the State Department of Health and the Kentucky Medical Association, was instrumental in the enactment of strong public health laws; organized the various divisions of the state health department and secured adequate funds for its support from the state legislature. Continued the effective organization of the Kentucky Medical Association begun by his father.

WRITINGS: Numerous editorials and obituaries in *J. Ky. Med. Assoc.* and portions of public health *Bulletins. Course in Physical Education for the Common Schools of Kentucky* (1920); "Methods of Getting People to Build Privies," *Southern Med. J.* 15 (1922): 818-22. REFERENCES: E. F. Horine, "Arthur Thomas McCormack, 1872-1943," *Ky. Med. J.* 41 (1943): 289-290; *JAMA* 122 (1943): 1201; memorial issue, *Ky. Med. J.* 42 (Aug. 1944): 215-50; *NCAB*, 32: 495.

                                                                                    E. H. Conner

McCORMACK, JOSEPH NATHANIEL (November 9, 1847, near Howard's Mill, Ky.-May 4, 1922, Louisville, Ky.). *Physician; Medical organizer; Public health*. Son of Thomas, farmer and merchant, and Elizabeth (Brown) McCormack. Married Corinne Crenshaw, 1871; one child, Arthur T. McCormack (q.v.). EDUCATION: 1870, M.D., Miami University (Cincinnati, Ohio); 1871, intern, Cincinnati General Hospital. CAREER: Practiced medicine: 1871-75, Nelson County, Ky.; and 1876-83, Bowling Green, Ky.; on Kentucky State Board of Health: *post* 1879, member; 1883-1913, secretary; and 1914-22, state sanitary inspector; 1892, member, International Quarantine Commission; in American Medical Association: 1899-1913, chairman, Special Committee on Reorganization; 1902-7, member, House of Delegates; and 1910-13, member, Council of Health and Public Instruction. CONTRIBUTIONS: Overhauled Ky.'s archaic health laws and greatly improved its public health. Instrumental in securing a medical practice law (1888), licensure laws (1898, 1904), vital statistics law (1908), and a law combining health agencies (1918). Drafted the state's first sanitary code and conducted a statewide, sanitary-education campaign. Was very effective in extending public health reforms to the rural counties. Drafted a new constitution for the AMA that granted membership to physicians in good standing with their local society and created a strong new legislative body, the House of Delegates (1901). Spent next ten years establishing and strengthening county and state medical societies and winning support for the AMA and its journal; work was largely responsible for the rapid growth of the AMA in the early twentieth century.

WRITINGS: "A Plea for Unification and Uniform Organizations of State and County Societies," *Med. Record.* 65 (1904): 104-6; "What the People Should Know About the Doctors and What the Doctors Should Know About Themselves," *Alabama Med. J.* 19 (Dec. 1906): 7; "The New Gospel of Health and Long Life," *Ky. Med. J.* 21 (Jan. 1923): 26. REFERENCES: James G. Burrow, *AMA, Voice of American Medicine* (1963), 28, 36-51; *DAB*, 11: 606-7; John H. Ellis, *Medicine in Kentucky* (1977), 51-57; *JAMA* 78 (1922): 1475; Miller, *BHM*, p. 70.

S. Galishoff

McCREADY, BENJAMIN WILLIAM (October 28, 1813, New York, N.Y.-August 9, 1892, New York). *Physician; Industrial hygiene.* Son of Thomas and Margaret (Miller) McCready. Married Margaret Doyle; Jane Gall; four children. EDUCATION: Studied medicine with John Brodhead Beck, N.Y.; 1835, M.D., College of Physicians and Surgeons (Columbia); c. 1836, house physician, New York Hospital. CAREER: *Post* c. 1837, practiced medicine, New York City; physician, Tombs prison; dispensary physician; at Bellevue Hospital: 1848-73, visiting physician; and 1874-92, consulting physician; founder and teacher, College of Pharmacy; at Bellevue Hospital Medical College: 1861, founder; and 1861-72, materia medica and therapeutics faculty; chief medical examiner, Washington Life Insurance Company (N.Y.). CONTRIBUTIONS: Wrote the first American work on occupational diseases (1837); dealt with 31 occupations divided into roughly four sections: out-of-doors employment, textile workers, various artisans and tradesmen, and professional and literary men. Concluded that most occupations were not intrinsically dangerous except for those trades where dust or vapors were inhaled or where toxic substances were handled, but that substandard housing, poor sanitation, lack of wholesome exercise, and other deleterious environmental conditions attendant upon a life of low wages were conducive to ill health. Treatise had little influence but is valued for the portrayal of the hazards faced by American workers at that time. Helped found the College of Pharmacy and the Bellevue Hospital Medical College. An authority on forensic medicine and often asked to testify in disputed will and insanity cases.

WRITINGS: "On the Influence of Trades, Professions, and Occupations in the United States in the Production of Disease," *Trans., Med. Soc. of the State of New York* 3 (1837): 91-150. REFERENCES: Carey P. McCord, "The Second Ramazzini Oration. Benjamin William McCready, M.D. (1813-1892) and His Essay. . . ," *Industrial Med.* 16 (Nov. 1947): 535-38; *On the Influence of Trades. . .with an Introductory Essay by Genevieve Miller* (1943); *NCAB*, 9: 364.

S. Galishoff

McDOWELL, EPHRAIM (November 11, 1771, Rockbridge Co., Va.-June 25, 1830, Danville, Boyle County, Ky.). *Physician; Abdominal surgery.* Son of Samuel, soldier, surveyor, and jurist, and Mary (McClung) McDowell. Married Sarah Hart Shelby, December 29, 1802; six children. EDUCATION: c. 1786-90, studied medicine under Alexander Humphreys, Staunton, Va.; 1792-94, University of Edinburgh, Scotland; 1793-94, studied anatomy and surgery under John Bell, Edinburgh. CAREER: Became a busy practitioner in Danville, where he gained a reputation for surgical skills and was widely consulted by physicians and patients throughout Ky. and adjacent states. Known to have successfully performed amputations, herniotomies, vesicolithotomies and ovariotomies; 1819-29, served on Board of Trustees, Centre College, Danville. CONTRIBUTIONS: Known to have taught medicine to apprentices or office pupils (James McDowell, William A. McDowell and Alban Gilpin Smith [q.v.]); December 25, 1809, introduced ovariotomy to the world as a successful operation for treatment of ovarian tumors and performed the operation at least twelve times.

WRITINGS: "Three Cases of Extirpation of Diseased Ovaria," *Eclectic Repertory and Analytical Rev.* (Phila.) 7 (1817): 242; ibid, 9 (1819): 546; rep. in *Medical Classics* 2 (1938): 642. REFERENCES: *BHM* (1975-79), 81; (1980), 26; *DAB*, 6, pt. 2: 27-79; S. D. Gross, "Ephraim McDowell," *Lives of Eminent Am. Physicians and Surgeons* (1861), 207-30; E. F. Horine, "The Stagesetting for Ephraim McDowell, 1771-1830," *Bull. Hist. Med.* 24 (1950): 149; Miller, *BHM*, pp. 70-71; *NCAB*, 5: 148; A. Schachner, *Ephraim McDowell 'Father of Ovariotomy' and Founder of Abdominal Surgery* (1921).

E. H. Conner

McDOWELL, JOSEPH NASH (April 1, 1805, Lexington, Ky.-September 25, 1868, St. Louis, Mo.). *Surgeon.* Son of John and Lucy (Lagrand) McDowell. Married Amanda Virginia Drake, c.1827; four children. EDUCATION: 1825, M.D., Transylvania University, Lexington, Ky. CAREER: Professor of anatomy: 1825-26, Transylvania University; 1826, Jefferson Medical College, Philadelphia; and 1835-39, Cincinnati Medical College; 1840-61, professor of anatomy and surgery and dean, medical department, Kemper College, later Missouri Medical College, St. Louis; 1861-65, surgeon, Confederate Army; 1865-68, professor of surgery and dean, Missouri Medical College. CONTRIBUTIONS: Noted for role in founding Missouri Medical College, the first medical school west of the Mississippi River. A skilled surgeon and widely renowned as a teacher of anatomy. Excelled, however, as an orator and polemicist, both useful tools in the medical wars of the nineteenth century. In these conflicts, was most noted for assistance to brother-in-law Daniel Drake (q.v.), in Cincinnati, Ohio, and for the fierce rivalry that grew up in St. Louis between McDowell's school and the rival St. Louis Medical College of Dr. Charles Alexander Pope (q.v.).

REFERENCES: *BHM* (1964-69), 168; (1970-74), 114; Marjorie Fox Grisham, "Joseph Nash McDowell and the Medical Department of Kemper College, 1840-1845," *Bull. Missouri Hist. Soc.* 12 (1956): 358-71; Otto Juettner, *Daniel Drake and His Followers* (1909), 192-94; Miller, *BHM*, p. 71; Cynthia DeHaven Pitcock, "Doctors in Controversy," *Missouri Hist. Rev.* 60 (1966): 336-49; Robert E. Schlueter, "Joseph Nash McDowell (1805-1868)," *Washington Univ. Med. Alumni* 1 (1937-38): 9-14.

D. R. Sneddeker

MACFADDEN, BERNARR (August 16, 1868, Mill Spring, Mo.-October 12, 1955, Jersey City, N.J.). *Author; Publisher; Personal hygiene*. Son of William R., farmer, and Mary (Miller) Macfadden. Married Tilley Fountaine; Marguerite Killy, 1901, one child; Mary Williamson, 1913, seven children; Jonnie Lee, 1948. EDUCATION: Grade school only. CAREER: Series of odd jobs, including farm laborer, delivery boy, printer's assistant; built himself up with dumbbells; taught gymnastics, academies in Ill. and Mo.; professional wrestler; 1894, set up exercise studio, New York City; 1899, began to publish *Physical Culture* magazine; 1901, established physical culture sanitaria, N.Y., N.J., Mich., Ill., and health food restaurants; 1919, began publishing *True Story* magazine; 1924-32, published *New York Evening Graphic* newspaper; 1924-41, head of Macfadden Publications. CONTRIBUTIONS: Called a prophet of the early twentieth-century wave of health-fad reform in America, with emphasis on exercise, rest, fresh air, almost meatless diet, abstinence from alcohol, coffee, or tobacco. Advocated long fasts, barefoot walking, and only natural cures for illness. Supported chiropractors and naturopaths and thereby received opposition from the medical profession. His magazines popularized and spread the morality of the "roaring 20s" to the working classes. A Barnumlike character boosting his every move, like the contest for Great Britain's perfect woman (1913); the winner was Mary Williamson, whom he soon married and who gave birth to seven of his children. Charged by Anthony Comstock for obscenity (1905), arrested (1907) for circulating obscene material through the U.S. mails (copies of *Physical Culture* magazine including article informing men how they contracted venereal disease), found guilty, fined $2,000, and sentenced to two years in prison; President William H. Taft granted clemency in response to a deluge of letters from subscribers to Macfadden's magazines.

WRITINGS: Wrote more than 100 books, including five-volume encyclopedia (1911-12), constantly updated. All writings for a popular audience. REFERENCES: *DAB*, Supplement 5: 452-54; M. Fishbein, *Medical Follies* (1925); W. H. Taft, "Bernarr Macfadden," *Missouri Hist. Rev.* (Oct. 1968).

M. Kaufman

MACFARLANE, CATHARINE (April 7, 1877, Philadelphia, Pa.-May 27, 1969, Philadelphia). *Physician; Obstetrics; Gynecology; Oncology*. Daughter of John James, school principal and later librarian, and Henrietta Ottinger (Huston) Macfarlane, schoolteacher. Never married. EDUCATION: 1895, certificate in biology, University of Pennsylvania; 1898, M.D., Woman's Medical College of Pennsylvania; 1899, intern, Woman's Hospital of Philadelphia; postgraduate study, Johns Hopkins University (gynecological urology); Royal Charité, Berlin (obstetrics); Frauenklinik, University of Vienna (gynecology); Radium Hemmet, Stockholm (radiology). CAREER: All of her career was spent in Philadelphia, at the Woman's Medical College of Pennsylvania: advanced from instructor in obstetrics (1898) to professor of gynecology (1922); 1942, research professor of gynecology; 1940, served briefly as interim dean of the college; and 1946, became vice-president, Board of Corporators; simultaneously with faculty appointments, held appointments at a number of hospitals in the city and engaged in the private practice of gynecology. CONTRIBUTIONS: Best known for her Cancer Control Research Project. With two colleagues, Faith Fetterman, M.D., and Margaret Castix Sturgis, M.D., established a cancer-screening project (1938) in the Department of Gynecology, Woman's Medical College of Pennsylvania. This project, the first of its kind in Pa., was designed to detect early signs of uterine cancer. The study involved conducting pelvic examinations every six months on 1,319 presumably well women who volunteered to participate. Conceived as a five-year study, the screening continued for 15 years with a permanent facility and detection program being established at the college (mid-1950s). In addition to doing cancer research, spoke out on the issue of birth control, appearing on the platform with Margaret Sanger (q.v.) at the first Pennsyvania State Conference on Birth Control, Philadelphia (1922), and was active in supporting women in the medical profession, serving as president, American Medical Women's Association (1936), and vice-president, Medical Women's International Association (1937-47). First woman member (1932), College of Physicians of Philadelphia, and first woman president (1943), Obstetrical Society of Philadelphia.

WRITINGS: *Reference Hand-Book of Gynecology for Nurses* (1908; 6th ed., 1934); numerous articles in the field of obstetrics and gynecology, especially detection and treatment of cancer of the uterus. "The Treatment of Pre-Cancerous Lesions of the Cervix," *Surgical Clinics of North Am.* (1939); "An Experiment in Cancer Control," *Am. Gyn. & Obst. J.* (1940); "Control of Cancer of the Uterus: Report of a 10 Year Experiment," *JAMA* (Jun. 23, 1948). A complete list of her publications is in the Archives and Special Collections on Women in Medicine, the Medical College of Pennsylvania, Philadelphia, Pa. REFERENCES: Macfarlane Papers are in the Archives and Special Collections on Women in Medicine, The Medical College of Pennsylvania, Philadelphia; R. B. Sturgis, "First Woman Fellow of the College of Physicians of Philadelphia: Memoir of Catharine Macfarlane, 1877-1969," *Trans. and Studies of the Coll. of Physicians of Phila.*, 38 (1971): 157-160.

S. L. Chaff

McGEE, ANITA NEWCOMB (November 4, 1864, Washington, D.C.-October 5, 1940, Washington). *Physician: Military medicine.* Daughter of Simon, astronomer, U.S. Naval Observatory, and Mary Caroline (Hassler) Newcomb. Married William John McGee, geologist and anthropologist, 1888; two surviving children. EDUCATION: Private schools, Washington, D.C.; courses, Newnham

College, Cambridge, England, and the University of Geneva, Switzerland; 1892, M.D., Columbian University (later George Washington); 1892, postgraduate studies, Johns Hopkins University. CAREER: 1892-96, medical practice, Washington, D.C.; withdrew from practice to do original studies, becoming a secretary of the American Association for the Advancement of Science, recording secretary of the Women's Anthropological Society of America, and surgeon-general of the Daughters of the American Revolution (DAR); 1898, director, DAR Hospital Corps, receiving all applications for service as army nurses; 1898-1900, organized permanent Army Nurse Corps; 1904-5, served the government of Japan in the Russo-Japanese War, a "superior of nurses," reporting on hospitals in Japan, Manchuria, and Korea. CONTRIBUTIONS: Screened applicants for army nursing positions in the Spanish-American War, conflicting with Clara Barton (q.v.) and the American Red Cross, which considered that role to be one of its functions. Major role in organization of a permanent Army Nurse Corps (1901), which was to be led by a graduate nurse (the latter provision was pushed through by her opponents, who resented her for her antagonism to the Red Cross). Resigned after selecting her successor. Buried with military honors in the Arlington National Cemetery.

WRITINGS: Articles in the *Trained Nurse and Hosp. Rev.* 1898-1907; papers in the Library of Congress and the National Archives, *Washington, D.C.* REFERENCES: *BHM* (1964-69), 168; *Am. Men of Sci.* (1938); Emma R. McGee, *Life of W. J. McGee* (1915); *NCAB*, 10: 350; *Notable Am. Women*, 2: 464-6.

M. Kaufman

McGEE, LEMUEL C. (August 2, 1904, New Boston, Tex.-Feb. 18, 1975, Wilmington, Del.). *Physician; Internal and industrial medicine.* Son of Thomas L., photographer, and Elizabeth Murrell. Married Mary Virginia Provence, 1936; two children. EDUCATION: 1924, A.B., Baylor University, Waco, Tex.; 1927, Ph.D. (biochemistry and physiology), University of Chicago; 1929, M.D., Rush Medical College; intern: 1930, Baylor University Hospital, Dallas, Tex.; and 1931, Presbyterian Hospital, Chicago, Ill. CAREER: 1932-34, private practice in internal medicine; 1932-34, instructor in physiology and pharmacology, Baylor University College of Medicine, Dallas (half-time); 1935-39, chief of internal medicine, Golden Clinic, Davis Memorial Hospital, Elkins, W.Va.; 1939-40, research fellow in medicine and biochemistry, School of Medicine, Harvard University and Peter Bent Brigham Hospital; 1940-69, medical director, Hercules Powder Co., Wilmington; 1949-58, visiting professor of industrial medicine, University of Pennsylvania School of Medicine. CONTRIBUTIONS: A nationally recognized expert in industrial medicine, authored 88 articles in medical and scientific journals and a standard text on industrial medicine. Governor of Del. for the American College of Physicians (1948-57); vice president, American College of Physicians (1957-58); president, Delaware Academy of Medicine (1952-54), and Medical Society of Delaware (1960-61); fellow, College of Physicians, Philadelphia (1945).

WRITINGS: *Student Manual of Industrial Medicine* (1950); 88 articles in journals.

REFERENCES: Lewis B. Flinn, "Memoirs of Lemuel C. McGee," *Delaware Med. J.* (May 1975): 234-35; *Wilmington Morning News*, March 1, 1975.

W. H. Williams

McGILLYCUDDY, VALENTINE TRANT O'CONNELL (February 14, 1849, Racine, Wis.-June 6, 1939, San Francisco, Calif.). *Physician; Surgery.* Son of Daniel and Johanna (Trant) McGillycuddy. Married Fanny E. Hoyt, 1875. EDUCATION: 1867, University of Michigan; 1869, M.D., Detroit College of Medicine; 1869-70, postgraduate work, Michigan State University. CAREER: 1871-75, topographical engineer and acting physician, U. S. Survey of Great Lakes and Brit.-Am. Boundary Line; 1875, topographer, Jenney-Newton Survey of the Black Hills; 1876-79, surgeon, U.S. Second Cavalry; 1879-86, Indian agent, Pine Ridge Indian Reservation, Dakota Territory; 1892-97, dean, South Dakota School of Mines; 1898-1912, supervising medical inspector, Pacific Coast and Mountain division, Mutual Life Insurance Co. of New York; 1912, moved to California. CONTRIBUTIONS: While Indian agent, personally quelled an uprising instigated by Chief Red Cloud of the Oglala Sioux (c. 1881) and organized the first Indian Police. Delegate to the S. Dak. Constitutional Convention and signatory of the state constitution (1889). Set up a temporary clinic (1890) to aid both Indian and white victims of the Wounded Knee Massacre.

REFERENCES: *Heroes without Glory: Some Good Men of the Old West* (1965); Julia B. McGillycuddy, *McGillycuddy Agent* (1941); *Who Was Who in Am.*, 4: 637.

D. W. Boilard and P. W. Brennen

McGRAW, THEODORE ANDREWS (November 11, 1839, Detroit, Mich.-September 6, 1921, Detroit). *Physician; Surgery.* Son of Alexander C., shoe manufacturer and officer of several medical institutions, and Susana (Walker) McGraw. Married Alice Simpson, 1866; two children. EDUCATION: Mr. Bacon's School, Detroit; 1859, A.B., University of Michigan; studied medicine, University of Bonn; 1863, M.D., College of Physicians and Surgeons (N.Y.). CAREER: 1863-65, assistant surgeon, U.S. Army; at Detroit Medical College and its successor, Detroit College of Medicine: 1868-1914, founding professor of surgery; and 1881-98, president; 1887, president, Michigan State Medical Society; vice-president, American Medical Association and American Surgical Association; surgeon, Harper and St. Mary's hospitals, Detroit. CONTRIBUTIONS: Pioneer of thyroid surgery. Developed "McGraw ligature," a rubber ligature for use in intestinal surgery. Leader in Detroit medical education.

WRITINGS: "Upon the Use of the Elastic Ligature in the Surgery of the Intestines," *JAMA*, 16 (1891): 685-94. Writings listed in *Index Catalogue*, 2nd series, 10:19. REFERENCES: *JAMA*, 77 (1921): 956; Kelly and Burrage (1928), 785-86; Michigan State Med. Soc., *J.* 20 (1921): 429, 476-80; *NCAB*, 20: 176; *Who Was Who in Am.*, 1: 813; Frank Woodford and Philip P. Mason, *Harper of Detroit* (1964), 304-5.

M. Pernick

McGUIRE, HUNTER HOLMES (October 11, 1835, Winchester, Va.-September 19, 1900, Richmond, Va.). *Physician; Surgeon.* Son of Dr. Hugh Holmes, physician, and Mrs. Ann Elizabeth (Moss) McGuire. Married May Stuart, 1866; nine children. EDUCATION: Premedical education, Winchester Academy; 1855, M.D., Winchester Medical College; 1858-59, further medical studies, Philadelphia, Pa.; 1860, M.D., Medical College of Virginia. CAREER: 1857-58, professor of anatomy, Winchester Medical College; 1860, quiz instructor, University of Louisiana; 1861-65, medical director, Confederate Army of the Shenandoah and Confederate Army of Northern Virginia; 1865-78, professor of surgery, Virginia Medical College; president: 1875, Association of Medical Officers of the Army and Navy of the Confederate States; 1880-81, Medical Society of Virginia; 1886, American Surgical Association; 1889, Southern Surgical Association; and 1892, American Medical Association; 1893-1900, president and professor, University College of Medicine, Richmond. CONTRIBUTIONS: Medical director, Confederate Armies, and personal physician to Stonewall Jackson; was at Jackson's side at his death. Helped establish the Confederate Ambulance Corps and initiated the practice of freeing captured Union medical officers (1861-65). Did pioneering surgical work; famous for his abdominal and genital-urinary surgery; expert on gunshot wounds. Described many of his surgical techniques in articles (1861-1900). Helped found the University College of Medicine, Richmond, a school with a three-year graded curriculum, the only one in the South at the time (1893). Founded St. Luke's Hospital, Richmond.

WRITINGS: "Clinical Remarks on Cancer of the Breast," *Trans. Med. Soc. of Virginia* 12 (1881); contributed to the American edition of Timothy Holmes, *System of Surgery, Theoretical and Practical,* 3 vols. (1881-82); contributed to John Ashburst's *Internat. Encyclopedia of Surg.,* 6 vols. (1881-86); "Operative Interference in Gun-Shot Wounds of the Peritoneum," *TAMA* 32 (1881); contributed to William Pepper, *System of Practical Medicine,* 5 vols. (1885-86); "The Last Wound of General Jackson," *Richmond Med. J.* 1 (1866): 403-12. REFERENCES: *BHM* (1970-74), 114; Wyndham Blanton, *Medicine in Virginia in the Nineteenth Century* (1933); *DAB,* 12: 59-60; Howard A. Kelly, *Cyclopedia of Am. Med. Biog.* (1912); Otis F. Manson, "Biographical Sketch of Dr. Hunter Holmes McGuire," *Virginia Med. Monthly* 4 (1877): 481-84; *NCAB,* 42: 120; W. L. Peple, "Hunter Holmes McGuire," *Surg. Gyn. & Obst.* 36 (1932): 114-18; James M. Phalen, "Surgeon Hunter H. McGuire, He Rode with Stonewall," *Military Surgeon* 89 (1941): 908-10.

P. Addis

McKAY, READ JENNINGS (February 6, 1843, St. Louis, Mo.-March 1, 1918, Wilmington, Del.). *Physician; Ophthalmology; Otology.* Son of Harrison B. and Sarah (Jennings) McKay. Married Mary Stuart Elliott, 1873; three surviving children. EDUCATION: 1861, A.B., Lincoln Academy, Lincoln, Mo.; 1867, M.D., Bellevue Medical College, N.Y.; 1871-72, studied in London and Paris. CAREER: 1873-77, assistant to chair of ophthalmology, Bellevue, New York City; private practice: 1873-77, New York City; and 1877-1918, Wilmington. CONTRIBUTIONS: During the nineteenth century, was the only oculist and aurist in Delaware. Wrote a number of papers on ophthalmology and otology. President, Medical Society of Delaware (1885) and New Castle County Medical

Society (1904). REFERENCES: Meridith I. Samuels, *Med. Soc. of Del., 150th Annual Session* (1939), 82-83.

W. H. Williams

McKEAN, ROBERT (July 13, 1732, Chester County, Pa.-October 17, 1767, Raritan Landing, N.J.). *Minister; Physician.* Son of William, taverner, and Letitia (Finney) McKean, taverner. Married Mabel Graham Antill, 1761; no children. EDUCATION: Tutored privately; studied medicine and theology under the Rev. Dr. Francis Alison; studied theology, England; 1760, M.A. (hon.), College of Philadelphia. CAREER: 1757-67, medical missionary, Society for the Propagation of the Gospel in Foreign Parts; pastor: 1757-63, Christ Church, New Brunswick, N.J.; and 1763-67, St. Peter's Church, Perth Amboy, N.J. CON-TRIBUTIONS: A "physician of bodies as well as the souls of men." Promoted zealously the science of medicine and played an important role in establishing professional standards for physicians. Helped found the Medical Society of New Jersey (1766), the first organization of its kind in the New World, and served as its first president (1766-67). REFERENCES: W. Northey Jones, *The History of St. Peter's Church in Perth Amboy*, 60-63; *N.J. Med. Rep.* 1 (1848): 171-72; Fred B. Rogers, "The Last Illness of Robert McKean (1732-1767)," *J. of the Med. Soc. of New Jersey* 54 (1957): 540-43; idem, "Robert McKean (1732-1767): First President of the Medical Society of New Jersey," in *Help-Bringers: Versatile Physicians of New Jersey* (1960), 21-32; William A. Whitehead, *Contributions to the Early History of Perth Amboy and Adjoining Country*, 225-91; Stephen Wickes, *History of Medicine in New Jersey, and of Its Medical Men, from the Settlement of the Province to A.D. 1800* (1879), 329-30.

W. Barlow

McKEE, WILLIAM HENRY (September 7, 1814, Raleigh, N.C.-April 24, 1874, Raleigh). *Physician.* Son of James and Priscilla (Macon) McKee. Married Susan E. Battle, 1842, four children; Eliza O. Nixon, 1854, one child. EDU-CATION: 1839, M.D., University of Pennsylvania. CAREER: c. 1829-37, clerk and then partner in a Raleigh pharmacy; 1840-74, private medical practice, Raleigh. CONTRIBUTIONS: Co-organizer (1849), first secretary (1849-52), and an early president (1857-59), North Carolina State Medical Society. Served for years as the society's representative to the AMA. Elected to first State Board of Medical Examiners (1859). President of Board of Directors of state institution for the deaf, dumb, and blind and as that institution's physician. REFERENCES: *Cyclopedia of Eminent and Representative Men of the Carolinas of the 19th Century* (1892): 239-41; *History of North Carolina* 5 (1919): 235-36.

T. L. Savitt

MACKENZIE, KENNETH ALEXANDER JAMES (January 13, 1859, Cumberland House, Manitoba, Canada-March 15, 1920, Portland, Oreg.). *Physician; Internist; Medical educator.* Son of Roderick, businessman, and Jane (Mackenzie) Mackenzie. Married Cora Hardy Scott, 1885; four children; Marion Higgins Brown, 1905. EDUCATION: 1881, M.D., McGill University; 1881-82, postgraduate study, Edinburgh, London, Paris, Berlin, and Vienna. CAREER:

1882-1920, practice, Portland; 1895-1920, chief surgeon, Oregon and Washington Railroad and Navigation Company; 1882-1920, medical staff, St. Vincent's Hospital, Portland; medical faculty: 1883-86, Willamette University medical department; and 1887-1911, University of Oregon; 1912-20, dean, University of Oregon Medical School. CONTRIBUTIONS: One of the first to realize that Oreg. needed a medical school as a part of the state university and helped organize the University of Oregon medical department (1887). One of the first faculty members of the institution. Under his leadership as dean, the school made progress in becoming a medical center. The state legislature increased appropriations dramatically, a merger with the Willamette University medical department occurred, and a competent full-time faculty was appointed. Admissions standards were raised, the curriculum made more rigorous, and the school received full accreditation. Obtained land for a new campus (1914), and the school was moved to its present location (1919). Gave seven acres of land to Multnomah County, and (1920) a county hospital and home for nurses was begun. Made first mention in medical literature of the use of oil in the pleural cavity to collapse the lung.

WRITINGS: "A Preliminary Report on a Method of Treating Empyema without Resort to Pneumothorax," *Trans., Am. Surg. Assoc.* 32 (1914): 655-58. REFERENCES: O. Larsell, *The Doctor in Oregon; Northwest Medicine* 19 (1920): 104-5; *Who Was Who in Am.*, 1: 763.

G. B. Dodds

McKENZIE, ROBERT TAIT (May 26, 1867, Almonte, Ontario, Canada-April 28, 1938, Philadelphia, Pa.). *Physician; Rehabilitation Medicine; Physical Education.* Son of William (minister) and Catherine (Shiells) McKenzie. Married Ethel O'Neal, 1907; no children. EDUCATION: Almonte High School; Ottawa Collegiate Institute; 1889, A.B., McGill University; 1892, M.D., McGill University; 1891, diploma, Harvard Summer School, physical education; 1892-93, intern, Montreal General Hospital. CAREER: 1895, house physician to governor-general of Canada; 1895-1904, medical director of physical training, demonstrator of anatomy, McGill University; 1904-37, faculty, University of Pennsylvania, director of physical education (1904-31), professor of physical therapy (1907-31?), research professor (1931-38); 1915-16, rehabilitation and physical medicine specialist, Royal (England) Army Medical Corps; 1900?-38, sculptor. CONTRIBUTIONS: Pioneer in rehabilitation medicine and physical education, established a special department of physical education at McGill (1895-1904), a new program in physical education at Pennsylvania (1904-7), and became first professor of physical therapy at any American university (1907). Developed and disseminated ideas on special therapy, methods of reeducation, and fashioning facial masks for reconstruction of the maimed through plastic surgery. Recognized as a leader in physical medicine by his peers. Served as president, American Academy of Physical Medicine, and similar professional organizations.

WRITINGS: *Exercise in Education and Medicine* (1909); *Reclaiming the Maimed* (1918). REFERENCES: *DAB*, Supplement 2, 417-18; Adelaide M. Hunter, "R. Tait McKenzie:

Pioneer in Physical Education'' (unpublished dissertation, Teachers College, Columbia University, 1950); *Who Was Who in Am.*, 1: 816.

T. L. Savitt

McKINNEY-STEWARD, SUSAN MARIA SMITH (1847, Brooklyn, N.Y.-1918, Xenia, Ohio). *Physician; Public speaker.* Daughter of Sylvanus, a successful farmer, and Anna Springsteel Smith. Married the Rev. William Guillard McKinney (d. 1895), two children; Rev. Theophilus G. Steward. EDUCATION: 1870, M.D., New York Medical College and Hospital for Women, where she became the first black woman to receive a degree from a medical college in N.Y. and the third black woman to receive a medical degree in the United States; 1887-88, postgraduate study, Long Island Medical College Hospital. CAREER: 1870-95, practiced medicine in Brooklyn—the first black woman to do so—and maintained a Manhattan office as well; 1881, participated in founding the Brooklyn Woman's Homeopathic Hospital and Dispensary (later renamed the Memorial Hospital for Women and Children) and remained a member of its staff until 1895; 1882, became a member of the medical staff, New York Medical College and Hospital for Women; physician, Brooklyn Home for Aged Colored People, and a member of their governing board (1892-95); during second marriage, to Theophilus Steward, a U.S. Army chaplain, traveled extensively with husband and practiced medicine in Nebr. and Mont.; 1898, moved to Ohio; 1898-1918, faculty member and resident physician, Wilberforce University in Xenia; lectured on a number of occasions about women in medicine in the United States; 1911, addressed the Interracial Congress in London, speaking on the topic of colored women in America. CONTRIBUTIONS: As a community leader and organizer, worked with both the young and the aged and especially women for whom she provided medical care and served as a dynamic role model.

WRITINGS: *Women in Medicine: A Paper Read Before the National Association of Colored Women's Clubs, Wilberforce, Ohio, August 6, 1914* (1914). Excerpts from her paper read at the Interracial Congress in London appear in *The Crisis* 3 (Nov. 1911). REFERENCES: Two articles by Leslie L. Alexander, M.D., provide information on the life and family of Dr. Susan Smith McKinney-Steward: *The Crisis* (Jan. 1980): 21-23; and *JNMA* (Mar. 1975), 173-75. Information on the life of Dr. McKinney-Steward is in the keeping of her great grandson, William S. McKinney, D.D.S.

S. L. Chaff

McLEAN, MARY HANCOCK (February 28, 1861, Washington, Mo.-May 17, 1930, St. Louis, Mo.). *Obstetrician and gynecologist.* Daughter of Dr. Elijah, physician, and Mrs. Mary (Stafford) McLean. EDUCATION: 1875-78, Lindenwood College; 1878-80, Vassar College; 1883, M.D., University of Michigan. CAREER: 1884, assistant physician, St. Louis Female Hospital; 1885, private practice of obstetrics and gynecology combined with public health work until her death in 1930. CONTRIBUTIONS: Despite obstacles facing women in nineteenth-century medicine, education and family connections helped obtain an appointment equivalent to an internship 40 years before such positions were generally available to women. First woman member, St. Louis Medical Society

(1885). Extensively involved in voluntary benevolence and public health activity, in addition to her private practice. Helped found the St. Louis YWCA (1905); Founded a free evening clinic for working women (by 1908). On the staff of several hospitals and served as an advisor to women physicians entering medical practice in St. Louis. In her later career, became active in missionary work in China; supported some 20 Chinese students through medical school. REFERENCES: Marion Hunt, "Woman's Place in Medicine: The Career of Dr. Mary Hancock McLean," *Missouri Hist. Soc. Bull.* 36 (1980): 4; Dr. Bertha Van Hoosen's autobiography, *Petticoat Surgeon* (1947), contains a personal view of Dr. McLean; Ann Andre-Johnson, *Notable St. Louis Women* (1914), contains an interview with her.

M. Hunt

MacLEOD, COLIN MUNRO (February 28, 1909, Port Hastings, Ontario, Canada-February 11, 1972, London, England). *Physician; Microbiology; Bacterial genetics; Immunology.* Son of John Charles and Lillian (Munro) MacLeod. Married Elizabeth Randol, 1938; one child. EDUCATION: 1932, M.D., McGill University; 1932-34, intern, Montreal General Hospital; 1934, went to the United States; 1941, naturalized. CAREER: 1934-41 medical staff, Rockefeller Institute Hospital; at New York University School of Medicine: 1941-56, microbiology faculty; and 1960-66, medicine faculty; at Army Epidemiological Board (later Armed Forces Epidemiological Board): 1941-46, director, Committee on Pneumonia; and 1946-55, president; 1944-46, chief, preventive medical section, Committee on Medical Research, Office of Scientific Research and Development; 1956-60, research medicine faculty, University of Pennsylvania Medical School; at New York City Health Research Council: 1958-60, executive secretary; and 1960-70, chairman; 1963-66, deputy director, Office of Science and Technology, Executive Office of the President; 1966-72, vice-president for medical affairs, Commonwealth Fund; 1970-72, president and scientific director, Oklahoma Medical Research Foundation. CONTRIBUTIONS: Worked with Oswald T. Avery (q.v.) in the advanced stages of his development of a serum treatment for pneumonia. Saw that sulfonamides were more effective in treating the disease and made important laboratory studies of their properties; described the first "sulfapyridine-fast" strain of pneumococcus, the occurrence of sulfonamide inhibitors, and the conditions most likely to lead to the emergence of resistant strains (1930s). Worked with Avery and Maclyn McCarty on their epochal studies of the transformation of pneumococcal types; showed that specific and inheritable changes could be induced in a bacterial cell to which deoxyribonucleic acid (DNA) derived from another cell had been introduced (1944). With Michael Heidelberger, showed that injection of purified polysaccharides of pneumococcus offered protection against epidemic pneumonia. Played a major role in the emergence of New York University Medical School as a first-rate institution. Heavily committed to government service during his last 30 years of life.

WRITINGS: "Metabolism of 'Sulfapyridine-Fast' and Parent Strains of Pneumococcus Type I," *Proc. Soc. for Experimental Biol. & Med.* 41 (1939): 215-18; "Studies on Chemical Nature of Substance Inducing Transformation of Pneumococcal Types; Induction of Transformation by Deoxyribonucleic Acid Fraction Isolated from Pneumococcus Type III," *J. of Experimental Med.* 79 (1944): 137-58 (with Oswald T. Avery and Maclyn McCarty); "Prevention of Pneumococcal Pneumonia by Immunization with Specific Capsular Polysaccharides," *ibid.* 82 (1945): 445-65 (with Michael Heidelberger, Richard G. Hodges, and William G. Bernhard). REFERENCES: *Am. Philos. Soc. Yearbook* (1972), 222-30; *McGraw-Hill Modern Men of Sci.* 2 (1966): 340-41; *N.Y. Times*, February 14, 1972; *Trans., Assoc. of Am. Physicians* 75 (1972): 31-32; *Who Was Who in Am.*, 5: 450.

S. Galishoff

McMASTER, PHILIP DURYEE (September 14, 1891, Philadelphia, Pa.-March 20, 1973, Mount Kisco, N.Y.). *Physician; Physiology; Immunology.* Son of John Bache, historian, and Gertrude (Stevenson) McMaster. Married Elizabeth Parsons Dwight, 1923; two children. EDUCATION: 1914, B.S., Princeton University; 1918, M.D., University of Pennsylvania; 1917-19, resident, University of Pennsylvania Hospital; 1929-30, research fellow in psychology, Harvard University. CAREER: 1918, U.S. Army; 1919-62, at Rockefeller Institute for Medical Research; during World War II, worked at the Office of Scientific Research and Development and at National Research Council. CONTRIBUTIONS: Did his first work in the laboratory of Peyton Rous (q.v.), where he devised methods for the intubation and sterile drainage of the gallbladders and bile ducts, which, in turn, enabled him to study the flow and formation of bile; revealed that the normal gallbladder rapidly concentrates hepatic bile but that the diseased organ cannot; provided a basis for diagnostic dye tests for the presence of gallstones and gallbladder disease. Later, with Robert Elman, established the origin and source of clinically and diagnostically important bile pigments; settled the question of the origin of urobilinuria, a condition in which bile reaches the intestines. Did last work, and was a pioneer, in the development of research methods concerning the formation of antibodies and their methods of combatting disease; with Stephen Hudack and later with John Kidd, investigated the physiology of the lymphatic system and the mechanics of lymph flow; demonstrated that bacterial and viral antibodies were first formed in the draining lymph nodes.

WRITINGS: "The Concentrating Activity of the Gall Bladder," *Proc., Soc. for Experimental Biol. & Med.* 17 (1920): 159 (with P. Rous); "A Method for the Permanent Sterile Drainage of Intra-abdominal Ducts, as Applied to the Common Duct," *J. of Experimental Med.* 37 (1923): 11 (with P. Rous); "Studies on Urobilin Physiology and Pathology. I. The Quantitative Determination of Urobilin," *ibid.*, 41 (1925): 503 (with R. Elman); "The Participation of Skin Lymphatics in Repair of the Lesions Due to Incisions and Burns," *ibid.*, 60 (1934): 479 (with S. S. Hudack); "Development of Antiviral Properties within Lymph Nodes," *Proc., Soc. for Experimental Biol. & Med.* 34 (1936): 547 (with J. G. Kidd). A bibliography is in *BMNAS*. REFERENCES: *BMNAS* 50 (1979): 287-308; *N.Y. Times*, March 21, 1973.

S. Galishoff

McNEILL, WILLIAM CLARENCE (February 16, 1878, Lake Waccamow, N.C.-April 11, 1964, Washington, D.C.). *Physician; Gynecologist; Teacher.*

Son of Henry Clay, undertaker and construction worker, and Lucy Alice (Reeves) McNeill. Married Mary Alice Wheeler, 1910; three children. EDUCATION: 1900, Howard Academy; 1904, M.D., Howard University. CAREER: 1904, assistant to secretary-treasurer, Howard Medical School; 1905-7, assistant surgeon, Freedmen's Hospital, Washington, D.C.; at Howard Medical School: 1907-20, secretary-treasurer; and 1910-43, professor of gynecology; 1904-50s, private practice, Washington, D.C. CONTRIBUTIONS: Fine and respected teacher at Howard for almost 40 years (1905-43) who developed reputation for noticing and financially helping many needy Howard medical students. A key figure in the operation of Howard, when, as secretary-treasurer, was executive officer of the medical school. Led campaigns to raise money for Howard Medical School from private sources to meet American Association of Medical Colleges accreditation standards (1911) and to match General Education Board gift (*post* World War I).

REFERENCES: W. Montague Cobb, "William Clarence McNeill, M.D., 1878-," *JNMA* 50 (1958): 314; Rayford Logan, *Howard University, The First Hundred Years* (1969); obituary, *JNMA* (1965): 71; unpublished autobiography in possession of family.

T. L. Savitt

MacNIDER, WILLIAM deBERNIERE (June 25, 1881, Chapel Hill, N.C.-May 31, 1951, Durham, N.C.). *Physician; Pharmacologist; Medical educator.* Son of Virgilius St. Clair, physician, and Sophia Beatty (Mallett) MacNider. Married Sarah Jane Foard, 1918; one child. EDUCATION: 1903, M.D., University of North Carolina; 1903, postgraduate training, University of Chicago and Western Reserve University. CAREER: 1905-50, at University of North Carolina: 1905-50, professor of pharmacology; 1905-37, 1940-43, head, Department of Pharmacology; and 1937-40, dean, Medical School. CONTRIBUTIONS: Established first Department of Pharmacology, University of North Carolina (1905). Associate editor for a number of years, *Proceedings of the Society for Experimental Biology and Medicine, Quarterly Journal of Alcohol Study,* and *Journal of Pharmacology and Experimental Therapeutics*. Internationally known for research on effects of toxic agents on kidneys and liver and on the process of aging. Member and officer of numerous medical and pharmacological organizations, including North Carolina Medical Society (1926). Promoted the needs of University of North Carolina Medical School throughout career, but especially during deanship (1937-40), particularly the expansion of the school to four years and the need for increased funding.

WRITINGS: Numerous articles. REFERENCES: Dorothy Long, ed., *Medicine in North Carolina* (1972); NCAB, 40: 153-54; *Who Was Who in Am.,* 3: 545.

T. L. Savitt

McQUARRIE, IRVINE (April 20, 1891, Silver Reef, Utah-September 9, 1961, Minneapolis, Minn.). *Pediatrician.* Son of Robert G. and Charlotte (Macfarlane) McQuarrie. Married Vira Perkins, 1912; three children. EDUCATION: 1915, A.B., University of Utah; 1919, Ph.D., University of California; 1921, M.D., Johns Hopkins; 1921-24, internship, Henry Ford Hospital, Detroit, Mich. CAREER:

1921-24, practice in Detroit; 1925-26, instructor of pediatrics, Yale University; 1926-30, associate professor of pediatrics, University of Rochester; 1930-55, professor and head, Department of Pediatrics, University of Minnesota; 1955-59, director of medical education, Kauikeolani Children's Hospital, Honolulu, Hawaii; 1959, moved to Berkeley, Calif.; 1939, visiting professor, Peiping University Medical College, China; 1947, study of medical education, research, and hospitals of Japan for the Rockefeller Foundation. CONTRIBUTIONS: Did important research on convulsions at Henry Ford Hospital. Editor-in-chief, *Brennemann's Practice of Pediatrics*. Was co-founder of the Society for Pediatric Research and the American Academy of Pediatrics.

WRITINGS: *Experiments on Nature and other Essays* (1944); articles in *J. of Children's Diseases* (1954) and *Acta Pediatrics* (1954). REFERENCES: *Who Was Who in Am.*, 4: 647; *N.Y. Times*, September 11, 1961, p. 27:5.

R. Rosenthal

MADDOCK, WILLIAM O. (November 25, 1923, Tacoma, Wash.-January 5, 1969, Anchorage, Alaska). *Physician; Endocrinology.* Son of Harold J. Maddock. Married Alice; five children. EDUCATION: University of Oregon School of Medicine: 1947, M.Sc.; and 1948, Ph.D., M.D.; consistently performed at head of class; 1949, intern, Detroit Receiving Hospital; 1950-52, fellowship in internal medicine. CAREER: Instructor, Wayne State University School of Medicine; October 1954-October 1956, with U.S. Army in Korea and Japan; 1956-58, associate professor of medicine, Wayne State University, Detroit, Mich.; 1958-69, private practice, Anchorage; served one term as chief of staff, Providence Hospital, Anchorage; director, Doctors' Clinic, Anchorage. As first editor of *Alaska Medicine*, the journal of the Alaska Medical Association, set a high standard of professional communication for colleagues to follow.

REFERENCES: *Alaska Med.* 11, no. 2 (Mar. 1969).

A.R.C. Helms

MAGHEE, THOMAS GILLISON (1842, Evansville, Ind.-September 29, 1927, Lander, Wyo.). *Physician; Surgeon.* Son of Joseph, physician, and Mary (Jacobs) Maghee. Married Mollie Williams (d. 1884), four sons. Evelyn Baldwin, 1885; one daughter. EDUCATION: Hanover College; 1868, M.D., Bellevue Hospital Medical College. CAREER: 1873, went to Wyo. as post surgeon, Fort Brown, now Fort Washakie near Lander; 1874, cited for gallantry in action during the Bates Battle against the Indians; 1878, resigned from the army and began practice, Green River, Wyo.; elected representative of Sweet Water County, Wyo., to the territorial legislature; 1880-1905, practice, Rawlins, Wyo.; 1905, returned to Lander and organized the Wyoming State Training School, later serving as its superintendent. CONTRIBUTIONS: A well-known dermatologist, credited with performing the first plastic surgery in the state of Wyo. When a sheepherder attempted suicide by firing a shotgun from below his chin, and the blast destroyed his face (1886), restored the face by forming new lips, nose, lower jawbone and chin. Kept photographic records of the surgery. REFERENCES: Hebard Collection, Coe Library, University of Wyoming, Laramie, Wyo.; *Rawlins Republican*, July 2, 1897, August 16, 1923.

A. Palmieri

MAGRUDER, GEORGE LLOYD (November 1, 1848, Washington, D.C.-January 28, 1914, Washington). *Physician; Materia medica and therapeutics*. Son of Thomas Contee, paymaster on the Washington aqueduct and Capitol extension, and disbursing officer under Quartermaster-Gen. M. C. Meigs, and Elizabeth Olivia (Morgan) Magruder. Married Belle Burns, November 22, 1882; two children. EDUCATION: 1868, A.B., Gonzaga College (Washington, D.C.); 1870, M.D., Georgetown Medical School; 1871, A.M., Gonzaga College. CAREER: 1871-73, professor of chemistry, Gonzaga College; at Georgetown Medical School: prosector of minor surgery and professor of materia medica (1883-96), dean and treasurer of the medical faculty, and emeritus professor of materia medica and therapeutics; practiced medicine in Washington from the time he graduated in medicine until his death; 1871-72, physician to the poor; 1883-87, physician to the police and fire departments; consulting physician to Providence and Emergency hospitals and member of the Board of Visitors, Government Hospital for the Insane (St. Elizabeth's). CONTRIBUTIONS: Very active in public health work in Washington, D.C., especially in regard to the water and milk supply. Began the campaign (1894) for a pure water supply by chairing the local medical society's committee on typhoid fever, which resulted in the building of a filtration plant. Helped to obtain a pure milk supply by securing an investigation by the Department of Agriculture (1906-7) into the water supplies of dairy farms that furnished milk to D.C.; the appointment of a milk commission for D.C. (1907); and an investigation by the Public Health Service and the Department of Agriculture of D.C.'s milk industry, which resulted in the publication of the Hygienic Laboratory's Bulletin 41, *Milk and Its Relation to Public Health*. A founder, Central Dispensary and the Georgetown University Hospital.

WRITINGS: "The Milk Supply of Washington, D.C.," *JAMA* 49 (1907): 1088-93; *The Dissemination of Disease by Dairy Products* (1910); *The Solution of the Milk Problem* (1913). Bibliography listed at the end of his biographical sketch in *Washington Med. Annals* 13 (1914): 206-9. REFERENCES: William B. Atkinson, ed. *Physicians and Surgeons of the U.S.* (1878), 369; *DAB*, 6, pt. 2: 204; Kelly and Burrage (1920), 755-56; D. S. Lamb et al., *History of the Medical Society of the District of Columbia, 1817-1909* (1909), 298-99.

R. A. Kondratas

MAHONEY, JOHN FRIEND (August 1, 1889, Fond du Lac, Wis.-February 23, 1957, Stapleton, N.Y.). *U.S. public health officer; Venereal disease*. Son of David, engineer, and Mary Ann (Hogan) Mahoney. Married Leah Ruth Arnold, 1926; two children. EDUCATION: 1910, S.B., Milwaukee University; 1914, M.D., Marquette University; intern: 1914-15, Milwaukee County Hospital; and 1915-16, Chicago Lying-in Hospital. CAREER: At U.S. Public Health Service: 1917, commissioned medical officer; 1925-29, adviser to the U.S. Foreign Service, Haiti, Ireland, England, and Germany, where he studied methods used in foreign countries to control syphilis; and 1929-49, director, Venereal Disease Research Laboratory, U.S. Marine Hospital, Staten Island (later U.S. Public Health Service Hospital); at New York City health department: 1949-54, commissioner; and 1954-57, director, Bureau of Laboratories; clinical syphilology faculty, New York University School of Medicine; dermatology faculty, College of Physicians and Surgeons (Columbia). CONTRIBUTIONS: Showed that sulfonamides could cure gonorrhea (1937). Discovered and perfected the penicillin treatment of syphilis (1943); replaced treatment with arsenical compounds and salvarsan that because they took about 18 months, were seldom completed. New therapy provided nearly 100 percent cure rate and took only two weeks.

WRITINGS: "Sulfanilamide Therapy in Hospitalized Gonorrhea," *Am. J. of Syphilis, Gonorrhea & Venereal Diseases* 22 (1938): 691-98 (with C. J. Van Slyke and J. Durward Thayer); "Penicillin Treatment of Early Syphilis. A Preliminary Report," *Venereal Disease Information* 24 (Dec. 1943): 355-57 (with R. C. Arnold and A. Harris); "The Use of Penicillin Sodium in the Treatment of Sulfonamide-Resistant Gonorrhea in Men," *Am. J. of Syphilis, Gonorrhea, & Venereal Diseases* 27 (1943): 525-28 (with Charles Ferguson, M. Buchholtz, and C. J. Van Slyke). REFERENCES: *JAMA* 164, no. 3 (1957): 313; *NCAB*, 47: 156; *N.Y. Times*, February 24, 1957; *Who Was Who in Am.*, 3: 548.

S. Galishoff

MAIN, JOHN HANSON THOMAS (November 13, 1813, Frederick County, Md.-September 30, 1891, Fort Smith, Ark.). *Physician; Surgeon.* Son of John W., farmer and Methodist preacher, and Susan (Mayne) Main. Married Isabella Armour, 1848; one daughter. EDUCATION: *Post* 1829, apprentice to Allen G. Miller, Richmond County, Ohio; 1836, M.D., Starling Medical College. CAREER: Private practice: 1836-37, Mansfield, Ohio; 1837-38, New Orleans, La.; and 1838-91, Fort Smith, Ark. CONTRIBUTIONS: Began practice at Fort Smith in a 12-foot-square log cabin as the first civilian physician on that U.S. Army post. Encouraged professional organization as a charter member, Crawford County Medical Society (1845), the Fort Smith Medical Association (1870), and the State Medical Society of Arkansas (1875); and as president, Crawford County Medical Society (1847) and, after a division of counties, Sebastian County Medical Society (1881). Promoted community development as Fort Smith alderman, (1840-54). Supplemented professional income by farming during first years of practice and eventually became wealthy owner of farm land, Fort Smith residences, the Main Hotel, and the Fort Smith Hospital and Free Dispensary, incorporated in 1882.

REFERENCES: Auxiliary to the Sebastian County Medical Society, *Physicians and Medicine: Crawford and Sebastian Counties* (1977), 454-57. Clara B. Eno, *History of Crawford County* (1955), 208.

D. Konold

MAJOR, RALPH HERMON (August 29, 1884, Clay County, Mo.-October 15, 1970, Kansas City, Kans.). *Physician; Historian.* Son of John Sleet, a banker, and Virginia (Anderson) Major. Married Margaret Norman Jackson,

1915; three children; after her death, Wanda E. Graham, 1967. EDUCATION: 1902, A.B., William Jewell; at Johns Hopkins: 1910, M.D.; and 1910-12, house officer; studied in Munich under Friedrich Müller and pathology under Orphuls at Stanford. CAREER: 1919-21, Henry Ford Hospital; at University of Kansas: 1921-50, chairman, Department of Internal Medicine; and 1950-55, chairman, Department of the History of Medicine. CONTRIBUTIONS: Authored 184 scientific and historical papers including some of the earlier clinical reports on the use of insulin. Among early graduates of Johns Hopkins who colonized academic departments across the United States. In his words, when he arrived on the medical campus of the University of Kansas (1914), the "total assets of the institution consisted of seven and one-half acres of land (not a bargain at any price), $95,000 invested in three buildings, and an annual budget of $30,000." When he became emeritus professor some 40 years later, University of Kansas had one of the better state-supported medical schools in the country. No small measure of credit can be traced directly to his talent and dedication. Early in life, developed a passion for the history of medicine, which was manifest both in writings and Oslerian approach to teaching medical history. Five years as chairman secured departmental status for the history of medicine at Kansas. President, American Association of the History of Medicine (1950-52).

WRITINGS: *Physical Diagnosis* first appeared in 1937, has been translated into six languages, and is now entering its ninth edition. *The Doctor Explains* (1931); *Classic Descriptions of Disease* (1932); *Disease and Destiny* (1936); *An Account of the University of Kansas School of Medicine* (1968). REFERENCES: *BHM* (1970-74), 116; Robert Hudson, "Ralph H. Major, 1884-1970," *Bull. Hist. Med.* 45 (1971): 283-86.

R. Hudson

MAJORS, MONROE ALPHEUS (October 12, 1864, Waco, Tex.-late 1960, Los Angeles, Calif.). *Physician*. Son of Andrew Jackson and Jane (Barringer) Majors. Married Georgia Groom, 1889, one child, divorced 1904; Estelle C. Bonds, 1909, two children. EDUCATION: 1878-83, preparatory school; Tillotson College and Normal School (Austin, Tex.); 1886, B.S., Central Tennessee College; 1886, M.D., Meharry Medical College. CAREER: 1886-1952, private practice: 1886, Brenham, Tex.; 1888-90, Los Angeles, Calif.; 1890- c. 1896, Waco; c. 1896-c. 1897, Decatur, Ill.; c. 1897-99, Indianapolis, Ind.; 1899-1901, Waco; and 1901-c. 1923, Chicago; 1887-88, taught school, rural Tex, to escape racial violence in Brenham and Dallas, Tex.; 1891-94, lecturer in hygiene and sanitation, Paul Quinn College, Waco; 1893, spent five months in Chicago working with local physicians at Provident Hospital and for Frederick Douglass; 1893-95, editor, *Texas Searchlight (Waco)*; 1898-99, associate editor, *Indianapolis Freeman*; 1908-11, editor, *Chicago Conservator*; 1925, lost most of his vision suddenly. CONTRIBUTIONS: Prime spirit and one of 14 founders of second oldest black medical association, the Lone Star State Medical, Dental and Pharmaceutical Society (1886). Practiced medicine for 66 years. Became first black to practice medicine west of the Rocky Mountains (1888) when he moved to Los Angeles to escape racial persecution in Tex. Edited and published newspapers and periodicals that often addressed racial problems (1893-1920s). Vocal participant in local politics and civic affairs on behalf of blacks and black rights throughout his career, which sometimes caused him severe problems but also won him respect. Built and operated a hospital for blacks in Waco (1893-96, 1899-1901). Worked on various medical and other civic committees for Chicago and Illinois. Wrote first nursery rhyme book for black children (1921), poems for the *Bee*, and articles for the *Chicago Defender*. Close friend of black poet Paul Lawrence Dunbar in Chicago.

WRITINGS: *Noted Negro Women* (1893); *First Steps and Nursery Rhymes* (1921); many newspaper and periodical articles. Writings listed in *WWICA* 6 (1941-43): 353. REFERENCES: W. Montague Cobb, "Monroe Alpheus Majors, 1864-," *JNMA* 47 (Mar. 1955): 139-41; Frank L. Mather ed., *WWCR* (1915), 183; obituary (very brief), *Jet* 19 (1961): 46; *WWICA* 6 (1941-43): 350, 353.

                                                                                            T. L. Savitt

MALL, FRANKLIN PAINE (September 28, 1862, Belle Plaine, Ia.-November 17, 1917, Baltimore, Md.). *Anatomist; Embryologist*. Son of Francis, farmer, and Louise Christine (Miller) Mall. Married Mabel S. Glover, 1895; two children. EDUCATION: Private school; 1883, M.D., University of Michigan Medical School; 1883-86, studied at Heidelberg and Leipzig, Germany, under physiologist K. F. W. Ludwig and embryologist Wilhelm His. CAREER: 1886-89, fellow and instructor in pathology, Johns Hopkins University Medical School; 1889-92, adjunct professor of vertebrate anatomy, Clark University; professor of anatomy: 1892-93, University of Chicago; and 1893-1917, Johns Hopkins Medical School; 1914-17, director, Department of Embryology, Carnegie Institute. CONTRIBUTIONS: Outstanding medical professor who contributed notably to transforming study of anatomy in the United States by introducing German methodology. Conducted fundamental research in the pathology of the human embryo and helped lay the foundations for the study of normal and pathological anatomy. Traced the origin of the thalmus gland. Added to knowledge of the structure and function of the intestines and developed concept of structural units within organs. Discovered the motor nerves of the portal system. Primary founder, *American Journal of Anatomy* (1901). Played a major role in the Association of American Anatomists. Helped organize the Association of Morphologists (1890). Co-editor, *Journal of Morphology* and *Anatomical Record*. Published over 60 papers in the fields of anatomy, physiology, and embryology.

WRITINGS: *A Study of the Causes Underlying the Origin of Human Monsters* (1908); *Manual of Human Embryology* (German ed., 1910-11; American ed., 1910-12, co-editor with Franz Keibel); *Contributions to Embryology*, 9 vols. (1915-20, co-editor with Franz Keibel). A bibliography is in *BMNAS*. REFERENCES: *BHM* (1975-79), 82; *BMNAS* 16 (1936): 65-122; *DAB*, 12: 220-21; *DSB*, 9: 55-58; G. Carl Huber, "Franklin Paine Mall, 1862-1917, In Memoriam," *Anat. Record* 14 (1918): 3-17; Kelly and Burrage (1920); Florence R. Sabin, *Franklin Paine Mall: The Story of a Mind* (1934); William Welch, et al., "Memorial Services in Honor of Franklin Paine Mall, Professor of Anatomy, Johns Hopkins University, 1893-1917," *Johns Hopkins Hosp. Bull.* 29 (1918): 109-23.

                                                                                            J. Duffy

MALLORY, FRANK BURR (November 12, 1862, Cleveland, Ohio-September 27, 1941, Brookline, Mass.). *Physician; Pathology.* Son of George, ship captain, and Anna (Faragher) Mallory. Married Persis McClain Tracy, 1893; two children. EDUCATION: Harvard University: 1886, A.B., and 1890, A.M., M.D.; 1890, intern, McLean Hospital (Waverly, Mass.); 1893, studied in Prague, Czechoslovakia, and Freiburg, Germany. CAREER: At Harvard University: 1890-91, assistant in histology; 1891-92, assistant in pathological anatomy, and 1894-1932, pathology faculty; 1894-1932, pathologist, Boston City Hospital; president: 1910, American Association of Pathologists and Bacteriologists; and 1910-11, American Association for Cancer Research. CONTRIBUTIONS: Leading American figure in histologic pathology during the first third of the twentieth century. Developed new, widely adopted staining methods and prepared the way for the development of histochemistry in pathology. Greatly increased the reliability of frozen tissue sections during surgery. Developed special histological methods for the study of cancer, which provided impetus to the classification and study of that disease. Added to knowledge of the pathological lesions of typhoid fever, epidemic cerebrospinal meningitis, diphtheria, and whooping cough. Nation's foremost authority on liver diseases, especially cirrhosis of the liver. Wrote highly regarded textbooks *Pathological Technique* (1897) and *The Principles of Pathologic Histology* (1914, with James H. Wright); former was one of the first adequately illustrated pathology textbooks and by 1923 had run through eight editions. Trained many persons who occupied chairs of pathology (1920s-40s). Helped found the American Association for Cancer Research and the American Association of Pathologists and Bacteriologists. Edited *Journal of Medical Research (post* 1923) and continued in that position when the name of the publication was changed to *American Journal of Pathology* (1925-40).

WRITINGS: "The Results of the Application of Special Histological Methods to the Study of Tumors," *J. of Experimental Med.* 10 (1908): 575-93; "Cirrhosis of the Liver—Five Different Types of Lesions from Which It May Arise," *Johns Hopkins Hosp. Bull.* 22 (1911): 69-75. REFERENCES: *DAB*, Supplement 3: 502-3; Miller, *BHM*, p. 67; *NCAB*, 33: 513-14; *Who Was Who in Am.*, 2: 342.

S. Galishoff

MALONEY, ARNOLD HAMILTON (July 4, 1888, Cocoye Village, Trinidad, British West Indies-August 8, 1955, Washington, D.C.). *Physician; Pharmacology.* Son of Lewis Albert, building contractor, grocery chain owner, and carriage builder, and Estelle Evetta (Bonas) Maloney. Married Beatrice Pocahontas Johnston, 1916; two children. EDUCATION: c.1909, B.A., Naparima College (Trinidad), affiliate of Cambridge University, England; c.1909-c.1910, Lincoln University (Pa.); c.1910, M.A., Columbia University; c.1915-1916, Syracuse University; c.1929, M.D., Indiana University School of Medicine; c.1931, Ph.D. (pharmacology), University of Wisconsin. CAREER: Before becoming a physician, held ministerial positions in Annapolis, Md.; Syracuse, N.Y.; and Indianapolis, Ind. (1911-22) and a professorship of psychology at Wilberforce University (1922-25); 1931-53, Department of Pharmacology, Howard University School of Medicine: 1931-32, associate professor; and 1932-53, professor and head; 1931-53, consultant in pharmacology, Freedmen's Hospital. CONTRIBUTIONS: Performed research in various areas of pharmacology, particularly on the action of picrotoxin as an antidote to CNS depression from high doses of barbiturates. He and Joseph L. Johnson were (in 1931) the second and third blacks to earn both the M.D. and Ph.D. degrees. First black professor of pharmacology in United States.

WRITINGS: More than 50 articles and several nonmedical books. "Barbiturate-Coriamystin Antagonism," *Proc. Soc. for Experimental Biol. & Med.* 34 (1936): 591-93; "The Protective Action of Picrotoxin in Prolonged Anesthesia," *Am. J. of Surg.*, n.s., 34 (1936): 571-80. Some writings listed in *WWICA* 7 (1950): 351; and in *NUC-Pre-1956*, 357: 652. Most are listed in W. Montague Cobb, *The First Negro Medical Society* (1939), 110-12. REFERENCES: W. Montague Cobb, "Arnold Hamilton Maloney, M.D., 1888-1955," *JNMA* 47 (1955): 424-26; Arnold H. Maloney, *Amber Gold, An Adventure in Autobiography* (1946); *WWAPS* 1 (1938): 757; *WWICA* 7 (1950): 351.

T. Savitt

MANN, FRANK CHARLES (September 11, 1887, Decatur, Ind.-September 30, 1962, Rochester, Minn.). *Physiologist.* Son of Joseph E. and Louisa (Kiess) Mann. Married Velma J. Daniels, 1914; three children. EDUCATION: Decatur High School; 1907, B.S., Marion Normal College; Indiana University: 1911, A.B.; 1913, M.D.; and 1914, M.A. CAREER: At Indiana University: 1908-12, teaching fellow in physiology; and 1913-14, instructor in experimental surgery; 1914-52, chief, Division of Experimental Surgery and Pathology, Mayo Foundation; 1914-48, director, Mayo Foundation Institute of Experimental Medicine; 1927-52, professor of experimental surgery, Mayo Foundation. CONTRIBUTIONS: Authority on physiology of the liver, gastro-intestinal surgery, and surgery of kidneys and blood vessels. Achieved international recognition for work on removal of the liver. Established the crucial role of the liver in supplying glucose for the remainder of the body in a fasting state. Demonstrated role of the liver in urea formation. Established the extrahepatic formation of bile pigment. Made important contributions to the pathogenesis of peptic ulcer, pancreatitis, cholecystitis, and other gallbladder diseases. Did homologous transplantation of intact mammalian heart (1933). President, American Physiological Society (1936-37).

WRITINGS: Author or co-author of more than 400 papers. REFERENCES: *BMNAS*, 38: 161-204; *N.Y. Times*, October 2, 1962, p. 39: 2; *Who Was Who in Am.*, 4: 609.

R. Rosenthal

MANNING, ISAAC HALL (September 14, 1866, Pittsboro, N.C.-February 12, 1946, Chapel Hill, N.C.). *Physician; Medical educator; Physiology; Internal medicine.* Son of John and Louisa (Hall) Manning. Married Martha Battle Lewis, 1906, some children; Mary Best Jones, 1911, some children. EDUCATION: 1886, B.A., University of North Carolina; 1894-95, University of North Carolina; 1897, M.D., Long Island College Hospital. CAREER: 1899-1901, surgeon, Atlantic Coast Line Railroad; at University of North Carolina School of Medicine: 1901-39, professor of physiology and bacteriology (emeritus 1939-46); and 1905-

33, dean. CONTRIBUTIONS: As dean, built the University of North Carolina Medical School from a small developing institution into a strong, reputable facility with firm funding, good equipment, and fine faculty, although never succeeded in convincing the legislature to expand the school from a two to a full four-year curriculum. Promoted and developed the Hospital Saving Association (1935), an early prepayment health plan in N.C., and served as its first president (1935-41) and then medical director (1941-46). President, North Carolina Medical Society (1933-34). REFERENCES: Dorothy Long, ed., *Medicine in North Carolina* (1972), 234-35, 373-97; *Who Was Who in Am.*, 2: 344.

T. L. Savitt

MARCH, ALDEN (September 20, 1795, Sutton, Mass.-June 17, 1869, Albany, N.Y.). *Physician; Anatomy; Surgery; Medical education.* Son of Jacob, farmer, and Eleanor (Moore) March. Married Joanna P. Armsby, 1824; four children. EDUCATION: 1818, studied medicine with William Ingalls, Boston, Mass.; 1820, M.D., Brown University; 1841, 1848, 1856, studied medicine, Europe. CAREER: 1814-17, ran his father's farm; 1817, schoolteacher, Hoosick, N.Y.; 1820-38, practiced medicine, operated private school of anatomy, Albany; 1824-38, anatomy and physiology faculty, Vermont Academy of Medicine, Castleton, Vt.; at Albany Medical College (later merged with Fairfield Medical School to become Albany Hospital and Medical College): 1830-34, founder and anatomy and operative surgery faculty; and 1839-69, founder and surgery faculty; president: 1832, 1833, Medical Society of the County of Albany; 1857, New York State Medical Society; and 1864, American Medical Association. CONTRIBUTIONS: Organized the Albany Medical College (1839). One of the first persons in the United States to teach anatomy by dissection. Conducted free surgical clinics attended by students, where he performed a great variety of operations. Modified and devised several surgical procedures and instruments, including an improved splint for use in hip diseases, improved forceps for harelip operation, a new instrument for removing urinary calculi, and instruments for the removal of dead bone.

WRITINGS: *A Lecture on the Expedience of Establishing A Medical College and Hospital in the City of Albany* (1830); *Coxalgia or Hip Disease* (1853); *Improved Forceps for Hare-Lip Operation. . .* (1855). REFERENCES: *DAB*, 12: 268; Emerson Crosby Kelly, "The Doctors March to Armsby of Albany," *Bull. Hist. Med.* 30 (1956): 32-37; Kelly and Burrage (1928), 808-9; *NCAB*, 2: 445; *Who Was Who in Am.*, Hist. Vol.: 402.

S. Galishoff

MARINE, DAVID (September 20, 1880, Whiteleysburg, Md.-November 26, 1976, Lewes, Del.). *Pathologist.* Son of David and Nancy (Baynard) Marine. Married Mary Elizabeth Nuttle, 1923; one son. EDUCATION: Western Maryland College: 1900, A.B.; and 1906, A.M.; 1905, M.D., Johns Hopkins University; December 1913-May 1914, studied with Theodore Kocher, Berlin. CAREER: At Western Reserve University: 1905-6, demonstrator in pathology; 1906-7, demonstrator in neuro-pathology; 1906-10, lecturer; 1910-12, assistant professor;

and 1912-15, associate professor; 1920-38, assistant professor, College of Physicians and Surgeons, Columbia University; 1920-45, director, Laboratory of Montefiore Hospital, New York City; retired to Rehoboth Beach, Del. CONTRIBUTIONS: Determined that iodine was necessary to thyroid function; suggested that Grave's disease be treated with iodine and that iodine be used in goiter prophylaxis. Described cyanide-goiter. Credited with the initial understanding of the cause and the means of prevention of endemic goiter.

WRITINGS: "The Relation of Iodine to the Structure of the Thyroid Gland," *Arch. Int. Med.* 1 (1908): 349-84 (with W. W. Williams); "Further Observations on the Relation of Iodine to the Structure of the Thyroid Gland in the Sheep, Dog, Hog and Ox," *Arch. Int. Med.* 3 (1909): 66-77 (with C. H. Lenhart); "Further Observations on the So-Called Thyroid Carcinoma of the Brook Trout (Salvelinus Fontinalis) and Its Relation to Endemic Goiter," *J. of Experimental Med.* 13 (1911, with C. H. Lenhart); "The Pathological Anatomy of Exophthalmic Goiter," *Arch. Int. Med.* 8 (Sept. 1911): 265-316 (with C. H. Lenhart); "The Prevention of Simple Goiter in Man," *J. Lab. and Clin. Med.* 3 (1917): 40-48 (with O. P. Kimball), first in a series of six papers of that title; "The Prevention of Goiter," *Public Health, Mich.* 9 (1923): 23-24. REFERENCES: *BHM* (1975-79), 83; Lawrence A. Kohn, "The Midwestern American 'Epidemic' of Iodine-Induced Hyperthyroidism in the 1920s," *Bull. of the N.Y. Acad. of Med.* 52 (Sept. 1976): 770-81 (contains excellent references); Josip Matovinovic, "David Marine (1880-1976): Nestor of Thyroidology," *Perspectives in Biol. Med.* (Summer 1978): 565-89; J. H. Means, *The Association of Physicians: Its First Seventy-Five Years* (1961); *NCAB,* F: 484; G. N. Stewart, ed., *The Prevention of Simple Goiter: Studies by David Marine, C. H. Lenhart, O. P. Kimball and J. M. Rogoff* (1923).

G. P. *Jenkins*

MARRIOTT, W[ILLIAMS] McKIM (March 5, 1885, Baltimore, Md.-November 11, 1936, San Francisco, Calif.). *Pediatrician; Biochemist.* Son of James Hamilton Wilson and Lucretia (Williams) Marriott. Married Elizabeth D. Robinson, 1911; two children. EDUCATION: 1904, B.S., University of North Carolina; 1910, M.D., Cornell, with graduate work in biochemistry. CAREER: At Washington University School of Medicine: 1910-12, instructor, Department of Biochemistry; and 1913-14, assistant, Department of Pediatrics; 1914-17, instructor and associate in pediatrics, Johns Hopkins Medical School; 1917-36, chairman, Department of Pediatrics, Washington University School of Medicine; and physician-in-chief, St. Louis Children's Hospital; 1923-36, dean, Washington University School of Medicine; 1936, dean and professor of research medicine, University of California Medical School, San Francisco. CONTRIBUTIONS: Made major advances in the understanding of infant feeding and metabolism, the effects of acidosis, and dehydration in diseases of infants and children. First interest was in biochemistry, and this laid the basis for his later clinical discoveries. A student of Philip Shaffer, (q.v.) in St. Louis, Mo., and John Howland (q.v.) in Baltimore, trained many leading pediatricians, including his successor as chairman of pediatrics, Dr. Alexis F. Hartmann (q.v.). Despite the fact that reputation as a pediatrician per se was slight, was appointed to organize the full-time Department of Pediatrics, Washington University (1917), and, in addition, served as dean, medical school (1923-36).

WRITINGS: "Acidosis Occurring with Diarrhea," *Am. J. of Diseases of Children* 11 (1916): 309 (with John Howland); "The Pathogenesis of Certain Nutritional Disorders," *Trans., Am. Pediat. Soc.* 31 (1919): 34; "Anhydremia," Harvey Lecture, *Physiol. Rev.* 3 (1923): 275; "Newer Aspects of Acidosis," *JAMA* 91 (1928): 1695 (with A. F. Hartmann); *Infant Nutrition* (Text) (1930); "Observations on Nature and Treatment of Diarrhea and Associated Systemic Disturbances," *J. Pediat.* 3 (1933): 181 (with A. F. Hartmann and M. E. Senn). REFERENCES: *DAB*, Supplement 2: 432-33; *NCAB*, 36: 140; obituary, *J. Pediat.* (Dec. 1936): 861; Borden S. Veeder, "W. McKim Marriott," *J. Pediat.* (1938): 619-26; idem, "Williams McKim Marriott," *Pediatric Profiles* (1955): 218-28, reprinted from *J. Pediat.* 47, no. 6 (1955): 791-801.

M. Hunt

MARSHALL, CLARA (May 8, 1847, London Grove Township, Chester County, Pa.-March 13, 1931, Bryn Mawr, Pa.). *Physician; Educator.* Daughter of Pennock and Mary (Phillips) Marshall, rural reformist Quaker stock on both sides. Did not marry. EDUCATION: 1875, M.D., Woman's Medical College of Pennsylvania (WMCP); 1876, additional study, Philadelphia College of Pharmacy. CAREER: 1874, appointed instructor in pharmacy, WMCP, while still a student; 1876 appointed professor of materia medica and general therapeutics, as the college's board sought to fill-out the faculty with women; although her precocious appointment was questioned by some of the faculty, held the chair until 1905; 1888, appointed dean of the college, serving until 1917; maintained a private practice in central Philadelphia, Pa.; seems not to have been active in civic or Quaker affairs, but joined (or rejoined) a Philadelphia meeting "by application" late in her life (1924). CONTRIBUTIONS: Somewhat sternly but effectively guided the WMCP through the critical "Flexnerian" years and beyond, maintaining more than acceptable standards despite limited resources—so that the school emerged as the only surviving women's medical college. Initiated successful moves to build a hospital wholly controlled by the college, an indispensible accomplishment. Did no notable scientific work.

WRITINGS: *The Woman's Medical College of Pennsylvania: An Historical Outline* (1897); about eight to ten papers and case reports (mostly gynecologic) in various journals, some listed in a useful compilation of early articles by women physicians in her *Woman's Medical College.* REFERENCES: No full account of her life, but many letters and other materials are in the Archives and Special Collections on Women in Medicine, Medical College of Pennsylvania, Philadelphia; *DAB*, 6, pt. 2: 307-8; *Notable Am. Women*, 2: 501-2.

S. J. Peitzman

MARSHALL, E[LI] KENNERLY, JR. (May 2, 1889, Charleston, S.C.-January 10, 1966, Baltimore, Md.) *Physiologist; Pharmacologist; Renal function; Chemotherapy.* Son of Eli Kennerly, merchant, and Julia Irene (Brown) Marshall. Married Alice Berry Carroll, 1917; three children. EDUCATION: 1908, B.S., College of Charleston; at Johns Hopkins: Ph.D., 1911, M.D., 1917; 1912, studied in Germany. CAREER: At Johns Hopkins: 1911-14, physiological chemistry faculty; 1914-19, pharmacology faculty; 1921-32, physiology faculty; and 1932-55, pharmacology and experimental therapeutics faculty; 1919-21, pharmacology faculty, Washington University. CONTRIBUTIONS: One of the principal architects of modern chemotherapy and a leading investigator of renal physiology. Devised a method for the determination of urea in biological fluids (1913). Illuminated the processes of filtration, reabsorption, and secretion in the formation of urine and the role played by the convoluted tubules; one of the first demonstrations of a specific kidney function (1923). Established a method for determining the absorption, distribution, and excretion of sulfanilamide in animals and man (late 1930s); led to the establishment of rational dose schedules for these drugs. Produced an intravenous sulfonamide, sodium sulfapyridine. Developed a drug that remains in the intestinal tract, sulfaguanidine, which is credited with saving Port Moresby, New Guinea, from Japanese capture by controlling an epidemic of dysentery among Australian soldiers. The leader of a medical team established during World War II to develop better means of treating malaria; succeeded in defining the role of the four-amino and eight-amino quinolines in human malaria. Devised method to measure cardiac output in a living animal not under anesthesia (1926); subsequently developed a method for man using nitrous oxide and ethylene, which was widely employed until it was superseded by cardiac catheterization. Discovered the part played by anoxia in respiratory depression (1936); discovery revealed the danger of carbon dioxide narcosis when oxygen is administered to patients with chronic pulmonary or cardiac disease.

WRITINGS: "The Mechanism for the Elimination of Phenolsulphonepthalein by the Kidneys. A Proof of Secretion by the Convoluted Tubules," *Johns Hopkins Hosp. Bull.* 34 (1923): 1 (with J. L. Vickers); "Studies on the Cardiac Output of the Dog. I. The Cardiac Output of the Normal Unanesthetized Dog," *Am. J. of Physiol.* 77 (1926): 459; "Depression of Respiration by Oxygen," *J. of Pharmacology and Experimental Therapeutics* 57 (1936): 437 (with Morris Rosenfeld); "Bacterial Chemotherapy. The Pharmacology of Sulfanilamide," *Physiol. Rev.* 19 (1939): 240; "Sulfanilylguanidine: A Chemotherapeutic Agent for Intestinal Infections," *Johns Hopkins Hosp. Bull.* 67 (1940): 163-68 (with A. C. Bratton, H. J. White, and J. T. Litchfield). REFERENCES: *BHM* (1976), 21; A. McGehee Harvey, *Adventures in Medical Research*, 396-400; Thomas H. Maren, "Eli Kennerly Marshall, Jr., 1889-1966," *Johns Hopkins Hosp. Bull.* 119 (Oct. 1966): 247-54; *N.Y. Times*, January 12, 1966; *Who Was Who in Am.*, 4: 613.

S. Galishoff

MARSHALL, HUBERT (December 27, 1905, Mingo, W. Va.-May 12, 1976, Morgantown, W.Va.). *Physician.* Son of F. Piatt, farmer, and Mary Ellen (Beaty) Marshall. EDUCATION: Davis and Elkins College; at University of Louisville: 1928, A.B.; and 1932, M.D.; internship, Louisville Hospital. CAREER: 1933-34, practice, Davis Memorial Hospital, Elkins, W.Va.; 1934-49, U.S. Army surgeon; 1951-69, area administrator, District 31, U.S. Mine Workers Association Health and Retirement Fund; 1933-34, private practice, Elkins. CONTRIBUTIONS: Developed rural health clinics and group practice to see that miners in rural areas had health care. Helped develop Fairmont Clinic and Golden Clinic. Under his direction, paraplegics and amputees were sent to the Institute of Physical Medicine and Rehabilitation, N.Y., and Henry Kaiser Institute, Orange, N.J. Went into the hills to find people who needed assistance; arranged funding for transportation to assure rehabilitation for the disabled. Interested in equitable payment for doctors' services. Instrumental in obtaining the use of Intermittent Positive Pressure breathing equipment for home use.

K. Nodyne and R. Murphy

MARSHALL, HYRUM LEO (September 10, 1884, Tooele, Utah-October 11, 1972, Napa, Calif.). *Physician.* Son of Henry, farmer, and Rhoda (Pickett) Marshall. Married Lucille Rogers, 1918; three children. EDUCATION: 1908, A.B., University of Utah; 1909-10, University of Utah Medical School; 1914, M.D., Columbia University College of Physicians and Surgeons; 1915-17, intern, several N.Y. hospitals; 1918, studied at Trudeau Sanatorium; 1930, M.S., public health, University of Michigan. CAREER: 1917-19, Naval Medical Corps; 1918, helped fight flu epidemic in N.Y. harbor; 1919-50, director, University of Utah Student Health Service; at University of Utah Medical School: 1921-43, professor, physical welfare; and 1945-46, 1949-50, acting dean; 1951-54, director, public health and medical services, Trust Territory, Pacific Islands; 1955-64, planning coordinator, new University of Utah medical complex; 1947-50, director, National Tuberculosis Association; 1937-40, member, Board of Trustees, Utah State Hospital Association; president: 1942-43, Utah State Public Health Association; and 1948, American College Health Association. CONTRIBUTIONS: Organized the Student Health Services, University of Utah (1921). Mobilized financing for the new University of Utah medical complex.

WRITINGS: "Screwworm Fly in Utah," *Rocky Mt. Med. J.* 41 (Jul. 1944): 478-80 (with D. T. Jones); "Malaria in Utah," *ibid.*, 45 (Jun. 1948): 469-72 (with D. M. Rees); "Changing Horizons in College Health Services," Presidential Address, *Proc. Am. Student Health Assoc. Bull.* 29 (1948): 7-10. REFERENCES: *Who's Important in Med.* (1952), 644.

H. Bauman

MARTIN, FRANKLIN HENRY (July 13, 1857, Ixonia, Wis.-March 7, 1935, Phoenix, Ariz.). *Physician; Editor; Surgical gynecology.* Son of Edmond, farmer, and Josephine (Carlin) Martin. Married Isabelle Hollister, 1886; no children. EDUCATION: 1880, M.D., Chicago Medical College (now medical department, Northwestern University); c. 1881, house officer, Mercy Hospital (Chicago, Ill.). CAREER: c. *post* 1882, practiced medicine, Chicago; 1883-88, surgical staff, South Side Dispensary; 1886-88, surgery faculty, Polyclinic Hospital Medical School, Chicago; *post* 1887, gynecological staff, Woman's Hospital; 1888, organizer with W. F. Coleman, Post-Graduate Medical School and Hospital; on Council of National Defense: 1916-21, member, Advisory Committee, and 1917-19, chairman, General Medical Board; 1917-19, Medical Corps, U.S. Army; president: 1919, American Gynecological Society; 1921, Gorgas Memorial Institute of Tropical and Preventive Medicine; and 1928-29, American College of Surgeons. CONTRIBUTIONS: One of the first Americans to practice aseptic surgery. Reduced the mortality in operations for uterine fibroid by devising a procedure for tying off the uterine arteries to cause atrophy of the fibroid (1892). Pioneered the surgical removal of the bladder by transplanting the ureters in the colon (1899). Founded and edited *Surgery, Gynecology and Obstetrics* (1905-35), one of the leading surgical journals of the world, to which he added the *International Abstract of Surgery* (1913). Organized the Clinical Congress of Surgeons of North America (1910); three years later was merged into the American College of Surgeons, which he largely created and in whose affairs he played a prominent role. Founded Charity Hospital (1887) and Gorgas Memorial Institute of Tropical and Preventive Medicine (1921, Panama). Helped edit *American Journal of Obstetrics and Gynecology* and *Chicago Medical Recorder*. Oversaw the mobilization of physicians, surgeons, and dentists during World War I.

WRITINGS: *Treatment of Fibroid Tumors of the Uterus* (1897); *A Treatise on Gynecology* (1903). REFERENCES: *DAB*, Supplement 1: 542-43; Miller, *BHM*, p. 68; *NCAB*, C: 372; *Who Was Who in Am.*, 1: 782.

S. Galishoff

MARTIN, HENRY NEWELL (July 1, 1848, Newry, County Down, Ireland-October 27, 1896, Burley-in-Wharfedale, Yorkshire, England). *Physiologist; Cardiac physiology.* Son of Congregational minister and schoolmaster. Married Hetty (Cary) Pegram, 1878; no children. EDUCATION: University of London: 1871, M.B.; and 1872, D.Sc.; Cambridge University: 1874, B.A.; 1875, D.Sc.; and 1877, M.A. CAREER: 1870, demonstrator to instructor of psychology, Michael Foster, Trinity College, Cambridge, England; assistant to T. H. Huxley in biology course, Royal College of Science (South Kensington, England); 1874, fellow, Trinity College; 1876-93, biology faculty, Johns Hopkins University; 1893-96, in England because of ill health; 1890, president, American Society of Naturalists. CONTRIBUTIONS: Helped establish physiology as an independent science without regard to its applications to medicine. A founder, American Physiological Society, and editor, British *Journal of Physiology*. Developed a method for isolating and perfusing a mammalian heart to study the effects on it of variables such as temperature, alcohol, and arterial and venous pressure. Laid down broad foundations for instruction and research in experimental biology. Founded and edited *Studies from the Biological Laboratory of the Johns Hopkins University* (1877-93). Wrote several well-regarded textbooks, including *A Course of Practical Instruction in Elementary Biology* (1875, with T. H. Huxley), *The Human Body* (1881), and *Handbook of Vertebrate Dissection* (1881, with William Moale).

WRITINGS: "On a Method of Isolating a Mammalian Heart," *Studies from the Biological Lab. of the Johns Hopkins Univ.* 2 (1882): 213-33; "The Direct Influence of Gradual Variations of Temperature upon the Rate of Beat of the Dog's Heart," *Physiological Trans. of the Royal Soc. of London* 174 (1883): 663-88. Article reprinted as *Physiological Papers*, Memoirs from the Biological Laboratory of the Johns Hopkins

University 3 (1895). REFERENCES: *BHM* (1964-69), 175; (1974-79), 84; *DAB*, 12: 337-38; *DSB*, 9: 142-43; Clark A. Elliott, *Biog. Dictionary of Am. Sci.* (1979), 170-71; *NCAB*, 12: 113.

S. Galishoff

MARTLAND, HARRISON STANFORD (September 10, 1883, Newark, N.J.-May 1, 1954, New York, N.Y.). *Physician; Pathology; Industrial medicine; Forensic medicine.* Son of William Harrison, physician, and Ida (Bucklish) Martland. Married Myra C. Ferdon, 1910; two children. EDUCATION: 1901, A.B., Western Maryland College; 1905, M.D., College of Physicians and Surgeons (Columbia); 1905-6, intern, New York City Hospital, Welfare Island; 1907-8, studied at Russell Sage Institute of Pathology, Blackwells Island, N.Y. CAREER: 1909-53, pathological staff, Newark City Hospital; and pathologist, Newark; during World War I, U.S. Army Medical Corps, Bellevue Medical College unit, in charge of the military hospital in Vichy, France, and later consulting pathologist, Vanderbilt Hospital, Paris; 1925-27, county physician, Essex County, N.J.; 1927-53, chief medical examiner, Essex County; *post* 1933, forensic medicine faculty, New York University-Bellevue Medical Center; 1945-46, pathology and bacteriology faculty, Essex College of Medicine, Essex County; for 18 years, director, Dazian Foundation for Medical Research, New York City. CONTRIBUTIONS: Established the professional medical examiner system, Essex County. Best known for studies of the effects of radioactive material on the human body; showed that several women who worked in a N.J. watch factory applying luminous paint to watch dials had died from cancer caused by minute traces of radioactive substances in paint; subsequently designed protective devices for employees on the Manhattan Project at Oak Ridge, Tenn., where the atomic bomb was being developed, as a result of which only two workers died from the enormous amount of radiation produced there. Showed that punch drunkenness in prize fighters is a medical ailment caused by rupture of tiny blood vessels in the brain as occurs in other types of concussion. Demonstrated that most deaths from syphilitic heart disease result from lesions of the aorta and aortic valves rather than from myocardial lesions. Established the lethal effects of beryllium poisoning, which led to regulatory reforms governing the use of the mineral in industrial processes.

WRITINGS: "Some Unrecognized Dangers in the Use and Handling of Radioactive Substances," *Proc., N.Y. Pathological Soc.* 25 (1925): 87-92; "Cardiac Syphilis (Syphilitic Aortitis)," *J. of the Med. Soc. of New Jersey* 24 (1927): 689-701; "Punch Drunk," *JAMA* 91 (1928): 1103-7; "Recent Progress in Medical-Legal Field in United States," *Proc. Institute of Med., Chicago* 9 (1933): 261-78; "Occupational Beryllium Poisoning in New Jersey," *J. of the Med. Soc. of New Jersey* 45 (1948): 5-14 (with H. A. Brodkin and H.S. Martland, Jr.). A bibliography is in Samuel Berg, *Harrison Stanford Martland, M.D.; the Story of a Physician, a Hospital, an Era* (1978). REFERENCES: Berg, *Harrison Stanford Martland; Current Biog.* (1940), 565-66; *NCAB*, 44: 502-3; *N.Y. Times,* May 2, 1954.

S. Galishoff

MASON, JAMES TATE (May 20, 1882, Lahore, Orange County, Va.-June 20, 1936, Seattle, Wash.). *Surgeon.* Son of Claiborne Rice Tate, physician, and

Mary Moore (Woolfolk) Mason. Married Laura DeWolfe Whittlesey, 1912; three children. EDUCATION: Locust Dale Military Academy; 1905, M.D., University of Virginia; 1905-6, intern, Philadelphia Polyclinic; 1906-7, resident, Philadelphia Municipal Hospital. CAREER: 1907, ship's doctor on ship to Seattle; 1908-9, assistant physician, Pacific Coast Coal Company, Black Diamond, Wash., and then Franklin, Wash.; 1909-36, general surgical practice, Seattle; 1911-14, King County coroner; 1916-20, superintendent, King County Hospital. CONTRIBUTIONS: Founded Mason Clinic (1918) and became its surgeon-in-chief. Established (with seven associates) the Virginia Mason Hospital (1919), at which he served as chief surgeon until death. This hospital became one of the leading general hospitals in the Northwest. A leading national specialist in goiter surgery. Elected president, AMA (1935).   REFERENCES: *NCAB*, 26: 447; Edgar I. Stewart, *Washington, Northwest Frontier* 4 (1927): 547; *Who Was Who in Am.*, 1: 786; *Who's Who in Am. Med.* (1925), 1004.

T. L. Savitt

MATAS, RUDOLPH (September 12, 1860, Bonnet Carre, St. John's Parish, La.-September 23, 1957, New Orleans, La.). *Physician; Surgery.* Son of Narciso Hereu, physician, and Teresa (Jordá) Matas. Married Adrienne (Goslee) Landry, 1895; no children. EDUCATION: 1876, graduated, College of St. John, Matamoros, Mexico; 1880, M.D., medical department, University of Louisiana (later Tulane University); c. 1878-80, undergraduate intern, Charity Hospital, New Orleans. CAREER: 1879-82, at National Board of Health: 1879, medical clerk; laboratory assistant; and interpreter, Yellow Fever Commission, Havana, Cuba; 1881, medical inspector, Vicksburg, Miss.; 1881, suppression of yellow-fever epidemics, Brownsville, Tex. and Mier, Mexico; *post* 1881, practiced medicine, New Orleans; at Tulane University: 1885-95, anatomy faculty and 1894-1927, surgery faculty; surgical staff: 1894-1928, Charity Hospital; and 1904-35, Touro Infirmary, New Orleans; 1916-17, organizer and director, Base Hospital 24 (Tulane Unit); 1917-18, director, New Orleans School for Intensive Surgery War Training, Medical Reserve Corps, U.S. Army; president: 1894-95, Louisiana State Medical Association; 1909, American Surgical Association; 1911, Southern Surgical Association; 1920, American Association for Thoracic Surgery; and 1924-25, American College of Surgeons. CONTRIBUTIONS: A pioneer in vascular surgery. Developed a simple and safe method of treating an aneurysm by means of an intrasaccular suture; became known as the Matas operation (1888-1902). Developed a test to determine the adequacy of the collateral circulation before performing surgery of the great blood vessels (1900-1914). Extended the work of William Halsted (q.v.) in using cocaine in local and regional anesthesia (1886-1902). Introduced the concept of continuous intravenous drip of saline solution and other fluids for the treatment of shock, hemorrhage, and collapse. Devised surgical techniques and apparatus to keep the lungs inflated in intrathoracic operations. Employed naso-gastric tube drainage and developed a method of continuous drainage of the duodenal tube. Endowed the library at Tulane Medical School, which was named in his honor. Edited *New Orleans Medical and Surgical*

Journal (1883-85). Helped organize the New Orleans Polyclinic, the first postgraduate medical school in that city, and was a founding fellow, American College of Surgeons.

WRITINGS: "Traumatic Aneurism of the Left Branchial Artery. . . ," *Med. News* 53 (1888): 462-66; "Intralaryngeal Insufflation for the Relief of Acute Surgical Pneumothorax. . . ," *JAMA* 34 (1900): 1371-75, 1468-73; "Local and Regional Anesthesia with Cocaine and Other Analgesic Drugs. . . ," *Phila. Med. J.* 6 (1900): 820-43; "Surgery of the Vascular System," in William W. Keen (q.v.), *Surgery, Its Principles and Practice*, 5 (1910); ". . . Testing the Efficiency of the Collateral Circulation as a Preliminary to the Occlusion of the Great Surgical Vessels," *Trans. Am. Surg. Assoc.* 28 (1910): 4-54. REFERENCES: *BHM* (1964-69), 176; (1975-79), 84; (1980), 27; Isidore Cohn, *Rudolph Matas (1860-1957). A Biography of One of the Great Pioneers in Surgery* (1960); Miller, *BHM*, pp. 68-69; *NCAB*, 47: 148-49; *Who Was Who in Am.*, 3: 561.

S. Galishoff

MATHER, COTTON (February 12, 1662 or 1663, Boston, Mass.-February 13, 1727 or 1728, Boston). *Protestant clergyman; Author; Inoculation.* Son of Increase, clergyman and president of Harvard College, and Maria (Cotton) Mather. Married Abigail Phillips, 1686; Elizabeth (Clark) Hubbard, 1703; Lydia (Lee) George, 1715; 15 children. EDUCATION: 1678, B.A., Harvard College; studied medicine. CAREER: c. 1680, assisted father at Second Church, Boston; 1685, ordained; 1685-1727 or 1728, minister, Second Church; 1690-1703, fellow, Harvard College; distinguished clergyman and scholar. CONTRIBUTIONS: Played a major role in introducing inoculation in the Western world. Prevailed upon a local physician, Zabdiel Boylston (q.v.), to employ inoculation during a severe smallpox epidemic that afflicted Boston (1721), after having learned of its successful use in the Middle East in the *Transactions of the Royal Society of London* and from an African slave he owned. In the following year, published a statistical proof of inoculation's effectiveness in preventing deaths from smallpox, which led to its widespread adoption in America and Europe.

WRITINGS: *An Account. . . of Inoculating the Smallpox. . .* (1722). REFERENCES: Otho T. Beall, Jr., and Richard H. Shryock, *Cotton Mather: First Significant Figure in American Medicine* (1954); *BHM* (1964-69), 176; (1970-74), 119; John B. Blake, *Public Health in the Town of Boston, 1630-1822* (1959), 52-73; *DAB*, 12: 386-89; Clark A. Elliott, *Biog. Dictionary of Am. Sci.* (1979), 172; *Who Was Who in Am.*, Hist. Vol.: 408.

S. Galishoff

MATHEWS, JOSEPH McDOWELL (May 29, 1847, New Castle, Ky.-December 21, 1928, Los Angeles, Calif.). *Physician; Proctology.* Son of Caleb Moffatt, judge, and Frances S. (Edwards) Mathews. Married Sallie E. Berry, 1877. EDUCATION: 1867, M.D., University of Louisville; 1877, studied colonic and rectal surgery, St. Mark's Hospital (London). CAREER: 1867-76, practiced medicine with W. B. Oldham, New Castle; 1877-1912, practiced medicine, Louisville, Ky., specializing in proctology; 1877-78, surgery faculty, Louisville Hospital College of Medicine; at Kentucky School of Medicine: 1878-95, surgery faculty; and *post* 1882, proctology faculty; president: 1898, Kentucky State Board of Health; 1897-98, American Medical Association; and 1899, American Proctologic Society. CONTRIBUTIONS: America's first proctologist and the first orthodox physician anywhere in the world to limit practice to rectal diseases. Took proctology out of the hands of quacks and charlatans and placed it on a firm, scientific basis. Introduced British surgical methods for the treatment of diseases of the colon and rectum. Exerted a conservative influence in rectal surgery; opposed most radical operations because of their demonstrated failure to save or prolong life. Lacking modern diagnostic and laboratory tools, developed the art of manual diagnosis of rectal diseases to a high level of sophistication. Wrote *Treatise on Diseases of the Rectum, Anus and Sigmoid Flexure* (1892), the first proctology textbook by an American allopathic physician. Organized the American Proctologic Society (1899). Started *Mathews' Medical Quarterly* (1894), first journal on proctology in United States.

WRITINGS: "Some Observations after One Thousand Operations for Hemorrhoids," *JAMA* 11 (1888): 766; "Our Diagnostic Resources in Rectal and Allied Diseases," ibid., 21 (1893): 725; "Is Total Extirpation of the Rectum Ever Justifiable?" ibid., 25 (1895): 94. A bibliography is in Curtice Rosser, "The First Proctologist: the Life and Writings of Joseph McDowell Mathews," *Trans., Am. Proctological Soc.* (1946). REFERENCES: Morris Fishbein, *History of the AMA* (1947), 677-78; Miller, *BHM*, p. 69; *NCAB*, 13: 18-19; Rosser, "First Proctologist," pp. 429-49; *Who Was Who in Am.*, 4: 619.

E. H. Conner

MATSON, RALPH CHARLES (January 21, 1880, Brookville, Pa.-October 26, 1945, Portland, Oreg.). *Surgeon; Pulmonologist.* Son of John, farmer, and Minerva (Brady) Matson. Married Adeline Ferarri, 1907; Chiara De Bona, 1923; no children. EDUCATION: 1902, M.D., University of Oregon Medical School; 1906-7, postgraduate study, Cambridge University, and St. Mary's Hospital (London): 1902-5, intern and resident, Good Samaritan Hospital, Portland; postgraduate study: 1911-12, University of Berlin, University of Vienna, and Academy of Medicine (Dusseldorf, Germany); and 1923-25, Victoria Park and St. Mary's hospitals (London) and the University of Vienna. CAREER: 1905-45, practice, Portland; 1906-45, medical faculty, University of Oregon; 1906-45, medical staff, Good Samaritan Hospital, Portland; 1912-25, co-medical director, Portland Open Air Sanitarium; 1916, Harvard University surgical unit with the British Expeditionary Forces; 1917, Royal Army Medical Corps; 1917-20, U.S. Army Medical Corps; 1939-40, president, American College of Chest Physicians; 1941-45, editor-in-chief, *Diseases of the Chest*. CONTRIBUTIONS: International authority on tuberculosis and chest surgery. Contributed to the creation of a modern Multnomah County tuberculosis sanitarium. Led campaign of public information about tuberculosis. In the war, devised a new method of irrigating wounds. Pioneer in thoracic surgery. Originated electro-surgical method of cutting adhesions in artificial pneumothorax.

WRITINGS: "Operative Collapse Therapy in the Treatment of Pulmonary Tuberculosis," *Western J. of Surg.* 38 (1930): 662-79, 743-54; 39 (1931): 13-24; "Total Removal of the Right Lung for Bronchogenic Carcinoma,'' *Diseases of the Chest* 4 (Jun. 1938): 43-46 (with J. M. Roberts and M. Bisaillon); ''Evaluation of Various Surgical Procedures in the Treatment of Pulmonary Tuberculosis,'' *ibid.*, 12 (1946): 40-47 (with W. S. Conklin and S. Domm). REFERENCES: O. Larsell, *The Doctor in Oregon* (1947); *NCAB*, D: 386-87; James T. Speros, ''Ralph Charles Matson: 1880-1945,'' *Diseases of the Chest* 11 (1945): 687-88; John E. Tuhy, *Annals of the Thoracic Clinic*.

G. B. Dodds

MATSON, RAY WILLIAM (January 21, 1880, Brookville, Pa.-September 12, 1934, Portland, Oreg.). *Surgeon; Pulmonologist*. Son of John, farmer, and Minerva (Brady) Matson. Married Carolyn Holmes; no children. EDUCATION: 1902, M.D., University of Oregon Medical School; 1902-5, intern and resident, Good Samaritan Hospital, Portland; postgraduate study: 1909, 1914, 1920, 1925, University of Vienna; 1909, University of London; and 1919, University of Paris. CAREER: 1905-34, practice, Portland; 1906, city health officer and city physician, Portland. 1907-43, medical staff, Portland Open Air Sanitarium; 1917-19, U.S. Army Medical Corps; 1903-34, medical faculty, University of Oregon Medical School; 1930-34, surgical consultant, U.S. Veterans Administration Hospital, Portland. CONTRIBUTIONS: International authority on tuberculosis. Primarily interested in early diagnosis and collapse therapy and a pioneer in the latter field. Also pioneered in oleothorax in the United States and wrote a classic account in that field and in phrenic neurectomy. Translated Alfred Wolff-Eisner's *Clinical Immunity and Sero-Diagnosis* from the German.

WRITINGS: ''End Results of 600 Cases of Pulmonary Tuberculosis Treated by Artificial Pneumothorax,'' *Am. Rev. of Tuberculosis* 9 (1924): 294-336 (with R. C. Matson and M. Bisaillon); ''Observations Concerning the Contralateral Lung in Pulmonary Tuberculosis Treated by Artificial Pneumothorax,'' *ibid.*, 10 (1925): 562-82 (with R. C. Matson and M. Bisaillon); ''Oleothorax,'' *ibid.*, 25 (1932): 419-68. REFERENCES: Allen K. Krause,''Ray William Matson: 1880-1934,'' *Am. J. of Tuberculosis* 31 (1935): 250-53; John E. Tuhy, *Annals of the Thoracic Clinic*.

G. B. Dodds

MAURY, RICHARD BROOKE (February 15, 1834, Georgetown, D.C.-March 7, 1919, Memphis, Tenn.). *Physician*; *Gynecology*. Son of Richard Brooke, private secretary to President James Monroe and first clerk, U.S. Department of the Navy, and Ellen (Magruder) Maury. Married Jane S. Ellett, 1861, six children; Jennie B. Poston, 1876, three children. EDUCATION: 1851-52, University of Virginia, M.D., 1857; 1858, M.D., University of New York; 1859, intern, Bellevue Hospital, N.Y. CAREER: 1859, due to pulmonary disease, went to Port Gibson, Miss., to regain health; 1861-65, Civil War, surgeon for the 28th Mississippi Calvary, Confederate States of America; in charge of military hospitals, Brookhaven and Lauderale Springs, Miss., and Greenville, Ala.; 1867, moved from Port Gibson to Memphis, limiting private practice to gynecology after 1885; 1884, established Drs. Maury and Robert Wood Mitchell's Sanatorium for the Diseases of Women, providing an operating room where major gynecological surgery was performed; first training school for nurses in Memphis was established by Dr. Maury; 1892, organized the Lucy Brinkley Hospital for Women, now a part of Memphis Methodist Hospital; at Memphis Medical College: 1869, professor of physiology; and 1871-73, professor of theory and practice of medicine; 1885-97, professor of gynecology, Memphis Hospital Medical College; 1870-71, president, Memphis Board of Education; 1877, became member, first Tennessee State Board of Health; 1906, president, American Gynecological Association; 1903, retired and devoted last years to various public services; 1911, organized West Tennessee Audubon Society and served several years as president; led movement to establish public recreational areas in the city. CONTRIBUTIONS: Achieved benefits in the health of women as an early specialist in gynecology. Improved abdominal surgery. Developed hospital facilities for women. Established first nurses training program in the area. Participated in medical teaching in gynecology. Made several contributions to public health as a member, Tennessee State Board of Health. Last years devoted to public service.

WRITINGS: Published about 38 articles, mainly in medical journals, the most important relating to tubal or ectopic pregnancy, diagnosis, and operative therapy. REFERENCES: Lee R. Brown, "Richard Brooke Maury (1834-1919)," *Trans. Am. Gyn. Soc.* 44 (1919): 373-76; *NCAB*, 14: 240; W. S. Speer, *Sketches of Prominent Tennesseans* (1888), 77-79.

                                                                                      S. R. Bruesch

MAXCY, KENNETH FULLER (July 27, 1889, Saco, Maine-December 12, 1966, Baltimore, Md.). *Physician; Epidemiology.* Son of Frederick Edward, physician, and Estelle Abbey (Gilpatric) Maxcy. Married Gertrude Helene McClellan, 1918; three children. EDUCATION: 1911, A.B., George Washington University; 1915, M.D., Johns Hopkins University; 1915-17, intern and resident, Johns Hopkins Hospital; 1921, D.P.H., Johns Hopkins School of Hygiene and Public Health. CAREER: 1917, medical staff, Henry Ford Hospital; 1918, U.S. Army Medical Corps; 1919-29, hygienic laboratory, U.S. Public Health Service; 1929-36, bacteriology and preventive medicine faculty, University of Virginia; 1936-37, public health and preventive medicine faculty, University of Minnesota; 1938-54, bacteriology and public health faculty, Johns Hopkins School of Hygiene and Public Health; 1937-40, 1942-45, 1948-52, scientific director, International Health Division, Rockefeller Foundation; 1943, member, United States of America Typhus Commission. CONTRIBUTIONS: Discovered that a mild form of typhus that was endemic in parts of the southeastern United States was not spread by body lice as is classical typhus; concluded on the basis of laboratory and epidemiological studies that the disease, endemic or murine typhus, was transmitted to man by rat fleas, whose host provided a natural reservoir of infection (1925-26). During World War II, collaborated in a field study of "scrub typhus" (tsutsugamushi disease) in New Guinea; resulted in a complete understanding of the disease and better control methods. Organized and directed investigations of poliomyelitis; argued persuasively that it was transmitted primarily by direct contact rather than by water, sewage, or insect vectors, as was commonly believed (1940s). Edited the seventh and eighth editions of Milton Rosenau's (q.v.) *Preventive Medicine and Hygiene* (1951, 1956). Made valuable studies of malaria, hepatitis, and meningococcal meningitis.

WRITINGS: "Clinical Observations on Endemic Typhus (Brill's Disease) in the Southeastern United States," *Public Health Reports* 41 (1926): 1213-20; "An Epidemiological Study of Endemic Typhus (Brill's Disease) in the Southeastern United States, . . ." ibid., (1926): 2967-95; "Hypothetical Relationship of Water Supply to Poliomyelitis," *Am. J. of Public Health* 33 (1943): 41-45; "Tsutsugamushi Disease (Scrub Typhus, Mite-borne Typhus) in New Guinea," ibid., 35 (1945): 1121-30 (with others). Writings are listed in *BMNAS*. REFERENCES: *BMNAS* 42 (1971): 161-73; Philip E. Sartwell, "Why We Are Here: A Tribute Presented at the Dedication of the Kenneth F. Maxcy Laboratories," *Am. J. of Epidemiology* 89 no. 5 (May 1967): 503-7; *Who Was Who in Am.*, 4: 621-22.

S. Galishoff

MAY, FREDERICK (November 16, 1773, Boston, Mass.-January 23, 1847, Washington, D.C.). *Physician; Obstetrics.* Son of Col. John May, distinguished Boston merchant. Married; many children. EDUCATION: 1792, A.B., Harvard College; Harvard University: 1795, M.B.; and 1811, M.D. CAREER: *Post* 1795, Washington, D.C., practice, one of the first physicians to practice in that area; 1823-39, professor of obstetrics, medical department, Columbian College (later George Washington University); 1832, physician to the Eastern Cholera Hospital. CONTRIBUTIONS: Very influential, popular, and skillful obstetrician with an enormous practice. Scholarly man and brilliant lecturer. Incorporator of the Medical Society of the District of Columbia and its third president (1833-48). President, Medical Association of the District of Columbia (1847). Member, Pathological Society of Washington and first Board of Health.

WRITINGS: "An Inaugural Dissertation on the Animating Principle, or Anima Mundi; How Afforded and How Acting in Man; and How Acted upon in That Disease Commonly Denominated, Tetanus or Lock-jaw. . ." (Thesis, Harvard, 1795). REFERENCES: *Boston Med. and Surg. J.* 36 (1847): 249-52; S. C. Busey, *Personal Reminiscences* (1895), 124-25; Kelly and Burrage (1920), 770; D. S. Lamb et al., *History of the Medical Society of the District of Columbia, 1817-1909* (1909), 218.

R. A. Kondratas

MAYNARD, DAVID SWINSON (March 22, 1808, Castleton, Vt.-March 13, 1873, Seattle, Wash.). *Physician.* Married Lydia A. Rickey, 1828, two children, divorced, 1852; Catherine Broshears, 1853. EDUCATION: Castleton Medical School: apprentice, Dr. Theodore Woodward (q.v.), professor; and before 1828, M.D. CAREER: Early 1830s-50, practiced medicine, Cleveland, Ohio; early 1830s-37, co-founded and taught, Cleveland's first medical school; 1849-50, treated numerous cases of cholera, Cleveland and Oregon Trail; 1850, traveled from Ohio to Wash. State; 1850-73, practiced medicine, Seattle. CONTRIBUTIONS: One of Seattle's first and leading physicians and settlers. Promoted Seattle and Wash. Territory financially, medically, and governmentally. Founded Seattle's first hospital (1863). One of the state's and city's leading citizens. REFERENCES: Thomas W. Prosch, *David S. Maynard and Catherine T. Maynard, Biographies of Two* *of the Oregon Immigrants of 1850* (1906); idem, "Dr. D. S. Maynard, The Pioneer Physician of Seattle," *Northwest Med.* 2 (1904); short biographical sketch, in Clarence B. Bagley, *History of Seattle* 2 (1916): 828-29; Bill Speidel, *Doc Maynard: The Man Who Invented Seattle* (1978).

T. L. Savitt

MAYO, CHARLES HORACE   (July 19, 1865, Rochester, Minn.-May 26, 1939, Chicago, Ill.). *Physician; Surgery.* Son of William Worrall (q.v.), physician, and Louise Abigail (Wright) Mayo. Brother of William James Mayo (q.v.). Married Edith Graham, 1893; eight children. EDUCATION: Chicago Medical College (later Northwestern University): 1888, M.D.; and 1904, M.A.; 1888, postgraduate study, New York Polyclinic and New York Post-Graduate medical schools; *post* c. 1889, annual study leaves in United States and abroad. CAREER: 1889-1929, surgeon and associate chief of staff, Mayo Clinic; surgery faculty: 1919-36, University of Minnesota Medical School; and 1915-1936, Graduate School of the University of Minnesota (Mayo Foundation); 1900-1902, member, Minnesota State Board of Health and Vital Statistics; 1912-37, health officer, Rochester; president: 1911-1912, Society of Clinical Surgery; 1914-15, Clinical Congress of Surgeons of North America; 1916-17, American Medical Association; and 1924-25, American College of Surgeons; 1924-32, editorial board, *Archives of Clinical Cancer Research.*
See **MAYO, WILLIAM JAMES** for further information.

MAYO, WILLIAM JAMES   (June 29, 1861, Rochester, Minn.-July 28, 1939, Rochester). *Physician; Surgery.* Son of William Worrall (q.v.), physician, and Louise Abigail (Wright) Mayo. Brother of Charles Horace Mayo (q.v.). Married Hattie M. Damon, 1884; five children. EDUCATION: 1883, M.D., University of Michigan; 1884, certificated, New York Post-Graduate Medical School; 1885, M.D., New York Polyclinic Medical School; *post* c. 1889, annual study leaves, United States and abroad. CAREER: 1883-88, practiced medicine with father, Rochester; 1889-1928, surgeon and associate chief of staff, Mayo Clinic; 1892-99, member, Minnesota State Board of Health; president: 1905-6, American Medical Association; 1911-12, Society of Clinical Surgery; 1913-14, American Surgical Association; 1918-20, American College of Surgeons; and 1925-26, Congress of American Physicians and Surgeons. CONTRIBUTIONS: Made the Mayo Clinic one of the world's foremost centers for surgical care, training, and research. Provided surgical treatment for appendicitis, gallstones, stomach ulcers, goiter, and other diseases of internal organs for the inhabitants of Rochester's rural hinterland following the acceptance of Listerian antiseptics (1880s). Studied and improved the methods of other surgeons. Made many innovations of their own, with "Dr. Will" excelling in abdominal surgery and "Dr. Charlie" in surgery of the thyroid gland. Donated over $2,500,000 to establish the Mayo Foundation for Medical Education and Research in affiliation with the graduate school of the University of Minnesota (1915). Provided one of the first degree programs in graduate medical education and was especially renowned for its excellence in surgery. Through the work of the Mayo Clinic, popularized the idea of cooperative, private medical practice. Took in numerous associates in surgery and medicine who were given the opportunity to travel, study, and do their own research. Brought to bear in the treatment of each patient the resources of a well-equipped, multispecialty clinic. Excellent results obtained and desirable work conditions at the clinic demonstrated the advantages of group practice in private medical care.

WRITINGS: W. J. Mayo, "Malignant Diseases of the Stomach and Pylorus," *Trans. Am. Surg. J. Assoc.* 18 (1900): 97-123; idem, "An Operation for the Radical Cure of Umbilical Hernia," *Annals of Surg.* 34 (Jan. 1901): 276-80; *William J. Mayo and Charles H. Mayo, A Collection of Papers Published Previous to 1909* (1912); C. H. Mayo, "Enterostomy and the Use of the Omentum in the Prevention and Healing of Fistula," *Annals of Surg.*, 66 (Nov. 1917): 568-70. Partial bibliographies are in *Physicians of the Mayo Clinic and the Mayo Foundation* (1937), 921-37, 942-59. REFERENCES: *BHM* (1964-69), 178; (1970-74), 120; (1975), 16; (1977), 22; (1978), 20; (1980), 28; *DAB*, Supplement 2: 438-41; Miller, *BHM*, p. 70; *NCAB*, 30: 1-3; *Who Was Who in Am.*, 1: 794.

S. Galishoff

MAYO, WILLIAM WORRALL (May 31, 1819, Manchester, England-March 6, 1911, Rochester, Minn.). *Physician; General surgery.* Son of James and Ann (Bousal) Mayo. Married Louise Abigail Wright, 1851; four children. Father of William James and Charles Horace Mayo (q.v.). EDUCATION: Early education at Owens College, where he studied physics and chemistry with John Dalton; 1845, immigrated to the United States; 1854, M.D., University of Missouri; 1870-71, postgraduate study, Bellevue Hospital Medical College. CAREER: 1845-47, taught physics and chemistry, New York City; 1847-49, apprentice with Dr. Eleazar Deming, Lafayette, Ind.; 1850-54, assistant to Dr. John Hodges, University of Missouri Medical School; medical practice: 1854-55, LaPorte, Ind.; and 1855-96, Rochester; 1863, provost surgeon for southern Minn., U.S. Army; *post* 1885, medical staff, St. Mary's Hospital (Rochester); active in local and state politics. CONTRIBUTIONS: With his sons, William J. (q.v.) and Charles H. (q.v.), developed the Mayo Clinic, a group surgical practice that became famous the world over (*post* 1883). A pioneer in abdominal surgery in the United States. Helped found the Minnesota State Medical Society (1868) and was its president (1873).

WRITINGS: Mainly papers to the *Trans. Minn. State Med. Soc.* REFERENCES: *BHM* (1964-69), 177-78; (1970-74), 120; (1978), 20; *DAB*, 12: 466-67; Kelly and Burrage (1928), 821; Miller, *BHM*, pp. 69-70; *NCAB*, 19: 241.

S. Galishoff

MEAD, KATE CAMPBELL HURD (April 6, 1867, Danville, Quebec, Canada-January 1, 1941, Haddam, Conn.). *Gynecologist; Historian.* Oldest child of Edward Payson, physician, and Sara Elizabeth (Campbell) Hurd. Married William Edward Mead, 1893; no children. EDUCATION: 1888, M.D., Woman's Medical College of Pennsylvania; 1888-89, intern, New England Hospital for

Women and Children; 1889-90, postgraduate clinic work, Paris, Stockholm, London; 1890-93, postgraduate courses, Johns Hopkins Medical School; 1904, clinics, Vienna. CAREER: 1890-93, medical director, Bryn Mawr School for Girls, Baltimore, Md.; following marriage, moved to Middletown, Conn., and engaged in private practice; 1907-25, consulting gynecologist, Middlesex Hospital, of which she was an incorporator; 1923-24, president, the American Medical Women's Association. CONTRIBUTIONS: Left practice (1925) to travel and begin pioneering historical studies of women in medicine. Maintained an interest in social welfare. Established (with Alice Hall) an evening dispensary "for Working Women and Girls" while in Baltimore (1891). Later helped arrange milk stations and district nursing associations in Conn.

WRITINGS: "Is Infant Mortality an Index to Social Welfare?" *Woman's Med. J.* 27 (1917): 10; "Amalgamation, Not Segregation," *Bull. Med. Women's Nat. Assoc.* 4 (1923): 42; *Medical Women of America* (1933); *History of Women in Medicine from the Earliest Times to the Beginning of the Nineteenth Century* (1938; only first volume published; ms. of second volume at Schlesinger Library, Radcliffe College, Cambridge, Mass.); articles on medical history. REFERENCES: Dorothy I. Lansing, "Kate Hurd Mead, M.D., and Her Prestigious Lectures in the History of Medicine," *J. Am. Med. Women's Assoc.* 33 (1978): 116-23; Esther P. Lovejoy, "Kate Hurd Mead," *Bull. Hist. Med.* 10 (1941): 314-17; *NCAB*, 38: 490; *Notable Am. Women, 1607-1950*, 2: 241-42; Rosemary Stevens, "The Changing Idea of a Medical Specialty [The Kate Hurd Mead Lecture]," *Trans. and Studies of the Coll. of Physicians of Phila.*, 5th Series, 2 (1980): 159-77.

S. J. Peitzman

MEIGS, ARTHUR VINCENT (November 1, 1850, Philadelphia, Pa.-January 1, 1912, Philadelphia). *Physician; Pediatrics.* Son of John Forsyth (q.v.), M.D., and Ann Wilcocks (Ingersoll) Meigs. Married Mary Roberts Browning, October 16, 1878; three sons. EDUCATION: University of Pennsylvania: 1866, A.B., and 1871, M.D.; 1871-72, postgraduate study, Vienna; 1872-74, resident physician, Pennsylvania Hospital. CAREER: 1874-1912, private practice, Philadelphia; 1881, visiting physician, Pennsylvania Hospital; and attending physician, Sheltering Arms (home for foundlings) and Children's Hospital; in College of Physicians: 1885, fellow; 1904-7, president; 1889, elected to American Philosophical Society. CONTRIBUTIONS: Greatest contribution was accurate chemical analysis of human and cow's milk to make it more suitable for infant consumption.

WRITINGS: *Milk Analysis and Infant Feeding* (1885); *The Origin of Disease* (1897). REFERENCES: *DAB*, 6, pt. 2: 502-3; A. Levinson, "The Three Meigs and Their Contributions to Pediatrics," *Annals of Med. Hist.* 10 (1928): 138-48; Edward B. Meigs, "Memoir of Arthur Vincent Meigs, M.D.," *Trans. Coll. of Physicians of Phila.*, 3rd series, 36 (1914); *NCAB*, 25: 181.

T. E. Cone, Jr.

MEIGS, CHARLES DELUCENA (February 19, 1792, St. George, Bermuda-June 22, 1869, Hamanassett, Delaware County, Pa.). *Physician; Obstetrics and gynecology.* Son of Josiah and Clara (Benjamin) Meigs. Married Mary Montgomery, 1815; unknown number of children. EDUCATION: 1809, A.B., University of Georgia; 1809-12, apprentice to Dr. Thomas Fendall, Augusta, Ga.; 1817, M.D., University of Pennsylvania. CAREER: 1815-16, practiced, Augusta; 1817-61, practiced, Philadelphia, Pa.; *post* 1826, edited *The North American Medical and Surgical Journal*; 1837, a founder, Preston Retreat; 1841-61, professor of obstetrics and diseases of women and children, Jefferson Medical College. CONTRIBUTIONS: Leader in American obstetrics. Did much to elevate standards of care and the practice of obstetrics. Known for violent opposition to the use of anesthesia in childbirth, the practice of oöpherectomy, and the concept of the transmission of puerperal sepsis. Described cardiac thrombosis with embolism as cause of death in labor. Popular teacher with flamboyant style. Had wide influence through lectures and writings; however, following death, influence was short-lived.

WRITINGS: *The Philadelphia Practice of Midwifery* (1838); *Females and Their Diseases. . .*, 4 eds. (1848); "The Heart Clot," *Med. Examiner* 5 (1849): 141-52; *Obstetrics: The Science and the Art* (1849); *On the Nature, Signs, and Treatment of Childbed Fevers. . .* (1854). REFERENCES: *DAB*, 6: 503-4; A. Levinson, "The Three Meigs and Their Contribution to Pediatrics," *Annals of Med. Hist.* 10 (1928): 138-48; John Forsyth Meigs, "Memoir of Charles D. Meigs, M.D.," *Trans. Coll. of Physicians of Phila.*, n.s., 4 (1873): 417-48; *NCAB*, 6: 390; W. Robert Penman, "Charles Delucena Meigs, M.D.; An Assessment of His Role in Philadelphia Obstetrics," *Trans. and Studies of the Coll. of Physicians of Phila.*, 4th series, 43 (1976): 121-24; Herbert Thoms, "Charles Delucena Meigs," *Am. J. of Obstet. Gynecol.* 31 (1936): 1049-55.

L. D. Longo

MEIGS, JOHN FORSYTH (October 3, 1818, Philadelphia, Pa.-December 16, 1882, Philadelphia). *Physician; Diseases of women and children.* Son of Charles Delucena (q.v.), and Mary (Montgomery) Meigs. Married Ann Wilcocks Ingersoll, October 17, 1844; eight children. EDUCATION: 1838, M.D., University of Pennsylvania; 1838-40, resident physician, Pennsylvania Hospital; 1840-41, studied in Paris with Velpeau and Louis. CAREER: 1841, started to practice medicine, Philadelphia, in father's house. 1843-54, taught obstetrics and the practice of medicine and diseases of children, Philadelphia Association for Medical Instruction; 1859-81, physician, Pennsylvania Hospital; visiting physician, Children's Hospital; and consulting physician, Women's Hospital; fellow, Philadelphia College of Surgeons; member, American Philosophical Society. CONTRIBUTIONS: A prominent physician, best known for his work on pediatrics which went through seven editions (1848-76).

WRITINGS: *A Practical Treatise on the Diseases of Children* (1848); *A History of the First Quarter of the Second Century of Pennsylvania Hospital* (1877). REFERENCES: *DAB*, 6, pt. 2: 505-6; A. Levinson, "The Three Meigs and Their Contributions to Pediatrics," *Annals of Med. Hist.* 10 (1928): 138-48; A. V. Meigs, "Memoir of J. Forsyth Meigs, M.D." *Trans. Coll. of Physicians of Phila.*, 3rd series, 1 (1884); T. G. Morton and Frank Woodbury, *The History of the Pennsylvania Hospital* (1895); *NCAB*, 25: 100.

T. E. Cone, Jr.

MELTZER, SAMUEL JAMES (March 22, 1851, Ponevyezh, Russia-November 7, 1920, New York, N.Y.). *Physician; Physiology; Pharmacology.* Son of Simon, teacher, and Taube (Kowars) Meltzer. Married Olga T. Levitt, 1870; two children. EDUCATION: 1882, M.D., University of Berlin; 1883, went to the United States. CAREER: 1883-1904, practiced medicine, New York City; 1904-19, physiology and pharmacology staff, Rockefeller Institute for Medical Research; member, two national commissions on resuscitation, and chairman, third commission; president, half dozen or more medical societies. CONTRIBUTIONS: Observed that in swallowing, reflex stimulation of inspiratory muscles is accompanied by reflex inhibition of respiratory muscles and vice versa (1889); theorized that this reciprocal action occurred in all antagonistic muscles; developed the idea still further into a general physiological principle that formed the theoretical basis of all his scientific work. Showed that magnesium salts produced a state of unconsciousness and muscle relaxation, leading to their use in the treatment of tetanus (1905). With John Auer (q.v.), developed the technique of intratracheal insufflation, a new method of artificial respiration, in which air is blown through a tube inserted into the trachea. By adding an anesthetic agent to the air stream, thoracic surgeons were able to operate without fear of collapsing the lungs (1910); led to the discovery of pharyngeal insufflation, a method of artificial respiration intended for use by laymen in cases of accidents and drownings; because apparatus designed to resuscitate victims required training to operate, use was limited to industrial plants. Developed hypothesis that bronchial asthma is related to anaphylaxis and occurs when there is a severe allergic reaction (1910). With his daughter, Clara, demonstrated that under certain circumstances adrenalin could have long-lasting effects on the blood vessels and the muscles of the iris. Introduced the engineering term "factors of safety" to describe the reserve powers of body mechanisms (1906). Played a leading role in the establishment of professional societies and journals devoted to experimental medicine.

WRITINGS: "Inhibition," *N.Y. Med. J.* 69 (1899): 661-66, 699-703, 739-43; "Physiological and Pharmacological Studies of Magnesium Salts," *Am. J. of Physiol.* 14 (1905): 366-88; 15 (1906): 387-405; 16 (1906): 233-51 (with John Auer); "The Method of Respiration by Intratracheal Insufflation. . .," *Med. Record* 77 (1910): 477-83; "Bronchial Asthma as a Phenomenon of Anaphylaxsis," *JAMA* 55 (1910): 1021-25. A bibliography is in *BMNAS*. REFERENCES: *BHM* (1975-79), 85; (1980), 28; *BMNAS* 21 (1926): 15-23; *DAB*, 12: 519-20; *DSB*, 9: 265-66; Kelly and Burrage (1928), 830-32; *NCAB*, 15: 354; *Who Was Who in Am.*, 1: 829.

S. Galishoff

MENDEL, LAFAYETTE BENEDICT (February 5, 1872, Delhi, N.Y.-December 9, 1935, New Haven, Conn.). *Physiological chemist; Nutrition.* Son of Benedict, merchant, and Pauline (Ullman) Mendel. Married Alice Relaine Friend, 1917; no children. EDUCATION: Yale University: A.B., 1891; Ph.D., 1893; 1895-96, studied physiology and chemistry at universities of Breslau and Freiburg. CAREER: 1893-1935, physiological chemistry faculty, Yale University; director, Russell Sage Institute for Pathology; member, council on pharmacy and chemistry, American Medical Association; research associate, Carnegie Institution of Washington; member, educational advisory board, John Simon Guggenheim

Medical Foundation; president, American Society of Biological Chemistry (1911); first president, American Institute of Nutrition (1933-34). CONTRIBUTIONS: In conjunction with Thomas B. Osborne (q.v.) made epochal discoveries about the chemical composition of food proteins and their biological value in nutrition and the role of hitherto unknown accessory food factors—vitamins—in health and disease. Demonstrated that proteins in which there is a shortage or absence of certain amino acids, notably lysine and typtophan, are incapable of sustaining growth and cannot be synthesized by the animal organism but must be provided by the animal's food. Equally far-reaching, showed that trace amounts of previously unidentified organic substances (vitamins) are essential to health. Found that butter fat contains an organic substance soluble in fat, now known as vitamin A, without which rats cannot thrive; same discovery had been submitted for publication a few weeks earlier by Elmer V. McCollum (q.v.) at the University of Wisconsin who is therefore regarded as the discoverer of vitamin A. Also found that milk contained a water-soluble substance, now known as vitamin B, that is essential for maintenance and growth. Helped edit several publications including the *Journal of Biological Chemistry* (1911-35), "Scientific Monographs" of the American Chemical Society (1920-35), and the *Journal of Nutrition* (1928-35).

WRITINGS: *Feeding Experiments with Isolated Food-substances*, 2 pts., Carnegie Institution of Washington Publication No. 156 (1911); *Changes in the Food Supply and Their Relation to Nutrition* (1916); *Nutrition, the Chemistry of Life* (1923); a bibliography is in *BMNAS*, 18 (1937). REFERENCES: *DAB*, Supplement 1: 549-50; *DSB*, 9: 284-86; *NCAB*, 26: 424-25; *Who Was Who in Am.*, 1: 829.

S. Galishoff

MENDENHALL, DOROTHY REED (September 22, 1874, Columbus, Ohio-July 31, 1964, Chester, Conn.). *Physician; Public health.* Daughter of William Pratt, shoe manufacturer, and Grace (Kimball) Reed. Married Charles Elwood Mendenhall, 1906; four children. EDUCATION: 1895, B.L., Smith College; 1900, M.D., Johns Hopkins University; 1901, internship in pathology, Johns Hopkins University, with Dr. William Osler (q.v.); 1902, resident, New York Infirmary for Women and Children; 1903-6, resident physician, Babies Hospital of New York. CAREER: 1914-35, field lecturer, Department of Home Economics, University of Wisconsin; 1917-36, medical officer, U.S. Children's Bureau; 1936, after husband's death, withdrew from public life. CONTRIBUTIONS: Did early research on the cause of Hodgkin's disease and was instrumental in calling governmental attention to the problems of maternal and child health. Demonstrated (1901) that Hodgkin's disease was not a form of tuberculosis but that a specific cell was a distinctive characteristic of the disease. Helped establish some of the first infant welfare clinics in Wis. (1914-30). Efforts were rewarded (1937) when Madison achieved recognition as the city with the lowest infant mortality rates in the United States. Work with the Children's Bureau called attention to high infant and maternal mortality. Pointed out the prevalence of malnutrition among children and studied the deleterious effects of excessive medical intervention in childbirth.

WRITINGS: "On the Pathological Changes in Hodgkin's Disease with Especial Reference to Its Relation to Tuberculosis," *Johns Hopkins Hosp. Reports* 10, no. 3 (1902): 133-96; "Prenatal and Natal Conditions in Wisconsin," *Wisconsin Med. J.* 25 (1917): 353-69; six chapters in *Child Care and Child Welfare: Outline for Study* (1929). Writings listed in *Notable Am. Women* and Author Catalog, *N.Y. Acad. of Med.*, vol. 26. REFERENCES: Jean Bergman, "Dorothy Reed Mendenhall," State Historical Society of Wisconsin Women's Auxiliary, *Famous Wisconsin Women* 6 (1976): 48; Gena Corea, "Dorothy Reed Mendenhall: Childbirth Is Not a Disease," *Ms. Magazine* 2 (Apr. 1974): 98-104; *Notable Am. Women, The Modern Period*, 468-70.

C. O. Borst

MENNINGER, CHARLES FREDERICK (July 11, 1862, Tell City, Ind.-November 28, 1953, Topeka, Kans.). *Physician*. Son of August V., miller, and Katherine (Schmidberger) Menninger. Married Flora Vesta Knisely, 1885 (d.1945); three sons; Pearl Boam, 1948. EDUCATION: 1882, A.B., Central Normal College of Danville, Ind.; M.A., Campbell College, Holton, Kans; 1889, M.D., Hahnemann Medical College, Chicago, Ill.; 1908, M.D., Kansas Medical College, Topeka. CAREER: Began medical career as a practitioner, Topeka; 1900, broke with homeopathic training to such an extent that he was elected president, Shawnee County Medical Society; 1908, visited Mayo Clinic and resolved to duplicate that accomplishment in Topeka; 1919, with return of son Karl from Boston, Mass., established the Menninger Diagnostic Clinic; joined by another son, William C., the emphasis of the clinic increasingly became psychiatric. CONTRIBUTIONS: Menninger Foundation was established (1941) to enhance psychiatric education and research. Menninger Sanitarium was added to the Foundation (1945), and by 1954, when the new Charles Frederick Menninger Memorial Hospital opened, organization had attained worldwide fame. Reported 10 percent of all psychiatric residents in the United States were enrolling in the Menninger Foundation (1955). Story is remarkable as that of a modestly educated physician who could defer to the drive and ambition of two talented sons, even though that meant giving up his vision of a multiple specialty clinic along the lines of Mayo's. In the process, oversaw the development of an international center of psychiatry. REFERENCES: *BHM* (1970-74), 121; (1975-79), 86; *DAB*, Supplement 5: 483-84; Walker Winslow, *The Menninger Story* (1956).

R. Hudson

MENNINGER, WILLIAM CLAIRE (October 15, 1899, Topeka, Kans.-September 6, 1966, Topeka). *Physician; Psychiatry*. Son of Charles Frederick (q.v.) and Flora Vesta (Knisely) Menninger; brother of Karl Menninger. Married Catherine Louisa Wright, 1925; three children. EDUCATION: 1919, A.B., Washburn College, Topeka; 1922, M.A., Columbia University; 1924, M.D., Cornell University Medical School; 1924-25, internship in medicine and surgery, Bellevue Hospital, N.Y.; 1927, training in psychiatry, St. Elizabeth's Hospital, Washington, D.C.; 1934-35, training in psychoanalysis, Chicago Psychoanalytic Institute. CAREER: 1917-18, 2nd lieutenant, U.S. Army; 1926-66, at Menninger Clinic, Topeka, founded by father and brother in 1919: 1926-27, practiced internal medicine; 1927-66, practiced psychiatry; 1930-45, medical director, Menninger Sanitarium; 1941-46, secretary, and 1946-66, general secretary, Menninger Foundation; 1946-66, professor of psychiatry, Menninger School of Psychiatry; 1942-46, in U.S. Army Medical Corps: 1943-46, director, Neuropsychiatry Consultants Division, Office of the Surgeon General; 1946-66, brigadier general, U.S. Army Reserve; 1947-66, professor of clinical psychiatry, University of Kansas; 1948-49, president, American Psychiatric Association; in American Psychoanalytic Association: 1947-49, president; and 1949-51, counsellor. CONTRIBUTIONS: Early studies (1923-26) in physiology. "Sales manager for psychiatry": stressed increased access to psychiatric treatment for all parts of American society; directed expansion of psychiatric services at the Menninger Clinic and, through work with the Army Neuropsychiatry Consultants Division, promoted this expansion throughout the United States. Also promoted increase in number of physicians trained in psychiatry, primarily through Menninger Clinic and consulting work after World War II. Very active in boy scouting, at least in part for its role in developing mental hygiene.

WRITINGS: More than 200 papers on psychiatric topics. *Juvenile Paresis* (1936); *Fundamentals of Psychiatry* (1943); *Psychiatry: Its Evolution and Present Status* (1948); *Psychiatry in a Troubled World: Yesterday's War and Today's Challenge* (1948); *You and Psychology* (1948), with Muroe Leaf. Many of his papers have been reprinted in Benard H. Hill, ed., *Psychiatrist for a Troubled World: Selected Papers of William Claire Menninger* (1967). REFERENCES: Henry W. Brosin, "A Biographical Sketch," in Hill, *Psychiatrist for a Troubled World*; *Current Biog.* (1945), 400-402; Albert Deutsch, "The Menningers of Topeka," *Survey Graphic* 36 (1947): 475-77, 500-503; *NCAB*, H: 53-54; *NUC Pre-1956 Imprints*, 376: 318-20; *N.Y Times*, September 7, 1966, pp. 1, 41; *N.Y. Times Magazine*, November 6, 1955, pp. 13 ff.; L. Rangell, "William C. Menninger (1899-1966)," *J. Am. Psychoanalytic Assoc.* 15 (1967): 923-29; David Shakow, "The Development of Orthopsychiatry: The Contributions of Levy, Menninger, and Stevenson," *Am. J. of Orthopsychiatry* 38 (1968): 804-9; *Time* (October 25, 1948), cover story.

M. M. Sokal

MERGLER, MARIE JOSEPH (May 18, 1851, Mainstockheim, Bavaria-May 17, 1901, Los Angeles, Calif.). *Physician; Surgeon; Obstetrics and gynecology.* Daughter of Francis R., physician, and Henriette (von Ritterhausen) Mergler. Never married. Immigrated with family to Cook County, Ill., 1853. EDUCATION: 1869, Cook County Normal School; 1872, State Normal School, Oswego, N.Y.; 1879, M.D., Woman's Medical College, Chicago, Ill.; 1880-81, studied pathology and clinical medicine, Zurich. CAREER: 1881, established general medical practice, Chicago, but soon developed an interest in obstetrics and gynecology and that same year became surgical assistant to William H. Byford (q.v.), Woman's Hospital of Chicago; until 1890, served as an adjunct professor of gynecology, Woman's Hospital, when she succeeded Byford in the chair of gynecology; at Woman's Medical College: *post* 1882, professor of materia medica; 1885, secretary of the faculty, and 1899, dean; 1882, became the second woman named to the staff of Cook County Hospital; 1886, became attending surgeon, Woman's Hospital; 1890, appointed gynecologist, Wesley Hospital; 1895, became head physician and surgeon, Dr. Mary H. Thompson's Hospital for Women and Children; 1895-1901, professor of gynecology, Post-Graduate Medical School of Chicago. CONTRIBUTIONS: One of the most highly esteemed women in American medicine in the late nineteenth century. A good diagnostician and an excellent surgeon, especially in the field of abdominal surgery, was devoted to teaching and medical practice and was especially concerned with advocating medical education for women.

WRITINGS: *A Guide to the Study of Gynecology* (1891); "Diseases of the New Born," *An American Textbook of Obstetrics* (1895, with Charles W. Earle). Numerous articles on gynecological subjects for state and local medical publications. Served for a number of years on the editorial staff, *Medical Woman's Journal*. REFERENCES: Chicago Medical Society, *History of Medicine and Surgery, and Physicians and Surgeons of Chicago* (1922), 149-150; *DAB*, 6, pt. 2: 550-51; Eliza M. Mosher, "The History of American Medical Women," *Med. Woman's J*. (Jan. 1923); *Notable Am. Women, 1607-1950*, 529-30; F. M. Sperry, comp., *A Group of Distinguished Physicians and Surgeons of Chicago (1904), 110-13*.

                                                                                          V. Drachman

MERIWETHER, CLINTON PALMER (May 8, 1867, Batesville, Ark.-November 2, 1919, Little Rock, Ark.). *Physician; Tuberculosis*. Son of William Douglas, merchant, and Sarah Eleanor (Bradley) Meriwether. Married Myrtle Sharum, 1894; two children. EDUCATION: 1888, M.D., Missouri Medical College; 1900, one term, Bellevue Hospital Medical College. CAREER: Private practice: 1888-98, Walnut Ridge, Ark.; 1898-99, U.S. Army Medical Corps; 1900-7, Tucson, Ariz.; and 1907-17, Little Rock, Ark.; 1911-12, medical faculty, University of Arkansas Medical Department; 1917-19, U.S. Army Medical Corps. CONTRIBUTIONS: Edited *Monthly Bulletin of the Arkansas Medical Society* (1909-13). Secretary, Arkansas Medical Society (1911-19). Medical aide to Ark. Governor Charles H. Brough during World War I; advised Brough in the establishment of a state Medical Advisory Board to supervise selective draft physical examinations. Supported the establishment of the Arkansas Association for the Relief and Control of Tuberculosis; led its successful drive for legislation (1909), creating the Arkansas Tubercular Sanitarium; served on the Sanitarium's Board of Trustees until health failed from tuberculosis (1919).   REFERENCES: Weston A. Goodspeed, *The Province and the States*, 3 (1904): 366.

                                                                                          D. Konold

MERRICK, MYRA (KING) (1825, Leicester, England-November 10, 1899, Cleveland, Ohio). *Physician; Homeopath; Obstetrics*. Daughter of Richard and Elizabeth King. Married Charles H. Merrick, 1848; one child. EDUCATION: 1851, apprenticed under Dr. Levi Ives, New Haven, Conn; 1852, M.D., Central Medical College (Eclectic), Rochester, N.Y. CAREER: August 1852, established medical practice, Cleveland; during the Civil War, moved practice to Lorain, Ohio, and collected and distributed supplies to the northern soldiers; 1868, founded the Cleveland Homeopathic Hospital College for Women, serving as professor of obstetrics and president; 1878, founded the Women's and Children's Free Medical and Surgical Dispensary, which later evolved into Woman's General Hospital. CONTRIBUTIONS: First woman to practice medicine west of the Allegheny Mountains. Supported other women in their efforts to obtain a medical education and medical experience and sought to provide medical care for needy women and children in a dignified and sympathetic way. REFERENCES: Marion Noville Gibbons, "A Woman Carries the Caduceus—Myra K. Merrick," in Howard Dittrick, comp., *Pioneer Medicine in the Western Reserve* (1932); Glen Jenkins, "Women Physicians and Woman's General Hospital," in Kent L. Brown, ed., *Medicine in Cleveland and Cuyahoga County, 1810-1976* (1977); "Pioneer Medical Women of Cleveland and the Story of the Women's and Children's Free Medical and Surgical Dispensary," *J. Am. Med. Women's Assoc.* 6 (May 1951): 186-89; Bertha L. Selmon, "The Homeopathic Medical College for Women: Cleveland: 1868-1870," *Med. Women's J.* 53 (Apr. 1946): 29-32.

G. P. Jenkins

MERRITT, JOHN WEBSTER (August 11, 1906, Gainesville, Fla.-October 4, 1963, Jacksonville, Fla.). *Physician; History*. Son of Claude F., civil engineer, and Maude (Webster) Merritt. Married Daphne Elise Davis, 1947; two sons. EDUCATION: 1929, B.S. in Pharmacy, University of Florida; 1933, M.D., The Johns Hopkins University; 1933, resident, Harvard Service, Boston City Hospital. CAREER: Upon completion of residency, returned to Jacksonville and entered practice; stayed there for remainder of life except for one year (1941-42) as medical officer, U.S. Army Medical Corps, Camp Blanding, Fla.; 1936-55, staff, Riverside Hospital. CONTRIBUTIONS: Especially noted for interest in the medical history of Fla., a field in which he was a pioneer. Collection of Floridiana included 979 bound volumes, as well as thousands of letters, pamphlets, maps, and manuscripts, most relating to medical history. Through determined search, accumulated a complete set of Florida Medical Association *Proceedings, Transactions, Journal*, to replace the only extant set, destroyed by fire (1901).

WRITINGS: Nineteen historical articles for *J. Fla. Med. Assoc.*, 13 of which related to medical history of Jacksonville and Duval County, Fla. These articles were later revised and published in *A Century of Medicine in Jacksonville and Duval County* (1949), 201 pp. Similar articles relating to medical history of St. Augustine, Fla., and Gainesville were published in *J. Fla. Med. Assoc.* In addition, published nine articles on medical science as well as other items reflecting his thinking on medical deontology and philosophy. REFERENCES: Dr. J. Webster Merritt Memorial Collection, Haydon Burns (Public) Library, Jacksonville; William M. Straight, "Florida's Medical Historian—J. Webster Merritt," *J. Fla. Med. Assoc.* 66, no. 8 (Aug. 1979): 860-65; *Times-Union* (Jacksonville), October 6, 1963.

E. A. Hammond

MESERVE, CHARLES FRANCIS (July 15, 1850, North Abington, Mass.-April 20, 1936, Raleigh, N.C.). *Educator*. Son of Charles and Susanna (Blanchard) Meserve. Married Abbie Mary Whittier, 1878 (d. 1898); one child; Julia

Frances Philbrick, 1900; no children. EDUCATION: 1874, Coburn Classical Institute, Waterville, Maine; 1877, A.B., Colby College. CAREER: *Post* 1869, teacher, East Stoughton, Mass., public schools; principal: 1877-85, Rockland (Mass.) High School; and 1885-89, Oak Street School, Springfield, Mass.; 1889-94, superintendent and special disbursing agent, Haskell Institute, Lawrence, Kans. (a federal government Indian industrial training school); 1894-1919, president, Shaw University, Raleigh, N.C., 1919-36, trustee, Shaw University. CONTRIBUTIONS: As second president, Shaw University, oversaw the growth and development of Leonard Medical School, one of a handful of black medical colleges in the United States. Helped many financially poor students make their way through Leonard and into practice. Also made decision (1918) to close Leonard when financial support failed. Spent much time and effort fund raising. A co-organizer of the Capon Springs (W. Va.) conference (1898), which developed into the annual conference "Education for the South." Investigated workings of Dawes Commision (1896) for Indian Rights Association of Philadelphia.

WRITINGS: Many articles and reports on black education. REFERENCES: *Biog. Dictionary of Am. Ed.* (1978) 2: 890-91; *NCAB*, 26: 355-56; *Twentieth Century Biographical Dictionary of Notable Americans*, 7: unpaginated; *Who Was Who in Am.*, 1: 834.

T. L. Savitt

MEYER, ADOLF (September 13, 1866, Niederweningen, Switzerland-March 17, 1950, Baltimore, Md.). *Physician; Psychiatrist; Neurologist.* Son of Rudolf, Zwinglian Protestant minister, and Anna (Walder) Meyer. Married Mary Potter Brooks, 1902; one child. EDUCATION: Early education, Zurich gymnasium; 1890, passed Swiss examination to practice medicine; 1890-92, studied in various European cities; 1892, M.D., University of Zurich. CAREER: 1892, went to the United States; 1892-95, neurology faculty, University of Chicago; 1893-95, pathology staff, Illinois Eastern Hospital for the Insane, Kankakee, Ill.; 1895-1902, pathologist and later director of clinical and laboratory work, Worcester (Mass.) Insane Hospital; 1895-1902, psychiatry faculty, Clark University; 1902-10, director, Pathological (later Psychiatric) Institute, New York State Hospitals; psychiatry faculty: 1904-9, Cornell University Medical School; and 1910-41, Johns Hopkins Medical School; 1910-41, director, Henry Phipps Psychiatric Clinic. CONTRIBUTIONS: Propounded the doctrine of psychobiology, the belief that human behavior is integrated at a symbolic level, as opposed to the mind-body separation then widely accepted by psychologists. Viewed psychiatric disorders as unsuccessful adjustment patterns rather than as distinct disease entities of organic or hereditary origins. Believed that in most cases effective treatment could be provided by changing the patient's environment. Stressed the importance of a uniform method of compiling case histories, which he abetted in his classic work *Critical Review of the Data and General Methods and Deductions of Modern Neurology* (1898). Integrative, pluralistic approach made Americans receptive to the promise of dynamic psychiatry and prepared them to accept psychoanalysis and psychosomatic medicine. Helped Clifford Beers (q.v.) establish and name the mental hygiene movement (1909). Transformed N.Y. State's insane asylums into modern mental hospitals; fought to have social workers added to their staffs and to have follow-up care after discharge. Did important scientific work in neuroanatomy and neuropathology. Organized a model program of psychiatric research and teaching at Johns Hopkins and the Phipps Clinic, which set a standard for other medical schools and institutions. Trained many of the nation's leading clinical psychologists and psychiatrists. A founder, American Psychoanalytical Association and American Board of Psychiatry and Neurology (1934).

WRITINGS: "Fundamental Concepts of Dementia Praecox," *British Med. J.* 2 (1906): 757-60; "The Relation of the Auditory Center to Aphasia," *Trans. Assoc. of Am. Physicians* 23 (1908): 116-23; "Objective Psychology or Psychobiology with Subordination of the Medically Useless Contrast of Mental and Physical," *JAMA* 65 (1915): 860-63. Writings are in Eunice E. Winters ed., *The Collected Papers of Adolf Meyer* (1950-52). REFERENCES: *BHM* (1964-69), 182; (1975-79), 86; (1980), 28; *DAB*, Supplement No. 4: 569-72; Theodore Lidz, "Adolf Meyer and the Development of American Psychiatry," *Am. J. Psychiatry* 123 (1966): 320-32; Miller, *BHM*, p. 74; *NCAB*, 38: 45-46; *Who Was Who in Am.*, 2: 371.

S. Galishoff

MEYER, KARL FRIEDRICH (May 19, 1884, Basel, Switzerland-April 27, 1974, San Francisco, Calif.). *Pathologist; Veterinary science; Virology; Epidemiology.* Son of Theodor, merchant, and Sophie (Lichtenhahn) Meyer. Married Mary Elizabeth Lindsay, 1913, one child; Marion Lewis, 1960. EDUCATION: Zurich University: 1905, A.B., 1909, D.V.M.; and 1924, Ph.D.; postgraduate study, universities of Munich, Paris, Zurich, and Bern. CAREER: 1908-10, pathologist, Transvaal Department of Agriculture (South Africa); 1910, went to the United States; 1922, naturalized; 1910-13, pathology and bacteriology faculty, University of Pennsylvania; 1911-13, director, Laboratory and Experimental Farm, Pennsylvania Livestock Sanitary Board; at University of California: 1913-14, 1924-48, bacteriology and protozoology faculty; 1936-39, director, Public Health Curricula; 1948-54, experimental pathology faculty; and *post* 1960, history of health sciences faculty; at George Williams Hooper Foundation for Medical Research (University of California): 1915-24, tropical medicine staff, 1921-24, acting director; and 1924-54, director; *post* 1920, consultant, California Department of Public Health and Southern Pacific Railroad; 1926-30, director, Laboratory for Research in the Canning Industries; 1940-54, public health faculty, University of Southern California. CONTRIBUTIONS: Ranks alongside Theobald Smith (q.v.) as one of America's two greatest microbiologists. Demonstrated that Bang's disease of cattle and a human disease reported from Malta by David Bruce were caused by organisms of the same genus, which he named Brucella, in honor of Bruce (1920); alerted the medical community to the public health threat posed by brucellosis, which led to the development (by 1940) of an effective national control program. Isolated the viruses of eastern and western equine encephalitis and helped develop vaccines against the disease, which he predicted would be spread to man by insect vectors (1913, 1930). Developed the flash sterilization method of canning and a "fakeproof" system of testing that practically eliminated the danger of botulism in commercial canning (early 1920s). Identified a baffling form of pneumonia as psittacosis, or parrot fever; showed that it occurred in many species of birds and therefore renamed it ornithosis (1933-43); helped devise methods of using tetracyclines to control the disease in humans and in turkeys. Called attention to the many dangerous zoonoses that exist in the animal kingdom. Demonstrated that there is a reservoir of sylvatic plague in numerous species of wild rodents. During World War II, was largely responsible for the decision of the armed services to develop a killed plague vaccine instead of a live, attenuated strain, a decision that later events have justified. Helped establish the effectiveness of antibiotic therapy for both bubonic and pneumonic plague.

WRITINGS: "A Comparison of the Morphologic, Cultural, and Biochemical Characteristics of *B. abortus* and *B. melitensis*. Studies of the genus Brucella nov. gen.," *Internat. J. of Infectious Diseases* 27 (1920): 173-84 (with E. B. Shaw); "The Animal Kingdom—A Reservoir of Disease," *Proc., Institute of Medicine of Chicago* 8 (1931): 234-61; "The Preventive Measures of the State of California against Botulism," *J. Preventive Med.* 5 (1931): 261-93; "Plague Immunization. I. Past and Present Trends," *J. Infectious Diseases* 129, Supplement (May 1974): S13-S18. REFERENCES: *Current Biog.* (1952), 416-19; *N.Y. Times*, April 29, 1974; James H. Steele, "Karl Friedrich Meyer," *J. Infectious Diseases* 129, Supplement (May 1974): S3-S9; *Who Was Who in Am.*, 6: 282.

                                                                                              S. Galishoff

MEYER, WILLY (July 24, 1858, Minden, Germany-February 24, 1932, New York, N.Y.). *Physician; Surgery*. Son of Abraham and Bertha (Simon) Meyer. Married Lilly Ottilie Maass, 1885; four children. EDUCATION: Studied at the universities of Bonn and Erlangen; University of Bonn: 1880, M.D.; and 1880-83, assistant to Trendelenburg, surgical clinic. CAREER: *Post* 1884, practiced medicine, New York City; 1886-93, clinical surgery faculty, Woman's Medical College; surgical staff: 1886-1923, New York Skin and Cancer Hospital; 1884-1923, Lenox Hill Hospital; and 1887-1923, Post Graduate Hospital; 1922-23, president, American Association for Cancer Research. CONTRIBUTIONS: Made contributions in many areas of surgery and was one of the early pioneers of thoracic surgery. Published (1884) the first description of Trendelenburg's elevated pelvic position for the performance of certain pelvic and abdominal operations. Simultaneously with William Halsted (q.v.), originated (1894) the radical operation for cancer of the breast. Introduced in the United States many advances made by European physicians, including cystoscopy (1887), catheterization of the ureters in the male with the aid of the electric cystoscope (1896), and Bottini's operation for hypertrophy of the prostate gland (1897). An early advocate of the controlled pressure chamber for thoractomy, especially the negative-pressure cabinet introduced by Johann von Mikulicz-Radecki and Ernst F. Sauerbruch, and had a double chamber built at German Hospital. Founded the

New York Society for Thoracic Surgery and the American Association for Thoracic Surgery.

WRITINGS: "Ueber die Nachbehandlung des hohen Steinschnittes sowie über Verwendbarkeit desselben zur Operation von Blasenscheidenfisteln," *Archiv fuer Klinische Chirurgie* 31 (1884): 494-525; "An Improved Method of the Radical Operation for Carcinoma of the Breast," *Med. Record* 46 (Dec. 15, 1894): 746-49; "Pneumectomy with the Aid of Differential Air Pressure, an Experimental Study: The New Type of Apparatus Used," *JAMA* 53 (Dec. 11, 1909): 1978-87; "Impermeable Cardiospasm Successfully Treated by Thoracotomy and Esophagoplication. Abstract," *Annals of Surg.*, 53 (Feb. 1911): 293-94. REFERENCES: *NCAB*, C: 480-81; obituary, *Trans., Am. Surg. Assoc.* 50 (1932): 546-48; Mark M. Ravitch, *A Century of Surgery*, 2 vols. (1981); *Who Was Who in Am.*, 1: 836.

S. Galishoff

MIDDLETON, PETER (Scotland, England-January 9, 1781, New York, N.Y.). *Physician; Medical historian.* Married Susannah (Nicholls) Burges, 1776; one child. EDUCATION: 1752, M.D., University of St. Andrews (Scotland). CAREER: *Post* 1752, practiced medicine, New York City; 1756, surgeon-general, Crown Point expedition, French and Indian War; King's College (now Columbia University): 1767-70, physiology and pathology faculty; 1770-73, materia medica faculty; and 1773, governor; 1774, medical staff, New York Hospital; 1767-70, president, St. Andrew's Society of New York City. CONTRIBUTIONS: One of the most eminent physicians in the American colonies in the mid-eighteenth century. With John Bard (q.v.), made one of the first recorded dissections of a human body for purposes of anatomical instruction (1752 or later). Helped found the medical school of King's College and was one of the six physicians appointed to professorships when the school opened (1767). Wrote *A Medical Discourse, or an Historical Inquiry into the Ancient and Present State of Medicine* (1769), which, aside from Benjamin Franklin's brief account of the development of Pennsylvania Hospital, written in 1754, was the first American contribution to medical history. An incorporator of New York Hospital (1771). REFERENCES: *BHM* (1974-79), 86; *DAB*, 12: 602-3; Kelly and Burrage (1920), 789-90; W. B. McDaniel II, "The Beginnings of American Medical Historiography," *Bull. Hist. Med.* 26 (1952): 45-53; Miller, *BHM*, p. 74; *Who Was Who in Am.*, Hist. Vol.: 427.

S. Galishoff

MIDDLETON, WILLIAM SHAINLINE (January 7, 1890, Norristown, Pa.-September 9, 1975, Madison, Wis.). *Physician; Medical education.* Son of Daniel Shephard, grocer, and Ann Sophia Holstein (Shainline) Middleton. Married Maude H. Webster, September 30, 1921, (d. 1968); Ruth Addams, June 14, 1973; no children. EDUCATION: 1911, M.D., University of Pennsylvania; 1911-12, internship, Philadelphia General Hospital. CAREER: 1912-63, faculty, University of Wisconsin Medical School: 1912-15, instructor in clinical medicine; 1915-25, assistant professor; 1925-33, associate professor; 1933-60, professor; and 1935-55, dean; 1955-63, director of medical services, U.S. Veteran's Administration (VA); 1964-70, consultant in research and education, Veteran's Administration, Madison, Wis.; visiting professor: 1940, University of Michigan; 1941, University of Oregon Medical School; 1941, University of Illinois; 1951, University of Pennsylvania; and 1963, University of Oklahoma. CONTRIBUTIONS: As director of medical services, VA, maintained a high quality of medical care by frequently inspecting VA facilities and by building VA hospitals adjacent to medical schools. An exceptional teacher and diagnostician, who, as second dean of the University of Wisconsin Medical School, broadened the curriculum and established new chairs in biophysics and the history of medicine. An avid medical historian, became president, American Association for the History of Medicine (1934), and delivered the association's Garrison Lecture (1965). In addition to receiving six honorary doctorates and several honorary fellowships, was elected president, Central Society of Clinical Research (1933) and American College of Physicians (1950).

WRITINGS: Listed in William S. Middleton, "Collected Papers," *Wisconsin Med. J. 63* (1964): 548-53. Historical essays collected in *Medical History Essays* (1965) and *Values in Modern Medicine* (1972). REFERENCES: Paul F. Clark, *The University of Wisconsin Medical School: A Chronicle, 1848-1948* (1967); Chauncey D. Leake, "William Shainline Middleton, 1890-1975," *Bull. Hist. Med.* 50 (1976): 128-32, which includes a list of his medico-historical publications; *NCAB*, 58: 261.

S. E. Lederer

MILLER, [MANIA] HENRY, JR. (November 1, 1800, Glasgow, Barren County, Ky.-February 18, 1874, Louisville, Ky.). *Obstetrician; Teacher.* Son of Henry Miller. Married Clarissa Robinson, 1824; six children. EDUCATION: Educated in common schools of hometown; 1817-19, began study of medicine with Drs. Robert P. Gist and Absolom Bainbridge, Glasgow; 1819-20, 1821-22, Transylvania University medical department, Lexington, Ky.; M.D., 1822; c. 1823, attended course of lectures, Philadelphia, Pa., probably at a private school of anatomy. CAREER: 1820-21, practiced in partnership with Bainbridge, Glasgow; 1823, appointed demonstrator in anatomy, Transylvania University Medical Department; resigned without teaching; practiced medicine: 1824-27, Glasgow; and 1827-35, Harrodsburg, Ky.; 1835, invited to Louisville to assist in forming a faculty for the Louisville Medical Institute; 1837-46, professor of obstetrics and diseases of women and children, Louisville Medical Institute; 1846-58, professor of obstetrics, University of Louisville medical department; 1858-67, private practice, Louisville; 1859, elected president, American Medical Association; professor of medical and surgical diseases of women: 1867, University of Louisville medical department; and 1869-74, Louisville Medical College. CONTRIBUTIONS: An excellent anatomist and operator, was always interested in improvements in diagnosis and medical and surgical management of disorders and diseases in patients. One of the first in Ky. to adopt the vaginal speculum for use in the diagnosis and treatment of gynecologic disorders. First to use anesthesia in obstetrics in his community and a strong advocate of its proper use. Performed ovariotomy six times with only one death. Obtained the charter for the Louisville Medical College (1869). An exemplary physician and professor who taught and practiced without participating in the petty political, personal and professional bickerings that consumed so much of the time of his contemporaries. Co-editor, *Louisville Journal Medicine and Surgery* (1838).

WRITINGS: *Theoretical and Practical Treatise on Human Parturition* (1849); *Principles and Practice of Obstetrics* (1858). No complete bibliography has been published, but 16 of his publications are listed in *Index Catalogue*. REFERENCES: *DAB*, 6 pt. 2: 626; E. S. Gaillard, "The Life of Dr. Henry Miller," *Richmond & Louisville Med. J.* 13 (1872): 129; H. M. Goodman, "Henry Miller, M.D.," *J. Ky. Med. Assoc.* 15 (1917): 99; S. D. Gross, E. S. Gaillard, and J. M. Keller, "Memoir of Henry Miller, M.D.," *TAMA* 26 (1875): 441; *NCAB*, 12: 229.

E. H. Conner

MILLER, THOMAS (February 18, 1806, Port Royal, Va.-September 20, 1873, Washington, D.C.). *Physician; Anatomist*. Son of Thomas Roy, who worked for the Navy Department, and Sally (Attaway) Miller. Married Virginia C. Jones, 1833; eight children. EDUCATION: Received early education at the Washington Seminary (later Gonzaga College); medical studies with Dr. Edward Cutbush and Dr. Henry Huntt; 1829, M.D., University of Pennsylvania. CAREER: 1830, with six others, founded a teaching institution, Washington Medical Institute; 1832, began teaching a course in practical anatomy; 1839-59, professor of anatomy, medical department, Columbian College (later George Washington University); attending surgeon, Washington Infirmary, and on consulting staff, Providence Hospital and Children's Hospital. CONTRIBUTIONS: Major contributions in the area of public health, especially sanitary reform and vital statistics. As president, Board of Health (1846-55), worked zealously to get the reluctant municipal authorities to enact ordinances that gave the board some authority to declare nuisances and power to abate them. Originated the movement to establish and enforce a system of registration of births and deaths in D.C. A founder, Medical Association of the District of Columbia (1833), and later president (1873). First president, Pathological Society of Washington (1841). Worked hard to help establish the Government Hospital for the Insane (St. Elizabeth's).

WRITINGS: *Introductory Lecture on Anatomy* (1840). REFERENCES: S. C. Busey, *Personal Reminiscences* (1895), 169-74; Kelly and Burrage (1920), 794-95; D. S. Lamb et al., *History of the Medical Society of the District of Columbia, 1817-1909* (1909), 226-27; *NCAB*, 2: 146; *TAMA* 25 (1874): 523-24.

R. A. Kondratas

MILLER, WILLIAM SNOW (March 29, 1858, Sterling, Mass.-December 26, 1939, Madison, Wis.). *Physician; Anatomy; Medical history*. Son of William and Harriet Emily (Snow) Miller. Married Carrie M. Bradley, 1881 (d. 1901), Alice L. Burdick, 1912; no children. EDUCATION: 1879, M.D., Yale University; 1880s, worked in pathology with Frances Delafield (q.v.) at the College of Physicians and Surgeons in New York and in chemistry with Benjamin Silliman (q.v.) at Yale; also engaged in medical practice; 1890-92, fellow, Clark University; 1895-96, University of Leipzig; 1906-7, fellow, Johns Hopkins University. CAREER: 1889-92, pathologist, City and Memorial hospitals, Worcester, Mass.; at University of Wisconsin: 1892-95, instructor of vertebrate anatomy;

1895-1904, assistant professor of anatomy; 1904-16, associate; 1916-24, professor; and 1924-39, professor emeritus; 1918-19, lecturer in medicine, Johns Hopkins University. CONTRIBUTIONS: Attained distinction in the teaching and study of anatomy, particularly in the minute anatomy of the lung where his researches gained him international recognition. Pioneer in the establishment of medical history as an academic discipline in the United States, primarily through founding (1909) at the University of Wisconsin a medical seminar that spurred development of comparable activities at other universities. Active collector of classic medical works that form basis of University of Wisconsin's present extensive rare book collection.

WRITINGS: "Abraham Chovet," *Annals of Med. Hist.* 8 (1926): 375-93; "William Beaumont and His Book," *ibid.*, n.s., 1 (1929): 155-79; "William Beaumont, M.D.," *ibid.*, n.s., 5 (1933): 28-51; *The Lung* (1937). Writings listed in *The William Snow Miller Festschrift* (1928), 83-85. REFERENCES: *DAB*, Supplement 2: 457-9; William S. Middleton, "Doctor William Snow Miller and His Seminar," *Bull. Hist. Med.* 8 (1940): 1067-72; *NCAB*, 38: 263.

W. J. Orr, Jr.

MILLS, CHARLES KARSNER (December 4, 1845, Philadelphia, Pa.-May 28, 1931, Philadelphia). *Physician; Neurology.* Son of James and Lavinia Ann (Fitzgerald) Mills. Married Clara Elizabeth Peale, 1873; four children. EDUCATION: 1864, graduated, Central High School, Philadelphia; University of Pennsylvania: 1869, M.D.; and 1871, Ph.D. CAREER: 1862-63, Union army; 1864-66, teacher; 1871-73, general practice; 1874, became chief, clinic for nervous diseases, University Hospital, Philadelphia; 1877, appointed neurologist, Philadelphia Hospital; 1877-1931, at University of Pennsylvania: 1877-1893, successively lecturer in electrotherapeutics and lecturer in neuropsychiatry; 1893-1901, professor of mental diseases and medical jurisprudence; 1901-3, clinical professor of nervous diseases; 1903-15, professor of neurology; and 1915-31, professor emeritus; 1883-98, professor of diseases of the mind and nervous system, Philadelphia Polyclinic; 1891-1902, clinical professor of nervous diseases, Woman's Medical College of Pennsylvania; 1887, 1924, president, American Neurological Association. CONTRIBUTIONS: Founded (1883) Philadelphia Neurological Society. Took part in several important cases in medical jurisprudence, examining, among others, Charles J. Guiteau (1881) and Harry K. Thaw (1924). Studied cerebral localization, particularly with regard to motor and sensory centers. Reported clinical studies of injuries extensively.

WRITINGS: More than 350 articles on medical topics; many articles on medical biography, medical history, and philosophy of neurology. *First Lessons in Physiology and Hygiene* (1883; rev. ed., 1885), reissued as *Physiology and Hygiene: With Special Reference to Alcohol, Tobacco, and Other Narcotics* (1904): *The Nursing and Care of the Nervous and the Insane* (1887; 3rd ed., with the assistance of Nathaniel S. Yawger, 1915); *The Nervous System and Its Diseases: A Practical Treatise on Neurology for the Use of Physicians and Students* (1898). REFERENCES: *DAB*, 13: 3-4; Miller, *BHM*, p.

75; *NCAB*, B: 331-32; *NUC Pre-1956 Imprints*, 385: 4-9; *N.Y. Times*, May 29, 1931; *Semi-Centennial Volume of the American Neurological Association, 1875-1924* (1924).

M. M. Sokal

MILLS, HIRAM FRANCIS (November 1, 1836, Bangor, Maine-October 4, 1921, Hingham, Mass.). *Hydraulic and sanitary engineer.* Son of Preserved Brayton, physician, and Jane (Lunt) Mills. Married Elizabeth Worcester, 1873. EDUCATION: 1856, C.E., Rensselaer Polytechnic Institute. CAREER: 1856-67, railroad and hydraulic engineer, N.Y. and New England; *post* 1868, consulting engineer, ten states and Mexico; *post* 1868, engineer, Essex Company, Lawrence, Mass.; and Locks and Canals Company, Lowell, Mass.; 1886-1914, member, Massachusetts State Board of Health; and chairman, committee on water supply and sewage; *post* 1901, consulting engineer, (Boston, Mass.) Metropolitan Water and Sewerage Board. CONTRIBUTIONS: Initiated and directed research on water and sewage treatment methods that helped bring about a marked decline in deaths from water-borne diseases. Helped organize the Lawrence Experiment Station which became world-famous for its research in water and sewage purification; constructed a slow-sand filter at Lawrence that greatly lowered the city's typhoid death rate (1893); provided first example of the ability of sand filters to protect urban water supplies, thereby beginning a new era in municipal sanitation. Prepared the sewage plan adopted by the Boston Metropolitan Water and Sewerage Board, which became a model of regional sanitary planning.

WRITINGS: *Flow of Water in Pipes* (1923, published posthumously). REFERENCES: *DAB*, 13: 8; *NCAB*, 12: 71; *Who Was Who in Am.*, 1: 846.

S. Galishoff

MILLSPAUGH, JOSEPH GILLISPIE (February 19, 1851, Battle Creek, Mich.-January 31, 1927, Monrovia, Calif.). *Physician; Surgeon.* Son of Jacob and Mary Ann (Dicker) Millspaugh. Married Anna Zang, 1879; three children. EDUCATION: Hope College: 1872, A.B.; and 1874, M.A.; 1876, M.D., University of Michigan; 1877, MDCM, Columbia University. CAREER: Physician and surgeon: 1877-83, Battle Creek, Mich.; and 1883-91, Park River, Dak. Territory; 1888-90, president, North Dakota Medical Association; 1889-91, superintendent, North Dakota State Board of Health; physician and surgeon: 1891-92, Superior, Wis.; and 1892-1927, Little Falls, Minn.; president, Upper Mississippi Medical Society. CONTRIBUTIONS: Considered the "father" of the North Dakota Medical Association; organized initial meeting and served as the first president. First superintendent of public health, N.Dak. REFERENCES: James Grassick, "Joseph Gillispie Millspaugh: First President of the North Dakota Medical Association," *J.-Lancet* 51 (1931); idem, *North Dakota Medicine: Sketches and Abstracts* (1926), 75-83; *Little Falls Transcript* (Minn.), February 1, 1927, p. 1.

L. Remele

MILROY, WILLIAM FORSYTH (December 28, 1855, York, N.Y.-September 24, 1942, Hollywood, Calif.). *Physician; Internal medicine.* Son of James, farmer, and Sarah Ann (Cullings) Milroy. Married Lillian Barton, April 26, 1886; two children. EDUCATION: State Normal School, Geneseo, N.Y.; 1879, University of Rochester; 1880, Johns Hopkins University; 1882, M.D., College of Physicians and Surgeons of New York; 1882-84, intern, Charity and Maternal hospitals in New York City. CAREER: 1884-1933, medical practice, Omaha, Nebr.; 1884-1933, professor of clinical medicine, Omaha Medical College and its successor, University of Nebraska College of Medicine; president: 1885-87, board of trustees, Omaha Medical College; 1890, Omaha-Douglas County Medical Society; 1916, Nebraska State Medical Society; 1918, Missouri Valley Medical Society; and 1923, Nebraska Children's Home Society; 1923, vice-president, American Therapeutic Society. CONTRIBUTIONS: Published an article (1892), "An Undescribed Variety of Hereditary Oedema," which William Osler (q.v.) named "Milroy's disease"; continued this study for 35 years. Outstanding teacher and a contributor to the literature of internal medicine and public health. Contributed to the scholarly record of the history of medicine and medical education in Nebr. Active in professional organizations, often assuming the role of conciliator.

WRITINGS: "The Aetiology and Course of Pulmonary Consumption as Influenced by the Climate and Soil of Eastern Nebraska," *Med. Record* 32, no. 18 (Oct. 29, 1887): 563-66; "Typhoid Fever and Water Supply in Omaha," *The Omaha Clinic* 2, no. 1 (Apr. 1889): 1-11; "An Undescribed Variety of Hereditary Oedema," *N.Y. Med. J.* 56 (Nov. 5, 1892): 505-8; "Chronic Hereditary Edema," *JAMA* 91, no. 16 (Oct. 20, 1928): 1172-75. REFERENCES: Archives, University of Nebraska Medical Center Library of Medicine, Omaha, Nebr.; S. M. Baldwin and R. M. Baldwin, *Nebraskana* (1932), 831; *NCAB*, 31 (1944): 337-38; A. T. Tyler and E. F. Auerbach, *History of Medicine in Nebraska* (1977, enlarged by B. M. Hetzner), 218.

B. M. Hetzner

MINOKA-HILL, LILLIE ROSA (August 30, 1876, St. Regis Reservation, N.Y.-March 18, 1952, Fond du Lac, Wis.). *Physician.* Daughter of Joshua Allen, Philadelphia, Pa., physician, and a Mohawk woman. Married Charles Abram Hill, 1905; six children. EDUCATION: 1895, diploma, Grahame Institute, Philadelphia; 1899, M.D., Woman's Medical College of Pennsylvania; 1900, intern, Woman's Hospital, Philadelphia. CAREER: 1900-1905, private practice, Philadelphia; after marriage to Hill, an Oneida, moved to Oneida, Wis., and withdrew from formal medical practice while continuing a small unofficial practice among neighbors and relatives; 1916, upon death of husband, financial circumstances forced her to resume full-time medical practice and she established a clinic in her home; patients, poor themselves, usually paid her in kind; 1934, after sitting for a Wis. medical license federal government also reimbursed her for some services; 1946, following a heart attack, limited practice to the clinic. CONTRIBUTIONS: The sole trained physician in Oneida (*post* 1917). Not only tended the medical problems of Oneidas and non-Oneidas but taught nutrition, sanitation, and general preventive medicine. Community works won her many accolades: Oneida tribe adopted her; Indian Council Fire named her outstanding

American Indian of the Year (1947); and State Medical Society awarded her an honorary lifetime membership (1949). Grateful patients erected a monument in her honor outside Oneida. REFERENCES: Victoria Brown, "Dr. Rose Minoka Hill," *Uncommon Lives of Common Women* (1975), 65-66; idem, "An Indian Physician Remembers. . .," *The Crusader* 43, no. 5 (May 1951): 8-9; *Notable Am. Women: The Modern Period* (1980), 481-83.

R. D. Apple

MINOT, CHARLES SEDGWICK (December 23, 1852, West Roxbury, Mass.-November 19, 1914, Milton, Mass.). *Biologist; Anatomy; Embryology.* Son of William and Katherine (Sedgwick) Minot. Married Lucy Fosdick, 1889; no children. EDUCATION: 1872, B.S., Massachusetts Institute of Technology; 1873-76, studied biology, physiology, zoology, and morphology, Harvard University, and in Paris, France, and Leipzig and Würzburg, Germany; 1878, D.Sci., Harvard University. CAREER: 1878-80, private biological research; at Harvard University: 1880-83, oral pathology and surgery faculty, dental school; 1883-1905, histology and embryology faculty, medical school; and *post* 1905, comparative anatomy faculty; 1912-13, exchange professor, universities of Berlin and Jena; president: 1894, American Society of Naturalists; 1900, American Association for the Advancement of Science; and American Association of Anatomists. CONTRIBUTIONS: Broadened the study of anatomy in the United States to include embryology, histology, and physical anthropology. Investigated the biological aspects of growth and aging, especially changes in cell structure from birth to death. Collected over 1900 vertebrate embryos that he cut into sections, numbered, and cataloged providing a sort of encyclopedia of vertebrate development for students and scientific investigators. Invented (1886) the automatic rotary microtome for sectioning vertebrate embryos. Made a microscopic study of the structure of the human placenta and described the blood channels in the liver which he named "sinusoids." Principal scientific contribution was *Human Embryology* (1892), a summation of all extant knowledge concerning human development together with a presentation of the most important areas of research for that science.

WRITINGS: "A Theory of the Structure of the Placenta," *Anatomischer Anzeiger* 6 (1891): 125-31; "A Bibliography of Vertebrate Embryology," *Memoirs of the Boston Soc. of Natural Hist.* 4, no. 11 (1893): 487-614; *Laboratory Textbook of Embryology* (1903); *The Problem of Life, Growth, and Death* (1908). A bibliography is in *BMNAS*, 14 (1920): 263-85. REFERENCES: *DSB*, 9: 416; Kelly and Burrage (1928), 849-51; Frederic T. Lewis, "Charles Sedgwick Minot," *Anatomic Record* 10 (1915-16): 133-64; *Who Was Who in Am.*, 1: 848.

S. Galishoff

MINOT, GEORGE RICHARDS (December 2, 1885, Boston, Mass.-February 25, 1950, Brookline, Mass.). *Physician and medical educator; Hematology.* Son of James Jackson, physician, and Elizabeth (Whitney) Minot. Married Marian Linzee Weld, 1915; three children. EDUCATION: Harvard University: 1908, A.B., and 1912, M.D.; 1912-13, house officer, Massachusetts General

Hospital; 1913-14, resident, Johns Hopkins Hospital. CAREER: 1914-15, medicine and physiology faculty, Johns Hopkins Medical School; medical staff: 1915-23, Massachusetts General Hospital; 1923-28, Peter Bent Brigham Hospital; and 1923-28, Collis P. Huntington Memorial Hospital; 1915-48, medicine faculty, Harvard Medical School; 1928-48, director, Thorndike Memorial Laboratory of Boston City Hospital. CONTRIBUTIONS: With William P. Murphy, demonstrated that pernicious anemia, a hitherto invariably fatal disease, could be cured by liver feedings for which they shared the 1934 Nobel Prize in medicine or physiology with George H. Whipple (q.v.); collaborated in the development of an effective liver extract (1927) and the identification—by others—of the active agent, vitamin B^{12}. Changed the focus of hematological research from descriptive morphological classifications to physiological studies of the blood, its creation and destruction. Did important research on blood transfusion, coagulation, and platelets. With Clark W. Heath, showed that hypochromic anemia could be treated with iron (1931-32). Demonstrated that the absence of a plasma globulin prevented normal blood-clotting, which later proved of great importance in the treatment of hemophilia (1946). Made authoritative studies of the effects of X-ray therapy on blood-cell production in chronic leukemia and lymphoid tumors. At The Thorndike, directed the first clinical research laboratory to be established in a municipal hospital; trained hundreds of students there, many of whom became professors in medical schools in the United States and abroad.

WRITINGS: "Lymphatic Leukemia: Age Incidence, Duration, and Benefit Derived from Irridation," *Boston Med. and Surg. J.* 174 (May 11, 1916): 667-74; "Treatment of Pernicious Anemia by a Specialist Diet," *JAMA* 87 (1926): 470-76 (with W. P. Murphy); *Pathological Physiology and Clinical Description of the Anemias* (1936, with William B. Castle); "The Relation of Certain Fractions of the Plasma Globulins to the Coagulation Defect in Hemophilia," *Blood* 1 (1946): 166-72 (with Jessica H. Lewis et al.). A bibliography is in *BMNAS*. REFERENCES: *BHM*, no. 5 (1964-69): 184; *BMNAS* 45 (1974): 337-83; *DAB*, Supplement 4: 580-83; *DSB*, 9: 416-17; Miller, *BHM*, p. 75; F. M. Rackemann, *The Inquisitive Physician* (1956); *Who Was Who in Am.*, 2: 376.

                                                                                              S. Galishoff

MINTON, HENRY McKEE (December 25, 1870, Columbia, S.C.-December 29, 1946, Philadelphia, Pa.). *Physician.* Son of Sawyer Theophilus and Jennie (McKee) Minton. Married Edith G. Wormley, 1902. EDUCATION: 1887-91, Phillips Exeter Academy; 1906, M.D., Jefferson Medical College; 1891-92, Law School, University of Pennsylvania; 1895, Ph.G., Philadelphia College of Pharmacy. CAREER: 1895-1902, drug business, Philadelphia; 1906-46, medical practice, Philadelphia; 1920-44, superintendent, Mercy Hospital, Philadelphia; 1915-46, staff member, Henry Phipps Institute (tuberculosis). CONTRIBUTIONS: Operated first black-owned drug store in Philadelphia (1895-1902). First pharmacist for first black hospital in Philadelphia (Douglass Hospital, 1895). Second superintendent of one of the most important hospitals in the history of blacks in medicine, Mercy Hospital, Philadelphia (1920-44). Organized first black medical fraternity (1904), Sigma Pi Phi (called the Boule). Disseminated public health information in Philadelphia. Wrote about black history. Supervisor, Negro Tuberculosis Bureau, Philadelphia (1923-44).

WRITINGS: "The Part the Negro Is Playing in the Reduction of Mortality," *Hosp. Soc. Serv.* 10 (1924): 1016. REFERENCES: W. Montague Cobb, "Henry McKee Minton, 1870-1946," *JNMA* 47 (1955): 285-86; *WWCR*, p. 193; *WWICA* 6 (1941-43): 367-68.

T. L. Savitt

MITCHELL, JOHN KEARSLEY (May 12, 1793, Shepherdstown, Va. [now in W.Va.]-April 4, 1858, Philadelphia, Pa.). *Physician; Chemist; Author.* Son of Alexander, physician, and Elizabeth (Kearsley) Mitchell. Married Sarah Matilda Henry, 1822; nine children, including Silas Weir Mitchell (q.v.). EDUCATION: Graduated, University of Edinburgh; 1819, M.D., University of Pennsylvania. CAREER: 1819-22, ship's surgeon on voyages to China and East Indies; 1822-58, practiced medicine, Philadelphia; at Philadelphia Medical Institute: 1824, medicine and physiology faculty; and *post* 1826, chemistry faculty; 1833-38, chemistry faculty, Franklin Institute; 1841-58, theory and practice of medicine faculty, Jefferson Medical College; medical staff, Pennsylvania Hospital and Philadelphia city hospital; wrote several books of poems, conducted chemical experiments, and was a popular lecturer on scientific subjects. CONTRIBUTIONS: First American to describe neuropathic arthritis (1831). Published *On the Cryptogamous Origin of Malarious and Epidemic Fevers (1849)*, in which, on *a priori* grounds, argued that a *contagium vivum* was responsible for these diseases.

WRITINGS: "On a New Practice in Acute and Chronic Rheumatism," *Am. J. of Med. Sci.* 8 (1831); 55-64; Silas Weir Mitchell, ed., *Five Essays by John Kearsley Mitchell, M.D.* (1859). A description of his writings in *Index Catalogue* also is in *J. Hist. Med. & Allied Sci.* 20 (1965). REFERENCES: *DAB*, 13: 54-55; Raymond N. Doetsch, "Mitchell on the Causes of Fevers," *Bull. Hist. Med.* 38 (1964): 241-59; Michael Kelly, "John Kearsley Mitchell (1793-1858) and the Neurogenic Theory of Arthritis, A Reappraisal," *J. Hist. Med. & Allied Sci.* 20 (1965): 151-56; Kelly and Burrage (1928), 853; Miller, *BHM*, p. 75; *NCAB*, 9: 346; *Who Was Who in Am.*, Hist. Vol.: 431.

S. Galishoff

MITCHELL, ROBERT WOOD (August 26, 1831, Madison County, Tenn.-November 2, 1903, Memphis, Tenn.). *Physician; Public health.* Son of Gen. Guilford Dudley, state (Miss.) militia officer, merchant, and schoolteacher, and Mary (Wood) Mitchell. Married Rebecca Park, 1872; no children. EDUCATION: Literary education, Centenary College, Jackson, Miss., but left school at 16 to clerk in a drug store; c. 1853, began the study of medicine under his brother-in-law, Dr. A. W. Washburne, near Yazoo City, Miss.; 1856, M.D., University of Louisiana (now Tulane). CAREER: 1857, became secretary, Memphis Board of Health; during Civil War: 1861, commissioned assistant surgeon, 15th Tenn. Infantry Regiment, Confederate States of America; later in 1861, became surgeon, 13th Tenn. Infantry Regiment, rising to division surgeon in the army of Tenn.; 1865, returned to Memphis; 1868, entered into a partnership with Dr. Richard Brooke Maury (q.v.); early in 1878, appointed president, Memphis

Board of Health, resigned, and became medical director, Howard Association of Memphis, during the yellow-fever epidemic; served similarly in the 1879 epidemic; 1879, appointed by President Rutherford B. Hayes to the National Board of Health; 1879, member, special committee that made a sanitary survey of Memphis in the autumn. CONTRIBUTIONS: Received national recognition for the effective leadership provided as medical director, Howard Association, during the yellow-fever epidemics (1878-79). Served on the National Board of Health as well as other boards and committees (1880s, 1890s) in connection with public health affairs.

WRITINGS: Few, mainly concerned with yellow fever and other public health topics. REFERENCES: W. S. Speer, *Sketches of Prominent Tennesseans* (1888), 556-58.

S. R. Bruesch

MITCHELL, S[ILAS] WEIR (February 16, 1829, Philadelphia, Pa.-January 4, 1914, Philadelphia). *Physician; Novelist; Poet; Neurology*. Son of John Kearsley (q.v.), physician, and Sarah Matilda (Henry) Mitchell. Married Mary Middleton Elwyn, 1858; two children. Mary Cadwalader, 1875; one child. EDUCATION: c. 1844-47, University of Pennsylvania; 1850, M.D., Jefferson Medical College; 1850-51, study in Europe. CAREER: 1851, began general practice; c. 1861-65, Union army surgeon in Civil War; in decades after the war, gained recognition and acclaim as an important neurologist, therapist, critic of mental asylums, poet, and novelist; while he remained a practitioner, was always engaged in research, making contributions to medical literature in many different fields; professor at the Philadelphia Polyclinic and College for Graduates in Medicine; closely associated with the Philadelphia Orthopedic Hospital and Infirmary for Nervous Diseases; for more than 40 years, helped to make it into a center for the treatment of nervous disorders; trustee, University of Pennsylvania; fellow and president, College of Physicians of Philadelphia; member of numerous American and European scientific societies, notably, National Academy of Science, French Academy of Medicine, Royal Medical Society of Norway, Academy of Sciences of Sweden, and Royal Academy of Medicine of Rome. CONTRIBUTIONS: Helped establish neurology as a medical specialty; began study of peripheral nerve injuries during Civil War. Research and writings ranged over a wide spectrum of neurological and related subjects including red neuralgia, the physiology of the cerebellum, sleeping disorders, ailuophobia (cat fear), weather conditions and nerve injury and disease, erythromelalgia, causalgia, the psychological effects of amputations, reflex paralysis, and snake venoms. Introduced inhalations of nitrite of amyl to check epileptic seizures and used freezing sprays to reduce pain and local spasm. Gained international attention for "rest cure," a mode of treatment that involved rest in bed, massages, a rich and full diet, isolation, and avoidance of disturbing events. A major critic of asylums and institutional psychiatry.

WRITINGS: About neurology: *Lectures on the Diseases of the Nervous System, Especially in Women* (1881); *Clinical Lessons on Nervous Diseases* (1895); *Injuries of Nerves and Their Consequences* (1972). About the rest cure: *Wear and Tear, or Hints for the*

Overworked (1871); *Fat and Blood: An Essay on the Treatment of Certain Forms of Neurasthenia and Hysteria* (1884). About criticism of mental institutions: "Address Before the Fiftieth Annual Meeting of the American Medico-Psychological Association, Held in Philadelphia, May 16, 1894," *J. of Nervous and Mental Disease* 21 (1894): 413-37. See also *A Catalogue of the Scientific and Literary Work of S. Weir Mitchell, Annotated by the Author* (1894). REFERENCES: *BHM* (1964-69), 184; (1970-74), 123; (1975-79), 87; *DAB*, 13: 62-65; Ernest Earnest, *S. Weir Mitchell, Novelist and Physician* (1950); Kelly and Burrage (1928), 854-57; Miller, *BHM*, pp. 75-76; *NCAB*, 9: 346; Richard D. Walter, *S. Weir Mitchell, M.D.—Neurologist* (1970).

L. V. Bell

MITCHILL, SAMUEL LATHAM (August 20, 1764, North Hempstead, L.I., N.Y.-September 7, 1831, New York, N.Y.). *Physician, scientist, and statesman.* Son of Robert, Jr., farmer, and Mary (Latham) Mitchill. Married Catherine (Akerly) Cock, 1799; two adopted daughters. EDUCATION: Tutored in classics by Rev. Leonard Cutting, professor of classical literature at King's College; apprenticed in medicine under maternal uncle, Dr. Samuel Latham; 1781-83, apprenticeship under Dr. Samuel Bard (q.v.); 1783-86, M.D., with high honors, University of Edinburgh; 1786-87, traveled through Europe; 1787, studied law with Robert Yates. CAREER: Entered practice of medicine; 1788, one of U.S. commissioners at Fort Stanwix who negotiated the purchase of the Iroquois lands of western N.Y.; 1790-92, 1797-99, N.Y. State Assembly; at Columbia College: 1792-95, professor of botany; and 1792-1801, professor, natural history, chemistry, and agriculture; 1801-4, 1809-13, U.S. House of Representatives; 1804-9, U.S. Senate; at College of Physicians and Surgeons: 1808-20, professor of natural history; and 1820-26, professor of materia medica and botany; vice-president: 1826-27, Rutgers Medical College, New York City; and 1827-30, Rutgers Medical Faculty of Geneva College, N.Y. CONTRIBUTIONS: The outstanding American scientist of his time. Labored to lay the foundations of all of the natural sciences in this country; first descriptive geology of N.Y. State; pioneer study of American fishes; explained and taught the chemical theories of Lavoisier. A founder (1797) and editor-in-chief, *Medical Repository*, first medical journal published in the United States. Devoted to the needs of American sailors and merchant seamen. Fought for sanitary reform, changes in quarantine laws, and harbor improvements. Founder (1817), Lyceum of Natural History of New York, which developed into the American Museum of Natural History and the New York Academy of Sciences.

WRITINGS: "A Sketch of the Mineralogical History of the State of New York," *Medical Repository* (1798-1801), 1: 279-303, 445-52; 3: 325-35; 5: 212-15; "Fishes of New York," *Trans., Literary and Philosophical Soc. of N.Y.* 1 (1815):355-492. Writings listed in *A Scientist in the Early Republic* (1934), 141-50; N. Y. Acad. of Med., *Author Catalog* 26 (1969): 867-72; Royal Society of London, *Catalog of Scientific Papers (1800-1863)* 4 (1879). REFERENCES: Alan D. Aberbach, "Samuel Latham Mitchill: A Physician in the Early Days of the Republic," *Bull. N.Y. Acad. of Med.* 40 (1964): 501-10; *BHM* (1964-69), 184; *DAB*, 7, pt. 1: 69-71; Courtney Robert Hall, *A Scientist in the Early Republic, Samuel Latham Mitchill, 1764-1831*; *NCAB*, 4: 409.

R. E. Batt

MOEUR, BENJAMIN BAKER (December 22, 1869, Decherd, Tenn.-March 16, 1937, Tempe, Ariz). *Physician*. Son of John Baptist, physician, and Esther Kelly (Knight) Moeur. Married Honor G. Anderson, June 15, 1896; four children. EDUCATION: 1896, M.D., Arkansas Industrial University (now University of Arkansas). CAREER: After a brief stay in Tombstone, Ariz., moved to Tempe, where he practiced medicine for the rest of his life. CONTRIBUTIONS: Physician for Arizona State University. Member, Arizona Constitutional Convention of 1910. Governor of Arizona (1933-37). While governor, conducted free medical clinic in the rotunda of the capitol.   REFERENCES: *Arizona Republic* (Phoenix), March 17 and 18, 1937; *NCAB*, 28: 422; *Who Was Who in Am.*, 1: 852.

J. S. Goff

MONETTE, JOHN WESLEY (April 5, 1803, Staunton, Va.-March 1, 1851, Washington, Miss.). *Physician*; *Historian*. Son of Dr. Samuel and Mrs. Mary (Wayland) Monette. Married Cornelia Jane Newman, 1828; ten children. EDUCATION: Chillicothe (Ohio) Academy; 1825, M.D., Transylvania University. CAREER: Until 1821, lived with family in Chillicothe, Ohio, when the family moved to Washington, Miss.; after graduating from medical school, practiced in Washington, where he had ample opportunity to observe and become an authority on yellow fever; investments in cotton and lands enabled Monette to accumulate a fortune sufficient to devote much of his time to literary and scientific studies; in addition to medical interests, devoted time and energy to natural history; 1824, wrote paper "Causes of the Variety of the Complexion and the Form of the Human Species," which antedated Darwin's *Origin of Species* by some 35 years; another paper of significance was "Essay on the Improbability of Spontaneous Production of Animals and Plants"; greatest literary undertaking was the writing of an elaborate two-volume work about the history and geography of the Mississippi Valley; mayor and councilman, Washington, Miss. CONTRIBUTIONS: Made careful investigation of yellow-fever epidemics that struck Natchez and Washington, Miss. Read paper before Jefferson College (1837) that suggested the use of quarantines in restricting the disease. Technique was employed in the New Orleans, La., epidemic of 1841. Became recognized as an authority on yellow fever, and wrote many articles on the disease, including a series in the *Western Journal of Medicine and Surgery* (1842-43). Another medical contribution that indicates pioneer work was an article in the *Western Medical Journal* referring to the use of oil of turpentine as an external irritant, particularly in the treatment of typhus fever.

WRITINGS: *An Account of the Epidemic of Yellow Fever That Occurred in Washington, Mississippi, in the Autumn of 1825* (1827); *Oil of Turpentine as an External Irritant* (1827); *Observations on the Epidemic of Yellow Fever of Natchez and the Southwest* (1842). REFERENCES: *DAB*, 7 pt. 1: 85; Miller, *BHM*, p. 76; John A. Milne, "Early Mississippi Physicians," *J. of Mississippi Hist.* 18 (Jul. 1956): 157-74; *NCAB*, 15: 4; Franklin L. Riley, "Life and Literary Services of Dr. John W. Monette," *Publications of the Mississippi Hist. Soc.* 9 (1906): 199-237.

M. S. Legan

MONTEZUMA, CARLOS (1865, Central Ariz.-January 31, 1923, Fort McDowell Indian Reservation, Ariz.). *Physician; Internist.* Born "Wassaja," a Yavapai Indian. Taken prisoner in 1872 and sold for $30 to C. Gentile, who took him to Chicago and raised him. Married Marie Keller, 1913; no children. EDUCATION: 1884, B.S., University of Illinois; 1889, M.D., Chicago Medical College. CAREER: 1889-96, physician, U.S. Indian service, variously assigned in N.Dak., Nev., Wash., and at Carlisle Indian School, Pa.; 1896-1922, practice, Chicago, Ill.; 1896-1914, associated with Dr. Fenton B. Turck in his clinic (stomach and intestinal diseases) at Post-Graduate Medical School, Chicago; 1904-6, instructor in medicine, College of Physicians and Surgeons, Chicago; 1922, contracted tuberculosis, declined all medical aid, and returned to the reservation. CONTRIBUTIONS: Advocate of Indian rights. Prominent Chicago physician. REFERENCES: *Arizona Republican* (Phoenix), February 2 and 5, 1923; Bert Robinson, "The Great Yavapai," *Arizona Highways* (Aug. 1952); *Who Was Who in Am.*, 1: 855.

J. S. Goff

MOORE, AARON McDUFFIE (September 6, 1863, Columbus County, N.C.-April 29, 1923, Durham, N.C.). *Physician.* Son of Isreal, farmer, and Eliza Moore. Married Catie S. Dancy, 1889; two children. EDUCATION: Normal schools, Lumberton and Fayetteville, N.C.; 1888, M.D., Leonard Medical College. CAREER: 1888-1923, medical practice, Durham; 1898-1923, North Carolina Mutual Life Insurance Company: co-founder, secretary-treasurer, medical director, and (later) president; 1901-23, founder and superintendent, Lincoln Hospital, Durham. CONTRIBUTIONS: Durham's first black physician (1888). After helping to launch a black pharmacy in Durham (1895), assisted in numerous black business ventures. Strong believer in black self-help movement and did what he could to aid it. Raised funds from white Durham community to found Lincoln Hospital (1901) and Colored Library (1913). Greatly assisted N.C. state rural school movement for blacks (1914-23) and Tuskegee fund raising efforts. Served as chairman, Board of Trustees, Shaw University, for ten years; gave large sums and left $5,000 to school upon death. Provided medical care and more to all who needed it in his rounds. Worked hard to improve all aspects of life in Durham black community and was revered for it. Crossed racial barriers in dealings with whites. Strong leader in North Carolina Mutual Life Insurance Company (1900-23).   REFERENCES: John A. Kenney, *The Negro in Medicine* (1912), 15-16; Frank L. Mather, ed., *Who's Who* (1915), 195; obituary, *JNMA* 16 (1924): 72-74; private papers, Manuscript Division, Duke University Library, Durham; Walter B. Weare, *Black Business in the New South—A Social History of the North Carolina Mutual Life Insurance Company* (1973), 29-30, 45-49, 52-57.

T. L. Savitt

MOORE, CARL VERNON (August 21, 1908, St. Louis, Mo.-August 13, 1972, Manistee, Mich.). *Physician; Hematology.* Son of Carl Vernon, a policeman, and Mary (Kemp) Moore. Married Dorothy Adams, May 25, 1935; one child. EDUCATION: 1928, A.B., Elmhurst College, Elmhurst, Ill.; 1932, M.D., Washington University, St. Louis; 1931-33, house officer, Barnes Hospital, St. Louis; 1934-35, National Research Council Fellow in Medicine, Ohio State University, Columbus, Ohio. CAREER: Ohio State University: 1935, instructor, medical research; and 1936-38, assistant professor of medicine; at Washington University: 1938-72, Department of Medicine, faculty; 1952-55, dean; and 1964-65, vice-chancellor for medical affairs. CONTRIBUTIONS: Major research interest was the metabolism of iron. Over the course of career, carried out and directed a long series of investigations of the absorption, use and excretion of iron. First to suggest that serum iron was transport iron (1937) and established the greater absorbability of ferrous over ferric iron compounds (1944). One of the first to use radioactive iron to study the absorption of iron from both plant and animal foods (1946, 1951). Later work in this field helped to show the value of iron-fortified bread. A pioneer in therapy with radioactive phosphorous for polycythemia vera (1944) and the first to use folic acid in treating macrocytic anemia of pregnancy.

WRITINGS: "The Mechanism of Iron Transportation: I, Chemical Methods and Normal Values for Plasma Iron and 'Easily Split-Off' Blood Iron," *J. Clin. Invest.* 16 (1937): 613 (with W. B. Arrowsmith, J. J. Quilligan, and J. T. Read); "Absorption of Ferrous and Ferric Radioactive Iron by Human Subjects and Dogs," *ibid.*, 23 (1944): 755 (with R. Dubach, V. Minnich, and H. K. Roberts); "Observations on the Absorption of Iron from Foods Tagged with Radioiron," *Trans. Assoc. of Am. Physicians* 64 (1951): 245 (with R. Dubach). Writings listed in *BMNAS*. REFERENCES: *BHM* (1975-79), 88; Elmer Brown, "Carl Vernon Moore," *Progress in Hematology* (1972), v-viii; William H. Daughaday, "In Memoriam: Carl V. Moore, M.D.," *Am. J. Med.* 54 (1973): 140-42; W. J. Harrington et al., "Carl V. Moore (1908-1972)," *Blood* 30 (1972): 771-75; *NCAB*, 57: 305-6.

D. R. Sneddeker

MOORE, EDWARD MOTT (July 15, 1814, Rahway, N.J.-March 3, 1902, Rochester, N.Y.). *Surgeon; Medical educator.* Son of Lindley Murray, teacher, and Abigail Lydia (Mott) Moore. Married Lucy Richard Prescott, 1847; eight children. EDUCATION: Attended Rensselaer School (Troy, N.Y.); 1833-35, apprentice to Dr. Anson Coleman of Rochester; 1835, College of Physicians and Surgeons of Columbia University; 1838, M.D., University of Pennsylvania; 1838-40, intern at Blockley Hospital and Frankford Lunatic Asylum. CAREER: 1840-42, medical practice at Rochester, N.Y.; 1842-53, professor of surgery, Vermont Medical College at Woodstock, teaching surgery at the Berkshire Medical Institution, Pittsfield; 1852-53, professor of anatomy, Buffalo University;

1853-56, professor of surgery, Starling Medical College, Columbus, Ohio; 1856-82, professor of surgery, University of Buffalo; 1882, returned to Rochester for medical and surgical practice; served as member of Rochester Board of Health, and as first president of the New York State Board of Health, which he helped organize. CONTRIBUTIONS: Well-known surgeon and educator. Served as president of the American Medical Association (1890), the American Surgical Association, and the New York State Medical Society (1874). Completed original studies of fracture of the collarbone, humerus, elbow joint, and Colles' Fracture.

WRITINGS: Various papers, including "Gangrene and Gangrenous Diseases," *International Encyclopaedia of Surgery*, 2 (1882) and an essay on "Dislocations" in *A Reference Handbook of Medical Sciences*, 2 (1886). REFERENCES: *DAB*, 7, pt. 1:119-20; *JAMA*, March 15, 1902; Kelly and Burrage (1928), 863-64.

M. Kaufman

MOORE, PHOEBIA G. (March 6, 1872, Mannington, W.Va.-June 4, 1953, Fairmont, W.Va.). *General physician*. Daughter of Theophilus Moore. EDUCATION: Fairmont Normal School and West Virginia University Medical School; 1903, M.D., Bennett Medical School, Chicago, Ill. CAREER: Practiced medicine, Mannington, W.Va. CONTRIBUTIONS: Notable work during the 1917 flu epidemic and after disastrous tornado struck Mannington (June 23, 1944). Work in medical education of farm women. Held a camp for the education of women every year at Jackson's Mill, W.Va.

WRITINGS: *Interesting Daughters of West Virginia* (with Ethel Clark Lewis). REFERENCES: *Better Times* (Monongalia County), January 30, 1980; Arthur Prichard, "Phoebia Moore, M.D., First Woman to Study Medicine at West Virginia University," *Goldenseal* 5 (Oct.-Dec. 1979); Edward J. Van Liere and Gideon S. Dodds, *History of Medical Education in West Virginia* (1965).

K. Nodyne and R. Murphy

MOORE, SAMUEL PRESTON (1813, Charleston, S.C.-May 31, 1889, Richmond, Va.). *Surgeon-general of the Confederate Army*. Son of Stephen West and Eleanor Screven (Gilbert) Moore. Married Mary Augusta Brown, 1845. EDUCATION: 1834, M.D., Medical College of South Carolina. CAREER: 1835-61, medical service, U.S. Army; served on the western frontiers, in Fla., N.Y., and La. and, during the Mexican War, along the Rio Grande River; 1861-65, surgeon-general, Confederate Army; *post* 1866, abandoned medical practice and became active in promotion of education and agriculture. CONTRIBUTIONS: Despite acute shortages of drugs, supplies, and skilled physicians, effectively managed the medical service of the Confederate Army. Obtained medicines from plants indigenous to the South. Established examining boards to weed out incompetents. Adopted the one-story pavilion hospital, which was soon copied by the Union Army and was used by the military until World War I. Reorganized the Confederate medical service along the lines obtaining in the U.S. Army. Organized and was president of the Association of Army and Navy Surgeons of the Confederate States (1863). Began and directed the publication of *Confederate States Medical and Surgical Journal* (January 1864-February 1865).

WRITINGS: *Manual of Military Surgery* (1863). REFERENCES: *DAB*, 13: 137-38; Kelly and Burrage (1928), 865; *NCAB*, 18: 311; J. I. Waring, *History of Medicine in South Carolina* (1967).

S. Galishoff

MOORMAN, LEWIS J. (February 9, 1875, near Leitchfield, Ky.-August 1954, Oklahoma City, Okla.). *Physician.* Son of Lemuel and Martha Elizabeth Moorman. Married Mary Davis Christian, April 27, 1909; three children. EDUCATION: 1898, B.S., Georgetown (Ky.) College; 1901, M.D., University of Louisville; postgraduate work: 1903, New York Polyclinic; and 1909, University of Vienna. CAREER: 1901-7, practice, Jet, Okla.; 1907, moved to Oklahoma City, where he practiced medicine; 1942-54, editor-in-chief, *Journal of the Oklahoma State Medical Association*; on medical faculty, Epworth College of Medicine, Oklahoma City, when it merged with Oklahoma University School of Medicine (1910): 1910-25, professor of physical diagnosis; 1925, appointed professor of clinical medicine; and 1931-35, dean. CONTRIBUTIONS: Nationally known specialist on tuberculosis and chest diseases and chairman of the group of AMA physicians who studied health conditions among Navajo-Hopi Indians. President, Oklahoma State Medical Association (1919-20), American Trudeau Society, National Tuberculosis Association, Oklahoma City Academy of Medicine.

WRITINGS: Interest in the history of medicine led to role in founding the Oklahoma City unit of History of Medicine, organizing a collection of memorabilia from fellow physicians throughout the state. In addition to writing many articles, wrote several books, including *Tuberculosis and Genius* and autobiography, *Pioneer Doctor*. REFERENCES: Mark R. Everett, *Medical Education in Oklahoma: The University of Oklahoma School of Medicine and Medical Center, 1900-1931* (1972); R. Palmer Howard, "Nominations for the All American Medical Hall of Fame," *Journal of the Oklahoma State Medical Association* 72, no. 7 (March 1979): 202-5; Lewis J. Moorman, *Pioneer Doctor* (Norman, Okla.: 1951); "L. J. Moorman" file, History of Medicine Collection, University of Oklahoma Health Sciences Center Library, Oklahoma City, Okla.

V. Allen

MORGAN, JOHN (June 10, 1735, Philadelphia, Pa.-October 15, 1789, Philadelphia). *Physician; Surgeon; Medical educator.* Son of Evan, ironmonger and realtor, and Joanna (Biles) Morgan. Married Mary Hopkinson, 1765; no children. EDUCATION: Reverend Finley's Nottingham Academy; 1757, A.B., College of Philadelphia; medical apprentice of John Redman (q.v.); 1760-63, student at London and Edinburgh; 1763, M.D., University of Edinburgh; 1763-65, postgraduate studies, Paris and Italy. CAREER: 1765, returned to Philadelphia and began medical practice; 1765, appointed professor of theory and practice of physic, College of Philadelphia; 1775-77, director-general of hospitals and physician-in-chief, Continental Army; 1773-83, senior medical officer, Pennsylvania Hospital. CONTRIBUTIONS: A founder of the first medical school in America, as well as the American Philosophical Society and the College of Physicians of Philadelphia. Endeavored to improve the quality of medical care given to members of the Revolutionary army, but removed without reason and felt disgraced, withdrawing from public life. His library was the start of the Library of the College of Physicians.

WRITINGS: *A Discourse upon the Institution of Medical Schools in America* (1765); *A Recommendation of Inoculation According to Baron Dimsdale's Method* (1776); *A Vindication of His Public Character in the Station of Director-General of the Military Hospitals...* (1777). REFERENCES: *Appleton's CAB*, 4: 401; *BHM* (1964-69), 188-89; (1970-74), 125; (1975-79), 89; *DAB*, 7: 172-75; F. P. Henry, *Standard History of the Medical Profession in Philadelphia* (1897); Kelly and Burrage (1920); Miller, *BHM*, pp. 76-77; W. F. Norris, *Early History of Medicine in Philadelphia* (1886); J. Whitfield Bell, Jr., *John Morgan: Continental Doctor* (1965).

D. I. Lansing

MORGAN, THOMAS HUNT (September 25, 1866, Lexington, Ky.-December 4, 1945, Pasadena, Calif.). *Zoologist; Geneticist.* Son of Charlton Hunt, insane asylum director, and Ellen Key (Howard) Morgan. Married Lillian V. Sampson, 1904; four children. EDUCATION: State College of Kentucky: 1886, B.S.; and 1888, M.S.; 1890, Ph.D., Johns Hopkins University. CAREER: 1891-1904, biology faculty, Bryn Mawr College; 1904-28, experimental zoology faculty, Columbia University; *post* 1928, director, Kerckhoff Laboratories of Biological Sciences, California Institute of Technology; 1910-12, president, Society for Experimental Biology and Medicine. CONTRIBUTIONS: Awarded the 1933 Nobel prize in medicine or physiology for clarification of the laws and mechanisms of heredity. First native-born American and first nonphysician to receive the award. Did initial and last research in experimental embryology. Studied sex determination, differentiation of structures, regeneration, evolution, and adaptation. Became interested in genetics (c. 1907) and started studying the vinegar fly, *Drosophilia melanogaster* (commonly called fruit fly). Found a white-eyed mutant to be a sex-linked recessive trait carried by genes located in a particular chromosome. Developed numerous hybrids in the following years and discovered unexpectedly that Mendel's laws were valid. Developed the first general theory of the transmission mechanism of heredity which he summarized in *The Mechanism of Mendelian Heredity* (1915, co-authored with Alfred H. Sturtevant, Hermann J. Muller [q.v.], and Calvin B. Bridges). Book established the main tenets of modern genetics: that genes, the invisible physical units of heredity, are arranged in linear order on chromosomes; that they are held together in a number of linkage groups; and that there is interchange, or crossing over, in the same linkage group, the frequency being proportional to the distance between the genes involved. Trained and worked with many of the nation's leading geneticists.

WRITINGS: *The Physical Basis of Heredity* (1919); *The Theory of the Genes* (1926); *The Scientific Basis of Evolution* (1932); *Embryology and Genetics* (1933). A bibliography is in *BMNAS*. REFERENCES: G. E. Allen, *T. H. Morgan...* (1978); *BHM* (1964-69), 189; (1970-74), 125: (1976), 22: (1978), 21; (1980), 29; *BMNAS* 33 (1954): 283-325; *DAB*, Supplement

3: 538-41; *DSB*, 9: 515-26; I. Shine and S. Wrobel, *T. H. Morgan*. . . (1976); *Who Was Who in Am.*, 12: 382-83.

S. Galishoff

MORMAN, WILLIAM DANIEL (December 20, 1901, Augusta, Ga.-October 9, 1951, St. Louis, Mo.). *Otolaryngologist.* Son of W. D., minister, and Mattie Morman. Married Verneeda Williams, 1947. EDUCATION: 1925, B.S., Morehouse College; 1929, M.D., Howard University; 1929-30, intern, St. Louis City Hospital #2; 1942, postgraduate course (Rosenwald Fund Fellowship) in thoracic surgery, University of Pennsylvania. CAREER: 1931-45, hygiene inspector, St. Louis public schools; 1934-51, staff, at Homer G. Phillips Hospital, St. Louis, 1934-51, associate director, Department of Otolaryngology; and 1941-51, associate chief of staff; ?-1956, head, Department of Otolaryngology, St. Mary's Infirmary and People's Hospital, St. Louis. CONTRIBUTIONS: Held many positions of importance in NMA and in St. Louis medical circles. Would have been next president-elect of NMA (1951). In NMA: Board of Trustees (1937-49); secretary, House of Delegates (1936-37); secretary, board (1947-49); and chair, ENT Section (1946-51). On executive boards, at various times, of Homer G. Phillips, St. Mary's, and People's hospitals, St. Louis. He and Walter A. Younge were first black physicians elected to St. Louis Medical Society (1949). Diplomate, American Board of Otolaryngology (1940). Fellow, American Academy of Otology, Rhinology and Laryngology (1941) and American College of Surgeons (1948). Secretary (1932-38) and president (1938), Mound City Medical Forum. President, Missouri Pan-Medical Association (1944). Civil rights activist and recognized community leader in St. Louis. Worked with St. Louis University and several St. Louis hospitals to solve racial problems of physicians and patients.

REFERENCES: W. Montague Cobb, "William Daniel Morman, M.D., 1901-1951," *JNMA* 51 (1959): 66; obituary, *JNMA* 44 (1952): 70-72.

T. L. Savitt

MORRELL, JOSEPH ROWLAND (December 7, 1879, Logan, Utah-July 5, 1974, Ogden, Utah). *Industrial surgeon; Public health.* Son of Joseph, merchant, and Margaret (Rowland) Morrell. Married Jeannette McKay, 1907; five children. EDUCATION: 1895-96, Utah Agricultural College, Logan; 1904, M.D., Rush Medical College; 1904-6, intern, Cook County Hospital, Chicago, Ill.; 1910-11, postgraduate study, University of Vienna. CAREER: 1911-45, staff, Thomas D. Dee Memorial Hospital, Ogden; 1911-45, division surgeon, Denver and Rio Grande Railroad, Union Pacific Railroad, and Southern Pacific Railroad; 1922, 1924, president, Utah State Medical Association; 1923-45, member, Utah State Board of Health (chairman, 1936-45); 1923-45, member, Utah Board of Medical Examiners (chairman, 1940-45); 1945, after retiring, surgery on his hip for arthritis was successful and enabled him to serve as head of the Medical Dispensary, Ogden Defense Depot (1956-67). CONTRIBUTIONS: Promoted public health legislation and the enforcement of codes during long tenure on the Utah State Board of Health.

WRITINGS: "Acute Anterior Poliomyelitis with Report of Some Unusual Cases,"
Northwest Med. 15 (Jan. 1917): 9-11; *Utah's Health and You. A History of Utah's Public
Health* (1956). REFERENCES: *WWAPS* 1 (1938): 854.

H. Bauman

MORSE, JOHN FREDERICK (December 27, 1815, Essex, Vt.-December
31, 1874, San Francisco, Calif.). *Physician.* Son of Elijah Morgan, farmer and
natural healer, and Hannah Morgan (Curtiss) Morse. Married Rebecca Lockwood
Cannon, October 14, 1843, four children; Caroline F. Lowney, January 16,
1854, five children. EDUCATION: 1844, M.D., University of New York. CAREER:
1849, following brief period of practice, Brooklyn, N.Y., arrived in Sacramento,
where he practiced medicine, helped organize the local medical society (1850),
and edited the *Daily Sacramento Union*; practice, San Francisco, and professor
of theory and practice of medicine, medical department, University of the Pacific;
1864-70, professor of clinical medicine and diagnosis, Toland Medical College;
1870, reorganized medical department, University of the Pacific, unable to teach
due to poor health. CONTRIBUTIONS: Founder and editor, *California State Medical
Journal* (1856). A founding member, San Francisco County Medical Society,
and its president.   REFERENCES: Henry Harris, *California's Medical Story* (1932),
374-77.

Y. V. O'Neill

MORTON, SAMUEL GEORGE (January 26, 1799, Philadelphia, Pa.-May
15, 1851, Philadelphia). *Physician; Naturalist; Ethnologist; Anatomy.* Son of
George and Jane (Cummings) Morton. Married Rebecca Grellet Pearsall, 1827;
eight children. EDUCATION: 1817, began medical studies with Joseph Parrish,
Philadelphia; 1820, M.D., University of Pennsylvania; 1823, M.D., University
of Edinburgh. CAREER: *Post* 1824, practiced medicine, Philadelphia; 1829, physician to almshouse; *post* 1830, lectured at Philadelphia Association for Medical
Instruction, associated with Joseph Parrish; 1839-43, anatomy faculty, medical
department, Pennsylvania (Gettysburg) College, Philadelphia; 1849, president,
Academy of Natural Sciences of Philadelphia; father of invertebrate paleontology
in the United States; made extensive comparative studies of human crania and
wrote about the origin and physical characteristics of the different races. CON-
TRIBUTIONS: Wrote *Illustrations of Pulmonary Consumption* (1834), the first
book on the subject to appear in the United States, in which he recommended
fresh-air treatment of the disease. Published an American editon of John Mack-
intosh, *Principles of Pathology and Practice of Physics* (1836). Most important
medical contribution was *Human Anatomy, Special, General, and Microscopic*,
written in 1849.

WRITINGS: "Observations on Cornine," *Phila. J. of the Med. and Physical Sci.* 11
(1825): 195-98. REFERENCES: *BHM* (1974-79), 89; *DAB*, 13: 265-66; *DSB*, 9: 540-41;

Clark A. Elliott, *Biog. Dictionary of Am. Sci.* (1979), 186; Kelly and Burrage (1928), 874-77; *NCAB*, 10: 265-66; *Who Was Who in Am.*, Hist. Vol.: 441.

S. Galishoff

MORTON, WILLIAM THOMAS GREEN (August 9, 1819, Charlton, Mass.-July 15, 1868, New York, N.Y.). *Dentist; Discoverer of ether anesthesia.* Son of James, farmer, and Rebecca (Needham) Morton. Married Elizabeth Whitman, 1844; five children. EDUCATION: Northfield Academy; 1840, graduate of Baltimore College of Dental Surgery; 1844-45, Harvard Medical School. CAREER: Left family farm at age 17 and, after business failures in Boston, Mass., studied dentistry; 1842-43, dental practice, Boston, associated with Horace Wells (q.v.). After partnerships dissolved in 1843, stayed in Boston and became a highly successful dentist. CONTRIBUTIONS: After various experiments, devised a method of inducing anesthesia with sulphuric ether and applied it successfully for a dental extraction on Eben Frost. Two weeks later, (October 16, 1846), was allowed by Dr. John C. Warren (q.v.) to administer ether to Gilbert Abbott, a young printer who had an uneventful and painless ligation of a vascular tumor of the neck performed at Massachusetts General Hospital. Patented the procedure and equipment for the inhalation of "Letheon" and immediately found himself embroiled in a bitter dispute over the discovery of anesthesia that lasted until his death, bringing about complete destruction of his practice, near poverty, disappointment and enmity. Improved crude methods of attaching false teeth.

WRITINGS: *Morton's Letheon* (1846); *Remarks on the Proper Mode of Administering Sulphuric Ether by Inhalation* (1847); *On the Loss of the Teeth and the Modern Way of Restoring Them* (1848). REFERENCES: *BHM* (1964-69), 189; (1970-74), 126; *DAB*, 7 pt. 1: 268-71; Miller, *BHM*, pp. 77-78; *NCAB*, 8: 332; N. P. Rice, *Trials of a Public Benefactor* (1859); G. S. Woodward, *The Man Who Conquered Pain* (1962).

G. C. Sanchez

MOSHER, ELIZA MARIA (October 2, 1846, Cayuga County, N.Y.-October 16, 1928, Murray Hill, N.Y.). *Physician; Hygiene; Women's education.* Daughter of Augustus, farmer, and Maria (Sutton) Mosher. Never married. EDUCATION: 1862, Friends Academy (Union Springs, N.Y.); studied medicine: 1869, New England Hospital for Women and Children (Boston, Mass.); 1870-71, with Lucy E. Sewall; and at the Woman's College of New York Infirmary; 1875, M.D., University of Michigan; 1879-81, studied medicine, London and Paris. CAREER: 1875-77, medical practice (with Elizabeth Hait Gerow), Poughkeepsie, N.Y.; at Massachusetts State Reformatory for Women: 1877-79, resident physician; and 1881-83, superintendent; 1883-87 (with Lucy Hall), resident physician and associate professor of physiology and hygiene, Vassar College; 1886-95, 1902-28, medical practice, Brooklyn, N.Y.; 1895-1901, dean of women, professor of hygiene, and woman's physician, University of Michigan; 1905-28, editor, *Medical Woman's Journal.* CONTRIBUTIONS: An early woman graduate of the University of Michigan's pioneering co-educational but sex-segregated medical school; the first dean of women and first female professor in the undergraduate college of the university. Introduced a program of regular physical examinations and mandatory exercise for college women thereby blunting male criticisms that higher education was unhealthy for women but reinforcing the idea that women's health required special attention.

WRITINGS: "Habits of Posture a Cause of Deformity and Displacement of the Uterus," *N.Y. J. of Gyn. Obst.* 3 (1893): 962-77; *Med. Woman's J.* (1910-1928); *Health and Happiness: A Message to Girls* (1912); "The Human in Medicine, Surgery, and Nursing," *Med. Woman's J.*, 32 (May 1925): 117. Writings listed in *Index Catalogue*, 2nd series, 11: 118. REFERENCES: *DAB*, 13: 277-78; Dorothy Gies McGuigan, *A Dangerous Experiment: 100 Years of Women at the University of Michigan* (1970), 60-63; *Med. Woman's J.* 32 (May 1925): 117-54; 55 (Feb. 1948): 38-43; *Notable Am. Women*, 2: 587-89; typescript biography by Florence Hazzard, Michigan Historical Collections, Bentley Historical Library, Ann Arbor, Michigan; *Who Was Who in Am.*, 1: 873.

M. Pernick

MOSSELL, NATHAN FRANCIS (July 27, 1856, Hamilton, Ontario, Canada-October 27, 1946, Philadelphia, Pa.). *Physician; Surgeon (Genito-urinary).* Son of Aaron, brick manufacturer, and Eliza (Bowers) Mossell. Married Gertrude E. H. Bustill, 1881; two children. EDUCATION: 1879, A.B., Lincoln University, Pa.; 1882, M.D., University of Pennsylvania (first black graduate); 1884, A.M., Lincoln University; postgraduate study: Philadelphia Polyclinic Hospital; and early 1890s, Guy's, Queens College, and Saint Thomas hospitals, London. CAREER: 1881-82, associated with University of Pennsylvania Out-Patient Surgical Clinic; 1882-1933, private practice, Philadelphia; 1895-1933, medical director, Frederick Douglass Memorial Hospital, Philadelphia. CONTRIBUTIONS: Founded Frederick Douglass Memorial Hospital, Philadelphia (1895). Erected $100,000 building for hospital (1908) and raised money to pay for it (by 1915). Served NMA as co-founder (1895) and president (1907-8). Fought vigorously throughout life against racial barriers and discrimination. First black member, Philadelphia County Medical Society (1888).

WRITINGS: "The Modern Hospital: Its Construction, Organization and Management," *JNMA* 1 (1909): 94-102; "The Modern Hospital Largely Educational," *JNMA* 8 (1916): 133-35. Writings listed in *JNMA* 46 (1954): 128-30. REFERENCES: W. Montague Cobb, "Nathan Francis Mossell, M.D., 1856-1946," *JNMA* 46 (1954): 118-30; John A. Kenney, *The Negro in Medicine* (1912), 15; *WWCR* 1 (1915): 202; *WWICA* 6 (1941-44): 375.

T. L. Savitt

MOTEN, PIERCE SHERMAN (July 28, 1878, Winchester, Tex.-February 1, 1965, Birmingham, Ala.). *Physician.* Son of Pierce, farmer and businessman, and Amanda Moten. Married Evla Lee Moore Young, 1907; four children. EDUCATION: 1900, A.B., Tuskegee Institute; 1902, premedical courses, Walden University, Nashville, Tenn.; 1906, M.D., Meharry Medical College; 1898-1900, prescription clerk, Tuskegee, Ala.; 1900-1902, private premedical courses under Roscoe C. Bruce and George W. Carver, Tuskegee. CAREER: Private practice: 1906-12, Quincy, Fla.; and *post* 1913, Birmingham. CONTRIBUTIONS: Improved medical facilities of Birmingham to serve black population better:

organized, built, and operated 32-bed hospital for the Courts of Calanthe of Ala. (1920). Formed organization that was instrumental in establishing an emergency station (clinic) for expectant mothers (late 1920s); needed because overcrowded county hospital that served blacks often rejected expectant mothers. This emergency station developed into a pediatric, obstetrics, and gynecology clinic (Southside Clinic) in larger more permanent quarters. Following visits from national health leaders (1937), the Slossfield Center was established, which grew to provide full hospital services and a training facility for black physicians. As historian, Alabama State Medical Association, preserved information on blacks important in that state's medical past. Also served as officer in both that organization and the Birmingham Medical, Dental and Pharmaceutical Association. REFERENCES: ["Pierce S. Moten"], *JNMA* 53 (1961): 432-35; *WWICA* 6 (1941-44): 376.

T. L. Savitt

MOTT, VALENTINE (August 20, 1785, Glen Cove, Oyster Bay, Long Island, N.Y.-April 26, 1865, New York, N.Y.). *Surgeon; Pioneer vascular surgeon.* Son of Henry, physician, and Jane (Way) Mott. Married Louisa Dunmore Mums, 1819; nine children. EDUCATION: Private school, Newton, Long Island, N.Y.; 1804-7, apprentice to Valentine Seaman (q.v.); 1806, M.D., Columbia College; 1807-9, private pupil of Sir Astley Cooper, London; and studied medicine, University of Edinburgh. CAREER: 1809-11, lecturer and demonstrator of operative surgery, Columbia College; professor of surgery: 1811-13, Columbia College; 1813-26, College of Physicians and Surgeons, N.Y.; 1826-27, Rutgers Medical College of New Jersey; and 1827-30, Rutgers Medical Faculty of Geneva College, N.Y.; 1831-34, professor of operative surgery and surgical and pathological anatomy, College of Physicians and Surgeons; 1834-41, extended tour of Europe; 1841-50, professor of surgery and surgical anatomy and president of the faculty, University of the City of New York; 1850-52, third tour of Europe; 1852-65, emeritus professor of surgery, College of Physicians and Surgeons. CONTRIBUTIONS: Father of American vascular surgery. Achieved fame in America and Europe for ligation of great vessels for aneurysm. Ligated the innominate artery for aneurysm for the first time in the history of surgery (1818). Sir Astley Cooper said Mott had performed more of the great operations than any surgeon in history up to his time. Samuel D. Gross (q.v.) considered Mott the leading American surgeon of the first half of the nineteenth century. Remarkably successful in rhinoplasty and facial restoration from the mutilation caused by excessive doses of mercury (calomel). Outstanding teacher of surgery. One of the first surgeons in America to give clinical instruction. Deep sense of medical tradition; by his sacrifice of a barnyard rooster at the temple at Epidaurus symbolically imbued American medicine with the spirit of Aesculapius. College of Physicians and Surgeons of Columbia University honored him with the Valentine Mott Professorship of Surgery.

WRITINGS: "Reflections on Securing in a Ligature the Arteria Innominata," *Med. & Surg. Register* 1 (1818): 9-54; Alfred Velpeau, *New Elements of Operative Surgery* (1847, trans. P. S. Townsend, under supervision of, and with notes and observations by Mott); "Pain and Anesthetics," in *Military, Medical and Surgical Essays Prepared for the United States Sanitary Commission, 1862-1864* (1865). Writings listed in *Author Catalog*, New York Acad. of Med. 27: 466-69. REFERENCES: *BHM* (1970-74) 126; *DAB*, 7, pt. 1: 290-91. S. D. Gross, *Memoir of Valentine Mott, M.D., L.L.D.* (1868); C. R. Hall, "Valentine Mott: Nassau County Surgeon," *Nassau County Hist. J.* 16 (1955): 1-10; Miller, *BHM*, p. 78; *NCAB*, 6: 281; I. M. Rutkow, "Valentine Mott (1785-1865), the Father of American Vascular Surgery: A Historical Perspective," *Surgery* 85 (1979): 441-50.

R. E. Batt

MOULTRIE, JOHN, JR. (January 18, 1729, Charlestown, S.C.-March 19, 1798, England.) *Physician.* Son of Dr. John and Mrs. Lucretia Cooper Moultrie. Married Dorothy (Dry) Morton, 1753, one daughter; Eleanor Austin, 1762, four sons, two daughters. EDUCATION: Apprentice to father; 1746, began study at Edinburgh; 1749, first native-born American to graduate from Edinburgh. CAREER: 1750-67, practiced medicine, Charlestown, S.C.; 1756, justice of peace; 1760, representative in General Assembly; 1761, major of militia in the Cherokee War; 1764, appointed member of James Grant's Royal Council of East Florida, later president of council; 1771, appointed lieutenant governor in command of East Florida; obtained a vast number of acres, among these "Bella Vista," near St. Augustine, Fla.; 1783, England ceded Fla. to Spain, and Moultrie lost everything; 1784, moved to England. CONTRIBUTIONS: Prominent South Carolina physician.

WRITINGS: *Thesis on Yellow Fever, Based on His Observations During the Epidemic of 1745 in Charlestown* (1805), quoted frequently by Rene La Roche in his publication of 1855. REFERENCES: *DAB*, 13: 292-93; Joseph Johnson, *Traditions and Reminiscences Chiefly of the American Revolution in the South* (1851); J. G. Mumford, *A Narrative of Medicine in America* (1903); *South Carolina Am. & Gen. Gazette* (1771); James Thacher, *Am. Med. Biog.* (1828); Eleanor W. Townsend, *Annals of Med. Hist.* (1940); Joseph Ioor Waring, *History of Medicine in South Carolina, 1670-1825* (1964).

J. P. Dolan

MOURITZ, ARTHUR ALBERT ST. MAUR (May 1856, London, England?-December 1, 1943, Honolulu, Hawaii). *Physician.* Son of American father and French mother. Married Arnita Cardet, June 1885; three children. EDUCATION: Age 16, began medical studies at Oxford University; 1879, licentiate, Royal College of Physicians, London, and Royal College of Surgeons, England; attended Cambridge University and studied under Jean Martin Charcot at Paris Academy. CAREER: Before 1883, in the British Navy; served two years as ship's surgeon on sailing clippers and steamers of the Dutch India Company on the South American run; 1883, arrived in Honolulu; 1883, secretary, Board of Health; 1884-87 appointed by Board of Health as physician for leper settlement, Kalaupapa, Molokai, and rest of the island of Molokai; 1893-95, expert observer of Goto method of treating leprosy; 1888-1905, at Mapulelu, Molokai, government physician for all of the island of Molokai, except Kalaupapa, while carrying on a private practice; 1905, moved to Kilauea, Kauai; 1907, moved to Honolulu and maintained private practice until his death. CONTRIBUTIONS: Did research and writing on infectious diseases and his book on leprosy is a collector's item.

WRITINGS: *Tragedy of the Careless* (1906); *Path of the Destroyer* (1916); *Brief World's History of Influenza* (1920); *Conquest of Smallpox* (1924); *Brief World History of Leprosy* (1943). REFERENCES: *Hawaii Med. J.* (1944): 202; *Honolulu Advertiser*, December 2, 1943; *Honolulu Star-Bulletin*, December 1, 1943.

J. A. Breinich

MOURSUND, WALTER HENRIK (August 13, 1884, Fredericksburg, Tex.-April 2, 1959, Houston, Tex.). *Physician; Educator; Administrator*. Son of Albert W., lawyer and judge, and Henrikke (Mowinkle) Moursund. Married Freda Adelaide Plate, June 24, 1907; three children. EDUCATION: 1906, M.D., medical department, University of Texas, Galveston, Tex. CAREER: 1906-11, general practice, Fredericksburg, Seguin, Marion, Lavernia, and Sulphur Springs, Tex.; 1911, joined faculty, Baylor University College of Medicine, Dallas, Tex., as assistant in bacteriology and pathology; 1917-18, captain, director, Eighth Corps area laboratory, Fort Sam Houston, Tex.; at Baylor University College of Medicine: 1911-43, faculty, teaching physiology, pathology, bacteriology, and hygiene; and 1923-43, 1943-53, dean; 1943-59, professor of hygiene and preventive medicine; 1943-59, dean emeritus and director of endowment. CONTRIBUTIONS: Dean and professor, Baylor University College of Medicine, for 30 years during reorganization struggles in Dallas and after the 1943 move to Houston, 10 years in developing the Texas Medical Center.

WRITINGS: *History of Baylor University College of Medicine, 1900-1953* (1956); "Medicine in Greater Houston, 1836-56" (with Mildred Moursund Essig, ed.), manuscript, Houston Academy of Medicine-Texas Medical Center Library, Houston, Tex. REFERENCES: John S. Chapman, *University of Texas Southwestern Medical School. . .* (1976); *JAMA* 170 (1959): 987; N. D. Macon, *John Freeman and His Friends* (1973); *Texas State J. of Med.* 55 (1959): 394; *Who Was Who in Am.*, 3: 956.

J. P. Morris

MULLER, HERMANN JOSEPH (December 21, 1890, New York, N.Y.-April 5, 1967, Indianapolis, Ind.). *Geneticist; Evolution; Eugenics*. Son of Hermann J., manufacturer, and Frances Louise (Lyons) Muller. Married Jessie Marr Jacobs, 1923, one child; Dorothea J. Kantorowicz, 1939, one child. EDUCATION: Columbia University: 1910, B.A.; 1911, M.A.; and 1916, Ph.D. CAREER: 1915-18, biology faculty, Rice Institute; zoology faculty: 1918-20, Columbia University; and 1920-32, Texas University; 1932, studied in Berlin with N. W. Timofeeff-Ressovsky; 1933-36, geneticist, U.S.S.R. Academy of Sciences (Moscow and Leningrad); 1937-40, member, Institute of Animal Genetics, University of Edinburgh; 1941-45, biology faculty, Amherst College; *post* 1945, zoology faculty, Indiana University. CONTRIBUTIONS: Awarded the 1946 Nobel Prize in physiology or medicine for work, done mainly in the 1920s, on the mutagenic effect of X-rays in Drosophilia. As a graduate student, made major contributions to Thomas H. Morgan's (q.v.) studies, which established the basic principles of modern genetics (1910-15). Recognized that the individual gene is the basis of life and biological evolution since it alone in the body can reproduce itself and undergo inheritable changes. With Edgar Altenburg, designed quantitative studies of rates of mutation in fruit flies under both natural and artificial conditions; found that X-rays can increase the mutation rate as much as 150 times and produce a variety of anatomical changes (1927); filled in a gap in Darwin's theory of evolution by natural selection by demonstrating the existence of numerous random (nonadaptive) mutations; showed that mutations occur as the result of alterations within individual genes and chromosome breakage; led to the development of radiation genetics, which has aided in the mapping of chromosomes and the study of the chemical constituents of cells. An outspoken opponent of Lysenko's theory that acquired characteristics could be inherited (1930s). Stressed the importance of minimizing human exposure to ionizing radiation of any kind; argued for restraint in the use of medical X-rays and opposed the development and testing of nuclear weapons. Was concerned that conditions of modern life were causing the creation of a large pool of defective and inferior genes; therefore advocated that the sperm of men of outstanding quality be frozen for use in artificial insemination after their deaths.

WRITINGS: *The Mechanism of Mendelian Heredity* (1915, with T. H. Morgan et al.); "Artificial Transmutation of the Gene," *Sci.* 66 (1927): 84-87; *Out of the Night: A Biologist's View of the Future* (1935). Writings are listed in *BMFRS*. REFERENCES: *BHM* (1970-74), 127; (1975), 17; *Am. Philos. Soc. Yearbook, 1967*, pp. 137-42; *BMFRS* 14 (1968): 349-89; *DSB*, 9: 564-65; *Who Was Who in Am.*, 4: 687.

S. Galishoff

MUMFORD, JAMES GREGORY (December 2, 1863, Rochester, N.Y.-October 18, 1914, Clifton, N.Y.). *Physician and author; Surgery; Medical history.* Son of George Elihu and Julia Emma (Hills) Mumford. Married Helen Sherwood, 1892; no children. EDUCATION: 1885, graduated, Harvard College; 1890, M.D., Harvard Medical School; 1890-91, house officer, Massachusetts General Hospital. CAREER: 1891-1912, practiced medicine, Boston, Mass.; lecturer, Harvard Medical School; ?-1912, surgical staff, Massachusetts General Hospital; 1912-14, physician-in-chief, Clifton Springs Sanitarium (N.Y.). CONTRIBUTIONS: Wrote several books about surgery, including *Clinical Talks on Minor Surgery* (1903); *Surgical Aspects of Digestive Disorders* (1905, with A. K. Stone); *Some End Results of Surgery* (1908); and a textbook, *The Practice of Surgery* (1910). Was equally known for writings about the lighter side of medicine, including *Surgical Memoirs and Other Essays* (1908) and *A Doctor's Table Talk* (1912). Early in career became interested in medical history and wrote *A Narrative of Medicine in America* (1903). Edited *The Harvard Medical School*, by Thomas Francis Harrington, 3 vols. (1905).

WRITINGS: *One Hundred Surgical Problems: The Experiences of Daily Practice Dissected and Explained* (1911). REFERENCES: *DAB*, 13: 324-25; Kelly and Burrage (1928), 884-86.

S. Galishoff

MUNSON, ENEAS (June 13, 1734, New Haven, Conn.-June 16, 1826, New Haven). *Clergyman; Physician.* Son of Benjamin, mechanic and schoolmaster, and Abigail (Punderson) Munson. Married Susanna Howell, 1761, nine children; Sarah (Sanford) Perit, 1804. EDUCATION: 1753, B.A., Yale College; 1753-55, studied divinity either in New Haven or Northampton, Mass., and was licensed to preach; 1756-58, studied medicine under Dr. John Darbie, Oyster Ponds, Long Island, N.Y. CAREER: 1753-55, taught school in Northampton; 1755, domestic chaplain for the Gardiner family on Long Island while serving in the army; practiced medicine: 1758-60, Bedford, N.Y.; and 1760-1826, New Haven. CONTRIBUTIONS: A founder, Connecticut Medical Society (1792), and its first vice-president. On the death of Dr. Leverett Hubbard, first president, was chosen to succeed him in office (1794-1801). Society conferred the honorary degree of M.D. (1794). When the Yale Medical School was organized (1813), was asked to fill the professorship in materia medica and botany. Although he performed no duties, retained the title of professor of materia medica and botany until death. Represented New Haven in the Connecticut General Assembly (1778-81).

WRITINGS: Two articles, a "Case of Lock'd Jaw, Successfully Treated by Electricity" and a report about expectorating calculi during attacks of hemoptysis sustained by a Mr. Caleb Hotchkiss in *Cases and Observations by the Med. Soc. of New Haven* (1788); "A letter on the Treatment Most Successful in the Cure of the Yellow Fever, in New Haven, in 1794," in a *Collection of Papers on the Subject of Bilious Fevers*, by Noah Webster (1796). REFERENCES: *Appleton's CAB*, 4: 462; Creighton Baker, M.D., "The Founding of the New Haven County Medical Association," *Conn. State Med. J.* 5 (Mar. 1941): 180-84; George Blumer, "Some Remarks on 'Cases and Observations, by the Medical Society of New Haven County,' " in Herbert Thoms, ed., *Heritage of Connecticut Medicine* (1942), 10-23; F. B. Dexter, *Yale Biographies and Annals* 2: 311-13; Kelly and Burrage (1928), 888-89; *NCAB*, 13: 420; J. Quen, "Dr. E. Munson," *J. Hist. Med.* 31 (1976): 307-19; George O. Sumner, M.D., "Early Physicians in Connecticut," *Conn. State Med. J.* 6 (Jun. 1942): 459-75.

J. W. Ifkovic

MUNSTERBERG, HUGO (June 1, 1863, Danzig, Germany-December 16, 1916, Cambridge, Mass.). *Psychologist.* Son of Moritz, lumber merchant, and Anna Munsterberg. Married Selma Oppler, 1887. EDUCATION: University of Geneva; 1885, Ph.D., University of Leipzig, Germany; 1887, M.D., University of Heidelberg, Germany. CAREER: 1887-92, lecturer, Freiberg, Germany; 1892-95, went to United States to head the psychology laboratory, invited by William James; 1895-97, returned to Freiberg; 1897-1916, professor of psychology, Harvard. CONTRIBUTIONS: Work in psychology helped pave the way for the use of psychology in industry, medicine, and education. Pioneered in applied psychology. Criticized widely for published support of Germany in the beginning of World War I.

WRITINGS: *Psychology and Industrial Efficiency* (1913); *Grundzuge der Psychotechnik* (1914); *Psychology and Social Sanity* (1914). See *DAB*, 7: 339, for listing of publications. REFERENCES: *DAB*, 7: 339; M. Hale (Ph.D. diss., University of Maryland, 1977); M. Munsterberg, *Hugo Munsterberg: Life and Work* (1922); *J. of Applied Psychology* (Jun. 1917); *NCAB*, 13: 85.

M. Kaufman

MURPHY, JAMES BUMGARDNER (August 4, 1884, Morgantown, N.C.-August 24, 1950, Bar Harbor, Maine). *Physician; Pathology; Oncology.* Son of Patrick Livingston, physician, and Bettie Wadell (Bumgardner) Murphy. Married Ray Slater, 1919; two children. EDUCATION: 1905, B.S., University of North Carolina; 1909, M.D., Johns Hopkins University; 1909-10, medical intern, Pathological Institute, New York State Hospitals on Ward's Island, New York City. CAREER: 1910-50, at Rockefeller Institute for Medical Research: *post* 1923, in charge of Laboratory of Cancer Research; 1917-19, Army Medical Corps, attached to surgeon-general, Washington, D.C., where he directed the organization of mobile medical laboratories in France and the training of their personnel; 1921-22, president, American Association for Cancer Research; 1922-30, commissioner, New York State Board of Charities; member: 1929-45, Board of Directors, American Cancer Society; 1937-44, Advisory Council, National Cancer Institute; and 1945-50, Committee on Growth, National Research Council; trustee: Memorial Hospital, N.Y.; Roswell Park Memorial Institute, Buffalo, N.Y.; and Jackson Memorial Laboratory, Bar Harbor. CONTRIBUTIONS: Developed improved methods for studying malignancies and for doing viral research. Produced one of the earliest applications of lyophilization, a freezing and drying process that insures the elimination of all living cells, to biological research. Perfected the technique of growing a chicken tumor virus in fertilized eggs. Helped explain the body's resistance to foreign-tissue grafts and helped elucidate the role of lymphocyte in immunological reactions and resistance to cancer and tuberculosis. Made pioneering studies of tumor inhibitors and the cause of cancer. Played an active role in educating the public on the need for early diagnosis and treatment of cancer.

WRITINGS: *The Lymphocyte in Resistance to Tissue Grafting, Malignant Disease, and Tuberculosis Infection. An Experimental Study.* Rockefeller Institute for Medical Research, *Monograph No. 21* (1926); "The Transmission of an Induced Lymphatic Leukemia and Lymphosarcoma in the Rat," *Cancer Research* 1 (1941): 379-83 (with Ernest Sturm); "An Analysis of the Trends in Cancer Research," *JAMA* 120 (1942): 107-11; "The Adrenals and Susceptibility to Transplanted Leukemia of Rats," *Sci.* 98 (1943): 568-69; "The Cancer Control Movement," *N.C. Med. J.* 5 (Apr. 1944): 121-25. A bibliography is in *BMNAS*. REFERENCES: *BMNAS* 34 (1960): 183-203; *DAB*, Supplement 6: 615-17; *DSB*, 9: 586-87; *Who Was Who in Am.*, 3: 626.

S. Galishoff

MURPHY, JOHN BENJAMIN (December 21, 1857, Appleton, Wis.-August 11, 1916, Mackinac Island, Mich.). *Surgeon; Teacher.* Son of Michael, farmer, and Ann (Grimes) Murphy. Married Jeannette C. Plamondon, 1885; five children. EDUCATION: 1876, Appleton High School; 1877-78, apprentice to Dr. J. R. Reilly, Appleton; 1879, M.D., Rush Medical College; 1879-80, intern, Cook County Hospital; 1882-84, studied in Vienna, Austria and Berlin and Heidelberg, Germany. CAREER: Clinical surgery: 1892-1900, College of Physicians and Surgeons; surgery: 1901-5, 1908-16, Northwestern University Medical School; 1884-92, 1905-8, Rush Medical College; 1895-1916, surgical staff, Mercy Hospital. CONTRIBUTIONS: Performed the initial operation in early acute appendicitis (1889). Developed metallic device (''Murphy Button'') for anastomosing hollow viscera without sutures (1892). Successfully sutured femoral artery (1897). Pioneered in the use of nitrogen to collapse and splint the abscessed tuberculous lung (1898). Introduced the drip method of rectal, saline infusion in treatment of peritonitis. Studies on surgery of the spinal cord and peripheral nerves that paved the way for modern neurosurgery. Made major advances in bone, joint, and tendon surgery. Produced *Surgical Clinics of John B. Murphy, M.D.* (1912-13) and *Clinics of John B. Murphy, M.D.* (1914-16), forerunner of *Surgical Clinics of North America*. A major founder, American College of Surgeons (1913).

WRITINGS: "Cholecysto-Intestinal, Gastro-Intestinal, Entero-Intestinal Anastomosis, and Approximation without Sutures (Original Research)" *Med. Record* 42 (1892): 665-76; "Resection of Arteries and Veins Injured in Continuity—End-to-End Suture—Experimental and Clinical Research," ibid., 51 (1897): 73-88. REFERENCES: Leslie B. Arey, *Northwestern University Medical School, 1859-1959: A Pioneer in Educational Reform* (1959), 405-13; *Am. J. of Obstet.* 75 (1917): 299-305; *DAB*, 7, pt. 1: 353-54; Loyal Davis, *J. B. Murphy: Stormy Petrel of Surgery* (1938); Miller, *BHM*, p. 79; *NCAB*, 13: 602.

                                                                                    W. K. Beatty

MURRAY, PETER MARSHALL (June 9, 1888, Houma, La.-December 19, 1969, New York, N.Y.). *Physician; Obstetrics and gynecology*. Son of John L., longshoreman, and Louvinia (Smith) Murray. Married Charlotte Wallace, 1917; one child. EDUCATION: 1910, A.B., New Orleans University; 1914, M.D., Howard University; 1914-15, intern, Freedmen's Hospital, Washington, D.C.; postgraduate study in surgery and gynecology, New York Post-Graduate School (Columbia University) and New York University (Bellevue Hospital). CAREER: 1915-18, assistant to dean and assistant clinical professor of surgery, Howard University Medical School; 1918-20, assistant surgeon-in-chief, Freedmen's Hospital; 1917-18, medical inspector, D.C. public schools; 1921-67, private practice in obstetrics and gynecology, New York City; 1928-52, staff member, Harlem Hospital, rising from provisional assistant status to director, Gynecological Service; 1924-64 (various times), consulting gynecologist, Sydenham Hospital and St. Clare's Hospital. CONTRIBUTIONS: First black member of the AMA House of Delegates (1949-61). President, NMA (1932), and chairman, NMA Publication Committee (1942-57). First black president, Medical Society of County of New York, a constituent AMA society (1955-56). Member, Howard University Board of Trustees (1924-58). A leader in numerous national causes to further black improvement including black health and its professionals. Served Board of Trustees of SUNY system as chair, Committee on Medical Education, and member, Committee on Planning and Development. First black to obtain certification in gynecology from American Board of Obstetrics and Gynecology (1931). One of the first black physicians appointed to Executive Committee of a well-established, traditional voluntary hospital (Sydenham Hospital, New York City, 1944).

WRITINGS: Numerous, including "Gastric and Duodenal Ulcers, with Report of Two Cases," *JNMA* 14 (1922): 143-46; "Gynecological Morbidity and Mortality Analysis at Harlem Hospital, 1936," *N.Y. State J. of Med.* 38 (1938): 361-64. Writings listed in *JNMA* 59 (1967): 80. REFERENCES: W. Montague Cobb, "Peter Marshall Murray, M.D., 1888-," *JNMA* 59 (1967): 71-74, 80; Herbert M. Morais, *The History of the Afro-American in Medicine* (1976): 119-20, 121, 130, 133-35, 163; *N.Y. Times*, December 21, 1969, p. 63; *WWAPS* 1 (1938): 870; *WWICA* 7 (1950): 390.

T. L. Savitt

MUSSEY, REUBEN DIMOND (June 23, 1780, Pelham, N.H.-June 21, 1866, Boston, Mass.). *Surgeon.* Son of Dr. John M. and Mrs. Beulah (Butler) Mussey. Married Mary Sewall, c. 1806; Mehitabel Osgood, 1809, nine children. EDUCATION: Amherst (N.H.) Academy; Dartmouth College: 1803, A.B.; and 1805, M.B.; 1809, M.D., University of Pennsylvania; 1812, M.D., Dartmouth; 1809, M.A. (hon.), Harvard; 1854, LL.D. (hon.), Dartmouth. CAREER: Practiced: 1805-8, Ipswich, Mass.; and 1809-14, Salem, Mass., with Daniel Oliver (q.v.); 1814-38, professor of anatomy and surgery and of medical theory and practice, Dartmouth; 1836-38, lecturer, Fairfield Medical College, N.Y.; 1831-35, professor of surgery, Bowdoin College, Maine; professor of surgery: 1838-52, Medical College of Ohio, Cincinnati, Ohio; and 1851-57, Miami Medical College, Cincinnati; 1857, retired to Boston; president: 1824-34, New Hampshire Medical Society; and 1850, American Medical Association. CONTRIBUTIONS: Accomplished the second temporary ligation of both common carotid arteries in a successful attempt to cure an extensive scalp nevus (1827) and removed the clavicle and scapula in a two-stage operation (1831). Argued that drugs can be absorbed through the skin and, against Astley Cooper, that intracapsular fractures can reunite.

WRITINGS: Most of Mussey's pioneering operations are summarized in his "Cases and Observations," *Am. J. of Med. Sci.* 21 (1837): 377-98. Also *Essay on Ardent Spirits* (1835); *TAMA* 1 (1848): 222-24; "Fracture of the Neck of the Thigh Bones," *Am. J. of Med. Sci.*, n.s., 33 (1857): 299-313; *Health, Its Friends and Foes* (1862). REFERENCES: A. B. Crosby (q.v.), "Eulogy on Reuben Dimond Mussey," *Trans., N.H. Med. Soc.* (1869): 61-81; *DAB*, 7, pt. 1: 372-73; Fielding H. Garrison, *Introduction to the History of Medicine*, 4th ed. (1929), 502-3, 761; *NCAB*, 9: 91; Francis R. Packard, *History of Medicine in the United States 2* (1931): 809-11.

J. W. Estes

N

NEAL, JOSEPHINE BICKNELL (October 10, 1880, Belmont, Maine-March 19, 1955, New York, N.Y.). *Physician; Neurology.* Daughter of Alton J. and Mary (Alexander) Neal. EDUCATION: 1901, B.A., Bates College; 1910, M.D., Cornell University Medical College. CAREER: 1902-6, taught mathematics and science in high schools, Maine and N.H.; *post* 1913, practiced medicine, New York City, limiting practice to consultation in neurology beginning in 1918; at New York City Department of Health: *post* 1910, Meningitis Division, Research Laboratory; and 1937-44, associate director, Research Laboratory; 1914-20, medicine faculty, Cornell University Medical College; at College of Physicians and Surgeons (Columbia): 1922-27, medicine faculty; and 1929-44, neurology faculty; 1922-27, attending physician, Pediatric Tuberculosis Section, Vanderbilt Clinic; 1927-29, director, William J. Matheson Survey of Epidemic Encephalitis; *post* 1927, executive secretary, Matheson Commission for Encephalitis Research; 1929-32, secretary, International Commission for the Study of Infantile Paralysis; 1932-55, staff, Neurological Institute of New York. CONTRIBUTIONS: An authority on the diagnosis, treatment, and control of infectious diseases of the nervous system, especially poliomyelitis, meningitis, and encephalitis. Best known for work as director, William J. Matheson Survey of Epidemic Encephalitis (1927-29). Findings appeared in *Encephalitis: A Clinical Study* (1942), for which she wrote four of the nine chapters.

WRITINGS: Wrote about 75 articles on acute infections of the central nervous system for medical journals and was a contributor to Isaac Arthur Abt's *Pediatrics* and Frederick Tice's *Practice of Medicine*. REFERENCES: *DAB*, Supplement 5: 511-12; *NCAB*, E: 228-29; *N.Y. Times*, March 20, 1955; *Who Was Who in Am.*, 3: 632.

S. Galishoff

NEWTON, ROBERT SAFFORD (December 12, 1818, Gallipolis, Ohio-October 9, 1881, New York, N.Y.). *Physician (eclectic); Editor.* Son of John and ? (Safford) Newton. Married Mary M. Hoy, 1843, one ? child. EDUCATION:

Lewisburg, Va., and Gallipolis academies; studied medicine with a pharmacist-physician in Gallipolis; ?-?, no degree, Medical College of Ohio, Cincinnati; 1841, M.D., Louisville Medical College. CAREER: 1841-45, cancer specialist, Gallipolis; 1845-49, eclectic practitioner, Cincinnati; 1849-51, professor of surgery, Memphis Institute; 1851-62, professor of surgery (1851-53), then of medical practice and pathology (1853-62), Eclectic Medical Institute of Cincinnati; 1851-62, conducted a hospital and school, Newton's Clinical Institute, Cincinnati; 1852-62, editor, *Eclectic Medical Journal*; 1863-81, medical practice, New York, N.Y.: 1865-81, professor of surgery, Eclectic Medical College of the City of New York. CONTRIBUTIONS: A controversial leader in Eclectic medicine, used his pen and editorial skills regularly in the name of medical reform. Founded the *Eclectic Medical Journal* (1852) and edited it (1852-62) and numerous others, including *Western Medical News* (Cincinnati, 1851-59), *American Eclectic Medical Review* (New York, 1866-72), *Medical Eclectic* (New York, 1873-81). Wrote numerous books and articles on eclectic medicine and surgery. Originated the circular incision for removal of the breast. Pressed Union military authorities to improve medical and sanitary conditions (1861-63). Instituted successful movement for recognition of eclectic practitioners in the army. Organized Eclectic Medical Society of the State of New York (1863), helped found Eclectic Medical College of the City of New York (1865) and served as its president (1875-81).

WRITINGS: *American Dispensatory (Eclectic)*, with John King (1852); *The Eclectic Treatise on the Practice of Medicine* (1861). Writings listed in *Appleton's CAB*, 4, 510. REFERENCES: *DAB*, 13: 475-76; Kelly and Burrage (1920), 902; *Who Was Who in Am.*, Hist. Vol.: 378.

T. L. Savitt

NICHOLS, MARY SARGEANT (NEAL) GOVE (August 10, 1810, Goffstown, N.H.-May 30, 1884, London, England). *Woman's rights and health reformer*. Daughter of William A., ardent Democrat and Freethinker, and Rebecca R. Neal, Universalist. Married Hiram Gove, 1831, one child, divorced; Thomas Low Nichols, 1848, one child. EDUCATION: Self-taught. CAREER: 1837, opened girls' school, Lynn, Mass., and offered lectures on anatomy, physiology, and hygiene; 1838, gave a course of lectures on health and hygiene, Ladies Physiological Society, Boston, Mass.; after this successful course, embarked on a career devoted to health reform, lectured throughout the Northeast, and dedicated herself to helping women relieve themselves of the physical and mental suffering caused by their ignorance of health issues, especially in regard to sex; 1840, edited *Health Journal and Advocate of Physiological Reform*; 1843, established *Health Journal and Independent Magazine*; 1845, inspired by Henry Gardiner Wright, founded a water-cure house, New York City; 1850, established a second water-cure establishment, New York City; 1851, with the help of her husband, Thomas Nichols, established the American Hydropathic Institute, a short-lived co-educational, water-cure medical school; 1855, soon alienated from the other leaders of the water-cure movement because of their heretical social views, the Nicholses moved to Cincinnati, Ohio, where they continued to lecture and write about health reform in *Nichols' Journal of Health, Water-cure, and Human Progress.* CONTRIBUTIONS: In support of diet reform, dress reform, health education, woman's rights, and the relations of the sexes, anticipated many of the social reforms adopted long after her death.

WRITINGS: A leading contributor to the *Water-cure J.*, published "Lectures to Ladies on Anatomy and Physiology" (1842) and *Experience in Water-Cure* (1849); *A Woman's Work in Water-Cure and Sanitary Education* (1868). REFERENCES: *DAB*, 7, pt. 1: 495-96; *NCAB*, 13: 140; Thomas L. Nichols, *Forty Years of American Life*, 2 vols. (1864, and later eds.); idem, *Nichols' Health Manual: Being Also a Memorial of the Life and Work of Mrs. Mary S. Gove Nichols* (1887); *Notable Am. Women, 1607-1950*, 627-29; Bertha Monica Steans, "Two Forgotten New England Reformers," *New Eng. Q.* (Nov. 1933).

V. Drachman

NIXON, PAT IRELAND (November 29, 1883, Old Nixon, Guadalupe County, Tex.-November 18, 1965, San Antonio, Tex.). *Physician; Surgeon; Historian.* Son of Robert Thomas and Frances Amanda (Andrews) Nixon. Married Olive Gray Read, July 3, 1912; four sons. EDUCATION: 1900, graduated from Luling High School; 1902, maxima cum laude graduate, Bingham School, Ashville, N.C.; 1905, B.S., University of Texas; 1909, M.D., Johns Hopkins; 1909-11, intern, Johns Hopkins Hospital. CAREER: 1911, opened office, San Antonio, and practiced medicine there for more than 50 years. CONTRIBUTIONS: Dynamic leader in county, regional, and state medical societies and in public health reform and politics. Indefatigable public servant, medical editor, and author of scientific and historical topics. Oversaw creation of Texas Medical History Collection by the Texas Medical Association and the Texas State Historical Association. Author of medical history essays for *Handbook of Texas* (1952).

WRITINGS: *A Century of Medicine in San Antonio* (1936); *The Medical Story of Early Texas, 1528-1853* (1946); *A History of the Texas Medical Association, 1853-1953* (1953); *The Texas Surgical Society: The First Fifty Years* (1965, with R. S. Sparkman et al.). A bibliography is in Herbert H. Lang, ed., *Pat Nixon of Texas* (1979). Nixon's papers are at Trinity University, San Antonio. REFERENCES: *BHM* (1964-69), 195; *Handbook of Texas* 3 (1976); 654.

J. Morris

NOGUCHI, HIDEYA [b. NOGUCHI, SEISAKU] (November 24, 1876, Inawashiro, Japan-May 21, 1928, Accra, Ghana). *Physician; Microbiology.* Son of Sayosuke, farmer, and Shika Noguchi; Married Mary Dardis, 1912; no children. EDUCATION: 1897, M.D., Tokyo Medical College; 1899, went to the United States; 1903-4, fellow, State Serum Institute, Copenhagen. CAREER: Assistant: 1897-98, (Tokyo) General Hospital; and 1898-1900, Government Institute for Infectious Diseases; 1898-99, lecturer on pathology and oral surgery, Tokyo Dental College; 1899-1900, physician, International Sanitary Board, in charge of general hospital and bacteriological laboratory, New Chwang, China; 1901-3, pathology faculty, University of Pennsylvania; 1904-28, member, Rockefeller Institute for Medical Research (later Rockefeller University). CONTRIBUTIONS: Known for studies of infectious diseases, snake venoms, and serological techniques and for cultivation of various spirochetes. Work was of uneven quality; some aspects have proved enduring but others either were disproved or could not be duplicated. Found *Treponema pallidum* in the central nervous system of persons who had died from general paresis and tabes dorsalis, proving that the two were late stages of syphilis (1913). Made useful contributions to the serological diagnosis of syphilis (1900s). Demonstrated that Oroya fever, a severe systemic disease, and verruga peruana, a localized skin affliction, were both manifestations of infection with *Bartonella bacilliformis* (1925-27). Cultivated the organisms of relapsing fever and Vincent's angina. Believed he had grown the spirochete of syphilis and the microorganisms responsible for several other diseases, but work could not be replicated by other researchers. Mistakenly announced that yellow fever was caused by a spirochete, *Leptospira icteroides* (1920s) and died while attempting to prove it.

WRITINGS: *Snake Venoms* (1909); *Serum Diagnosis of Syphilis. . .*(1910); "A Method for the Pure Cultivation of Pathogenic Treponema Pallidum (*Spirochaeta Pallida*)," *J. of Experimental Med.* 14 (1911): 99-108; "A Demonstration of Treponema Pallidum in the Brain in Cases of General Paralysis," *ibid.*, 17 (1913): 232-38 (with J. W. Moore); "Etiology of Oroya Fever. . .," *ibid.*, 43 (1926): 851-64 (with T. S. Battistini). A bibliography was prepared by the Rockefeller Institute for Medical Research and is available in selected libraries in the United States, Japan, and Europe. REFERENCES: *BHM*(1970-74), 130; (1977), 24; (1980), 30; P. F. Clark, "H. Noguchi," *Bull. Hist. Med.* 33 (1959): 1-20; *DAB*, 13: 542-43; *DSB*, 10: 141-45; Miller, *BHM*, p. 80; *Who Was Who in Am.*, 1: 902.

S. Galishoff

NOON, ADOLPHUS H. (June 23, 1838, London, England-March 23, 1931, Nogales, Ariz.). *Physician.* Married Emma C. E. Slaughter; five children. EDUCATION: Studied medicine under Dr. John Eglinton Seaman, South Africa; study at the College of Physicians, San Francisco, Calif. CAREER: Served four years in the British Army, South Africa; 1864, went to the United States and lived in Utah; 1879, settled in Ariz. and founded town of Oro Blanco; private practice of medicine on his ranch and in Nogales, Ariz. CONTRIBUTIONS: First president, Santa Cruz County Medical Society. Mayor, Nogales. Member, Ariz. legislature (1901).

REFERENCES: James H. McClintock, *Arizona* (1916); *Nogales International*, March 25, 1931; *Portrait and Biog. Record of Arizona* (1901).

J. S. Goff

NORTH, CHARLES EDWARD (July 28, 1869, Scarborough, N.Y.-July 27, 1961, Montclair, N.J.). *Bacteriologist; Dairy industry sanitation pioneer.* Son of Charles Randolph and Anna Mary (Haight) North. Married Amelia Potter

Palmer, 1903; five children. EDUCATION: 1893, A.B., Wesleyan University; 1900, M.D., College of Physicians and Surgeons (Columbia); 1905, postgraduate work in bacteriology, Columbia University; 1909-10, postgraduate work in public health, Harvard University. CAREER: 1900-1904, manager, Purity Milk Company; 1905-8, bacteriologist, Lederle Laboratories; 1908, director of research on value of bacterial vaccines and Opsonic index; 1908-10, consulting bacteriologist, Jersey City Water Department; 1908-10, established clean milk supply for infant milk stations, New York Milk Committee; 1917, chairman, Mayor Mitchel Committee on Milk (N.Y.); executive-secretary, National Commission on Milk Standards; 1938, secretary, Grade A Milk Association. CONTRIBUTIONS: Educated farmers and dairy companies in methods of producing safe, wholesome milk. Demonstrated that it was the cleanliness of milking techniques and equipment that mattered most in keeping bacterial counts low and that simple, inexpensive sanitary practices, such as using covered milk pails, washing the udders, and having clean hands, would protect milk's purity. Persuaded dairy companies to adopt the label "Grade A" for milk that met the highest bacteriological, sanitary, and physical standards which dairymen could sell at a premium price; reforms greatly improved dairy sanitary conditions and nearly eliminated infant mortality attributable to the use of raw milk (1900-1930). Invented numerous processes and devices for pasteurization and for dehydration and reconstitution of milk products. Consultant to several cities in the areas of milk and water supplies.

WRITINGS: *The Grading of Milk as a Substitute for Dairy Inspection. Massachusetts Agricultural Board, Circular No. 61* (1916); *Farmer's Clean Milk Book* (1918); "Milk and Its Relation to Public Health," in Mazÿck P. Ravenel ed., *A Half Century of Public Health* (1921), 236-89. REFERENCES: Norman Myrick, "He Led the Way to Better Milk," *Am. Milk Rev.* 16 (Jul. 1954): 32-33; *N.Y. Times*, July 28, 1961; *Who Was Who in Am.*, 4: 707.

S. Galishoff

NORTH, ELISHA (January 8, 1771, Goshen, Conn.-December 29, 1843, New London, Conn.). *Physician; Ophthalmologist.* Son of Joseph, local practitioner and farmer, and Lucy (Cowles) North. Married Hannah Beach, 1797, eight children. EDUCATION: Studied medicine with his father until he went to Hartford to study with Dr. Lemuel Hopkins (q.v.); 1793-95, studied at the University of Pennsylvania, but did not graduate; 1813, Connecticut Medical Society conferred the degree of M.D. CAREER: 1795-1812, practiced medicine, Goshen; 1812-43, practiced general medicine and ophthalmology, New London. CONTRIBUTIONS: A pioneer in the study of vaccination. Seized upon the results of the work of Edward Jenner and applied them successfully in practice. The first physician in the United States to report a human case of cowpox (1801). Through efforts, the first kine-pox used for vaccination purposes was introduced into the city of N.Y. In association with Dr. Benjamin Waterhouse (q.v.) and others, efforts in demonstrating the value of vaccination played a significant role in the control and prevention of smallpox in this country. Author of the first volume on cerebrospinal meningitis to be found in medical literature. Established the first eye infirmary in the United States (1817), an institution that continued for 12 years. Early use of the clinical thermometer and his carrying out of postmortem examinations with careful notes of findings. Invented or improved several instruments, including the eyelid speculum, the combination of the trephine and trepan, and a new form of catheter.

WRITINGS: *A Treatise on a Malignant Epidemic Commonly Called Spotted Fever* (1811); *Outline of the Science of Life, Which Treats Physiologically of Both Body and Mind* (1829); *The Pilgrim's Progress in Phrenology*, by "Uncle Toby" (1836). Wrote several articles in medical and scientific journals, including "The Rights of Anatomists Vindicated," by "Vesalius" (1829) and "On a Fuel," *Am. J. of Sci. & Arts* 11 (1826): 67. See bibliography in H. C. Bolton, "Memoirs of Elisha North," in *Proc., Conn. Med. Soc.* 3, no. 4 (1882). REFERENCES: Daniel M. Albert, M.D., and Marvin L. Sears, M.D., "Dr. Elisha North and the First Eye Infirmary," *Am. J. of Ophthalmology* 71 (Feb. 1951): 578-87; *DAB*, 7, pt. 1: 559; Charles B. Graves, "Medicine in New London One Hundred Years Ago," in Herbert Thoms, ed., *Heritage of Connecticut Medicine* (1942), 76-91; Sebastian R. Italia, "Elisha North: Experimentalist, Epidemiologist, Physician, 1771-1843," *Bull. Hist. Med.* 31 (1957): 505-36; Kelly and Burrage (1920).

J. W. Ifkovic

NORTHCROSS, DAVID CANEEN (1876-January 3, 1933, Detroit, Mich.). *Physician; Hospital administrator*. Married Dr. Daisy L., c. 1914; three children. EDUCATION: College of St. Joseph, St. Joseph, Mo.; 1906, M.D., University of Illinois; 1913, M.D., Bennett Medical College, Chicago, Ill. CAREER: General practice: before 1917, Montgomery, Ala.; and 1917-33, Detroit, with Dr. Daisy L. Northcross; active in the Republican party. CONTRIBUTIONS: Despite having applied for staff privileges (1917), officials of Harper Hospital prohibited him from seeing or consulting a patient of his, except during visiting hours. At least partly in response, established Mercy General, Detroit's first black-run hospital, a proprietary institution administered by the Northcross family until his son, David C. Northcross Jr., M.D., retired in 1974. The Drs. Northcross and others organized Dunbar Hospital (later Parkside), the city's first black nonprofit hospital (1919). REFERENCES: *Am. Med. Directory* (1932); Burton Historical Collections, Detroit Public Library; *Detroit News*, August 24, 1928, p. 41; January 4, 1933, p. 3; *JNMA*, 61 (1969): 448-52; 55 (1963): 475-84; 25 (1933): 37.

M. Pernick

NOTT, JOSIAH CLARK (March 31, 1804, Columbia, S.C.-March 31, 1873, Mobile, Ala.). *Physician; Surgeon; Writer on anthropology*. Son of Abraham, judge and member of Congress, and Angelica (Mitchell) Nott. Married Sarah Chestnut Deas, 1832; eight children. EDUCATION: 1824, graduated from South Carolina College; studied medicine, office of Dr. James Davis, Columbia; 1825-26, College of Physicians and Surgeons, New York City; study under Dr. Valentine Mott (q.v.); 1827, M.D., University of Pennsylvania; 1827-28, intern, Philadelphia Alms House (Old Blockley); 1835-36, study in Europe. CAREER: 1829, demonstrator of anatomy, University of Pennsylvania; medical practice: 1829-34, Columbia; 1836-57, Mobile; 1857, accepted chair of anatomy, University of Louisiana; 1858, resumed practice, Mobile; 1859-61, professor of surgery, Medical College of Alabama, Mobile; 1861-65, medical director to Gen. Braxton Bragg's Army, Confederate States of America; 1867, practice, Baltimore, Md.; 1868-72, surgical practice, New York City. CONTRIBUTIONS: Helped organize the Mobile Medical Society (1841), serving as president (1843, 1856, 1866). First to remove the coccyx surgically (1844). Suggested that yellow fever was transmitted by insects (1848). With George A. Ketchum (q.v.), established a private infirmary for Negro patients (1848) known as Dr. J. C. Nott's Infirmary which continued to operate until after the Civil War. Helped organize the Medical College of Alabama (1859) and the New York Obstetrical Society.

WRITINGS: "Extirpation of the Os Coccygis for Neuralgia," *New Orleans Med. J.* 1 (1844): 58; "On the Pathology of Yellow Fever," *Am. J. of Med. Sci.*, n.s., 9 (1845): 277-93; "Yellow Fever Contrasted with Bilious Fever—Reason for Believing It a Disease of Sui Generis—Its Mode of Propagation—Remote Cause—Probably Insect or Animalicular Origin," *New Orleans Med. and Surg. J.* 4 (1848): 563-601; *The Physical History of the Jewish Race* (1850); *Types of Mankind* (1854); *Indigenous Races of the Earth* (1857). REFERENCES: W. Bean, "J. C. Nott," *Bull. N.Y. Acad. of Med.* 50 (1974): 529-35; *BHM* (1964-69), 195; (1970-74), 131; (1975-79), 92; E. B. Carmichael, "J. C. Nott," *Bull. Hist. Med.* 22 (1948); *DAB*, 13: 582-83; Miller, *BHM*, p. 80; *NCAB*, 19: 84.

S. Eichold

NOVY, FREDERICK GEORGE (December 9, 1864, Chicago, Ill.-August 8, 1957, Ann Arbor, Mich.). *Bacteriologist; Educator.* Son of Joseph, tailor, and Frances (Janota) Novy. Married Grace Garwood, 1891; five children. EDUCATION: University of Michigan: 1886, A.B.; 1887, M.A., and 1891, M.D.; studied: 1888, Berlin; 1894, Prague; and 1897, Paris. CAREER: At University of Michigan Medical School: 1886, organic chemistry faculty; 1887-1902, hygiene and physiological chemistry faculty; 1902-35, bacteriology faculty; 1902-35, director, Hygiene Laboratory; 1930-33, chairman, Executive Committee, and faculty; and 1933-35, dean; member; 1897-99, Michigan State Board of Health; and 1901, U.S. Commission to Investigate Plague. CONTRIBUTIONS: Through teaching, research, and development of ingenious methods of laboratory investigation, helped establish the discipline of bacteriology in the United States. With Victor Vaughan (q.v.), established what is believed to be the first formal laboratory course in bacteriology in an American university (1889). Studied the toxins produced by bacilli initially overestimating their importance in disease (1888-91). Developed the Novy Jar and other apparatus for the cultivation of anaerobic bacteria; discovered an anaerobic bacillus, *Clostridium novyi*, capable of causing malignant edema (1894). Served on the U.S. Commission to Investigate Plague which established the existence of the disease in San Francisco,

Calif. (1901). Established the first antirabies station in the United States in Ann Arbor (1903). Did his best-known scientific studies on trypanosomes and spirochetes; with Ward J. MacNeal, developed an artificial medium for the cultivation of trypanosomes *lewisi* and *brucei*, the first pathogenic protozoan to be grown *in vitro*; delineated the different relapsing fever spirochetes and discovered the organism responsible for American relapsing fever—*Spirocheta novyi* (1906); showed that spirochetes and trypanosomes are independent forms of life. Studied anaphylaxsis and confirmed the existence of anaphylotoxin, a histaminelike substance (1917). Investigated microbial metabolism; made especially noteworthy studies of the respiration of tubercle bacilli (1920s). Charter member, Society of American Bacteriologists, and fifth president (1904).

WRITINGS: "Ein Neuer Anaërober Bacillus des Malignes Oedems," *ZHI* 17 (1894): 209-33; *Laboratory Work in Bacteriology*, 2d. ed. (1898); "On Trypanosomes," *Harvey Lectures* 1 (1905-6): 33-72; "Relapsing Fever and Spirochetes," *Trans., Assoc. of Am. Physicians* (1906): 456-64 (with R. E. Knapp); "The Respiration of the Tubercle Bacillus," *Journal of Infectious Diseases* 36 (1925): 168-232 (with M. H. Soule). A bibliography is in *BMNAS*. REFERENCES: *BHM* (1976), 23; *BMNAS* 33 (1959): 326-50; *DSB*, 10: 154-55; Miller, *BHM*, pp. 80-81; *NCAB*, 54: 427-28; *Trans., Assoc. of Am. Physicians* 71 (1958): 35-37; *Who Was Who in Am.*, 3: 646.

S. Galishoff

NUTTALL, GEORGE HENRY FALKINER   (July 5, 1862, San Francisco, Calif.-December 15, 1937, Cambridge, England). *Physician; Immunology; Parasitology*. Son of Robert Kennedy, physician, and Magdalena (Parrott) Nuttall. Married Paula von Oertzen-Kittendorf of Mecklenburg, Germany, 1895; three children. EDUCATION: Studies in England, France, Germany, and Switzerland; 1884, M.D., University of California; 1885-86, study at Johns Hopkins University with H. Newell Martin (q.v.); 1886, study at Breslau, Poland; 1890, Ph.D. (zoology and physiology), University of Göttingen; 1890-93, assistant to William Welch (q.v.), Johns Hopkins; 1893-94, study at Göttingen, Germany; 1894-99, assistant to Max Rubner, Berlin Hygienic Institute. CAREER: 1899-1931, faculty, Cambridge University; 1920-37, director, Molteno Institute for Research in Parasitology; 1931-37, Emeritus Quick Professor, Cambridge University. CONTRIBUTIONS: Through wide-ranging scientific accomplishments and international contacts, promoted the study of the transmission, pathogenesis, and control of infectious, and especially parasitic, diseases (1888-1937). Discovered the bactericidal activity of defibrinated blood (1888) thereby stimulating the development of humoral immunology and therapeutic sera. With William Welch (1892), discovered the agent of gas gangrene (now, *Clostridium perfringens*). With Hans Thierfelder, conducted the first successful experiments on animals raised in aseptic conditions (1895-97). Elucidated the role of *Anopheles* in malaria in England (1897-1901). Made advances in piroplasmosis and other tick-borne diseases and in serology. Promoted hygienic measures for disease control.

WRITINGS: "Experimente über die bakterienfeindlichen Einflüsse des thierischen Körpers," *ZHI* 4 (1888): 353; "A Gas-Producing Bacillus (*Bacillus aerogenes capsulatus*

n. sp.) Capable of Rapid Development in the Blood Vessels after Death," *Johns Hopkins Hosp. Bull.* 3 (1892): 81; *Blood Immunity and Blood Relationship* (1904). Writings listed in *Parasitology*. REFERENCES: *BHM* (1970-74), 131; *Int. Cong. Hist. Med. 21st Siena, 1968* 2 (c. 1969): 1166-67; *J. Hyg.* 38 (1938): 129-40; Miller, *BHM*, p. 81; *Parasitology* 30 (1938): 403-18; *Sci.* 87 (1938): 337-38.

L. P. Rubin

NUTTING, M[ARY] ADELAIDE (November 1, 1858, Waterloo, Quebec, Canada-October 3, 1948, White Plains, N.Y.). *Leader in professional nursing and nursing education*. Daughter of Vespasian, county clerk of the Circuit Court, and Harriet Sophia (Peasley) Nutting, seamstress. EDUCATION: 1891, Johns Hopkins Hospital Training School for Nurses in Baltimore. CAREER: At Johns Hopkins Hospital Training School for Nurses: 1891-94, head nurse and then assistant superintendent of nurses; and 1894, appointed superintendent of nurses and principal of the training school; 1899-1907, part-time teacher in an experimental, one-year program, Teachers College, Columbia University; 1907, accepted a full-time professorship in institutional management, Teacher's College; 1910-retirement in 1925, appointed chair, Department of Nursing and Health, Teacher's College; 1903-21, chair, Education Committee, National League of Nursing Education. CONTRIBUTIONS: Devoted life to incorporating the education of nurses into universities. As head of the Training School for Nurses at Johns Hopkins Hospital, was responsible for several innovations including the development of a six-month preliminary program for nursing students. An active member, American Society of Superintendents of Training Schools for Nurses of the U.S. and Canada, serving as president (1896, 1909), vice-president (1897), and secretary (1903, 1904). Helped establish the *American Journal of Nursing (1900)*. Organized and was the first president, State Association of Graduate Nurses, Md. (1903). Helped draft Maryland's first nurse-practice law (1904).

WRITINGS: *History of Nursing* (1907-12, with Lavinia L. Dock); *Standard Curriculum for Schools of Nursing* (1917, with Education Committee, National League of Nursing Education); *Nursing and Nursing Education in the United States* (1923, with Rockefeller Foundation Committee); *Educational Status of Nursing* (1912); *A Sound Economic Basis for Schools of Nursing* (1926). REFERENCES: *DAB*, Supplement 4: 631-33; Stella Goostray, "Mary Adelaide Nutting," *Am. J. of Nursing* (Nov. 1958); *Notable Am. Women, 1607-1950*, 642-44; *N.Y. Times*, October 5, 1948; Ethel Johns and Blanche Pfefferkorn, *The Johns Hopkins Hospital School of Nursing, 1889-1949* (1954).

V. Drachman

O

O'DWYER, JOSEPH (October 12, 1841, Cleveland, Ohio-January 7, 1898, New York, N.Y.). *Physician; Pediatrics.* Married Catherine Begg; eight sons, four who survived to adulthood. EDUCATION: 1863, apprentice to a Dr. Anderson, London, Ontario, Canada; 1866, M.D., College of Physicians and Surgeons, N.Y. CAREER: 1866-68, resident physician, Charity Hospital, N.Y., on Blackwell's Island; 1868-69, examining physician, New York City Board of Charities and Corrections; 1868, began an obstetrical partnership practice; 1872-97, attending physician, New York Foundling Hospital; on medical faculty, Post-Graduate Medical School and Hospital and Bellevue Hospital Medical College. CONTRIBUTIONS: At a time when tracheotomy was the only, albeit ineffective, method of treating asphyxiation in diphtheria, developed and pioneered laryngeal intubation (1880-85). "O'Dwyer tubes" became widely used in cases of diphtheria before the availability of antitoxin (1895) and later for other conditions of laryngeal ulceration or stenosis. Helped to promote antitoxin therapy (1895-98); among the first to suggest mechanical ventilation for the management of pneumonia.

WRITINGS: "Intubation of the Larynx," *N.Y. Med. J.* 42 (1885): 145; *Diphtheria and Intubation in Croup* (1889, with C. E. Billington); "The Evolution of Intubation," *Trans Am. Pediat. Soc.* 8 (1896): 9. Writings listed in *Jahrb Kinderheilk* 51 (1900): 544-59, 722. REFERENCES: *DAB*, 7, pt. 1: 627-8; R. R. Gifford, "The O'Dwyer Tube: Development and Use in Laryngeal Diphtheria," *Clin. Pediat.* 9 (1970): 179-85; *Med. Record* 53 (1898): 361-64; *Münch med Wchnschr* 45 (1898): 337-38; *Pediatrics* 5 (1898): 95-97.

L. P. Rubin

OHAGE, JUSTUS (October 13, 1849, Hanover, Germany-December 26, 1935, St. Paul, Minn.). *Surgeon.* Son of Dr. George and Mrs. Ohage. Married Augusta Ensor, 1877; four children. EDUCATION: Gymnasium, Hanover, Germany; went to America to join Union forces in Union army during the Civil War; returned to Germany to continue education after being wounded in battle; 1870, stretcher bearer in the Franco-Prussian War; went to America again as medical assistant to the construction crew of the Topeka-Atchison Railroad; 1880, M.D., Missouri University; postgraduate studies, Goettingen, Kiel, and Berlin, Germany; Edinburgh, Scotland; and London, England. CAREER: 1881, began medical practice, St. Paul; 1899-1918, health officer, St. Paul; 1890-99, clinical professor of surgery, University of Minnesota. CONTRIBUTIONS: Did the first successful cholecystectomy in America at St. Joseph's Hospital, St. Paul (1888). As health officer of St. Paul, worked for pure food laws and compulsory vaccination. At the St. Louis World Fair of 1904, St. Paul was declared to be the "healthiest city in the world." President: Ramsey County Medical Society (1889-90) and Minnesota State Medical Society (1895).

REFERENCES: *BHM* (1970-74), 132; *Minnesota Med.* 69 (Feb. 1972): 86-91.

R. Rosenthal

O'LEARY, JAMES LEE (December 8, 1904, Tomahawk, Wis.-May 28, 1975, St. Louis, Mo.). *Neuroanatomist; Neurologist.* Son of James and Mary (Whelan) O'Leary. Married Nancy Blair, 1939; two children. EDUCATION: University of Chicago: 1925, B.S.; 1928, Ph.D. (anatomy); and 1931, M.D. CAREER: 1927-28, instructor, anatomy, University of Chicago; at Washington University School of Medicine: 1928-32, assistant professor, anatomy; and 1933-46, associate professor, anatomy; 1943-45, instructor and physician, U.S. Army, discharged as lieutenant colonel; at Washington University School of Medicine: 1946-62, professor of neurology; and 1963-71, chairman, Department of Neurology; chief of neurology, Barnes Hospital; 1971-75, professor emeritus and lecturer, neurology and experimental neurosurgery. CONTRIBUTIONS: During first decade at Washington University School of Medicine (1928-38), was a key member in a group of investigators who founded modern neurophysiology. By the early 1930s, the work of Joseph Erlanger, (q.v.) and Herbert Gasser, (q.v.) had been in St. Louis, which became the center of this research. In collaboration with George Bishop (q.v.) and Peter Heinbecker, developed a method for providing reliable peripheral nerve-stained sections for measurement and comparison with the action potentials recorded from the same nerves. Thus helped to establish the correlation between axon diameter and conduction velocity. During World War II, volunteered for service and directed efforts toward developing accepted criteria for using EEG in neurological diagnosis. On return to St. Louis, assumed the major responsibility for the development of training and clinical services in neurology, always sustaining the connection between basic and clinical research. In later years, published data on the cerebral cortex (with Sidney Goldring), on pain mechanisms (with Henry Schwartz), and on the clinical and encephalographic aspects of epilepsy. Elected president, American Neurological Association (1962), and received its Jacoby Award (1971). After retirement as the first chairman, Department of Neurology, Washington University School of Medicine, continued work on a full-time basis. Co-authored a book (with Sidney Goldring), *Science and Epilepsy*, published posthumously (1976).

WRITINGS: "The Function of the Non-Myelinated Fibers of the Dorsal Roots," *Am. J. of Physiol.* 196 (1933): 647-69 (with P. Heinbecker and G. Bishop); "Nature and Source of Fibres Contributing to the Saphenous Nerve of the Cat," ibid., 194 (1933): 23-35; "Pain and Touch Fibers in Peripheral Nerves," *Arch. of Neurology and Psychiatry* 29 (1933): 771-89; "Experimentally Derived Correlates Between ECG and Steady Cortical Potential," *J. Neurophysiol.* 14 (1951): 275-88. REFERENCES: W. M. Cowan, "James L. O'Leary," *Anat. Record* 192 (1978): 135-36.

M. Hunt

OLIVER, DANIEL (September 9, 1787, Salem, Mass.-June 1, 1842, Cambridge, Mass.). *Physician.* Son of Rev. Thomas Fitch and Mrs. Sarah (Pynchon) Oliver. Never married. EDUCATION: 1805, A.B., Harvard College; 1807, M.A., Dartmouth; 1810, M.D., University of Pennsylvania (and a correlate degree from Dartmouth). CAREER: 1810-15, practice, Salem, where first became associated with Reuben D. Mussey (q.v.); on the medical faculty: 1815-40, Dartmouth, lecturing on several topics, including medical jurisprudence and mental philosophy; and 1840-42, Medical College of Ohio, Cincinnati, Ohio, at Mussey's invitation. CONTRIBUTIONS: A leading teacher of several medical disciplines. Wrote a textbook of physiology that went through three editions.

WRITINGS: *First Lines of Physiology: Designed for the Use of Students of Medicine* (1835). REFERENCE: Kelly and Burrage (1928), 917; *NCAB*, 9: 92.

J. W. Estes

OLYPHANT, DAVID (1720, Pithearies, Scotland-1805, Newport, R.I.). *Physician; Surgeon.* Married Hannah Freeman, 1787; one son. EDUCATION: Obtained an M.D. in Scotland. CAREER: 1749, in Battle of Culloden; 1749, immigrated to S.C. and became surgeon to the independent companies of His Majesty's regular footsoldiers; operated hospital for blacks with Dr. Patrick Machie; 1755, began practice, St. George's Parish, Dorchester, S.C.; 1759, physician, Charlestown, S.C.; member, Committee of Correspondence to Charles Garth (London agent for S.C.); 1776, member, General Assembly and Legislative Council of the Province; and director-general of the hospitals, Southern Department; 1780, prisoner of war, after his exchange, appointed director of American Hospitals under Nathaniel Greene; became deputy director, Hospital of the Southern Army; 1783, resumed practice, Dorchester, and seat in the assembly, serving a total of 28 years; 1787, moved practice to R.I. CONTRIBUTIONS: Greatest contribution was to the British forces in the field of surgery on the battlefield. REFERENCES: J. I. Waring, *History of Medicine in South Carolina* (1964).

J. P. Dolan

OPIE, EUGENE LINDSAY (July 5, 1873, Staunton, Va.-March 12, 1971, Bryn Mawr, Pa.). *Physician; Pathology; Microbiology; Epidemiology.* Son of Thomas, physician, and Sallie (Harman) Opie. Married Gertrude Lovat Simpson,

1902, four children; Margaret Lovat Simpson, 1916. EDUCATION: Johns Hopkins: 1893, A.B.; 1897, M.D.; and 1897-98, medical house officer. CAREER: 1898-1904, pathology faculty, Johns Hopkins Medical School; at Rockefeller Institute for Medical Research (later Rockefeller University): 1904-10, member; 1928-32, Board of Scientific Directors; and 1941-70, guest investigator; 1907-10, pathology staff, Presbyterian Hospital (N.Y.); at Washington University Medical School; 1910-23, pathology faculty; and 1912-15, dean; 1917-19, U.S. Army Medical Corps; 1923-32, pathology faculty, University of Pennsylvania; at Henry Phipps Institute for the Study, Treatment and Prevention of Tuberculosis: 1923-32, director of laboratories; and 1942-46, acting director; 1932-41, pathology faculty, Cornell Medical College; 1932-41, pathology staff, New York Hospital; 1935-38, scientific director, International Health Division, Rockefeller Foundation; 1939, visiting professor, Peiping Union Medical College. CONTRIBUTIONS: Described the life cycles of the malarialike parasites found in the blood of Baltimore birds (1898). Discovered the occurrence of degeneration of the islets of Langerhans in diabetes and stated that it was the likely cause of the disease (1900). Developed the theory that obstruction at the point of union of the bile and pancreatic ducts could cause acute pancreatitis. Wrote *Diseases of the Pancreas* (1902), which became the standard text on the subject for more than three decades. During World War I, showed that vermin were spreading trench fever among Allied soldiers and provided methods for the control of the disease. Made extensive studies of tuberculosis in Philadelphia families and in rural-to-city migrants in Jamaica and China (1923-39). Demonstrated the value of X-ray examination in diagnosing asymptomatic tubercular lesions, the tuberculin test as an indicator of the onset of infection, and the sputum test as an index of the probability of tuberculosis transmission within a household. Made additional important discoveries about the etiology and communicability of tuberculosis. Undertook major studies of pneumonia, epidemic influenza, cancer, diseases of the liver, inflammation, allergy and immunology, and fluid movements across cell membranes. Played a leading role in the upgrading of Washington University Medical School. Trained many of the nation's leaders in experimental medicine and pathology.

WRITINGS: "On the Haemocytozoa of Birds," *J. of Experimental Med.* 3 (1898): 79-101; "On the Relation of Chronic Interstitial Pancreatitis to the Islands of Langerhans and to Diabetes Mellitus," ibid., 5 (1900-1901): 397-428; *Epidemic Respiratory Disease* (1921); "Present Concepts of Tuberculous Infection and Disease, Their Principles and Application," *Am. Rev. of Tuberculosis* 32 (1935): 617-30. A bibliography is in *BMNAS*. REFERENCES: *BHM* (1970-74), 132; *BMNAS* 47 (1974): 293-320; *McGraw-Hill Modern Med. of Sci.* 1 (1966): 360-61; Miller, *BHM*, p. 81; *NCAB*, 57: 249-50; *N.Y. Times*, March 13, 1971; John H. Talbott, *Biographical History of Medicine* (1970), 940-43; *Who Was Who in Am.*, 5: 546.

S. Galishoff

ORR, H[IRAM] WINNETT (March 17, 1877, West Newton, Pa.-October 11, 1956, Rochester, Minn.). *Orthopedic surgeon.* Son of Dr. Andrew Wilson, dentist, and Frances Josephine (Winnett) Orr. Married Grace Douglass, September 7, 1904; five children. EDUCATION: West Newton High School; 1882-85, University of Nebraska, studied medicine with his uncle, Hudson J. Winnett, M.D., in Lincoln, Nebr., during this time; 1895-99, M.D., University of Michigan; 1899, intern, Bellevue Hospital, New York City; 1904, Northwestern University, studied with Dr. John Ridlon. CAREER: 1899-1956, practice of medicine and orthopedic surgery, Lincoln; 1905, formulated legislation for establishment of the Nebraska Orthopedic Hospital; at Nebraska Orthopedic Hospital: 1906-17, assistant surgeon and superintendent; 1919-48, chief surgeon; and 1948-56, senior consultant; in Nebraska State Medical Society: 1919-20, president; and 1915-17, secretary; 1936, president, American Orthopedic Association; 1921-22, chairman, Orthopedic Section, AMA; at Medical Department, U.S. Army, Goldthwait Unit of Orthopedic Surgery, England, and Surgical Hospital Center, Savenay, France: 1917, captain; and 1919, lieutenant colonel; 1899-1906, editor, *Western Medical Review*; at University of Nebraska College of Medicine and its predecessor, Omaha Medical College: 1903-9, lecturer; 1909, adjunct professor; and 1910-16, assistant professor, history of medicine; 1908, chief medical inspector, Lincoln Public Schools; 1919-21, editor, *American Journal of Orthopedic Surgery*; 1923-56, chief consultant and chief orthopedic surgeon, Lincoln General Hospital, Bryan Memorial Hospital, and Veterans Administration Hospital, Lincoln. CONTRIBUTIONS: Devised the "Orr Method" for treating osteomyelitis, compound fractures, and other infected wounds while at Savenay, France. Advocate of drainage and rest in wound-healing. Developed replacement techniques and control of fragments in fractures by skeletal pin fixation in plaster of paris and other immobilizing devices.

WRITINGS: *Osteomyelitis, Compound Fractures and Other Infected Wounds* (1929); *Wounds and Fractures: A Clinical Guide to Civil and Military Practice* (1941); *On the Contributions of Hugh Owen Thomas, Sir Robert Jones and John Ridlon, M.D., of New York and Chicago, to Modern Orthopedic Surgery* (1949); *Selected Pages from the History of Medicine in Nebraska* (1952), 149-56. REFERENCES: S. L. Koch, "Dr. H. Winnett Orr, 1877-1956," *Bull., Am. Coll. of Surg.* 42 (1957): 118-21; *NCAB*, H (1952): 266-67; Personal papers, University of Nebraska Medical Center Library of Medicine, Omaha, Nebr.

B. M. Hetzner

ORR, THOMAS GROVER (May 9, 1884, Carrol County, Mo.-November 19, 1955, Kansas City, Kans.). *Surgeon*. Son of Thomas Albert, farmer and banker, and Mildred Jane (Cook) Orr. Married Irene Harris, 1913; one son. EDUCATION: 1907, A.B., University of Missouri; 1910, M.D., Johns Hopkins; 1910-12, internship, New York Hospital; 1912-13, house officer, St. Mary's Free Hospital for Children. CAREER: 1915, began practice of surgery, Kansas City; at the University of Kansas School of Medicine, with time out for service in the Medical Corps (1918-19): 1915-24, professor of bacteriology, instructor in surgery, assistant professor of surgery, and chief of the Surgical Outpatient

Clinic; and 1924-49, professor and chairman of surgery, remaining as active professor until 1954; 1951, became editor, *The American Surgeon*, and at various times served on the editorial boards of *Surgery, Quarterly Review of Surgery, International Record of Medicine,* and *General Practice Clinics*; original member, American Board of Surgery; governor, American College of Surgeons; and president, American Surgical Association and Western Surgical Association. CONTRIBUTIONS: Made original contributions to the field of clinical investigation, especially in amputations, electrolytes and fluid balance, intestinal obstruction and the hepato-renal syndrome.

WRITINGS: Authored or shared in 231 scientific articles. *Modern Methods of Amputation* (1926); *Operations of General Surgery* (1944). REFERENCES: Stanley R. Friesen, "Thomas Grover Orr and Clinical Investigation," *Am. J. of Surg.* 116 (1968): 634-40.

R. Hudson

ORTON, SAMUEL TORREY (October 15, 1879, Columbus, Ohio-November 17, 1948, Poughkeepsie, N.Y.). *Physician; Neuropathology; Psychiatry.* Son of Edward, geologist and first president, Ohio State University, and Anna Davenport (Torrey) Orton. Married Mary Pelton Follett, 1908 (d. 1926), three children; June Frances Lyday, 1928. EDUCATION: 1901, B.S., Ohio State University; 1905, M.D., University of Pennsylvania; 1906, A.M., Harvard University; 1913-14, postgraduate study with Alzheimer, Breslau, Poland. CAREER: Pathologist: 1907-8, Columbus (Ohio) State Hospital; and 1908-9, St. Ann's Hospital, Anaconda, Mont.; and public health officer, Anaconda; 1910-12, pathologist, Worcester (Mass.) State Hospital, and assistant, neuropathology, Harvard Medical School; 1912, lecturer in neurology, Clark University; 1913, first neuropathologist, Harvard Medical School; 1914-19, at Department for Mental Diseases, Institute of Pennsylvania Hospital, Philadelphia, Pa.: 1914-17, pathologist and clinical director; and 1918-19, scientific director; 1919-27, professor of psychiatry and director, State Psychopathic Hospital, University of Iowa; 1920-30, member, Editorial Board, *Archives of Neurology and Psychiatry*; 1927-28, president, American Psychiatric Association; 1927-28, vice-president, American Neurological Association; 1929-36, professor of neurology and neuropathology, College of Physicians and Surgeons, Columbia University; 1929-36, neuropathologist, New York Neurological Institute; 1930, president, Association for Research in Nervous and Mental Diseases; 1935, recipient, Thomas W. Salmon Award and Lectureship; 1936-48, private practice in treatment of language disabilities (handicapped by peptic ulcers); 1943, consultant in language disabilities, Institute of Pennsylvania Hospital, Philadelphia. CONTRIBUTIONS: While at Worcester State Hospital, developed technical methods of study of the brain. As the first director, new State Psychopathic Hospital in Iowa City, organized a mobile mental hygiene unit (1926, first mobile unit in Ia. and second in the United States). Here began lifelong interest in the study and treatment of speech, reading, and writing disabilities in children. The Orton Society for professionals (in neurology, pediatrics, psychiatry, education, social work, psychology, and so on) and parents interested in developmental dyslexia was founded (1949) and named in honor of Orton, pioneer and noted authority in the field.

WRITINGS: "Some Technical Methods for the Routine Examination of the Brain from Cases of Mental Disease," *Worcester State Hospital Papers* (1912-13), 85; "An Analysis of the Errors in Diagnosis in a Series of Sixty Cases of Paresis," *J. of Nervous and Mental Diseases* 40 (1913): 779; "Word-Blindness in School Children," *Arch. Neurol. Psychiat.* 14 (1925): 581; "Physiological Theory of Reading Disability and Stuttering in Children," *New England J. of Med.* 199 (1928): 1046; "Neurologic Basis of Elementary Education," *Arch. Neurol. Psychiat.* 21 (1929): 641; "Special Disabilities in Writing," *Bull. Neurol. Inst. N.Y.* 3 (1933): 1 (with A. Gillingham); *The Development of Speech Understanding in Relation to Intelligence* (1934); *Reading, Writing and Speech Problems in Children* (1937); "Symposium on Behavior Problems in Children," *J. Conn. Med. Soc.* 3 (1939): 6 (with E. Kahn et al.). REFERENCES: *Arch. Neurol. Psychiat.* 61 (1949): 459; *Cumulative Index Medicus*; Paul E. Huston, "The Iowa State Psychopathic Hospital (Part One)," *JAMA* 139 (1949): 243; *NCAB*, D: 117, 37: 417; *Quarterly Cumulative Index to Current Medical Literature*; *Palimpsest* 54 (Nov.-Dec. 1973): 11; ibid., "(Part Two)" 55 (Jan.-Feb. 1974): 18; *Who Was Who in Am.*, 2 (1943-50); *Who's Important in Med.* (1945), 1028; *Who's Who in Am. Med., 1925*; *WWAPS* 1 (1938).

R. E. Rakel

OSBORNE, JOHN EUGENE (June 19, 1858 or June 9, 1858, Westport, N.Y.-April 24, 1943, Rawlins, Wyo.). *Physician; Politician.* Son of John C., saddler, and Mary E. (Reil) Osborne. Married Selina Smith, November 9, 1907; one daughter. EDUCATION: 1880, M.D., University of Vermont. CAREER: c. 1880s, medical practice and later established a drug store, Rawlins; 1882-87, surgeon, Union Pacific railroad; invested heavily in land and livestock; was considered to have owned the largest sheep ranch in Wyo.; 1882, elected to the territorial legislature; 1888, appointed chairman, state penitentiary commission, and served as mayor, Rawlins; 1897-99, served in the 55th Congress; 1892-95, governor, Wyo.; 1913-16, first assistant U.S. secretary of state. CONTRIBUTIONS: A leading early politician in Wyo. Abandoned practicing medicine generally, but was still known (1901) as a consulting physician and surgeon. REFERENCES: Thomas S. Chamblin, ed., *Historical Encyclopedia of Wyoming* (1955), 143; Ichabod S. Bartlett, *History of Wyoming* 3 (1918): 8; *Laramie Boomerang*, November 2, 1896; *NCAB* 11: 482; *Rawlins Republican Bulletin*, April 27, 1943; *Sheridan Newspaper*, October 16, 1917; *Who Was Who in Am.*, 4: 724; *Wyoming State Tribune*, April 25, 1943.

A. Palmieri

OSBORNE, THOMAS BURR (August 5, 1859, New Haven, Conn.-January 29, 1929, New Haven). *Biochemist; Protein chemistry.* Son of Arthur Dimon, banker, and Frances Louisa (Blake) Osborne. Married Elizabeth Annah Johnson, 1886; two children. EDUCATION: 1886-1928, analytical chemist, Connecticut Agricultural Experiment Station; 1904-28, research associate, Carnegie Institution of Washington; 1910, president, American Society of Biological Chemists; 1923-28, research associate in biochemistry, Yale University; director, Second

National Bank of New Haven. CONTRIBUTIONS: World's foremost authority on the proteins of plant seeds. Described more than 30 seeds, beginning with the oat kernel (1891). Made hydrolic decompositions of purified proteins, which revealed that proteins formerly thought to be identical, although obtained from different plant species, could usually be distinguished from one another on the basis of their amino acid composition (1906-9). With Lafayette B. Mendel (q.v.), spent remainder of life studying the nutritive properties of various proteins. Demonstrated that the amino acid lysine was necessary for normal growth. Found that butter contained a fat-soluble organic substance essential in nutrition (1913), later designated as vitamin A. Same observation was made a little earlier by E. V. McCollum (q.v.), who was credited with the discovery. Studied the distribution of vitamins in natural foodstuffs and the effects of various diets on growth and health. Work was largely responsible for the introduction of liver oil and orange juice in the diets of children. Helped edit *Journal of Biological Chemistry*.

WRITINGS: *Protein of the Wheat Kernel* (1907); *The Vegetable Proteins* (1909); "The Influence of Butter Fat on Growth," *J. Biol. Chem.* 16 (Dec. 1913): 423-37 (with L. B. Mendel); "The Influence of Cod Liver Oil and Some Other Fats on Growth," *J. Biol. Chem.* 17 (1914): 401-8 (with Lafayette B. Mendel). A bibliography is in *BMNAS* 14 (1931): 261-304. REFERENCES: *BHM* (1970-74), 133; *DAB*, 14: 74-75; *DSB*, 10: 241-44; *NCAB*, 21: 356; Hubert Bradford Vickery, "Thomas Burr Osborne," *J. of Nutrition* 59 (1956): 1-26; *Who Was Who in Am.*, 1: 921.

                                                                                    S. Galishoff

OSGOOD, EDWIN EUGENE (January 25, 1899, Fall River, Mass.-October 22, 1969, Portland, Oreg.). *Physician; Hematologist; Medical educator*. Son of William Pleasants, clergyman, and Lydia Lee (Smith) Osgood. Married Grace Elizabeth Haines, 1925; Mabel Mary Wilhelm, 1934; five children. EDUCATION: 1916-18, McMinnville College; University of Oregon: 1923, A.B.; and 1924, A.M. and M.D.; Multnomah Hospital: 1924-25, intern; and 1925-26, resident; 1926, studied at Mayo Clinic; 1927-28, studied at University of Vienna and at clinics in Basel, Switzerland; Freiburg and Berlin, Germany; Copenhagen, Denmark; and London, England. CAREER: 1928-69, medical faculty, University of Oregon. CONTRIBUTIONS: An authority on leukemia. Established first short-term culture of human bone-marrow cells (1936). Initiated the treatment of chronic leukemia by means of titrated, regularly spaced, total body X-ray irradiation (1941). Established first successful culture of cells from human leukemic blood (1954). Proposed a theory of the etiology of cancer that suggested cancer was caused by the absence of chemicals that normally regulate human cell growth (1957). Completed the Osgood Growth Prediction Charts designed to predict a child's growth from any age to adulthood (1961). Directed the first research team to unwind a human chromosome (1963).

WRITINGS: "A New Permanent Standard for Estimation of Hemoglobin by the Acid Hematin Method," *J. Biol. Chem.* 57 (1923): 107-10 (with H. H. Haskins); "Tables for Calculation of Color Index, Volume Index and Saturation Index Based on Recently Determined Standards," *J. Lab. and Clin. Med.* 12 (1927): 899-906; *An Atlas of Hem-*

atology (1937, with Clarice M. Ashworth). REFERENCES: *NCAB*, 57: 68-69; *Who Was Who in Am.*, 5: 549.

G. B. Dodds

OSLER, WILLIAM (July 12, 1849, Bond Head, Tecumseh County, Ontario, Canada-December 29, 1920, Norham Gardens, Oxford, England). *Physician.* Son of Rev. Featherston Lake, Episcopalian minister, and Mrs. Ellen (Pickton) Osler. Married Grace Linzee Revere, 1892; one child. EDUCATION: 1867-68, Trinity College, Ontario; 1872, M.D., McGill University; 1872-74, studied in London, Berlin, and Vienna. CAREER: 1874-84, lecturer and professor, McGill Medical School; and pathologist and physician, Montreal General Hospital; 1884-89, professor of clinical medicine, University of Pennsylvania Medical School; 1889-1905, physician-in-chief, Johns Hopkins University Hospital; and professor of medicine, Johns Hopkins Medical School; 1905-19, Regius professor of medicine, Oxford University. CONTRIBUTIONS: Member, Johns Hopkins Medical School "Big Four," and the leading authority on medical science in his day. His clinic at Hopkins set the pattern for modern clinical teaching, and his students and disciples played leading roles in dozens of medical institutions. Contributed to the understanding of the cardiovascular system, typhoid fever, and relationship of gallstones to typhoid, malaria, pneumonia, and tuberculosis. Active leader in the public health movement. An inspiring leader and a gifted writer whose bibliography consists of 730 titles. Textbook, *Principles and Practice of Medicine* (1892) was the standard work for more than 40 years. The continued existence of Osler Clubs today bespeaks the dramatic impact of his personality and success as a teacher.

WRITINGS: *Principles and Practice of Medicine* (1892); *Modern Medicine, Its Theory and Practice*, 7 vols. (1907-10, edited with Thomas McCrae); *The Evolution of Modern Medicine* (1921). For complete list, see Minnie Wright Blogg, comp., *Bibliography of Sir William Osler, 1870-1919* (1919). REFERENCES: Walter R. Bett, *Osler: The Man and the Legend* (1951); Harvey W. Cushing, *The Life of Sir William Osler*, 2 vols. (1940); *BHM* (1964-69), 198-99; (1970-74), 133; (1975-79), 94; (1980), 30-31; *DAB*, 14: 83-87; Edith G. Gettings, *The Great Physician, A Short Life of Sir William Osler* (1931); Kelly and Burrage (1928), 921-93; Miller, *BHM*, pp. 82-87; Sir William Osler Memorial Number, *Canadian Med. Assoc. J.* (1920).

J. Duffy

OTTO, JOHN CONRAD (March 15, 1774, near Woodbury, N.J.-June 26, 1844, Philadelphia, Pa.). *Physician; Hemophilia.* Son of Bodo, physician, and Catherine (Schweighauser) Otto. Married Eliza Tod, 1802; nine children. EDUCATION: 1792, B.A., College of New Jersey (now Princeton University); 1792, apprentice to Benjamin Rush (q.v.); 1796, M.D., University of Pennsylvania. CAREER: *Post* 1796, practiced medicine, Philadelphia; physician: 1798-1803, Philadelphia Dispensary; and 1813-34, Pennsylvania Hospital; 1832, chairman, committee of 12 leading physicians appointed to deal with cholera epidemic in Philadelphia; at Philadelphia College of Physicians: 1819, member; many years, censor; and 1840-44, vice-president; many years, physician, Orphan Asylum, Magdalen Asylum. CONTRIBUTIONS: Made first definitive clinical diagnosis of hemophilia, noting that females are not affected but may transmit the disease to their male children (1803); was one of the earliest significant contributions to medical science by an American.

WRITINGS: "An Account of an Hemorrhagic Disposition Existing in Certain Families," *Med. Repository* 6 (1803): 1-4. REFERENCES: *DAB*, 14: 109-110; Kelly and Burrage (1928), 925-26; R. F. Stone, *Biog. of Eminent Am. Physicians and Surgeons* (1894), 360; John H. Talbott, *Biographical Hist. of Med.* (1970), 372-73; *Who Was Who in Am.*, Hist. Vol.: 460.

S. Galishoff

OWENS-ADAIR, BETHENIA ANGELINA (February 7, 1840, Van Buren County, Mo.-September 11, 1926, Portland, Oreg.). *Physician; Social reformer.* Daughter of Thomas, farmer, and Sarah (Damron) Owens. Married Legrand Hill, 1854, one child; John Adair, 1884, one child. EDUCATION: 1874, M.D., Eclectic Medical College; 1880, M.D., University of Michigan; 1880-81, postgraduate study and clinical work, University of Michigan; Chicago, Ill.; and Europe. CAREER: Practice: 1874-78, 1881-87, Portland; 1888-89, Warrenton, Oreg.; and 1899-1905, North Yakima, Wash.; 1906-26, worked as social reformer. CONTRIBUTIONS: One of the first women with a medical degree to practice in Oreg. Over the intense opposition of male physicians, established a successful practice in Portland, rural Oregon, and North Yakima. An active member, Oregon State Medical Society. Became interested in the causes of temperance and woman suffrage and was chairman of the health and hygiene departments, Women's Christian Temperance Union. After retirement, became the pioneer advocate of eugenical sterilization in the Pacific Northwest. In speeches, writings, and lobbying, worked for the cause until it became adopted. Proposed that the Oreg. legislature adopt a bill to sterilize (with some exceptions) criminals, epileptics, insane, and feeble-minded persons in state institutions (1907). Such a bill was vetoed by the governor (1909). Bill was passed, but was defeated in a referendum (1913). Sterilization bill became law, but was declared unconstitutional (1917); later one was adopted (1923; amended in 1925).

WRITINGS: *Some of Her Life Experiences* (1906); *Human Sterilization* (1910); *Human Sterilization: It's* (sic) *Social and Legislative Aspects* (1922). REFERENCES: O. Larsell, *The Doctor in Oregon* (1947); *Notable Am. Women*, 2: 657-59.

G. B. Dodds

P

PACKARD, FRANCIS RANDOLPH (March 23, 1870, Philadelphia, Pa.-
April 18, 1950, Philadelphia). *Physician; Otolaryngology; Medical history.* Son
of John Hooker, physician, and Elizabeth (Wood) Packard. Married Christine
B. Curwen, 1899; Margaret Horstman, 1906, four children. EDUCATION: University of Pennsylvania: 1889, graduated, biology department; and 1892, M.D.;
1892-93, postgraduate work with William Osler (q.v.), Johns Hopkins Hospital;
1893-95, resident, Pennsylvania Hospital. CAREER: 1895-1950, practiced medicine, Philadelphia; *post* 1898, confined to otolaryngology; c.1897-c.1930, otolaryngology faculty, Philadelphia Polyclinic and College for Graduates in Medicine
(later affiliated with University of Pennsylvania); 1898, first lieutenant and assistant surgeon, Second Regiment, Pennsylvania Volunteer Infantry, Spanish-
American War; 1917-18, officer, Medical Corps, U.S. Army, attached to Base
Hospital 10, France; 1918-19, chief consultant in otolaryngology, District of
Paris; president: 1930, American Laryngological Association; 1936, American
Otological Society; and 1931-33, College of Physicians of Philadelphia. CON-
TRIBUTIONS: A noted otolaryngologist whose accomplishments included a mas-
toid periosteal elevator that was widely used for many years and a popular
textbook. Better known as a founder of American medical historiography. Most
important work was *The History of Medicine in the United States* (1901; 2d ed.,
2 vols., 1931); approach was largely biographical and often failed to distinguish
between the important and the trivial, but contained a wealth of information and
succeeded in arousing interest in medical history where little had existed before.
Founded and edited *Annals of Medical History* (1917-1942).

WRITINGS: *Textbook of Diseases of the Nose, Throat and Ear. . .* (1909); *The School
of Salerno* (1920); *Life and Times of Ambroise Paré* (1921); *Some Account of the Pennsylvania Hospital. . . to . . . 1938* (1938). A bibliography is in *Bull. Hist. Med.* REF-
ERENCES: W. B. McDaniel, "Francis R. Packard and His Role in Medical Historiography,"

Bull. Hist. Med. 25 (1951): 66-85; Miller, *BHM*, p. 87; *NCAB*, 39: 106-7; *Who Was Who in Am.*, 3: 660.

S. *Galishoff*

PADGETT, EARL CALVIN (July 8, 1893, Greenleaf, Kans.-December 2, 1946, Kansas City, Mo.). *Plastic surgeon.* Son of John Manson, a banker, and Martha (McGinnis) Padgett. Married Winona Youman, 1921; three children. EDUCATION: 1916, B.S., University of Kansas; 1918, M.D., Washington University; 1919-22, house officer, Barnes Hospital, and then assistant to Dr. Vilray P. Blair (q.v.) in plastic surgery for two years. CAREER: 1925, a brilliant surgeon, joined the faculty of the University of Kansas and rose to clinical professor of plastic surgery (1936), a position he held until his death. CONTRIBUTIONS: Greatest contribution was his share of the Padgett-Hood dermatome. Conceived the idea of bringing and holding the skin to a smooth fixed surface so a blade could be passed at a controlled distance, resulting in a large skin graft of uniform thickness (1930). Device was perfected over a seven-year period in collaboration with a University of Kansas professor of engineering, George J. Hood, and used for the first time on January 11, 1938. Invention was widely acclaimed and heavily used during World War II. A priority fight erupted when Hood attempted to secure a patent on the dermatome. Many aspects of the story remain unresolved. It appears certain, however, that the basic idea was Padgett's. What is unclear is who deserves credit for the many changes involved as the dermatome evolved.

WRITINGS: In addition to some 65 articles mostly devoted to problems of plastic surgery, Padgett authored three books: *Surgical Diseases of the Mouth and Jaws* (1938); *Skin Grafting from a Personal and Experimental Point of View* (1942); *Plastic and Reconstructive Surgery* (1948, with Kathryn L. Stephenson). REFERENCES: Lynn D. Ketchum, "An Historical Account of the Development of the Calibrated Dermatome, " *Annals of Plastic Surg.* 1 (1978): 608-11;:Edward A. Kitlowski, "Earl C. Padgett, M.D.," *Plastic and Reconstructive Surg.* 2 (1947): 283-85; *NCAB*, 37: 549.

R. *Hudson*

PAINE, MARTYN (July 8, 1794, Williamstown, Vt.-November 10, 1877, New York, N.Y.). *Physician.* Son of Elijah, farmer, jurist, and U.S. senator, and Sarah (Porter) Paine. Married Mary Ann Weeks, 1825; three children. EDUCATION: Academy of Mr. Vase, Atkinson, N.H.; 1813, A.B., Harvard College; 1813-16, apprenticeship to John and John C. Warren (q.v.); 1816, M.D., Harvard University. CAREER: private practice: 1816-22, Montreal, Quebec, Canada; and 1822-77, New York City; at University Medical College, N.Y.: 1841-50, professor of institutes of medicine and materia medica; 1850-67, professor of therapeutics; and 1867-77, professor emeritus. CONTRIBUTIONS: An influential member of the N.Y. medical profession and one of the prime movers in the organization of the University Medical College (1838-41). Personally lobbied for the N.Y. State anatomy act of 1854 and credited by many with the success of the efforts to liberalize regulations surrounding dissection. Influence could also be used for conservative purposes, and it was probably his attack (1846) on Nathan Smith Davis (q.v.) and the idea of a national medical convention that convinced many physicians outside N.Y. to participate in meetings that led to the founding of AMA. Attacked the introduction of Pierre Louis's numerical method into medicine (1840) and Charles Lyell's concept of uniformitarian geology (1856). A popular teacher but continued to teach vitalistic physiology and antiphlogistic therapeutics throughout long teaching career. Influential textbooks extended the influence of these ideas beyond his immediate students.

WRITINGS: *Medical and Physiological Commentaries*, 3 vols. (1840-44); *Defense of the Medical Profession in the United States* (1846); *The Institutes of Medicine* (1847), nine editions during Paine's lifetime; *Materia Medica and Therapeutics* (1848), three editions in Paine's lifetime; *On Theoretical Geology* (1856). Many lectures and articles listed in the Index Catalogue. REFERENCES: *DAB*, 7 pt. 2: 153-54; Samuel Francis, "Biographical Sketches of Distinguished Living New York Physicians—Martyn Paine, M.D., LL.D.," *Med. Surg. Reporter* 15 (1866): 63-67; *NCAB*, 11: 551; "Prof. Martyn Paine, M.D.," *Med. Record* 12 (1877): 735.

D. C. Smith

PALMER, ALONZO BENJAMIN   (October 6, 1815, Richfield, N.Y.-December 23, 1887, Ann Arbor, Mich.). *Physician; Pathology; Medical education.* Son of Benjamin, farmer, and Anna (Layton) Palmer. Married Caroline Augusta Wright, 1843, no children; married Love M. Root, 1867, no children. EDUCATION: 1839, M.D., College of Physicians and Surgeons of the Western District of New York (Fairfield, N.Y.); 1847-48, 1848-49, postgraduate study, College of Physicians and Surgeons (N.Y.) and University of Pennsylvania; 1859, 1879, 1880, study in Europe. CAREER: 1839-50, practice of medicine, Tecumseh, Mich.; 1850-53, medical practice with Nathan S. Davis (q.v.), Chicago, Ill.; 1852-55, city physician, Chicago; at University of Michigan medical department: 1852, 1854-87, faculty; 1860-87, professor of pathology and the theory and practice of medicine; and 1875-79, 1880-87, dean; 1855-60, editor, *Peninsular Journal of Medicine*; 1860, vice-president, American Medical Association; 1861, surgeon, Second Michigan Infantry; 1864-67, professor of pathology, Berkshire Medical Institution (Pittsfield, Mass.); 1869-79, professor of the practice of medicine, Bowdoin College; 1872, president, Michigan State Medical Society. CONTRIBUTIONS: Created a regular program of clinical instruction at St. Mary's Hospital, Detroit, Mich., for University of Michigan medical students (1858) long before most other medical schools offered such a course; led the faculty support for creation of the first University-owned teaching hospital in the United States (1869); as dean, instituted one of the first successful three-year medical curricula (1880). Early recognized that alcohol was a depressant, not a stimulant, and opposed the medical use of both alcohol and opiates.

WRITINGS: *Four Lectures on Homeopathy* (1869); *The New Departure in Medical Teaching: A Lecture Delivered at the Beginning of the Course on Pathology* (1877); *A Treatise on the Science and Practice of Medicine, or, the Pathology and Therapeutics of Internal Diseases*, 2 vols. (1882); *A Treatise on Epidemic Cholera and Allied Diseases*

(1885). Writings listed in Love Palmer, *Memorial of Alonzo Benjamin Palmer, M.D.* (1890), 166-67. REFERENCES: *DAB*, 14: 175; Burke Hinsdale, *History of the University of Michigan* (1906), 226; Kelly and Burrage (1928), 932-33; Corydon La Ford, *A Memorial Discourse on the Life and Services of Alonzo Benjamin Palmer* (1888); Palmer, *Memorial of Alonzo Benjamin Palmer*; *Representative Men of Michigan: American Biographical History of Eminent and Self-Made Men* (1878), district 2: 57-58; Wilfred Shaw, *The University of Michigan: An Encyclopedic Survey* (1951), pt. 5; *Who Was Who in Am.*, Hist. Vol.: 463.

M. Pernick

PALMER, BARTLETT JOSHUA (September 10, 1881, What Cheer, Ia.-May 27, 1961, Sarasota, Fla.). *Chiropractor*. Son of Daniel David (q.v.), chiropractor, and Lavina (McGhee) Palmer. Married Mabel Heath, 1904; one child. EDUCATION: High school, Davenport, Ia.; 1902, D.D., Palmer School of Chiropractic, Davenport. CAREER: 1902-61, practitioner and teacher of chiropractic (Palmer School of Chiropractic). CONTRIBUTIONS: Leading developer of chiropractic as an alternative system of healing. Pioneer in application of X-rays to chiropractic diagnosis. Inventor of neurocalometer (1922), dubious instrument for detecting subluxations of spinal column. President, International Chiropractic Association (1926-61).

WRITINGS: *The Philosophy and Principles of Chiropractic Adjustments* (1908); *The Tyranny of Therapeutical Transgressions* (1916); *Up from Below the Bottom* (1950). REFERENCES: Russell Gibbons, "Chiropractic History. Turbulence and Triumph," in *Who's Who in Chiropractic International, 1976-1978* (1977), 139-48; idem, *Chiropractic History: Lost, Strayed or Stolen* (1975); *NCAB*, 47: 566-67; obituary, *N.Y. Times*, May 28, 1961, p. 64.

J. C. Whorton

PALMER, DANIEL DAVID (March 7, 1845, Lake Skoogag, Canada, near Toronto, Ontario-October 20, 1913, Los Angeles, Calif.). *Physician*; *Chiropractor*. Son of Thomas and Catherine (McVay) Palmer. Married several times; last wife, Lavinia T. McGhee; son by this marriage was Bartlett Joshua Palmer (q.v.), who assumed management of Davenport, Ia., school. EDUCATION: Went to the United States at age 16 and taught school in Ill. and Ia.; in Burlington, Ia., educated in magnetic healing by Paul Coster. CAREER: Teacher and grocer before becoming a magnetic healer, 1883-95; 1895, moved to Davenport and attempted spinal adjustments while treating a patient for deafness; 1898, started Palmer School with one pupil; 1902, son graduated from his school; 1903, moved to Portland, Oreg. where he opened a school that closed in two years; 1906, returned to Davenport and was arrested for practicing medicine without a license; served six months in jail; 1906, moved to Oklahoma City, Okla., where he opened a school with a lawyer friend, Willard Carver; ended partnership with Carver and published his book of chiropractic; moved back to Portland, where he spent his time on publications. CONTRIBUTIONS: Simplified Andrew Still's (q.v.) theory of disease by confining treatment to spinal displacement—chiropractic. Theory was that body functions receive all vital forces through the nervous system and that disease can be treated by adjusting displaced or off-centerings (subluxations) of vertebra by hand pressure. Spinal manipulation is distinguished in chiropractic by suddenness and speed of the maneuver that prevents any control by the patient; this is called "dynamic thrust." Associates expanded his theory and used other therapeutic measures like diet and massage. Exponents who used other techniques were called "mixers"; the straights used only manipulation. Palmer's son B.J. led the "straights" from the Davenport school. B.J. expanded the profession and designed equipment like the neuro-calometer to locate "pinched" nerves. Eventually, the "mixers" dominated the chiropractic field and popularized the use of heat, massage, exercise, and the use of electricity as an adjunct to adjustments.

WRITINGS: *Text Book of the Science of Chiropractic* (1906); *Science, Art and Philosophy of Chiropractic* (1910). REFERENCES: *Chiropractic, State of the Art* (1981); *DAB*, 7: 177; Thorp McClusky, *Your Health and Chiropractic* (1957), 254.; *NCAB*, 18: 301.

R. Edwards

PALMER, ERROLL PAYNE (October 30, 1876, Church Hill, Miss.-February 6, 1955, Phoenix, Ariz.). *Physician; Surgeon.* Son of George Alfred, civil engineer, and Virginia (Payne) Palmer. Married Bertha Louise Schantz, 1907; seven children. EDUCATION: Chamberlin Hunt Academy, Port Gibson, Miss.; 1898, M.D., Barnes Medical College, St. Louis (now part of Washington University); 1909-10, study, universities of Berlin and Vienna, Royal College of Surgeons at St. Bartholomew's Hospital in London, Cornell University, N.Y.C. CAREER: 1900-1955, private practice, Phoenix. CONTRIBUTIONS: Considered the best and most noted surgeon in the community in his day; served as chief surgeon, St. Joseph Hospital, Phoenix. A founding member, American College of Surgeons, and governor of the organization (1923).

REFERENCES: *Arizona Republic* (Phoenix), February 7, 1960; *NCAB*, G: 339; Edward H. Peplow, Jr., *History of Arizona* (1955).

J. S. Goff

PALMER, THOMAS MARTIN (Jan. 6, 1821, Pendelton District, S.C.-June 3, 1895, Monticello, Fla.). *Physician (general practice); Hospital administrator; Druggist.* Son of Martin, wealthy planter, and Amelia (Miles) Palmer. Married sisters Jane Denham, 1847, four children; Jessie Denham, 1862. EDUCATION: Early education, schools of Monticello, Jefferson County, Fla; 1844, M.D., University of Maryland School of Medicine. CAREER: 1844-61, practice, Monticello; 1861, outspoken Secessionist, member of Florida Secession Convention, signer of Ordinance of Secession; 1861, surgeon, Second Florida Infantry Regiment; 1861-64, chief surgeon, Florida Hospital, near Richmond, Va.; 1864-65, chief surgeon, General Confederate Hospital, Richmond; 1865-93, practice and proprietor of drug store, Monticello; 1876, president, Florida Medical Association. CONTRIBUTIONS: Archetype of the successful country doctor of Fla. in mid-nineteenth century. Routine practice: delivering babies, treating fever victims, dressing wounds, and frequently employing his surgical skills. Highly esteemed by medical colleagues; beloved by citizens of community. Foremost advocate for improving quality of medical practice and raising standards for licensing physicians in Fla.; provided strong support for establishment and success of Florida Medical Association. First of 15 members of the Palmer family who became physicians.

WRITINGS: "The Medical History of Florida," *Proc., Fla. Med. Assoc.* (1877), 29-40. REFERENCES: *Family Friend* (Monticello), 1859-63; *Florida Sentinel* (Tallahassee), 1852-62; National Archives, Service Records, CSA, M251, Roll 40; Washington, D.C.; Theresa Yeager Palmer, comp., *The Palmer Physicians* (1966), 1-5; useful genealogical table appended to *Proc., Fla. Med. Assoc.* (1876).

E. A. Hammond

PANCOAST, JOSEPH (November 23, 1805, Burlington, N.J.-March 7, 1882, Philadelphia, Pa.). *Anatomist; Surgeon.* Son of John and Ann (Abbott) Pancoast. Married Rebecca Abbott, 1829. EDUCATION: 1828, M.D., University of Pennsylvania. CAREER: 1828, began medical and surgical practice, Philadelphia; 1831-38, conducted the Philadelphia School of Anatomy; 1835, elected physician, Philadelphia (Blockley) Hospital; 1838-45, visiting surgeon, Philadelphia Hospital; Jefferson Medical College: 1838-41, professor of surgery; 1841-74, professor of anatomy; 1854-64, surgical staff, Pennsylvania Hospital. CONTRIBUTIONS: Leading surgeon known for pioneering new operations, including ones for exstrophy of the bladder (1868), soft and mixed cataracts, empyema, occlusion of the nasal duct, and strabismus. Developed the plow and groove suture used in rhinoplasty. Originated an abdominal tourniquet (1860). Performed operation which cured some cases of tic douloureaux (1862).

WRITINGS: *Treatise on Operative Surgery* (1844, with two more editions). Also translated European works into English and edited Wistar and Horner's *System of Anatomy* (1839, 1843, 1846). REFERENCES: *DAB*, 7, pt. 2:198-99; Kelly and Burrage (1928), 934-35.

M. Kaufman

PAPANICOLAOU, GEORGE NICHOLAS (May 13, 1883, Kimi, Greece-February 19, 1962, Miami, Fla.). *Physician; Reproductive physiology; Exfoliative cytology.* Son of Nicholas, physician, and Mary (Critsutas) Papanicolaou. Married Mary A. Mavroyeni, 1910; no children. EDUCATION: 1904, M.D., University of Athens; 1910, Ph.D., University of Munich. CAREER: 1911, physiologist, Oceanographic Institute of Monaco; 1912-13, Medical Corps, Greek army; 1913, went to the United States; 1927, naturalized; *post* 1913, pathology staff, New York Hospital; 1914-61, anatomy faculty, Cornell Medical College; director, Papanicolaou Research Laboratory; and consultant, Papanicolaou Cytology Laboratory, Cornell Medical College; 1961, director, Papanicolaou Cancer Research Institute (Miami, Fla.). CONTRIBUTIONS: Pioneered the use of vaginal smears to study the guinea pig ovarian cycle; found that changes in the form of the epithelial cells could be correlated with the four stages of the animal's estrus cycle (1917); was used as a tool for measuring the sexual cycle of other laboratory animals and for determining the effects of the sex hormones. Studied the cytology of human vaginal fluid and found cancer cells in the smears of women with cervical cancer (1923); realized that this provided a means for diagnosing the disease but could not persuade physicians who continued to rely upon biopsy and endometrial curettage; gained the support of Joseph C. Hinsey, dean, Cornell Medical College, who (1940) encouraged Papanicolaou to devote his entire time to early cancer detection through recovery and identification of exfoliated cancer cells; led to authoritative publications on the subject (1940s and 1950s), which won acceptance for the eponymically-named Pap smear test as a routine screening technique; has led to sharp decline in deaths from cervical cancer, formerly the leading cause of cancer mortality in women. Extended technique to the diagnosis of cancer of other organs in which smears of exfoliated tissues could be made. Trained thousands of students in the microscopial detection of neoplastic disease.

WRITINGS: *Diagnosis of Uterine Cancer by the Vaginal Smears* (1943, with Herbert F. Traut); *The Epithelia of Women's Reproductive Organs* (1948, with Herbert F. Traut and Andrew A. Marchetti); *Atlas of Exfoliative Cytology* (1954). A bibliography is in D. Erskine Carmichael, *The Pap Smear: Life of George N. Papanicolaou* (1973). REFERENCES: *BHM* (1975-79), 95; Charles S. Cameron, "Dedication of the Papanicolaou Cancer Research Institute," *JAMA* 182 (1962): 556-59; *DSB*, 10: 291-92; Miller, *BHM*, p. 148; *NCAB*, 50: 52-53; *Who Was Who in Am.*, 4: 730-31.

S. Galishoff

PARK, ROSWELL (May 4, 1852, Pomfret, Conn.-February 15, 1914, Buffalo, N.Y.). *Surgeon.* Son of Rev. Roswell, minister and college president, and Mrs. Mary Brewster (Baldwin) Park. Married Martha Prudence Durkee, 1880; two sons. EDUCATION: Racine College (Wis.): 1872, B.A.; and 1875, M.A.; 1876, M.D., Northwestern University College of Medicine. CAREER: 1877-79, demonstrator of anatomy, Woman's Medical College of Chicago; 1879-82, adjunct professor of anatomy, Northwestern University; 1882, lecturer on surgery, Rush Medical College; 1883-1914, professor of surgery, University of Buffalo; and surgeon-in-chief, Buffalo General Hospital. CONTRIBUTIONS: Played a major role in the application of Listerian antiseptic techniques to American surgery, through writings and practices. Specialized in surgical pathology. A founder of the Gratwick Laboratory, which became the New York State Institute for the Study of Malignant Diseases. Attended President William McKinley when he was shot at the Pan-American Exposition in Buffalo (1901).

WRITINGS: *The Mutter Lectures on Surgical Pathology* (1892); *Surgery by American Authors* (1896); *An Epitome of the History of Medicine* (1897); *Principles and Practices of Modern Surgery* (1907). REFERENCES: *DAB*, 7: 207-8; Kelly and Burrage (1928), 936-37; *NCAB*, 8: 220; *N.Y. Times*, February 16, 1914; *Who Was Who in Am.*, 1: 934.

M. Kaufman

PARK, WILLIAM HALLOCK (December 30, 1863, New York, N.Y.-April 6, 1939, New York). *Physician; Microbiology; Public Health*. Son of Rufus, wholesale grocer, and Harriet Joanna (Hallock) Park. Never married. CAREER: 1883, A.B., College of the City of New York; 1886, M.D., College of Physicians and Surgeons (Columbia); 1886-89, intern, Roosevelt Hospital; 1889-90, studied at the University of Vienna. CAREER: 1890-c. 93, practiced medicine, New York City; 1893-1936, at Bureau of Laboratories, New York City Department of Public Health: 1910-36, director; at Bellevue Hospital Medical College (later New York University College of Medicine): 1895-97, contagious diseases faculty; 1897-1900, bacteriology and hygiene faculty; 1900-1933, bacteriology faculty; and 1933-37, preventive medicine faculty; *post* 1914, consulting bacteriologist, New York State Department of Health; *post* 1921, U.S. quarantine service; president: 1912, Society of American Bacteriologists; 1920, Society for Experimental Pathology; and 1923, American Public Health Association. CONTRIBUTIONS: Pioneered in applying bacteriological methods to improving the public health. Did most important work on diphtheria; demonstrated that the Klebs-Löffler bacillus, and not a protozoa as suggested by T. Mitchell Prudden (q.v.), was responsible for the disease; established the role of convalescent and well carriers in transmitting the disease and made physicians aware of the need for bacteriological examination of suspected cases; produced the first diphtheria antitoxin made in the United States, which was more potent than the European serums; initiated a comprehensive program of active immunization of New York City schoolchildren with toxin-antitoxin (1920); program was copied in cities all across the nation and led to the virtual eradication of diphtheria. Educated physicians and the public about the dangers of raw and dirty milk and succeeded (1914) in getting the health department to require compulsory pasteurization of nearly all of the city's milk supply. With A. R. Guerard, wrote *Bacteriology in Medicine and Surgery: A Practical Manual for Physicians, Health Officers and Students* (1899), an authoritative textbook that by 1939 had run through 11 editions.

WRITINGS: "Diphtheria and Pseudo-Diphtheria. A Report. . .on the Bacteriological Examination of 5,611 Cases of Suspected Diphtheria. . .,"*Med. Record* 46 (1894): 385-401 (with A. L. Beebe); *Public Health and Hygiene* (1920, editor and contributor); "Toxin-Antitoxin Immunization Against Diphtheria," *JAMA* 79 (1922): 1584-91; *Who's Who Among the Microbes* (1929, with Anna W. Williams). Most important writings are in Wade W. Oliver, *The Man Who Lived for Tomorrow: A Biography of William Hallock Park, M.D.* (1941), "References," 473-88. REFERENCES: *DAB*, Supplement 2: 513-14; *NCAB*, C: 314; *N.Y. Times*, April 7, 1939.

S. Galishoff

PARKER, PETER (June 18, 1804, Framingham, Mass.-January 10, 1888, Washington, D.C.). *Medical missionary; Diplomat*. Son of Nathan, farmer, and

Catherine (Murdock) Parker. Married Harriet Colby Webster, 1841; one child. EDUCATION: 1827-30, attended Amherst College; graduated from Yale University, 1831, studied theology at Yale Divinity School and was licensed to preach in 1833, M.D., 1834; ordained to the Presbyterian ministry, 1834. CAREER: 1834, appointed missionary physician to China by the American Board of Commissioners of Foreign Missions; 1834-35, maintained a dispensary in Singapore; 1835-55, operated a hospital in Canton; 1838, opened a hospital in Macao; 1844, secretary to Caleb Cushing when negotiating first treaty between United States and China; 1845, secretary to American delegation, during interims between commissioners was chargé d'affaires; 1855-57, American Commissioner and Minister to China; 1857-88, lived in Washington, D.C., involved in the affairs of the American Evangelical Alliance and the Smithsonian Institution. CONTRIBUTIONS: The first Protestant medical missionary to China. Operated a hospital in Canton for 20 years that specialized in ophthalmic treatment, especially the removal of cataracts. Instrumental in the organization of the Medical Missionary Society in China.

REFERENCES: *Bibl. Hist. Med.* (1964-69), 202; (1970-74), 136; (1975-79), 96; *DAB*, 14: 234-35; E.V. Gulick, *Peter Parker and the Opening of China* (1973); Miller, *BHM*, p. 88; *NCAB*, 10: 284-85; *Who Was Who in Am.*, Hist. Vol.: 465.

S. Galishoff

PARKER, WILLARD (September 2, 1800, Lyndeborough, N.H.-April 25, 1884, New York, N.Y.). *Physician; Educator; Surgery; Public health.* Son of Jonathan, farmer, and Hannah (Clark) Parker. Married Caroline Sarah Allen, 1831, two children; Mary Ann (Bissell) Coit, 1844, three children. EDUCATION: Harvard University: 1826, B.A.; and 1830, M.D.; 1827-29, house physician, U.S. Marine Hospital, Chelsea, Mass.; 1829-30, house surgeon, Massachusetts General Hospital; 1831, M.D., Berkshire Medical Institution; 1837-38, studied medicine in Paris. CAREER: 1830-33, anatomy and surgery faculty, Berkshire Medical Institution; 1834-36, anatomy faculty, Geneva Medical College; 1836-37, surgery faculty, Cincinnati Medical College; 1839-70, principles and practice of surgery faculty, College of Physicians and Surgeons (Columbia); 1865, president, New York State Inebriate Asylum at Binghampton; 1866, commissioner, New York Metropolitan Board of Health; and surgical staff, New York, St. Luke's, Roosevelt, and Mount Sinai hospitals; 1856, president, New York Academy of Medicine. CONTRIBUTIONS: An outstanding surgeon and teacher. Originated cystotomy for the treatment of chronic cystitis (1850). Ligated the subclavian artery for aneurysm on five occasions. First American to operate successfully for appendicitis (1864); advocated operating in the early stages of the disease before gross suppuration appeared. Active in public health and temperance movements. Secured the establishment of a hospital for infectious diseases in N.Y. that was named in his honor.

WRITINGS: "Cystitis; Lateral Operation on the Bladder, Death; Tuberculous Kidney," *N.Y. Med. J.*, n.s., 7 (Jul. 1851): 83-86; "Ligature of the Left Subclavian Inside the

Scalenus Muscle, Together with Common Carotid and Vertebral Arteries for Subclavian Aneurism. . . ,'' *Am. Med. Times* 8 (1864): 114-16; "An Operation for Abcess of the Appendix Vermiformis Caeci," *Med. Record* 2 (1867): 25-27. REFERENCES: William B. Atkinson, *Physicians and Surgeons of the U.S.* (1878), 482-83; *DAB*, 14: 242-43; Kelly and Burrage (1928), 939; *NCAB*, 9: 337; John H. Talbott, *Biographical History of Medicine* (1970), 559-61; *Who Was Who in Am.*, Hist. Vol.: 466.

S. Galishoff

PARMLY, ELEAZAR (March 13, 1797, Braintree Township, Orange County, Vermont-December 13, 1874, New York, N.Y.). *Dentist*. Son of Eleazer and Hannah (Spear) Parmly. Married Anna Maria Valk Smith, 1827; nine children. EDUCATION: 1810-12, attended school in Montreal, Canada; 1814-17, apprentice to Levi Spear Parmly, his brother, in Montreal (1814-15) and Quebec (1815-17); 1819, studied under J.F.C. Maury, Paris, France. CAREER: 1812-14, reporter, compositor, general assistant, *Canadian Courant*, Montreal; 1814, teacher, Orange County, Vermont; 1815-17, dental practice, Quebec; 1817-19, itinerant dentist, Ohio and Mississippi River settlements; 1819-21, dental practice, London, England; 1821-66, dental practice, New York City. CONTRIBUTIONS: A leading figure in the establishment of dentistry as a profession in America. Taught or worked with core of early dentists in New York City, including Solyman Brown and several of Parmly's relatives. Had one of the largest dental practices in the United States. Founded and served as first president of the first dental association (1834), the Society of Surgeon Dentists of the City and State of New York. Helped establish first dental periodical, the *American Journal of Dental Science*, and served on first editorial board. A founder of the American Society of Dental Surgeons (1840) and several times an officer. First president of the New York College of Dentistry (1866).

WRITINGS: *An Essay on the Disorders and Treatments of the Teeth* (1821). REFERENCES: *DAB*, 14: 251-52; *NCAB*, 28: 210-11; *Who Was Who in Am.*, Hist. Vol.: 395.

T. L. Savitt

PARRAN, THOMAS (September 28, 1892, St. Leonard, Md.-February 17, 1968, Pittsburgh, Pa.). *Physician; Public health administrator*. Son of Benjamin and Mary S. (Latimer) Parran. Married Angela Bentley Vandoren, 1918, four children; Buda Carroll Keller, 1930. EDUCATION: St. Johns College (Annapolis, Md.): 1911, B.A.; and 1915, M.A.; 1915, M.D., Georgetown University. CAREER: 1917-48, with U.S. Public Health Service: 1917-26, assigned mainly to rural sanitation and county health work; 1926-30, chief, division of venereal diseases; and 1936-48, surgeon-general; 1930-36, New York State Health Commissioner; 1946, president, United Nations Health Conference; 1948-58, first dean, University of Pittsburgh Graduate School of Public Health. CONTRIBUTIONS: Fought to eliminate the Victorian prudery that shrouded the nation's venereal disease problem. Inaugurated a national campaign to educate the public about venereal disease and persuaded universities to give the subject more attention in their teaching and research. Largely responsible for making the Wasserman test a requirement to obtain a marriage license. Encouraged adoption of the principles of anonymity, compulsory notification, and case-work investigation that together with the introduction of antibiotic therapy resulted in a sharp decline in the incidence of venereal disease (1940s and 1950s). Chief architect of American and international public health work in the post-World War II period. Oversaw the creation of the National Institutes of Health, which established the national government as the principal patron of health science research; prepared the way for the passage of the first Mental Health Act, the Hill-Burton Act (hospital construction), and the establishment of the Communicable Disease Center (later Center for Disease Control). Participated in the planning of the World Health Organization (1946).

WRITINGS: *Shadow on the Land* (1937); *Plain Words About Venereal Diseases* (1941). REFERENCES: *Current Biog.* (1940), 629-31; Bess Furman, *A Profile of the United States Public Health Service, 1798-1948* (1973), 389-462; *NCAB*, F: 436-37; *N.Y. Times*, February 17, 1968; *Trans., Assoc. of Am. Physicians* 83 (1970): 30-31; *Who Was Who in Am.*, 4: 734.

S. Galishoff

PARRISH, ISAAC (March 19, 1811, Philadelphia, Pa.-July 31, 1852, Philadelphia). *Physician; Ophthalmic surgery.* Son of Joseph, physician, and Susanna (Coxe) Parrish. Married Sarah Redwood Longstreth, 1834. EDUCATION: 1829, began medical studies with his father; 1832, M.D., University of Pennsylvania; 1831-32, intern, Blockley Hospital. CAREER: 1832-c.1852, practiced medicine, Philadelphia; 1834-52, surgical staff, Wills Hospital; active in prison reform and other social movements. CONTRIBUTIONS: Gave the first course in ophthalmic surgery at Wills Hospital (1839). Early suppporter of the use of ether and chloroform. First American to report formally a case of malignant melanoma.

WRITINGS: "Remarks on Spinal Irritation as Connected with Nervous Diseases," *Am. J. of Med. Sci.* 10 (1832): 294-314; "Case of Melanosis," ibid. 20 (1837): 266-68. REFERENCES: Kelly and Burrage (1920), 886; Willard L. Marmelzat, "The First Case of Malignant Melanoma Formerly Reported in America. . . ," *J. of Dermatologic Surg. and Oncology* 3 (1977): 30-31; *NCAB*, 12: 486; *Who Was Who in Am.*, Hist. Vol.: 467.

S. Galishoff

PARRISH, JOSEPH (November 11, 1818, Philadelphia, Pa.-January 15, 1891, Burlington, N.J.). *Physician.* Son of Joseph, physician, and Susanna (Cox) Parrish. Married Lydia Gaskill, 1840; three children. EDUCATION: Tutored privately; Philadelphia Quaker schools; Burlington Academy; 1844, M.D., University of Pennsylvania Medical School. CAREER: 1844-55, private practice, Burlington; 1856, medical faculty, Philadelphia Medical College; 1857-63, superintendent, Pennsylvania School for Feeble Minded Children; 1863-65, member, U.S. Sanitary Commission; 1867-74, head, Pennsylvania Sanitarium; 1872-74, head, Maryland Inebriate Asylum; 1875, resumed private practice, Burlington. CONTRIBUTIONS: Established (1847) and edited (1848-55) the *New Jersey*

Medical and Surgical Reporter, and *Transactions of the New Jersey Medical Society*, the first professional medical publication in the state. Founder (1870) and president (1872-91), American Association for the Study and Cure of Inebriety. Taught that inebriety was a disease and not a crime.

WRITINGS: *Alcoholic Inebriety from a Medical Standpoint* (1883); *Sanitary Commission Bulletin* (editor). REFERENCES: *Appleton's CAB*, 4: 659-60, D. C. English, "Joseph Parrish, M.D.," *Trans. Med. Soc. N.J.* (1891), 243-54; Kelly and Burrage (1928), 942; *NCAB*, 12: 486-87.

W. Barlow

PARSONS, MARY ALMERA (May 2, 1850, Colebrook, N.H.-January 12, 1944, Washington, D.C.). *Physician*. Daughter of Hezekiah III and Sarah M. (Bragg) Parsons. Never married. EDUCATION: 1870, graduated from the Robinson Female Seminary, Exeter, N.H.; 1874, M.D., Howard University. CAREER: General practitioner in D.C. for 60 years. CONTRIBUTIONS: Pioneering role in breaking down the barriers that barred women physicians in D.C. from the full privileges of their professional practice. Appealed to Congress to amend the charter of the Medical Society of the District of Columbia by changing the word *gentlemen* to *persons*, so that women physicians could be licensed. The amendment was approved (1875) and she, with Dr. Mary Spackman, became the first licensed women physicians in the District. Beginning in 1876, repeatedly applied for membership, Medical Society of the District of Columbia, and finally (1888) was the first woman admitted and the first woman elected vice-president (1901). A founder and first president (1909-13), Women's Medical Society of the District of Columbia. Appointed to the Committee of Women Physicians on the Council of National Defense during World War I. REFERENCES: Edith SeVille Coale, "Women Physicians of the District of Columbia," in John C. Proctor, ed., *Washington: Past and Present* 2 (1930): 656-58; D. S. Lamb et al., *History of the Medical Society of the District of Columbia, 1817-1909* (1909), 120, 330; obituary, *Washington Post*, January 14, 1944.

R. A. Kondratas

PARSONS, USHER (August 18, 1788, Alfred, Maine-December 19, 1868, Providence, R.I.). *Physician; Surgery*. Son of William, farmer, trader, and lumberman, and Abigail (Blunt) Parsons. Married Mary Jackson Holmes, 1822; one child. EDUCATION: 1807-12, studied medicine with various physicians in New England; 1812, licensed to practice medicine by Massachusetts Medical Society; 1818, M.D., Harvard Medical College. CAREER: 1812-23, Medical Corps, U.S. Navy, rising in rank from surgeon's mate to surgeon: 1812-13, in charge of sick and wounded at Black Rock; 1813, served with Commodore Perry, Battle of Lake Erie; 1813-23, assigned to various posts, including the Mediterranean Sea, Europe, and Charlestown Navy Yard (Mass.); anatomy and surgery faculty: 1820-22, Dartmouth Medical College; and 1822-28, Brown University; *post* 1823, practiced medicine, Providence; 1831-32, obstetrics faculty, Jefferson Medical College; 1837-40, president, Rhode Island Medical Society. CONTRIBUTIONS: Became a medical naval hero in the War of 1812 as a result of heroic and brilliant work in treating American wounded and sick at the Battle of Lake Erie. Published *The Sailor's Physician* (1820), a medical guide for ship physicians, which went through five editions in his lifetime. A founder, American Medical Association and its vice-president (1853). Helped establish Rhode Island Hospital and generally played an active role in the state's medical affairs.

WRITINGS: Won the Boylston Prize four times. Papers collected and published as *Boylston Prize Dissertations*: (1) Inflammation of the Periosteum; (2) Eneuresis Irritata; (3) Cutaneous Diseases; (4) Cancer of the Breast (1839); "Statistics of Large Surgical Operations," *Am. J. of Med. Sci.* 15-16 (Apr. 1848): 359-64. A bibliography is in *U.S. Naval Med. Bull.* 17 (1922): 423-60. REFERENCES: *BHM* (1970-74), 136; *DAB*, 14: 275-76; Kelly and Burrage (1928): 945-47; Miller, *BHM*, pp. 88-89; *NCAB*, 8: 204-5; *Who Was Who in Am.*, Hist. Vol.: 467-68.

S. Galishoff

PARVIN, THEOPHILUS (January 9, 1829, Buenos Aires, Argentina-January 29, 1898, Philadelphia, Pa.). *Physician; Obstetrics*. Son of Theophilus, minister, and Mary (Rodney) Parvin. Married Rachel Butler, 1853; three children. EDUCATION: 1847, B.A., University of Indiana; 1852, M.D., University of Pennsylvania; 1852, resident, Wills Eye Hospital, Philadelphia. CAREER: *post* 1852, practiced in Indianapolis, Ind.; 1864-69, professor of materia medica, Medical College of Ohio; 1869-76, professor of obstetrics, University of Louisville; 1867-69, edited *Western Journal of Medicine*; 1869-83, co-edited *American Practitioner*; professor of obstetrics and diseases of women and children: 1876-78, College of Physicians and Surgeons, Indianapolis; and 1878-82, Medical College of Indiana; professor of obstetrics: 1882-83, University of Louisville, Ky.; *post* 1883, Jefferson Medical College, Philadelphia, Pa. CONTRIBUTIONS: Prominent teacher of obstetrics. Pioneer in establishing hospital instruction in obstetrics for medical students. Championed application of ethical principles to questions of conscience and judgement. Obstetrical text and other writings remarkable for their sound doctrine and literary style. Founder, American Gynecological Society.

WRITINGS: *The Science and Art of Obstetrics*, 3 eds. (1886). REFERENCES: *DAB*. 7: 286; George Clark Mosher, "The Apostle of Casuistry in Medicine. An Idealization of Theophilus Parvin," *Am. J. of Obstet. Gynecol.* 13 (1927): 419-32; W. H. Parish, "In Memoriam Theophilus Parvin," *Trans. Am. Gyn. Soc.* 24 (1899): 511 ff.; Herbert Thoms, "Theophilus Parvin—An Important Influence in American Obstetrics and a Pioneer in Clinical Teaching," in *Chapters in American Obstetrics*, 2nd ed. (1961), 93-101.

L. D. Longo

PASSAVANT, WILLIAM ALFRED (October 9, 1821, Zelianople, Pa.-June 3, 1894, Pittsburgh, Pa.). *Philanthropist; Minister*. Son of Philip Louis and Zelie (Basse) Passavant. Married Eliza Walter, 1845; five children. EDUCATION: 1840, graduated from Jefferson College, Pa.; studied at Gettysburg Theological Seminary; 1843, ordained Lutheran minister. CAREER: Lutheran pastor: 1843-47, Canton, Md.; and c. 1848-94, First English Lutheran Church, Pittsburgh, Pa. CONTRIBUTIONS: After a visit to Kaiserwerth, Germany, deaconess institute (1846), began opening hospitals in America (Pittsburgh, 1848). Brought four deaconess nurses to Pittsburgh and to staff his hospitals in Milwaukee, Wis., and Chicago and Jacksonville, Ill., as well as orphanages in Rochester and Mt. Vernon, N.Y., and Boston, Mass. During the Civil War, deaconess nurses worked with Dorothea Dix (q.v.) in military hospitals. REFERENCES: *BHM* (1964-69): 203; *DAB*, 7: 289-90; G. H. Gerberding, *Life and Letters of W. A. Passavant* (1906).

M. Kaufman

PATRICK, HUGH TALBOT (May 11, 1860, New Philadelphia, Ohio-January 5, 1939, Chicago, Ill.). *Physician; Neurology.* Son of Abraham Westfall, lawyer, and Mary West (Talbot) Patrick. Married Fannie Gary, 1896; three children. EDUCATION: 1878-80, College of Wooster (Ohio); 1884, M.D., Bellevue Hospital Medical College; 1884-85, intern, Randall's Island Hospital, N.Y.; 1891-94, studied nervous and mental diseases in Europe. CAREER: 1886-1930, practiced medicine, Chicago; nervous and mental diseases faculty: 1895-1919, Medical School of Northwestern University; and *post* 1896, Chicago Polyclinic; 1907, president, American Neurological Association. CONTRIBUTIONS: Pioneered in the development of neurology in the Middle West. Best known as a clinical investigator who described with great clarity hysteria, traumatic neurosis, phobias, tics and chorea, branchial neuritis and sciatica, trifacial neuralgia, and other neurological disorders. Became the first editor, *Archives of Neurology and Psychiatry* (1919), which he made one of the premier journals in its field. For many years, edited the *Year Book of Nervous and Mental Diseases*.

WRITINGS: "The Technic and Results of Deep Injections of Alcohol for Trifacial Neuralgia," *JAMA* 58 (Jan. 20, 1912): 155-63; "Branchial Neuritis and Sciatica," *JAMA*, 69 (Dec. 29, 1917): 2176-79. A bibliography up to 1922 is in *Semi-Centennial Anniversary Volume of the American Neurological Association* (1924), 579. REFERENCES: *DAB*, Supplement 2: 515-16; *NCAB*, 30: 428-29; *Who Was Who in Am.*, 1: 941.

S. Galishoff

PATTISON, GRANVILLE SHARP (1791 or 1792, near Glasgow, Scotland-November 12, 1851, New York, N.Y.). *Physician; Anatomy.* Son of John Pattison. Survived by his wife, whose maiden name was Sharp; no children. EDUCATION: Educated at University of Glasgow; 1819, became member, Medico-Chirurgical Society of London, and fellow, Royal College of Surgeons; M.D., Jefferson Medical College. CAREER: 1818-19, assistant to Allan Burns, lecturer on anatomy, physiology, and surgery, Andersonian Institution (Glasgow); 1819-20, gave a series of private lessons in anatomy in Philadelphia; 1820-26, anatomy, physiology, and surgery faculty, University of Maryland; anatomy faculty: 1827-31, University of London; 1832-41, Jefferson Medical College; and 1841-51, University of the City of New York. CONTRIBUTIONS: One of the most successful teachers of anatomy in the first half of the nineteenth century; was especially renown for instruction in visceral and surgical anatomy and for demonstrations of their applications to the practice of medicine. Edited the second edition of Allan Burns's *Observations on the Surgical Anatomy of the Head and Neck* (1824). Edited the *American Medical Recorder* (1820) and the *Register and Library of Medical and Surgical Science* (1833-36). Co-edited the *American Medical Library and Intelligencer* (1836). Translated J. W. Masse's *Anatomical Atlas* and edited Jean Cruveilhier's *Anatomy of the Human Body.*

WRITINGS: *Experimental Observations on the Operation of Lithotomy* (1820). REFERENCES: *BHM* (1964-69), 205; *DAB*, 14: 311; Kelly and Burrage (1928), 950-51; "A Medical Duellist," *Annals of Med. Hist.*, 3rd series, 3 (1941): 82-83; Miller, *BHM*, p. 89; *NCAB*, 6: 69-70; *Who Was Who in Am.*, Hist. Vol.: 469.

S. Galishoff

PAUL, JOHN RODMAN (April 18, 1893, Philadelphia, Pa.-May 6, 1971, New Haven, Conn.). *Physician; Microbiology; Epidemiology.* Son of Henry Neill, lawyer, and Margaret Crosby (Butler) Paul. Married Mary Leita Harlan, 1922; no children. EDUCATION: 1915, A.B., Princeton University; 1919, M.D., Johns Hopkins Medical School; 1919-20, assistant pathologist, Johns Hopkins Medical School; 1920-22, intern, Pennsylvania Hospital. CAREER: 1922-28, director, Ayer clinical laboratory (Philadelphia); at Yale University Medical School: 1928-40, internal medicine faculty; and 1940-61, preventive medicine faculty; served on numerous committees for the U.S. Armed Forces, the National Foundation for Infantile Paralysis, the National Institutes of Health, and the World Health Organization. CONTRIBUTIONS: Using the approach of "clinical epidemiology," conducted important investigations of several microbial diseases. Undertook a systematic study of rheumatic fever in families in which he concluded that a streptococcus infection precipitated the disease (1928); proved hypothesis to the satisfaction of nearly all in his book *The Epidemiology of Rheumatic Fever* (1930). With W. W. Bunnell, developed a laboratory test for infectious mononucleosis on the basis of their discovery of heterophile antibodies in the sera of persons with the disease (1932). Demonstrated that serum hepatitis and infectious hepatitis were separate diseases and that the latter was transmitted by the fecal-oral route (1943). With James Trask (q.v.), organized the Yale Poliomyelitis Study Unit; discovered that the great majority of persons who are exposed to polioviruses have mild, unrecognizable cases but are infectious; found that polioviruses exist in at least two and maybe three serologic types. Pioneered in the field of serological epidemiology. Made a serologic study of the Egyptian population on the basis of which he concluded that exposure to polioviruses at a young age, as indicated by the presence of antibodies in the sera, accounted for that country's near absence of paralytic poliomyelitis; conversely, the sheltered populations of advanced countries were more susceptible (1943-44). Conducted a study of Alaskan Eskimos that indicated that a single exposure to a poliovirus type would confer lifelong immunity against that strain (1949); research gave support to those who wanted to develop a live, attenuated poliovirus vaccine.

WRITINGS: "The Presence of Heterophile Antibodies in Infectious Mononucleosis," *Am. J. of Med. Sci.* 183 (1932): 90-104 (with W. W. Bunnell); *Clinical Epidemiology* (1958); *A History of Poliomyelitis* (1971). Writings are listed in *BMNAS*. REFERENCES: *BMNAS* 47 (1975): 323-68; *McGraw-Hill Modern Men of Sci.* 1 (1966): 407-8; *N.Y. Times*, May 7, 1971; *Trans. Assoc. of Am. Physicians* 85 (1972): 40-43; *Who Was Who in Am.*, 5: 559.

S. Galishoff

PAYNE, HOWARD MARSHALL (August 18, 1907, Washington, D.C.-September 9, 1961, Boston, Mass.). *Physician; Internal medicine and chest diseases.* Son of John C. and Neenah (George) Payne. Married Kern Blackburn, 1934; two children. EDUCATION: 1928, A.B., Dartmouth College; 1929, education certificate, Dartmouth Medical College (first two years of medical school); 1931, M.D., Howard University; 1931-32, intern, Freedmen's Hospital; at Sea View Hospital, Staten Island, N.Y.: 1935-36, assistant resident in pathology; and 1936, resident in medicine (tuberculosis); 1937, General Education Board Fellow, Henry Phipps Institute (Philadelphia, Pa.). CAREER: 1932-58, private practice, Washington, D.C.; at Howard University Medical College: 1932-35, part-time clinical assistant in medicine; and 1937-58, medicine faculty (full professor in 1948); 1937-58, staff of Freedmen's Hospital (in charge of tuberculosis service *post* 1940); 1958-61, superintendent, Middlesex County Sanitarium, Waltham, Mass. CONTRIBUTIONS: Black leader in community and scientific work dealing with tuberculosis and chest disease in Washington, D.C. area. Helped obtain funds for, establish, and run as chief the Tuberculosis Annex of Freedmen's Hospital (1940-58). Published widely on tuberculosis. Served the Public Health Service on tuberculosis matters (1946-53), the National Tuberculosis Association (1946-52; president, 1951-52), and other national and international tuberculosis agencies. Part of Dean Numa P. G. Adams's program to rebuild and strengthen the Howard University Medical School (1930). A respected teacher and clinician.

WRITINGS: Published some 35 articles on all aspects of tuberculosis in numerous journals. Writings listed in *JNMA* 53 (1961): 655. REFERENCES: *JNMA* 53 (1961): 653-55; *WWICA* 7 (1950): 410-11.

T. L. Savitt

PEARCE, LOUISE (March 5, 1885, Winchester, Mass.-August 10, 1959, New York, N.Y.). *Pathologist; Laboratory investigator.* Daughter of Charles Ellis, tobacconist, and Susan Elizabeth (Hoyt) Pearce. Never married. EDUCATION: 1907, A.B. (physiology), Stanford; 1907-9, Boston University School of Medicine; 1912, M.D., Johns Hopkins Medical School; and intern, Johns Hopkins Hospital; 1913, fellow, laboratory of Simon Flexner (q.v.), Rockefeller

Institute for Medical Research. CAREER: Essentially entire career was at the Rockefeller Institute: *post* 1923, associate member; 1946-51, president, Woman's Medical College of Pennsylvania. CONTRIBUTIONS: With Wade Hampton Brown, developed tryparsamide for African Trypanosomiasis, and went to Belgian Congo (1920), where she confirmed its clinical efficacy. Did experimental biological studies of infectious and inherited diseases. Extensively studied experimental syphilis. Discovered a transplantable tumor. Studied hereditary diseases and defects in a large rabbit colony.

WRITINGS: *The Treatment of Human Trypanosomiasis with Tryparsamide* (1930); over 100 research papers, mostly in *J. of Experimental Med.*, some with Brown, Thomas M. Rivers, and others. Writings listed in *J. Path. Bact.* 82 (1961): 542-51. REFERENCES: Marion Fay, "Louise Pearce," *J. Path. Bact.* 82 (1961): 542-51; *Notable Am. Women, The Modern Period*, 531-32.

S. J. Peitzman

PEARL, RAYMOND (June 3, 1879, Farmington, N.H.-November 17, 1940, Hershey, Pa.). *Biologist; Statistician; Genetics.* Son of Frank, merchant, and Ida May (McDuffee) Pearl. Married Maud M. DeWitt, 1903; two children. EDUCATION: 1899, A.B., Dartmouth College; 1902, Ph.D., University of Michigan; 1905-6, studied at University of Leipzig, University College (London), and Naples Zoological Station, Carnegie Institution. CAREER: Zoology faculty: 1899-1906, University of Michigan; and 1906-7, University of Pennsylvania; 1907-18, biologist, Maine Agricultural Experiment Station; at National Research Council: 1916-18, member, Executive Committee, and chairman, Agricultural Committee; and 1919-35, member, Executive Board; 1917-19, chief, statistical division, U.S. Food Administration; at Johns Hopkins: 1918-25, biometry and vital statistics faculty, School of Hygiene and Public Health; 1919-35, statistician, Johns Hopkins Hospital; 1923-40, biology faculty, School of Medicine; and 1925-30, research professor and director, Institute of Biological Research. CONTRIBUTIONS: Through writing, teaching, and prosyletizing, won support for the use of statistical analysis in biology and medicine. Made pioneering studies of longevity and world population changes. Tried to answer the question why some persons lived longer than others; believed that an unhurried pace of living, moderate consumption of alcohol, intellectual work, and long-lived ancestors increased a person's chances of having a long life. An authority on the heredity and reproduction of poultry and cattle. Founded and edited the *Quarterly Review of Biology* (1926) and *Human Biology* (1929). Associate editor of several other journals.

WRITINGS: *Diseases of Poultry* (1915, with F. M. Surface and M. R. Curtis); *Modes of Research in Genetics* (1915); *The Biology of Death* (1922); *Introduction to Medical Biometry and Statistics* (1923); *The Natural History of Population* (1939). A bibliography is in *BMNAS* 22 (1943): 295-347. REFERENCES: *BHM* (1970-74), 138; *DAB*, Supplement

2: 521-22; *DSB*, 10: 444-45; *NCAB*, 15: 382; *N.Y. Times*, November 18, 1940; *Who Was Who in Am.*, 1: 949.

S. Galishoff

PECK, WASHINGTON FREEMAN (January 22, 1841, Galen, N.Y.-December 12, 1891, Davenport, Ia.). *Physician; Surgery.* Son of William H., farmer, and Alida (Hawes) Peck. Married Maria Purdy, 1865; three children. EDUCATION: 1860, first undergraduate house surgeon, Bellevue; and first medical student to combine lecture courses with hospital experience; 1863, M.D., Bellevue Hospital Medical College. CAREER: 1863-64, contract surgeon, U.S. Army (Lincoln General Hospital, Washington, D.C.); 1864-late 1880s, medical practice, Davenport; 1870-June 1891, first dean of the faculty and professor of surgery, State University of Iowa Department of Medicine; 1875-late 1880s, chief surgeon, Rock Island Railroad; 1890, delegate, International Medical Congress (Berlin, Germany) and International Surgical Congress (Birmingham, England); in Iowa State Medical Society: 1876, president; and 1885, vice-president; in AMA: 1882-83, chairman, Section on Surgery and Anatomy; and 1885, vice-president; fellow, American Surgical Association (membership was then limited to the top 100 surgeons). CONTRIBUTIONS: Secured the establishment of the medical school, Iowa City, Ia., at the University of Iowa (1868). Founder, with Sister Mary Barromeo, of Mercy hospitals, Davenport and Iowa City. Considered one of the top six American surgeons of his time, primarily because of skill in abdominal and pelvic operations, not often performed by surgeons of that time. It is often said that he remained skeptical of the "germ theory" and antiseptics throughout career; however, records of his operations and clinical procedures (*post* 1886) indicate that he had changed his mind.

WRITINGS: Published very few papers, although often read them at medical meetings. Especially noteworthy are presidential address to the Iowa State Medical Society (1876) and report as chairman of the AMA Section on Surgery (1883), a detailed account of the controversy then raging over the "germ theory" and the question of "antiseptic practice" in surgery. REFERENCES: Walter L. Bierring, *A History of the Department of Internal Medicine, State University of Iowa College of Medicine, 1870-1958* (1958); David S. Fairchild, *History of Medicine in Iowa* (1923); John T. McClintock, *Washington Freeman Peck* (1947); *One Hundred Years of Iowa Medicine, 1850-1950* (1950); University of Iowa Archives, Iowa City, Ia.

R. E. Rakel

PELL, THOMAS (1613, Southwyck, Sussex, England-September, 1669, Fairfield, Conn.). *Physician; Surgeon.* Son of Rev. John, scholar and schoolmaster, and Mrs. Mary (Holland) Pell. Married Lucy (French) Brewster. EDUCATION: Free School, Steyning, England; 1626-28, Magdalene College, Cambridge, England, entering at age 13; early 1630s, possibly learned surgery during military service in Holland; held no academic degrees. CAREER: As a boy, served as page to Prince Charles, and when Charles became King Charles I, was appointed gentleman of the bedchamber; 1629, left the Court and joined Sir Horace Vere's

Corps to fight in Holland, where he was commissioned an ensign; 1632, promoted to lieutenant after the siege of Maastricht; April 5, 1635, booked passage for New England on the ship ''Planter''; settled in Dorchester and then made his way to New Haven (Conn.) Colony; 1637-38, served as a lieutenant surgeon during the Pequot War; settled in Fairfield, where he owned considerable land; practiced medicine in New Haven; November 14, 1654, purchased a large tract of land from the Indians in what is now Westchester County, N.Y. In addition, the duke of York granted the land as an enfranchised township and manor; became lord of the manor of what is now Pelham and New Rochelle, N.Y. CONTRIBUTIONS: Considered Conn.'s first physician and surgeon because of service at Fort Saybrook. Practice, New Haven and Fairfield, further substantiates this honor. REFERENCES: Melville Roberts, M.D., ''Connecticut's First Surgeon: Thomas Pell,'' *Conn. Med.* 40 (Dec. 1976): 856-57; Melville Roberts, M.D., Juliet Vilinskas, M.D., and William C. Butterfield, M.D., ''Thomas Pell (1613-1669), Connecticut's First Physician and Surgeon,'' ibid., 37 (Jul. 1973): 363-64; Herbert Thoms, M.D., ''The Beginnings of Medical Practice in New Haven Colony,'' *Conn., State Med. J.* 4 (Nov. 1940): 639-44.

J. W. Ifkovic

PENNOCK, CASPAR WISTAR (July 2, 1799, Philadelphia, Pa.-April 16, 1867, Howellville, Pa.). Son of George and Sarah (Wistar) Pennock. Married Caroline Morris, 1833; one child. EDUCATION: 1828, M.D., University of Pennsylvania; 1830-33, studied in Paris. CAREER: Medical staff: 1828-29, *post* 1835, Philadelphia Almshouse Hospital; and *post* 1833, Philadelphia Dispensary. CONTRIBUTIONS: With William W. Gerhard (q.v.), studied the symptoms and pathological anatomy of typhus, differentiating it from typhoid fever. Devised a flexible-tube stethoscope to replace the stiff and awkward wood instrument used by Rene Laënnec (1839). Edited the treatise of Jean-Baptiste Bouillaud on the diseases of the heart (1837).

WRITINGS: *Observations on the Cholera of Paris* (1832, with W. W. Gerhard); ''Case of Anomalous Aneurysm of the Aorta Resulting from Effusion of Blood Between the Laminae Composing the Middle Coat of that Vessel,'' *Am. J. of Med. Sci.* 23 (Nov. 1838): 2-19. REFERENCES: *Appleton's CAB*, 4: 718; James Bordley and A. McGehee Harvey, *Two Centuries of American Medicine* (1976), 82; Kelly and Burrage (1928), 957.

S. Galishoff

PEPPER, WILLIAM (August 21, 1843, Philadelphia, Pa.-July 28, 1898, Pleasanton, Calif.). *Physician; Educator.* Son of William, physician, and Sarah (Platt) Pepper. Married Frances Sargeant Perry, 1873; four children. EDUCATION: University of Pennsylvania: 1862, graduated; and 1864, M.D.; 1864-65, resident physician, Pennsylvania Hospital; and visiting physician, Philadelphia Infirmary; 1871, studied methods of medical education in Europe. CAREER: Pathology and medical staffs: 1866-70, Pennsylvania Hospital; and 1867-71, Philadelphia Hospital; at University of Pennsylvania: 1865-68, morbid anatomy faculty; 1876-

84, clinical medicine faculty; 1880-94, provost; and 1884-98, theory and practice of medicine faculty; 1875-76, medical director, Philadelphia Centennial Exhibition; president: 1886, American Climatological Society; 1886, American Clinical Association; 1891, Association of American Physicians; and 1893, First Pan-American Medical Congress; made the University of Pennsylvania one of the nation's foremost medical centers; was deeply committed to programs of civic betterment in Philadelphia including, adult education, the Philadelphia Library, and the University Museum. CONTRIBUTIONS: One of the nation's most distinguished medical reformers in the late nineteenth century. At University of Pennsylvania, established the first teaching hospital in the United States directly associated with and staffed by the faculty of a university medical school (1874). Introduced a three-year graded curriculum (1877), an innovation soon followed by several of the nation's other better medical schools. Established and endowed the William Pepper Laboratory of Clinical Medicine (1894), the first laboratory in America for advanced clinical investigation into the etiology of disease. Described the malarial parasite (1867), called attention to the bone-marrow changes of pernicious anemia (1875), and outlined the treatment of tuberculosis that was adopted in the first decades of the twentieth century. Made many contributions to medical literature, including *A Practical Treatise on the Diseases of Children* (1870); *A System of Practical Medicine* (5 vols., 1885-86), issued under his editorship; and *Textbook of the Theory and Practice of Medicine* (2 vols., 1893-94). Best known for two addresses about *Higher Medical Education, the True Interests of the Public and the Profession* (1877, 1894), in which he discussed the changes needed in American medical education, which his reforms helped make possible in the following decades. Founded the *Philadelphia Medical Times* and was its editor (1870-71).

WRITINGS: *The Morphological Changes of the Blood in Malaria Fever* (1867, with Edward Rhoads and J. F. Meigs); "Local Treatment of Lung Cavities," *Am. J. of Med. Sci.* 69 (Jul. 1874): 253-56; "Progressive Pernicious Anaemia, or Anaematosis," ibid., 70 (1875): 313-47. REFERENCES: *DAB*, 14: 453-56; Kelly and Burrage (1928), 959-60; *NCAB*, 1: 345; Fred B. Rogers, "William Pepper, 1843-1898. . .," *J. of Med. Ed.* 34 (1959): 885-89; R. F. Stone, *Biog. of Eminent Am. Physicians and Surgeons* (1894), 380; *Who Was Who in Am.*, Hist. Vol.: 475.

S. Galishoff

PERKINS, ELISHA (January 16, 1741, Norwich, Conn.-September 6, 1799, New York, N.Y.). *Physician; Patent medicine.* Son of Dr. Joseph, physician, and Mrs. Mary (Bushnell) Perkins. Married Sarah Douglass, September 23, 1762; ten children. EDUCATION: Yale College. CAREER: 1759, began medical practice, Plainfield, Conn. CONTRIBUTIONS: Developed an antiseptic solution of sodium chloride and vinegar (1794) to treat scarlatina anginosa (a form of scarlet fever with a severe, irritated throat). Experimented with polished knife blade as an electric treatment for crippling diseases (1795); then experimented with metal tractors and was awarded (February 1797) U.S. patent for metallic tractors.

While doing surgery, observed that his metallic instrument caused muscles to contract. Developed metal rods sometimes with gold and silver points that, when drawn over the skin, drew off noxious electrical fluids. Claimed effective treatment of gout, pleurisy, and rheumatism. Sold metal rods at high prices, considering the cost of the metal in the tractors. When dismissed from the Connecticut Medical Society (1797), was given a year to justify his actions before final expulsion, but ignored the invitation. Treatment became a fad: "Perkinism." Benjamin Douglas Perkins, his son, publicized the treatment in London; tests demonstrated that painted wood rods produced the same effect, and Perkinism fell into disrepute.

WRITINGS: *The Influence of Metallic Tractors on the Human Body* (1798). REFERENCES: *BHM* (1964-69), 206; (1970-74), 139; (1975-79), 98; *DAB*, 7: 466-67; Howard Haggard, *Devils, Drugs and Doctors* (1931), 319-20; Stewart Holbrook, *Golden Age of Quackery* (1959), 40-42; Miller, *BHM*, p. 90; Jacques M. Quen, "Elisha Perkins, Physician, Nostrum-Vendor or Charlatan," *Bull. Hist. Med.* 37 (Mar.-Apr. 1963): 159-66.

R. Edwards

PERKINS, ROGER GRISWOLD (May 17, 1874, Schenectady, N.Y.-March 28, 1936, Providence, R.I.). *Pathologist; Preventive medicine; Public health.* Son of Maurice, professor of chemistry, Union College, and Anne Dunbar (Potts) Perkins. Married Edna Brush, 1905; four sons. EDUCATION: 1893, A.B., Union College; 1894, A.B., Harvard University; 1898, M.D., Johns Hopkins; 1898-1901, resident, Lakeside Hospital, Cleveland, Ohio; 1902-3, fellow, Rockefeller Institute. CAREER: 1901-30, professor of hygiene and preventive medicine, Western Reserve University Medical School; 1906-7, 1913-14, Cleveland city bacteriologist; 1914-23, chief, Bureau of Division of Health Laboratory; 1923-30, consultant to commissioner of health and director of laboratories; 1917-18, American Red Cross Commission to Rumania; 1918, medical associate to the scientific attaché, American embassy, Paris; 1919, director, Sanitation Division, American Red Cross Commission to the Balkan states. CONTRIBUTIONS: Eradicated typhoid in Cleveland (the first large city to chlorinate its water). Formed the Cleveland Health Council (1925). Established the Bureau of Laboratories, city of Cleveland. Introduced and maintained efficient food inspection. First described, with William T. Howard (q.v.), the streptococcus mucosus (pneumococcus, type III).

WRITINGS: "Bactericidal Action of the Blood Serum in Variola and in Varioloid," *J. of Med. Research* 10 (1903): 196-203 (with George O. Pay); "A Study of the Etiology of Variola" (with William Travis Howard) *Trans., Assoc. of Am. Physicians* 19 (1904): 383-404; "Typhoid Fever in Cleveland in 1911," *Cleveland Med. J.* 11 (1912): 816 (with T. S. Jackson), the first of an annual series published between 1912 and 1918; "Typhoid Fever in Cleveland, Ohio, for the Years 1918, 1919, and 1920," *Public Health Reports* 36 (May 20, 1921): 1095-1122; "Typhoid Fever in Cleveland, 1873-1926," *J. Preventive Med.* 1 (1927): 449-502. REFERENCES: *NCAB*, C: 172; 26: 448; Alphonso O. Okwuowulu, "Dr. Roger Griswold Perkins: The Man Who Took Typhoid Out of

Cleveland Water," *Bull. of the Cleveland Med. Library* 23 (Jun. 1977): 53-63; T. Wingate Todd, "The Physician as Anthropologist," *Sci.* 83 (Jun. 10, 1936): 588-90.

G. P. Jenkins

PERRY, JOHN EDWARD (April 2, 1870, Clarksville, Tex.-May 15, 1962, Houston, Tex.). *Physician; General practice.* Son of Anderson, slave and then farmer, and Louisa (White) Perry. Married Fredericka D. Sprague, 1912 (d. 1943), one child; Ora M. Brown, 1947, no children. EDUCATION: 1891, A.B.?, Bishop College, Marshall, Tex.; 1895, M.D., Meharry Medical College; 1897-98, Post-Graduate Medical School, Chicago, Ill., despite negative racial attitudes of instructors and students. CAREER: 1895, general practice, Mexico, Mo.; general practitioner: 1895-97, 1898-1903, Columbia, Mo.; and 1903-45, Kansas City, Mo.; 1945-62, active retirement in Houston. CONTRIBUTIONS: Moving force behind black hospital movement in central Midwest, especially in Kansas City and St. Louis, Mo. Founder (1910) and superintendent (1910-30) of what became Wheatley-Provident Hospital (1915), Kansas City, and chief of surgical service (1910-41), General Hospital No. 2, Kansas City, both black hospitals. Consultant to medical colleagues of central Midwest. President, NMA (1923). Chief concern was provision of adequate hospitals, both for black patients and for training of black physicians. Served on boards of Lincoln University (Mo.) (1921-41) and Meharry Medical College (1936-at least 1956). Involved in civic affairs such as Negro YMCA development in Kansas City.

WRITINGS: "Our Hospitals and Their Standardization," *JNMA* 14 (1922): 20-21; *Forty Cords of Wood: Memoirs of a Medical Doctor* (1947). Writings listed in *JNMA* 48 (1956): 296. REFERENCES: W. Montague Cobb, "John Edward Perry, M.D., 1870-," *JNMA* 48 (1956): 292-96; obituary notice, *JNMA* 54 (1962): 639; John E. Perry, *Forty Cords of Wood: Memoirs of a Medical Doctor* (1947); "Tribute to Dr. J. Edward Perry of Kansas City, Mo," *JNMA* 37 (1945): 101-2; *WWCR* 1 (1915): 215; *WWICA* 7 (1950): 414.

T. L. Savitt

PETER, ROBERT (January 21, 1805, Launceton, Cornwall, England-April 26, 1894, Lexington, Ky.). *Physician; Chemist; Educator.* Son of Robert and Johanna (Dawe) Peter. Married Frances Paca Dellam, October 6, 1835; eleven children. EDUCATION: Early education in England; c. 1819-27, worked in drug store of Charles Avery, Pittsburgh, Pa., and learned pharmacy and chemistry; was largely self-taught; 1827-28, Rensselaer Institute, Troy, N.Y.; 1832-34, studied medicine under L. P. Yandell (q.v.) and attended Transylvania University medical department, Lexington; 1832, M.D., Transylvania University. CAREER: 1817, went to the United States with his parents; landed at Baltimore, Md.; soon settled in Pittsburgh; after first becoming knowledgable in chemistry, developed an interest and proficiency in botany and established a Botanical Society in Pittsburgh; 1830-31, lectured on chemistry, Mechanics Institute and Western University of Pennsylvania, and taught chemistry to private classes in Pittsburgh; 1832, became lecturer in chemistry, Eclectic Institute of Lexington; at Transylvania University medical department: 1832-57, chemistry and pharmacy department; 1833-35, librarian; and 1841-57, dean; 1837-38, editor, *Transylvania Journal of Medicine and Associate Sciences*; 1850-53, professor of chemistry, Kentucky School of Medicine, Louisville; 1854-61, chemical assistant, first four geological surveys of Ky.; 1860, contributed to the geological surveys of Ark. and Ind.; 1862-65, acting assistant surgeon, U.S. General Hospital, to senior surgeon (major) of military hospitals of Lexington; 1865-78, professor of chemistry and experimental philosophy, Kentucky University, Lexington, into which Transylvania had been absorbed; 1878-87, professor of chemistry, Agriculture and Mechanical College, Lexington. CONTRIBUTIONS: Major contributions to medicine were as chemist, teacher, and administrator. Through efforts and diplomacy, Transylvania University and especially the medical department were funded and remained operational until 1859. Interested in the relation of the climate, topography, and chemical content of soils to epidemic disease and the formation of urinary calculi. As a means to elucidate these relationships, helped initiate the geological survey of Ky. and conducted numerous chemical analyses of the soils.

WRITINGS: "An Account of the Vegetable Alkalies, Including Their Therapeutic Action When Applied Internally, or by the Endermic Method," *Transylv. J. Med.* 7 (1834): 157-204; "Analysis of Three Urinary Calculi," ibid., n.s., 1 (1849): 209-25; "Remarks on Ozone and Its Supposed Influence in the Production of Epidemic Diseases, Especially Epidemic Cholera," ibid., n.s., 1 (1849): 148-57; *Transylvania University, Its Origin, Rise, Decline and Fall* (1896); *History of the Medical Department of Transylvania University* (1905). Writings listed in *Index Catalogue*, 1st series, 10 (1889), and 2nd series, 13 (1908). REFERENCES: A. H. Barkley, *Kentucky's Pioneer Lithotomists* (1913), 145-51; *DAB*, 7, pt. 2: 499-500; C. Kerr, *History of Kentucky* 4 (1922): 11-12; G. J. Munoff, "Dr. Robert Peter and the Legacy of Photography in Kentucky," *Register of the Ky. Hist. Soc.* 78 (1980): 208-18; *NCAB*, 4: 517; W. H. Perrin, ed., *History of Fayette County Kentucky* (1882), 208-18; W. B. Smith, "In Memoriam: Dr. Robert Peter," *Letters* (University of Kentucky) 1 (Aug. 1928): 34-40; J. D. Wright, Jr., "Robert Peter and Early Science in Kentucky" (Diss., Columbia University, 1955).

E. H. Conner

PETTIGREW, GEORGE ATWOOD (April 6, 1858, Ludlow, Vt.,-April 13, 1938). *Physician; Surgery*. Son of Josiah Walker and Susan Ann (Atwood) Pettigrew. Married Eudora Zulette Stearns, 1887; three children. EDUCATION: Black River Academy, Ludlow; 1879, Colby Academy, New London, N.H.; 1883, M.D., Dartmouth College. CAREER: 1883, began practice, Flandreau, S.Dak.; 1884-93, surgeon, Second Regiment of Dakota National Guards; 1885-89, surgeon-general, S.Dak.; 1897, appointed surgeon, First Regiment, South Dakota National Guards; and surgeon, Chicago, Milwaukee & St. Paul Railroad for six years; 1891, retired from active practice. CONTRIBUTIONS: Prominent in the development of eastern S.Dak. First surgeon-general, S.Dak. REFERENCES: George W. Kingsbury, *History of Dakota Territory*; *Memorial & Biographical Record-*

The Black Hills Region (1898), 314, 317; Doane Robinson, *History of South Dakota* 2 (1904): 1019-20; George Martin Smith, *South Dakota, Its History and Its People: Biographical* 4 (1915): 106; *Who Was Who in Am.*, 1: 965.

D. W. Boilard and
P. W. Brennen

PHARES, DAVID LEWIS (January 14, 1817, West Feliciana Parish, La.-September 19, 1892, Madison Station, Miss.). *Physician*. Son of William and Elizabeth (Starnes) Phares. Married Mary Armstrong Nesmith, 1836, eight children; Laura Blanche Duquercron, 1881; two children. EDUCATION: Louisiana State College: preparatory department; and 1837, A.B.; 1839, M.D., University of Louisiana medical department; 1840, A.M., University of Kentucky. CAREER: After completing undergraduate course, was offered a teaching position at Louisiana State College, but preferred to begin the study of medicine; upon graduation from medical school, was invited to remain as a member of the medical faculty, University of Louisiana, but declined to practice medicine, West Feliciana; moved to Whitestown (Newtonia), Wilkinson County, Miss., and practiced until 1880; 1842, erected buildings and opened Newton Female Institute; 1852, established Newton College; helped to establish the common school system in Miss.; was active figure in state politics and one of the leading spirits in the establishment of the Mississippi Agricultural and Mechanical (A&M) College; 1880-89, chair of biology, A&M College; 1889, moved to Madison Station, Miss., and resided there until death in 1892. CONTRIBUTIONS: Member, First Mississippi State Board of Health (organized, 1877). Recognized as an authority on the medical virtues of indigenous plants of the South. First to observe the medical properties of *gelsemium* and *viburnum*. President, Mississippi State Medical Association (1884-85).

WRITINGS: Numerous articles in local and state medical publications. REFERENCES: *BHM* (1975-79), 99; Kelly and Burrage (1928), 963-64; John A. Milne, "Early Mississippi Physicians," *J. of Mississippi Hist.* 18 (Jul. 1956): 157-74.

M. S. Legan

PHELPS, EDWARD ELISHA (April 24, 1803, Peacham, Vt.-November 26, 1880, Windsor, Conn.). *Physician; Surgeon*. Son of Dr. Elisha and Mrs. Susanna (Eastman) Phelps. Married Phoebe Foxcroft Lynn (or Lyon), 1830; one child. EDUCATION: 1822, Norwich, Vt., Military Academy; Dartmouth Medical School; 1825, M.D., Yale. CAREER: c. 1825-27, surveyed canals and plants of the Dismal Swamp in Va. and N.C.; 1828 until death, practiced in Windsor; 1835-37, professor of anatomy and surgery, University of Vermont; 1841-75, taught materia medica and therapeutics and the theory and practice of medicine, Dartmouth; 1861-65, U.S. Army surgeon; charter member, Connecticut Valley Medical Society, and one of its early presidents. CONTRIBUTIONS: Remembered chiefly as a medical educator and for long and enthusiastic service to the Dartmouth

Medical School. REFERENCES: William B. Atkinson, *Biographical Dictionary of Contemporary Am. Physicians and Surgeons*, 2nd ed. (1880), 527; Kelly and Burrage (1928), 964-65.

J. W. Estes

PHILLIPS, JOSIAH LAKE   (June 8, 1835, Farmington, Maine-June 12, 1882, Sioux Falls, S.Dak.). *Physician; Surgery.* Son of Allen Phillips, physician, and Annie (Croswell) Phillips. Married Harriet C. Dagette, 1867; seven children. EDUCATION: 1854, Bowdoin College; 1856, M.D., Rush College. CAREER: 1856, practice, Prairie du Chien, Wis.; 1857, moved to Dubuque, Ia.; 1857-61, justice of the peace, Sioux Falls, Dakota Territory; 1861-65, surgeon, 16th Iowa Infantry during the Civil War; 1869, permanently returned to Sioux Falls. CONTRIBU-TIONS: Helped establish the city of Sioux Falls, Dak. Territory, as part of the Western Town Company. First physician to go to Dak. Territory in a professional capacity. Performed the first known surgery in Dak. Territory, an amputation (1859). REFERENCES: Dana Bailey, *History of Minnehaha County, South Dakota* (1899), 663; Doane Robinson, *History of South Dakota* 2 (1904): 1516-17.

D. W. Boilard and
P. W. Brennen

PHYSICK, PHILIP SYNG   (July 7, 1768, Philadelphia, Pa.-December 15, 1837, Philadelphia). *Physician; Surgery.* Son of Edmund, receiver-general of Pennsylvania and agent for the Penn estates, and Abigail (Syng) Physick. Married Elizabeth Emlen, 1800; seven children. EDUCATION: 1785, B.A., University of Pennsylvania; 1785-89, studied medicine with Adam Kuhn (q.v.), Philadelphia, and John Hunter, London; 1790, house surgeon, St. George's Hospital, London; 1792, M.D., University of Edinburgh. CAREER: *Post* 1792, practiced medicine, Philadelphia; 1794, 1798, physician, Bush Hill (yellow fever) Hospital; surgical staff: 1794-1816, Pennsylvania Hospital; and 1800, almshouse infirmary; at University of Pennsylvania: 1800-1805, anatomy and surgery faculty; 1805-19, surgery faculty; and 1819-31, anatomy faculty; president: 1822, Phrenological Society of Philadelphia; and 1824, Philadelphia Medical Society. CONTRIBU-TIONS: Often referred to as "the father of American surgery." Devised numerous surgical procedures and instruments, including manipulation instead of mechanical traction in reduction of dislocations, new methods in treatment of hip-joint disease by immobilization, introduction of absorbable animal ligatures, needle forceps for tying deeply placed blood vessels, a long forceps snare and guillotine for tonsillectomy, and a new type of catheter for urinary tract surgery. Introduced the use of the seton for the treatment of disunited fractures of the humerus, developed an operation for artificial anus, invented guillotine tonsillotome, improved the operation for bladder stone, and was one of the first Americans to use the stomach pump for washing out the stomach.

WRITINGS: "Account of a New Mode of Extracting Poisonous Substances from the Stomach," *Eclectic Repertory and Analytical Review* 3 (1812-13): 111-13, 381-82; "A

Case of Fracture of the Bone of the Under Jaw, Successfully Treated with a Seton,"
Phila. J. of the Med. and Physical Sci. 5 (1822): 116-18; "Extracts from an Account of
a Case in Which a New and Peculiar Operation for Artificial Anus was Performed,"
ibid., 13 (1826): 199-202; "Description of a Forceps Employed to Facilitate the Extirpation of the Tonsil," *Am. J. of Med. Sci.* 2 (1828): 116-17. REFERENCES: L.R.C.
Agnew and G. F. Sheldon, "Philip Syng Physick. . .," *J. of Med. Ed.* 35 (1960): 541-
49; *BHM* (1970-74), 140; (1975-79), 99; *DAB*, 14: 554-55; Kelly and Burrage (1928),
965-66; Miller, *BHM*, p. 90; *NCAB*, 6: 391-92; John H. Talbott, *Biographical Hist. of
Med.* (1970), 370-71; *Who Was Who in Am.*, Hist. Vol.: 481.

S. Galishoff

PICOTTE, SUSAN LA FLESCHE (June 17, 1865, Macy, Nebr.-September
15, 1915, Walthill, Nebr.). *Physician.* Daughter of Joseph (Iron Eye), chief,
Omaha Indian Tribe, and Mary Gale La Flesche. Married Henry Picotte, 1894
(d. 1905); two children. EDUCATION: Father Hamilton's Presbyterian Mission
School, Macy; 1879-81, Elizabeth (N.J.) Institute for Young Ladies; 1886,
Hampton Normal and Agricultural Institute, Hampton, Va.; 1889, M.D., Woman's Medical College of Pennsylvania; 1889 (summer), intern, Woman's Hospital
in Philadelphia. CAREER: 1889-1906, physician, Omaha Agency School, and
government physician, Omaha Tribe; medical missionary, Women's National
Indian Association; 1906, delegate to Washington to obtain property rights for
Omaha and Winnebago Indians; 1913, established the first hospital and served
as health officer, Walthill. CONTRIBUTIONS: First Indian woman physician, devoted life to the welfare—physical, social, and economic—of the Omaha tribe.
As a member, State Federation of Women's Club Board, lobbied in the state
legislature and in Congress for better public health laws. Led a delegation to
Washington, D.C., to promote strict control of alcohol in regard to reservation
property. Represented her tribe in struggles with government bureaucracy. Said
to have treated every member of the Omaha tribe, saving many lives. A respected
practitioner in the white community as well. REFERENCES: N. K. Green, "Four
Sisters: Daughters of Joseph La Flesche," *Nebraska Hist.* 45 (Jun. 1964): 165-76; *Notable
Am. Women, 1607-1950*, 3: 65-66; personal correspondence, Archives, University of
Nebraska Medical Center Library of Medicine, Omaha.

B. M. Hetzner

PILCHER, LEWIS STEPHEN (July 28, 1845, Adrian, Mich.-December 24,
1934, Upper Montclair, N.J.). *Surgeon; Medical editor.* Son of Elijah Holmes,
minister, and Phebe Maria (Fisk) Pilcher. Married Martha Susan Phillips, 1870;
three children. EDUCATION: Graduated from Ann Arbor High School; 1862, A.B.,
University of Michigan; 1863, M.A.; 1866, M.D.; 1883-85, postgraduate study
in Europe. CAREER: 1864-65, Civil War service as a hospital steward; 1866,
medical practice, Flint and Detroit; 1866-67, practice in New York City; 1867-
72, served in the medical corps of the U.S. Navy; 1872-83, practice in Brooklyn;
1879-83, co-editor (with George S. Fowler), *Annals of Anatomy and Surgery*;
1885-1934, editor, *Annals of Surgery*; 1887-1907, staff of the Methodist Epis-

copal Hospital, Brooklyn; 1900-1908, staff, German Hospital of Brooklyn; served on medical and surgical staff of various hospitals in New York; 1885-95, professor of clinical surgery, New York Post-Graduate Medical School; 1913-28, member, New York State board of medical examiners. CONTRIBUTIONS: Edited until almost his 90th birthday America's leading surgical journal and the first in English devoted exclusively to surgery. President of the Medical Society of the State of New York (1892).

WRITINGS: *The Treatment of Wounds* (1883); *A List of Books by Some of the Old Masters of Medicine and Surgery, Together with Books on the History of Medicine and on Medical Biography* (1918); *A Surgical Pilgrim's Progress* (1925). REFERENCES: *DAB*, Supplement 1:599-600; *N.Y. Times*, December 25, 1934; Pilcher, *A Surgical Pilgrim's Progress* (1925); S. P. Rosenthal, "L. S. Pilcher: Editor, and Surgeon," *N.Y. J. of Med.*, 68 (1968): 684-86.

M. Kaufman

PINCUS, GREGORY GOODWIN (April 9, 1903, Woodbine, N.J.-August 22, 1967, Boston, Mass.). *Biologist; Endocrinology.* Son of Joseph William, teacher and editor, and Elizabeth Florence (Lipman) Pincus. Married Elizabeth Notkin, 1924; three children. EDUCATION: 1924, B.S., Cornell University; 1927, M.A., D.Sc., Harvard University; 1927-30, studied at Cambridge University and Kaiser Wilhelm Institute. CAREER: 1930-38, biology faculty, Harvard University; 1937-38, visiting investigator, Cambridge University; 1938-45, experimental zoology faculty, Clark University; at Worcester Foundation for Experimental Biology: 1944-56, co-founder and director of laboratories; *post* 1956, research director; 1944-51, physiology faculty, Tufts Medical School; *post* 1951, biology faculty, Boston University; served on many committees: National Institutes of Health, U.S. Public Health Service, and National Research Council. CONTRIBUTIONS: With Hudson Hoagland, established the Worcester Foundation for Experimental Biology, which became internationally famous for its investigations of steroid hormones and mammalian reproduction (1944). Made important discoveries concerning the effects, metabolism, and biosynthesis of steroid hormones. With Min Chueh Chang, began work (1950s) on the development of a birth-control pill. Discovered that several different progestin hormones prevented pregnancy in laboratory animals by inhibiting ovulation; in collaboration with John Rock extended studies to humans; conducted field tests of the hormones in pill form (1956); pill was made available to the public (1960) and has been used both to prevent pregnancy and to regulate the menstrual cycle. Founded the annual Laurentian Hormone Conference and edited the first 23 volumes of its proceedings, *Recent Progress in Hormone Research* (1946-67). Studied the role of hormones in diabetes, cancer, arthritis, schizophrenia, aging, and stress.

WRITINGS: *The Eggs of Mammals* (1936); "Studies of the Biological Activity of Certain 19-Nor Steroids in Female Animals," *Endocrinology* 59 (1956): 695-707 (with M. C. Chang et al.); *The Control of Fertility* (1965). Writings are listed in *BMNAS*. REFER

ENCES: *BHM* (1964-69), 209; (1970-74), 141; (1975-79), 99; *BMNAS* 42 (1971): 229-70; *Current Biog.* (1965), 314-16; *DSB* 10: 610-11; *McGraw-Hill Modern Men of Sci.* 2 (1966): 416-17; *N.Y. Times*, August 23, 1967; *Who Was Who in Am.*, 4: 754.

                                                                                          S. Galishoff

PINKHAM, LYDIA ESTES (February 9, 1819, Lynn, Mass.-May 17, 1883, Lynn). *Teacher; Housewife; Patent medicine manufacturer.* Daughter of William, shoemaker, and Rebecca (Chase) Estes. Married Isaac Pinkham, 1843; five children. EDUCATION: Graduated from Lynn Academy. CAREER: Schoolteacher to 1843; 1843-75, housewife; 1875, began manufacturing Lydia E. Pinkham's Vegetable Compound. CONTRIBUTIONS: When the family was reduced to poverty by the Panic of 1873, began manufacturing an herb medication which developed a reputation for curing "woman's weakness" and other female problems. By the 1890s, it was one of the most widely advertised patent medicines in America. REFERENCES: AMA, *Nostrums and Quackery* (1921); *DAB*, 7, pt. 2:624-25; Stewart Holbrook, *The Golden Age of Quackery* (1959); *The Life and Times of Lydia E. Pinkham* (1931); Sarah Stage, *Female Complaints: Lydia Pinkham and the Business of Women's Medicine* (1979).

                                                                                          M. Kaufman

PITCHER, ZINA (April 12, 1797, Sandy Hill, N.Y.-April 5, 1872, Detroit, Mich.). *Surgeon; Naturalist; Civic leader.* Son of Nathaniel, farmer, and Margaret (Stevenson) Pitcher. Married Anna Sheldon, 1824; two children; married Emily L. (Montgomery) Backus, 1867; one child. EDUCATION: Common schools, Washington County, N.Y.; studied science with Amos Eaton; Castleton Medical College (Vt.); 1822, M.D., Middlebury College (Vt.). CAREER: 1823-36, surgeon, U.S. Army; 1835-36, president, Army Medical Board; at Michigan Historical Society: 1822, founder; and 1836, librarian; 1836-72, medical practice and physician, St. Mary's Hospital, Detroit; 1837-52, founding member, Board of Regents, University of Michigan; 1838-51, president, Michigan Medical Society; 1840-42, 1843, mayor, Detroit; at *Peninsular Medical Journal*: 1853, cofounder; and 1855-58, editor; president: 1855-56, Michigan State Medical Society; and 1856, American Medical Association. CONTRIBUTIONS: As regent, University of Michigan, played the key role in establishing the medical department (1849). As mayor, established the Detroit public school system (1842). Nationally known naturalist, who collected and studied botanical, craniological, and fossil specimens and for whom several botanical species were named.

  WRITINGS: *An Address to the First Graduates of the Medical Department of the University of Michigan* (1851); "Indian Therapeutics," in Henry R. Schoolcraft, *Information Respecting the History, Condition, and Prospects of the Indian Tribes of the United States*, vol. 4 (1854). REFERENCES: *DAB*, 14: 636-37; Kelly and Burrage (1928), 970-71; *Michigan Univ. Med. J.* 3 (1872): 99-110; *NCAB*, 12: 214; *Representative Men of Michigan: American Biographical History of Eminent and Self-Made Men* (1878), district 1: 112; Wilfred Shaw, *The University of Michigan: An Encyclopedic Survey* (1951), pt. 5; *Who Was Who in Am.*, Hist. Vol.: 485.

M. Pernick

PITTENGER, FRED A. (October 15, 1875, Cordington, Ohio-February 13, 1964, Boise, Idaho). *Physician.* Son of Willis M., engineer, and Margaret (Kern) Pittenger. Married Alice Butterworth, 1902; one adopted daughter. EDUCATION: University of Iowa, four years, before enrolling in Chicago Homeopathic Medical College, M.D., 1899; intern, Chicago Homeopathic Hospital, two years, before enrolling in Northwestern University Medical College, M.D., 1904. CAREER: 1904-9, practice, Chicago, Ill.; 1909; settled in Boise, his boyhood home, where he practiced medicine. CONTRIBUTIONS: Leading Idaho physician, elected president of the Idaho State Medical Association (1924). City physician, Boise, for 12 years and surgeon, Idaho Soldiers Home, for 32 years. As a member, Idaho National Guard, served as Idaho surgeon-general (1912-13) and saw service on the Mexican border (1916) and at Fort Riley, Kans. (until 1919). REFERENCES: B. Defenbach, *Idaho: The Place and Its People* 2 (1933): 75; J. H. Hawley, *History of Idaho* 2 (1920): 195.

A. A. Hart

PITTMAN, NEWSOME JONES (August 9, 1818, Halifax County, N.C.-May 14, 1893, Tarboro, N.C.). *Physician; Surgeon.* Son of John, planter, and Mrs. Pittman. Married M. A. Pittman, two children; Mary Eliza Battle, two children. EDUCATION: 1839, M.D., University of Pennsylvania; 1850-53, studied medicine, Paris, Berlin, and London. CAREER: 1839-50, 1853-61, 1865-93, medical practice, Tarboro; 1861-65, surgeon, Confederate Army. CONTRIBUTIONS: Involved in numerous activities to promote the medical profession of N.C., including co-organizer (1849) and officeholder, North Carolina Medical Society and Edgecombe County medical society; co-organizer (1859) and member (1866-72), state medical examiners board; first vice-president, AMA (1877); delegate, AMA and North Carolina Medical Society to several international conferences; co-organizer, state board of health (1872-77). One of first strong advocates in N.C. for application of microscopy to pathology (1857) and a promoter of pathological anatomy (1851) in N.C.

WRITINGS: Several case reports in *Transactions* of North Carolina Medical Society. Writings listed in Dorothy Long, ed., *Medicine in North Carolina* 1 (1972): 185. REFERENCES: *Cyclopedia of Eminent and Representative Men of the Carolinas of the 19th Century* 2 (1892): 282-83; Long, *Medicine in North Carolina*, pp. 60-61, 77, 79, 110, 113, 584; obituary notice, *Trans., Med. Soc. of the State of N.C.* (1894), 193-4.

T. L. Savitt

PLUMMER, HENRY STANLEY (March 3, 1874, Hamilton, Minn.-December 31, 1936, Rochester, Minn.). *Internist; Endocrinologist.* Son of Albert, physician, and Isabelle (Steele) Plummer. Married Daisy Berkman, 1904; two adopted children. EDUCATION: Studied at the University of Minnesota for three years; 1898, M.D., Northwestern University. CAREER: 1898-1901, practice, Racine, Minn.; 1901-36, Mayo Clinic staff, Rochester, Minn.; and 1915-36, professor of medicine, Mayo Foundation, University of Minnesota. CONTRIBUTIONS: An early partner, Mayo Clinic; its X-ray pioneer. Also pioneered in the use of EKG in the study of heart conditions. Specialized in the investigation of exophthalmic goiter and later expanded research to thyroid diseases. Added to our knowledge of thyroid function. Helped to design the Mayo Clinic when its building was first constructed (1912) and again when the newer building was constructed (1929). Plummer Hall, where regular staff meetings are held, was named in his honor. REFERENCES: *DAB*, 11: pt. 2: 533-34; Helen Clapesattle, *The Doctors Mayo* (1941); *N.Y. Times*, January 2, 1937, p. 14:2; *Physicians of the Mayo Clinic* (1937); Proceedings of the Staff Meetings of the Mayo Clinic, July 6, 1938.

R. Rosenthal

POMEROY, JOHN (April 9, 1764, Middleboro, Mass.-February 19, 1844, Burlington, Vt.). *Physician; Educator*. Son of a farmer. Married Mary Porter, 1789; three children. EDUCATION: 1787, studied with Dr. Bradish, Cummington, Mass.; 1809, M.D. (hon.), University of Vermont. CAREER: 1779, Mass. militia; 1787, began medical practice, Cambridge, Vt.; 1792, moved to Burlington, where he remained for the rest of his life, although an invalid for the last five years; 1804-23, professor of medicine, University of Vermont. CONTRIBUTIONS: The most prominent physician of Burlington, began to take pupils before 1800. Petitioned the newly chartered University of Vermont to begin a course of instruction in medicine and (1804-23) served as professor, at first the only one, in his home and then in an office. University authorized use of some rooms for medical instruction in its only building (1815). Founding member, Vermont State Medical Society.

WRITINGS: Case reports and letters in manuscript: "Pomeroy Papers," Archives, University of Vermont, Burlington. REFERENCES: *J. Hist. Med.* (1949), 393-406; Martin Kaufman, *The University of Vermont College of Medicine* (1979), 5-20.

L. J. Wallman

POPE, CHARLES ALEXANDER (March 15, 1818, Huntsville, Ala.-July 5, 1870, Paris, France). *Surgeon*. Son of Benjamin S. and Eliza (Wyatt) Pope. Married Catherine O'Fallon, 1846; three children. EDUCATION: Green Academy, Huntsville; 1833-35, University of Alabama; apprentice to Drs. Thomas Fearn and Erskine, Huntsville; 1837-38, Cincinnati Medical College, Cincinnati, Ohio; 1839, M.D., University of Pennsylvania; 1839-40, studied in Paris. CAREER: 1841-43, private practice, St. Louis, Mo.; 1843-47, professor of anatomy and physiology, medical department, St. Louis University (St. Louis Medical College); at St. Louis Medical College: 1847-67, professor of surgery; and 1849-64, dean; committed suicide. CONTRIBUTIONS: The dynamic force behind the St. Louis Medical College, the second medical school established west of the Mississippi. With money provided by his father-in-law, John J. O'Fallon, supplied the school with its physical plant and built a free dispensary to provide care for the poor and clinical experience for the students. President, American Medical Association (1854). A founder, St. Louis Academy of Science (1856). One of the first surgeons in the region to limit his practice to surgery.

WRITINGS: Listed in Emmett Carmichael, "Charles Alexander Pope," *Annals of Med. Hist.* 3rd series, 2 (1940): 442-31. REFERENCES: Carmichael, "Charles Alexander Pope"; *NCAB* 12: 217.

D. R. Sneddeker

PORCHER, FRANCIS PEYRE (December 14, 1825, St. John's, Berkeley County, S.C.-November 19, 1895, S.C.). *Physician; Botany*. Son of Dr. William and Mrs. Isabella Sarah (Peyre) Porcher. Married Virginia Leigh; Margaret Ward. EDUCATION: Preparatory education, Mount Zion Academy; 1844, A.B., South Carolina College; 1847, M.D., Medical College of the State of South Carolina. CAREER: Began practice, Charleston, S.C.; 1852, established with Dr. Belin Flagg the Charleston Preparatory Medical School of the Medical College; lectured in Medical School on materia medica and therapeutics; became editor, *Charleston Medical Journal and Review*, serving for five years before the Civil War and resuming editorial activities with the new series that appeared after the war; surgeon and physician, marine and city hospitals; 1852, travelled extensively in Europe, visiting hospitals and clinics; during the Civil War, surgeon, Confederate Army, and served in the naval hospital, Norfolk, Va., and the South Carolina Hospital, Petersburg, S.C.; 1891, one of ten physicians from the United States selected to attend the International Medical Congress in Berlin; chosen as a delegate the following year but was unable to attend; 1892, elected president, section on general medicine, Pan American Congress. CONTRIBUTIONS: With Dr. J. J. Chisholm, opened a hospital for Negroes (1855) that was especially designed to care for the slaves from the plantations where suitable accommodations for the sick were lacking. During the Civil War, prepared a medical botany of the Southern states, *The Resources of the Southern Fields and Forests* (1863), which was highly acclaimed.

WRITINGS: *Illustrations of Disease with the Microscope: Clinical Investigations* (1861); several articles for *Med. News* (Philadelphia) and *Med. Record* (N.Y.). REFERENCES: *DAB*, 8, pt. 1:79-80; Miller, *BHM*, p. 91; *Southern J. of Med. & Pharm.* 2 (1847); *TAMA* 2 and 7 (1849, 1854); Joseph Ioor Waring, *A History of Medicine in S.C., 1825-1900* (1967).

J. P. Dolan

PORTER, HENRY RINALDO (February 13, 1848, Lee Center, N.Y.-March 3, 1903, Agra, India). *Physician; Surgeon*. Son of Henry N., physician, and

Helen (Polson) Porter. Married Lottie Viets, 1877; one child. EDUCATION: 1868-69, medical study with Dr. Henry N. Porter, Lee Center; 1872, M.D., Georgetown University. CAREER: In U.S. Army: 1872-75, acting assistant surgeon; and 1875-77, contract surgeon; 1875-1903, physician and surgeon, Bismarck, Dak. Territory, and N.Dak.; 1884-85, president, Missouri Medical Society (Bismarck, Dak. Territory); superintendent, Board of Health, Burleigh County, N.Dak. CONTRIBUTIONS: Noted military surgeon commended for gallantry during Apache Campaigns, Ariz. Territory (1872-1875). Gained national fame for gallantry during Little Big Horn fight (1876) in Mont. Territory, when he provided continuous service for 48 hours to defend perimeter maintained by survivors of Lt. Col. George Armstrong Custer's Seventh Cavalry. REFERENCES: *Bismarck Tribune*, March 5, 1903, p. 1; *Compendium of Hist. and Biog. of North Dakota* (1900), 160-65. Mentioned in nearly every history of the Battle of the Little Big Horn.

L. Remele

PORTER, JOSEPH YATES (October 21, 1847, Key West, Fla.-March 16, 1927, Key West). *Physician; State health officer.* Son of Joseph Yates and Mary A. (Randolph) Porter. Married Louise Curry, 1870; four children. EDUCATION: Orphaned before birth (father died two weeks before his birth); education entrusted to relatives; schools of Burlington, N.J.; 1870, M.D., Jefferson Medical College, Philadelphia, Pa. CAREER: 1870-73, acting assistant surgeon, U.S. Army, Ft. Jefferson (Dry Tortugas); 1875, reappointed, promoted to surgeon with captain's rank; 1880-89, service at Ft. Jefferson, Key West, Tampa, and Miami, Fla. and in Tex.; 1889-1917, health officer, Fla.; 1917, upon recommendation of Surg. Gen. William C. Gorgas (q.v.) reinstated in Army Medical Corps with rank of colonel; in this capacity, served at Ft. Jackson, S.C., and Camp Johnson, Fla.; 1919, returning to Key West, served without remuneration as city health officer and district health officer. CONTRIBUTIONS: Having survived an attack of yellow fever (1867) and having observed several deadly epidemics of the disease, became an authority on its prevention and treatment. Aware of the ineffectiveness of "shotgun quarantine," that is, localized restriction, labored long and diligently for a State Board of Health with power to coordinate preventive measures on a statewide basis. Officer in charge of federal relief services in the disastrous Jacksonville epidemic of 1888. Prime force behind establishment of State Board of Health (February 1889), having drafted the bill for legislative action. Responsible for creating six subordinate bureaus: Communicable Diseases (Field Service, Diagnostic Laboratories, Isolation Hospitals), Education, Child Welfare, Engineering, Vital Statistics, and Sanitary Science. President, Florida Medical Association (1886-87).

WRITINGS: "State Medicine," *Proc., Fla. Med. Assoc.* (1890), 62-74; "Looking Backward Over Fifty Years of Health Work in Florida," printed serially, *J. Fla. Med. Assoc.* (Jul., Aug., Sept., Oct., Nov., Dec., 1925, and Jan. 1926); "Additional Scraps from Memory's Storehouse of Sanitary Deeds in Florida During the Past Half Century," *ibid.* (Aug. 1926). REFERENCES: Frederick Eberson, "Yellow Fever Fighters: Dr. Joseph

Y. Porter, Dr. Isaac Hulse,'' *J. Fla. Med. Assoc.* 59 no. 8 (Aug. 1972): 22-29; *Proc., Fla. Med. Assoc.* (1875-1917); Rowland P. Rerick, *Memoirs of Florida* 2 (1902): 659-61; Wilson T. Sowder, ''Joseph Yates Porter, M.D.,'' *J. Fla. Med. Assoc.* 54 (Aug. 1967): 801-8; *Who Was Who in Am.*, 1: 984.

E. A. Hammond

PORTER, WILLIAM TOWNSEND (September 24, 1862, Plymouth, Ohio-February 16, 1949, Framingham, Mass.). *Physician; Physiology.* Son of Frank Gibson, physician, and Martha (Townsend) Porter. Married Alma Canfield Sterling, 1893; one child. EDUCATION: 1885, M.D., St. Louis Medical College (later Washington University); 1885-86, studied physiological chemistry, Philadelphia, and physiology, universities of Kiel, Breslau, and Berlin. CAREER: At St. Louis City Hospital: 1886-87, resident physician and acting superintendent; and for some time, in charge of medical and surgical work; 1887-93, physiology faculty, St. Louis Medical College; at Harvard University: 1893-1906, physiology faculty; and 1906-28, comparative physiology faculty. CONTRIBUTIONS: Established first physiology laboratory west of the Appalachian Mountains and introduced the use of laboratory experiments as a regular and important part of physiology instruction. Established the Harvard Apparatus Company (1901) to supply specialized physiological laboratory equipment at minimum cost to educational institutions. Made important studies of ventricular filling and pressure, control of respiration, coronary circulation, origin of the heartbeat, and the physical and mental development of children. Founded and edited *American Journal of Physiology* (1897-1914). During World War I, was chosen by the Rockefeller Foundation to do a study of the treatment of traumatic shock from which developed a personal account, *Shock at the Front* (1918), written for the general public.

WRITINGS: ''The Physical Basis of Precocity and Dullness,'' *Trans., Acad. of Sci. of St. Louis* 6 (1893): 160-81; ''On the Results of Ligation of the Coronary Arteries,'' *J. of Physiol.* 15 (1893-94): 121-38; *J. of Experimental Med.* 1 (1896): 46-70; *An Introduction to Physiology* (1901); *Physiology at Harvard* (1902); ''Traumatic Shock,'' *Harvey Lectures* 13 (1917): 21-43. REFERENCES: *DAB*, Supplement 4: 675-77; *NCAB* 15: 288; *Who Was Who in Am.*, 2: 428.

S. Galishoff

POST, GEORGE EDWARD (December 17, 1838, New York, N.Y.-September 29, 1909, Beirut, Lebanon). *Medical Missionary.* Son of Alfred Charles, surgeon, and Harriet (Beers) Post. Married Sarah Read, 1863; six children. EDUCATION: 1854, A.B., New York Free Academy (now College of the City of New York); 1860, M.D., New York University; 1861, graduate of Union Theological Seminary; 1863, D.D.S., Baltimore College of Dentistry. CAREER: 1861-63, Chaplain, 15th Regiment, New York Volunteers; 1863-67, medical missionary of American Board of Commissioners for Foreign Missions, Tripoli, Syria; 1868-1909?, professor of surgery and diseases of the eye and ear, then dean of medical school, Syrian Protestant College (now American University in Beirut); 1871-?, surgeon, Johanniter Hospital, Beirut. CONTRIBUTIONS: Served the medical and spiritual needs of many in the Near East (1863-1909). Taught western medicine to students in Arabic, even translating English texts in the basic and clinical sciences into Arabic. Performed a large number of major operations in his clinics. Raised money in United States to extend and endow work of the medical department. Edited *Al-Tabib*, an Arabic medical journal, for five years.

WRITINGS: In addition to Arabic translations and medical journal editing, wrote several botanical books and religious texts. REFERENCES: *DAB*, 15, 116-17; Kelly, *Cyclopedia Amer. Med. Biog.* (1912), 2: 280-81; *NCAB*, 13: 416; *Who Was Who in Am.*, 1: 985.

T. L. Savitt

POST, WRIGHT (February 19, 1766, North Hempstead, N.Y.-June 14, 1828, Throgg's Neck, N.Y.). *Physician; Surgery; Anatomy*. Son of Jotham and Winifred (Wright) Post. Married Mary Magdalen Bayley, 1790. EDUCATION: 1780-84, apprenticed to Richard Bayley (q.v.), N.Y.; 1784-86, studied medicine with John Sheldon and at the London Hospital; 1792, 1814, studied medicine, Europe, and collected anatomical specimens. CAREER: 1787, gave anatomy lectures, New York Hospital; *post* 1791, practiced medicine, N.Y., with his father-in-law Richard Bayley; 1792-1813, surgery faculty, medical department, Columbia University; 1792-1821, attending surgeon, New York Hospital; at College of Physicians and Surgeons: *post* 1813, anatomy and physiology faculty; and 1821-26, president. CONTRIBUTIONS: Helped introduce Hunterian methods and principles of surgery in the United States. Ligated the subclavian artery outside the scaleni muscles (1817). First person in America to ligate the femoral artery successfully for popliteal aneurysm according to John Hunter's method (1796) and the second to tie the external iliac artery for inguinal aneurism (1813). Created one of the nation's largest anatomical museums at Columbia.

WRITINGS: "A Case of Inguinal Aneurism," *Am. Med. and Philosophical Register*, 4 (1814): 443-53; "Case of Brachial Aneurism, Cured by Tying the Subclavian Artery above the Clavicle," *Trans., N.Y. Physio.-Med. Soc.* 1 (1817): 387-94. REFERENCES: *DAB*, 15: 121; Kelly and Burrage (1928), 980-81; *NCAB*, 9: 341.

S. Galishoff

POTT, JOHN (England ?-1642, Williamsburg, Va.). *Physician; Governor*. Thought to be the son of Henry and Grace Pott of "Harrop," Cheshire, England. Married Elizabeth? CAREER: 1621, arrived in Va. as physician general, Virginia Company; member, colonial Governor's Council; 1629-30, governor, Va. CONTRIBUTIONS: During tenure as governor, encouraged the passage of regulations to strengthen the colony's defenses and discouraged Lord Baltimore from attempting to place a Catholic settlement in Va. Suffered a number of political reverses. Arrested and tried for a series of crimes but was pardoned by the king. Later charged with treason, after attempting to overthrow Governor Harvey but was never tried. Although fame derives largely from political career, known as an able physician. Well respected for abilities in handling epidemic diseases and an expert in distilling water. REFERENCES: Wyndham Blanton, *Medicine in Virginia in the Seventeenth Century* (1930); *DAB*, 8, pt. 1: 123-24; I. N. Danforth, "Discussion of John Pott of Old Virginia," *Clin. Rev.* 19 (1903-4): 126-28; "John Pott Abstract of Virginia Land Patent," *Virginia Mag. of Hist. and Biog.* 1 (1893): 88-89; Howard A. Kelly, *Cyclopedia of Am. Med. Biog.* (1912); *NCAB*, 13: 383; "Several Early Physicians," *William and Mary Q.* 14 (1905): 96-100.

P. Addis

POTTER, ELLEN CULVER (August 5, 1871, New London, Conn.-February 9, 1958, Philadelphia, Pa.). *Physician; Gynecologist; Public health administration.* Daughter of Thomas W. and Ellen (Culver) Potter. Never married. EDUCATION: Following high school, studied art in academies in Boston, Mass.; New York City; and Norwich, Conn.; 1898-99, following a year in Europe, entered the Woman's Medical College of Pennsylvania, M.D., 1903; 1903-5, house officer, Philadelphia, first at the Woman's Hospital and then the new Hospital of the Woman's Medical College of Pennsylvania. CAREER: Until 1919, private practice, Germantown section of Philadelphia; won staff appointments to Germantown, Howard, Philadelphia General, and Woman's hospitals and the hospital of the Woman's Medical College of Pennsylvania; at Woman's Medical College of Pennsylvania: 1919-20, medical director; and for some years, clinical professor of gynecology. CONTRIBUTIONS: Engaged in social welfare activities even before medicine, had worked at the Morning Star Mission, N.Y.'s Chinatown (1895-96), and organized a settlement in the mill district of Norwich, Conn. (1895-97). Much later would give up private practice to become chief, Pennsylvania's Child Health Division (1920), and soon set up many new child health centers. Appointed secretary of welfare, commonwealth of Pa. (1923), supposedly becoming "the first woman to hold a state cabinet position." Increased the efficiency and scope of her department's work and initiated penal and other reforms. Director of medicine, Department of Institutions and Agencies of New Jersey (1930-46). Deputy commissioner for welfare (1946-49). Served on numerous commissions and as an officer of countless organizations, including presidency of the Medical Women's National Association (1929-30). Acting president, Woman's Medical College of Pennsylvania (1941-43).

WRITINGS: Numerous articles on social welfare and public health administration in various journals. REFERENCES: Article in *Public Health Admin. Rev.* 1 (1941): 351-57; obituary by F. Baumann, *J. Am. Med. Women's Assoc.* 13 (1958): 296-97. *DAB*, Supplement 6: 515-56; Correspondence, memorabilia, a typed bibliography, and many other items are in the Archives and Special Collections, Medical College of Pennsylvania, Philadelphia.

S. J. Peitzman

POTTER, NATHANIEL (1770, Easton, Md.-January 2, 1843, Baltimore, Md.). *Physician; Epidemiologist; Educator.* Son of Dr. Zabdiel, surgeon, and Mrs. Lucy (Bruff) Potter. Married twice, once to a Miss Ford; survived by two children. EDUCATION: Began college education in N.J.; 1796, M.D., University of Pennsylvania, where he was a student of Benjamin Rush (q.v.) for six years. CAREER: 1797, opened medical practice, Baltimore; 1801-9, secretary, Medical and Chirurgical Faculty of Maryland; 1802-5, attending physician, Baltimore General Dispensary; 1807-43, professor of theory and practice of medicine, College of Medicine, University of Maryland; 1811, editor, *Baltimore Medical and Philosophical Lyceum*; 1812, president, Baltimore Medical Society; 1812, 1814, dean, College of Medicine, University of Maryland; 1817, president, Medical Society of Maryland; 1840-43, editor, *Maryland Medical and Surgical Journal*; and attending physician, Baltimore Almshouse. CONTRIBUTIONS: Established noncontagiousness of yellow fever through self-inoculation (1797, 1798). A founder of the College of Medicine of Maryland (1807).

WRITINGS: *An Essay on the Medicinal and Deleterious Qualities of Arsenic* (1796); *A Memoir on Contagion, More Especially as it Respects the Yellow Fever. . .* (1818); edited, and adapted with notes, an American edition of John Armstrong's *Practical Illustrations of Typhus Fever. . .* (1821); edited, with S. Calhoun, George Gregory's *Elements of the Theory and Practice of Physic*, 2 vols., 2 eds. (1826, 1829); *Some Account of the Rise and Progress of the University of Maryland* (1838); *On the Locusta Septentrionales Americanae Decem Septimae* (1839); Writings listed in J. R. Quinan, *Medical Annals of Baltimore. . .* (1884), 148. REFERENCES: George H. Callcott, *History of the University of Maryland* (1982), 109-12; E. F. Cordell, *The Medical Annals of Maryland* (1891), 537; *DAB*, 15: 131-32; Kelly & Burrage (1928), 983-84; Miller, *BHM*, p. 91; *NCAB*, 5: 526; Quinan, *Medical Annals of Baltimore*, pp. 147-48; *Who Was Who in Am.*, Hist. Vol., 1607-1896: 492.

C. Donegan

POTTER, WILLIAM WARREN (December 31, 1838, Strykersville, N.Y.-March 14, 1911, Buffalo, N.Y.). *Physician; Obstetrician; Gynecologist; Editor.* Son of Lindorf, physician, and Mary Green (Blanchard) Potter. Married Emily A. Bostwick, 1859; three children. EDUCATION: Arcade and Genesee seminaries; Genesee College; apprentice to Dr. Lindorf Potter; 1859, M.D., University of Buffalo. CAREER: 1859-61, private practice, Cowlesville, N.Y.; 1861-65, surgeon, New York Volunteers; 1865-81, examining surgeon, Pension Bureau, Washington, D.C.; private practice, Mount Morris and Batavia, N.Y.; and medical staff, New York Institution for the Blind (Batavia); 1881-1911, private practice, Buffalo; editor: 1888-1911, *Transactions of the American Association of Obstetricians and Gynecologists*; and 1888-1911, *Buffalo Medical Journal*; 1891-1911, member and president (1897), New York State Board of Medical Examiners; 1895-99, president, National Confederation of Medical Examining and Licensing Boards; and medical staff, Women's Hospital, Buffalo General Hospital. CONTRIBUTIONS: A founder, American Association of Obstetricians and Gynecologists. Largely responsible for the establishment of the New York State Board of Medical Examiners (1891).

WRITINGS: *Observations on the Uterine Sound* (1886); *How Should Girls Be Educated* (1891); *Asepsis and Antisepsis as Applied in the Lying-In Chamber* (1892). REFERENCES:

Buffalo Med. J. 66 (1911): 502-3; *Express* (Buffalo), March 15, 1911; *JAMA* 56 (1911): 909; Kelly and Burrage (1928), 984-85; *Trans., Am. Assoc. of Obstetricians and Gynecologists* 24 (1911): 333-54.

D. O. Powell

POYNTER, CHARLES WILLIAM McCORKLE (July 16, 1875, Eureka, Ill.-October 25, 1950, Omaha, Nebr.). *Physician; Medical educator; Anatomist; Anthropologist.* Son of William Amos, farmer and governor, and Maria Josephine (McCorkle) Poynter. Married Clara Eliza Axtell, September 3, 1907; one child. EDUCATION: 1892, High School, Albion, Nebr.; 1898, B.S., University of Nebraska; 1902, M.D., University of Nebraska College of Medicine; intern, Bellevue Hospital, N.Y.; Lee's Clinic and Cook County Hospital, Chicago, Ill.; 1907-8, postgraduate study, Vienna, with Toldt Von Eiselberg; 1912, Harvard University. CAREER: 1892-93, 1895-96, teacher, Boone County, Nebr.; 1903-11, practice of medicine, Lincoln, Nebr.; at University of Nebraska College of Medicine, Lincoln: 1903-4, instructor of anatomy; 1906-7, adjunct professor of anatomy; 1908-9, assistant professor of anatomy; and 1910-12, professor of anatomy and chairman of the department; at University of Nebraska College of Medicine, Omaha: 1912-18, 1919-42, professor of anatomy and chairman of the department; 1918-19, 1929, acting dean; 1930-46, dean; and 1946-50, dean emeritus and director of anatomical research; in Association of American Medical Colleges: 1933-34, vice-president; 1935-39, Executive Council; and 1940-41, president. CONTRIBUTIONS: A basic scientist, devoted talents to teaching and administration of medical education. Outstanding professor of anatomy. Active in the Association of American Medical Colleges during a time when efforts were toward raising standards of medical education. Successful administrator of a medical college program during depression years and World War II. Provided substantial anthropological data concerning Indians of the Missouri River area.

WRITINGS: "A Study of the American Negro Brain," *J. of Comparative Neurology* 25 (Jun. 1915): 183-212 (with J. J. Keegan); "A Study of Nebraska Crania," *Am. Anthropology* 17 (1915): 509-24; "Arterial Anomalies Pertaining to the Aortic Arches and the Branches Arising from Them," *Nebraska Univ. Studies* 16 (Oct. 1916); "Some Observations on Wound Healing in the Early Embryo," *Anat. Rec.* 16 (Mar. 1919): 1-23; "Observations on the Palatine Tonsil," *Trans. Am. Acad. Ophthalmology* 25 (1920): 306-20; "Lens Antigen as a Factor in Congenital and Hereditary Eye Anomalies," *Am. J. of Ophthalmology* 8 (Mar. 1925): 184-92; (with E. V. Allen); "Concerning the Great Omentum," *Med. Clinics North America* 12 (Sept 1928): 499-505. Writings listed in the University of Nebraska Medical Center Library of Medicine, Omaha. REFERENCES: Archives, University of Nebraska Medical Center Library of Medicine, Omaha; *NCAB*, 39: 300.

B. M. Hetzner

PRESCOTT, SAMUEL CATE (April 5, 1872, South Hampton, N.H.-March 19, 1962, Boston, Mass.). *Bacteriologist; Food technology.* Son of Samuel Melcher, farmer and blacksmith, and Mary Emily (Cate) Prescott. Married Alice

D. Chase, 1910; three children. EDUCATION: 1894, S.B., Massachusetts Institute of Technology; 1900, studied in Berlin and Copenhagen. CAREER: 1894-95, chemist, Worcester (Mass.) Sewage Purification Works; at Massachusetts Institute of Technology: 1895-1914, biology faculty; 1914-32, biology and public health faculty; and 1932-42, dean, School of Science; 1902-9, bacteriology faculty, Simmons College; 1904-21, director, Boston Bio-Chemical Laboratory; director: 1914-17, research laboratory, United Fruit Company, Port Limon, Costa Rica; and 1918-19, Division of Dehydration, Bureau of Chemistry, U.S. Department of Agriculture; consultant in applied bacteriology to the food industry and for investigations of municipal water and milk supplies. CONTRIBUTIONS: Placed canning on a scientific basis by applying to it the principles of bacteriology; with William Lyman Underwood, isolated many of the bacteria responsible for spoilage in canned food and devised a practical method for sterilization (1897-98). Worked out the time-temperature requirements for boiling the cans and found solutions to many other technical problems of food production and preservation.

WRITINGS: *Food Technology* (1937, with Bernard E. Proctor); *Industrial Microbiology* (1940, with Cecil G. Dunn). REFERENCES: R.J.G. and M.S.P., "Famous Food Technologist to be Honored at National Meeting in Boston," *Food Technology* 7 (Apr. 1953): 8-12; *J. of Milk & Food Technology* 25 (Apr. 1962): 134-35; *NCAB*, 50: 294-95; *N.Y. Times*, March 21, 1962; *Who Was Who in Am.*, 4: 765.

S. Galishoff

PRESTON, ANN (December 1, 1813, Chester County, Pa.-April 18, 1872, Philadelphia, Pa.). *Physician; Educator*. Daughter of Amos, farmer, and Margaret (Smith) Preston. Never married. EDUCATION: West Chester Boarding school; 1852, M.D., Woman's Medical College of Pennsylvania; 1854, studied in Paris. CAREER: 1853-72, professor of physiology and hygiene, Woman's Medical College of Pennsylvania; at Woman's Hospital: 1861-72, founder and member, Board of Managers; and consulting physician; 1866-72, dean, Medical College of Pennsylvania. CONTRIBUTIONS: Pioneering woman physician, graduated in the first class of the Woman's Medical College of Pennsylvania. Chose medicine as a profession late in life (graduated at age 39). Founded Woman's Hospital to provide clinical experience to female medical students who were not allowed to take clinical lectures at other Philadelphia hospitals.

WRITINGS: *Reply to Preamble and Resolutions of the Philadelphia County Medical Society* (1867). REFERENCES: *Appleton's Cyclopedia*, 5: 112; Frederick P. Henry, *Standard Hist. of Med. Profession in Phila.* (1897); *BHM* (1964-69), 215; *DAB*, 8: 201-2; John S. Futhey and Gilbert Cope, *History of Chester County* (1881); Kelly and Burrage (1928), 990; Miller, *BHM*, p. 92; *NCAB*, 10: 467.

D. I. Lansing

PREVOST, FRANCOIS MARIE (c. 1764, Pont-de-Cé, France-May 18, 1842, Donaldsonville, La.). *Surgeon*. Son of Jean Pierre and Marie Anne (Kenotaire) Prevost. Married Marie Therese Burruchon, 1799, two children, one adopted;

Victorine Castellain, 1838. EDUCATION: M.D., University of Paris. CAREER: Practiced, Fort de Paix, Haiti, as the officier de Santé; c. 1800, fled the excesses of the Haiti slave insurrection and settled in Ascension Parish, La. a few miles up the river from New Orleans, La.; 1800-1842, practice, La. CONTRIBUTIONS: Performed the second Caesarean section in America (1822) on a slave woman in a dimly lit slave cabin, assisted by a slave woman. In four operations (1822-25), saved seven of eight lives. REFERENCES: *Am. J. of Med. Sci.* (Apr. 1878); *DAB*, 9: 209-10; John Duffy, *History of Medicine in Louisiana*, 1 (1958).

M. Kaufman

PRICE, JOSEPH (January 1, 1853, Rockingham County, Va.-June 6, 1911, Philadelphia, Pa.). *Surgeon; Obstetrics and gynecology.* Son of Joshua and Feby (Moore) Price. Married Louise Troth, 1887; seven children. EDUCATION: Fort Edward Collegiate Institute (N.Y.); Union College (Albany, N.Y.); 1877, M.D., University of Pennsylvania. CAREER:1877, ship surgeon; 1878, became head, obstetrical department, Philadelphia Dispensary, and created its gynecological department; 1887-94, resident physician, Preston Retreat (philanthropic maternity hospital); 1888, with Dr. C. B. Penrose, founded the Gynecean Hospital; 1891, founded the Joseph Price Hospital. CONTRIBUTIONS: A leading obstetrician and gynecologist in early Philadelphia; an early pioneer in tabulating the results of a specific surgical procedure. Surgical skill and innovative techniques helped make hysterectomy a safe operation. Taught physicians to save women from death caused by ruptured ectopic pregnancy. In the forefront of establishing hospitals, founding several, including the hospital bearing his name that became the largest private institution in the country for abdominal surgery. Taught the Mayo brothers surgical techniques. A founder, American Association of Obstetricians and Gynecologists, and president (1896).

WRITINGS: "Cleanliness and Maternities," *Med & Surg. Reporter* (Jul. 1890); "Retrospect of Abdominal Surgery," *Med. News* (Jun. 14, 1890); "Surgical Conception of Peritonitis," *Trans., Am. Assoc. Obstetricians and Gynecologists* (1891). Writings listed in Kelly and Burrage (1920). REFERENCES: *DAB*, 8: 213-14; Kelly and Burrage (1920); James W. Kennedy, *Practical Surgery of the Joseph Price Hospital* (1926); *NCAB*, 38: 378.

D. I. Lansing

PRIDE, MAYNARD PRINCE (June 1, 1914, Belpre, Ohio-August 6, 1973, Philadelphia, Pa.). *Physician.* Son of Eber, farmer, and Amy (Bradley) Pride. Married Frances Barnes, 1939; three children; Sue Randall, 1958; two children. EDUCATION: 1935, B.A., Marietta College; 1939, M.D., Western Reserve Medical School; 1939-46, intern and resident, University Hospital, Cleveland, Ohio. CAREER: Private practice, Morgantown W.Va., for 27 years; *post* 1960, surgery faculty, University of West Virginia School of Medicine. CONTRIBUTIONS: President, West Virginia Medical Association (1969). Member, West Virginia State Medical Licensing Board. Director, Federation of State Medical Boards. Worked to upgrade and modernize medical licensing procedures in W.Va. Member, comprehensive planning commission at the time the plans for the new Monongalia County Hospital were developed.

WRITINGS: "Plasma Volume Available (Thiocyanate) Volume and Total Circulating Plasma Proteins in Normal Adults," *Annals of Surg.* 121 (Mar. 1945): 352-60 (with C. E. Griffin et al.). REFERENCES: *NCAB*, 57: 718. Interviews with Mrs. Maynard Pride, and Dr. Reginald Krause of the University of West Virginia Medical School; clippings from the *West Virginia Med. J.*, at the medical library, University of W. Va. Med. School, Morgantown, W. Va.

K. Nodyne and R. Murphy

PRINCE, MORTON (December 21, 1854, Boston, Mass.-August 31, 1929, Boston). *Physician; Psychiatry.* Son of Frederick Octavius and Helen Susan (Henry) Prince. Married Fanny Lithgow Payson, 1885; two children. EDUCATION: 1871, graduated, Boston Latin School; 1875, A.B., Harvard College; 1879, M.D., Harvard Medical School; 1878-79, intern, Boston City Hospital; 1879-80, formal study, Vienna, Austria, and Strassburg, France, and informal study, Paris and Nancy, France. CAREER: 1881-86, at Boston Dispensary: 1881-82, district physician; and 1882-86, physician for diseases of the nervous system; 1882-1929, at Boston City Hospital: 1882-84, physician for diseases of the nose and throat; 1885-1913, physician for nervous diseases; and 1913-29, consulting physician; 1885-88, U.S. examining surgeon for pensions; 1895-98, instructor in neurology, Harvard Medical School; 1902-12, professor of nervous diseases, Tufts University Medical School; 1926-28, associate professor, abnormal and dynamic psychology, Harvard University; 1906-29, founder and editor, *Journal of Abnormal and Social Psychology*; service to American Neurological Association (president, 1911). CONTRIBUTIONS: Carried out extensive clinical studies in abnormal psychology and was best known for investigations of dissociation, particularly in relation to the case of "Christine L. Beauchamp." Led academic psychologists to realize the importance of "abnormal" psychology. Founded Harvard Psychological Clinic (1926).

WRITINGS: *The Nature of Mind and Human Automatism* (1885); *The Dissociation of a Personality: A Biographical Study in Abnormal Psychology* (1905; 2nd ed., 1908); *The Unconscious: The Fundamentals of Human Personality, Normal and Abnormal* (1914; 2nd ed., 1921); *The Psychology of the Kaiser: A Study of His Sentiments and His Obsessions* (1915). REFERENCES: *DAB*, 15: 230-32; Nathan G. Hale, Jr., *Psychotherapy and Multiple Personality: Selected Essays of Morton Prince* (1975), includes a bibliography of Prince, pp. 317-28; Otto M. Marx, "Morton Prince and the Dissociation of a Personality," *J. Hist. Behavioral Sci.* 6 (1970): 120-30; Miller, *BHM*, p. 92; Merrill Moore, "Morton Prince, M.D., 1854-1929," *J. of Nervous and Mental Diseases* 87 (1938): 701-10; Henry A. Murray, "Morton Prince: Sketch of His Life and Work," *J. of Abnormal and Social Psychology* 52 (1956): 291-95; *NCAB*, 25: 343-44; *NUC Pre-1956 Imprints, 471: 444-47; N.Y. Times*, September 1, 1929, sect. 2, p. 5.

M. M. Sokal

PROCTER, WILLIAM, JR. (May 3, 1817, Baltimore, Md.-February 9, 1874, Philadelphia, Pa.). *Pharmacist.* Son of Isaac and Rebecca (Farquhar) Procter.

Married Margaretta Bullock, 1849; Catherine Parry, 1864. EDUCATION: 1837, graduated, Philadelphia College of Pharmacy. CAREER: *Post* 1841, member, Commission on Revision of the U.S. Pharmacopoeia; 1844-74, owned and operated drugstore, Philadelphia; at Philadelphia College of Pharmacy: 1846-66, 1872-74, theory and practice of pharmacy faculty; 1851-53, trustee; 1855-57, corresponding secretary; and 1869-74, first vice-president; 1851, delegate, convention of pharmacists to fix standards for use by customs officials in drug inspection, New York City; 1862, president, American Pharmaceutical Association. CONTRIBUTIONS: Has been called the "father of American pharmacy." Edited the *American Journal of Pharmacy* (1850-71). Did extensive drug research; pioneered with ether and was one of the first to discover the salicylates of natural origin. Published the American edition of Francis Mohr and Theophilus Redwood's *Practical Pharmacy*. Helped found the American Pharmaceutical Association and was its first corresponding secretary (1852-57).

WRITINGS: Some 500 articles are in *J. of Pharmacy*. REFERENCES: George A. Bender, "The Father of American Pharmacy: William Procter, Jr. (1817-1874)," *Modern Pharmacy*, 41, no. 1 (1956), 4 p. insert; Ivor Griffith, "William Procter, Jr.—Father of American Pharmacy," *Am. J. of Pharmacy* 115 (Nov. 1943): 406-16; Miller, *BHM*, p. 92; *Who Was Who in Am.*, Hist. Vol.: 497.

S. Galishoff

PRUDDEN, T[HEOPHIL] MITCHELL (July 7, 1849, Middlebury, Conn.-April 10, 1924, New York, N.Y.). *Physician; Pathology; Bacteriology; Public health.* Son of George Peter and Eliza Anne (Johnson) Prudden. Never married. EDUCATION: Yale University: 1872, A.B., and 1875, M.D.; 1875-76, intern, New Haven Hospital; 1876-78, studied in Heidelberg and Berlin, Germany, and Vienna, Austria; 1882, 1885, studied in Germany. CAREER: At College of Physicians and Surgeons (Columbia): 1878-82, pathology and histology faculty, 1882-91, director, pathology and histology laboratory, and 1892-1909, pathology faculty; 1880-86, lecturer, normal histology, Yale University; 1901-24, member, Board of Scientific Directors, Rockefeller Institute; 1921-24, member, International Health Board, Rockefeller Foundation; consulting bacteriologist, New York City Board of Health; and member, New York State Public Health Council. CONTRIBUTIONS: Helped establish the discipline of pathology in the United States. With Francis Delafield (q.v.), wrote *A Handbook of Pathological Anatomy and Histology* (1885) which after many revisions was still widely used in American medical schools some 50 years later. One of the earliest bacteriological investigators in the United States. Played an active role in the development of the boards of health of New York City and N.Y. State.

WRITINGS: "Beobachtungen am Lebenden Knorpel," *Virchows Archiv für Pathologische Anatomie und Physiologie. . .*75 (1879): 1-14; *A Manual of Practical Normal Histology* (1882); *Dust and Its Dangers* (1890); "Studies on the Action of Dead Bacteria in the Living Body," *Med. Record* 53 (1891): 637-40, 697-707 (with Eugene Hodenpyl). A bibliography is in Lillian E. Prudden, ed., *Biographical Sketches and Letters of T. Mitchell Prudden, M.D.* (1927). REFERENCES: *BHM* (1970-74), 144; *DAB*, 15: 252-53;

DSB, 11: 175-77; Kelly and Burrage (1928), 996; *NCAB*, 9: 347; *Who Was Who in Am.*, 1: 999.

S. Galishoff

PURPLE, SAMUEL SMITH (June 24, 1822, Lebanon, N.Y.-September 29, 1900, New York, N.Y.). *Physician; Editor.* Son of Lyman Smith, shoemaker and tanner, and Minerva (Sheffield) Purple. Never married. EDUCATION: Apprentice to Dr. David Ransom, Earlville, N.Y.; 1842, Geneva Medical College; 1844, M.D., New York University Medical College. CAREER: 1844-1900, private practice, New York City; medical staff: 1844-46, Marion Street Maternity and New York Lying-in Asylum; and 1846-49, New York Dispensary; 1875-78, president, New York Academy of Medicine; editor: 1848-58, *New York Journal of Medicine*; and 1874-86, *New York Genealogical and Biographical Record.* CONTRIBUTIONS: A founder, New York Academy of Medicine and its library, to which he donated over 5,000 volumes of American medical journals.

WRITINGS: *Menstruation* (1846); *Contributions to the Practice of Midwifery and Forensic Medicine* (1853); *Medical Libraries* (1877). REFERENCES: *DAB*, 8: 269-70; Claude E. Heaton, "Samuel Smith Purple, 1822-1900," *Academy Bookman* 1 (1948): 3-5; Kelly and Burrage (1928), 997-98; *NCAB*, 6: 136; *N.Y. Genealogical and Biographical Rec.* 27 (1900): 1-6; *N.Y. Times*, October 1, 1900.

D. O. Powell

PURVIS, CHARLES BURLEIGH (April 14, 1842, Philadelphia, Pa.,-December 14, 1929, Boston, Mass.). *Surgeon; Medical educator.* Son of Robert, well-to-do benefactor, and Harriet D. Purvis. Married Ann Hathaway, 1871; two children. EDUCATION: 1860-63, Oberlin College; 1865, M.D., Wooster Medical College (now Western Reserve University); 1868, A.M., Howard University. CAREER: 1865-69, acting assistant surgeon, U.S. Army, Washington, D.C.; at Freedmen's Hospital, Washington, D.C.: 1869-81, assistant surgeon; and 1881-94, surgeon-in-chief; at Howard University Medical College: 1869-73, professor of materia medica and therapeutics; and 1873-1906, professor of obstetrics and gynecology; 1905-29, private practice, Boston, Mass. CONTRIBUTIONS: Second black faculty member, Howard University Medical College (March 15, 1869), and at any medical school. First and only Negro physician to attend a president (James A. Garfield, following assassination attack, 1881). One of three black physicians to be rejected for racial reasons from membership in a constituent society of the AMA (Medical Society of District of Columbia, 1869). Secretary, medical faculty (1873-96); president, medical faculty (1899-1900); and Board of Trustees (1908-26), Howard University. Major force in keeping Howard Medical School open during financial crisis (1873). Prevented closing of Freedmen's Hospital (1903). First Negro to serve on Board of Medical

Examiners, District of Columbia (1897-1904). REFERENCES: W. Montague Cobb, "Charles Burleigh Purvis," *JNMA* 45 (1953): 79-82; *Who Was Who in Am.*, 4: 769.

T. L. Savitt

PUSEY, WILLIAM ALLEN (December 1, 1865, Elizabethtown, Ky.-August 29, 1940, Chicago, Ill.). *Physician; Dermatology; Venereal disease; Radiology; Medical history.* Son of Robert Burns, physician, and Bell (Brown) Pusey. Married Sallie Warfield Cunningham, 1887; no children. EDUCATION: Vanderbilt University: 1885, A.B.; and 1886, A.M.; 1888, M.D., New York University; 1888-89, trained at the Skin and Cancer Hospital, N.Y.; 1889-90, 1891-92, studied dermatology, Europe; 1899, studied radiology, Europe. CAREER: *Post* 1893, practiced medicine, Chicago; 1894-1915, dermatology faculty, College of Physicians and Surgeons, Chicago (later affiliated with the University of Illinois); during World War I, chairman, committee on venereal disease control under the Surgeon General's Office; member: 1925-31, Executive Committee, National Research Council; and 1925-32, Commission on Medical Education; president: 1910, American Dermatological Association; and 1924, American Medical Association. CONTRIBUTIONS: A pioneer in the use of X-rays for the treatment of systemic malignancies (such as Hodgkin's disease) as well as for cutaneous diseases. With Eugene Wilson Caldwell, published *The Practical Application of the Roentgen Rays in Therapeutics and Diagnosis* (1903), which received worldwide attention. Introduced the use of solid carbon dioxide in dermatological treatment. Textbook *The Principles and Practice of Dermatology*, which appeared in 1907, went through four editions, the last appearing in 1924. Edited *Archives of Dermatology and Syphilology* (1920-37) and made it one of the best journals in its field. Promoted open discussion of syphilis and helped launch a vigorous campaign against the disease.

WRITINGS: "The Use of Carbon Dioxide Snow in the Treatment of Nevi and other Lesions of the Skin: A Preliminary Report," *JAMA* 49 (Oct. 19, 1907): 1354-56; *Syphilis as a Modern Problem* (1915); *A Doctor of the 1870's and 80's* (1932); *The History of Dermatology* (1933); *The History and Epidemiology of Syphilis* (1933). A bibliography is in *Archives of Dermatology and Syphilology* 35 (Jan. 1937). REFERENCES: *DAB*, Supplement 2: 546-47; *NCAB* 34: 135-36; *N.Y. Times*, August 31, 1940; *Who Was Who in Am.*, 1: 1001.

S. Galishoff

PUTNAM, CHARLES PICKERING (September 15, 1844, Boston, Mass.-April 23, 1914, Boston). *Pediatrician; Social welfare; Public health.* Son of Dr. Charles Gideon, physician, and Elizabeth Cabot (Jackson) Putnam (and grandson of James Jackson [q.v.]). Married Lucy Washburn, 1889; three children. EDUCATION: 1865, A.B., Harvard College; 1869, M.D., Harvard Medical School; postgraduate studies at Massachusetts General Hospital and in Germany. CAREER: 1871, began practice in Boston, eventually specializing in pediatrics and orthopedic surgery; 1873-79, lectured on the diseases of children at the

Harvard Medical School; 1871-73, physician to the Boston Dispensary, orthopedic surgeon from 1873-76; 1875, became physician to the Massachusetts Infants Asylum, chairman of its Board of Trustees (1898-1910). CONTRIBUTIONS: For many years, Boston's leading advocate of social welfare. A founder of the Boston Society for the Relief of Destitute Mothers and Infants (1873), which worked to keep mothers and children together, and president (1904-14). President, Associated Charities of Boston, when it was founded (1879), the nation's second such organization; chairman of various committees over the years until his death in 1914. Credited with reorganizing Boston's institutions for the care of delinquent children, the poor, and prisoners (1892-97); member of mayoral committees, chairman of the board of visitors, and advocate for the 1897 reorganization bill. Member of the Board of Children's Institutions (1897-1911) and chairman (1902-11). Helped James R. Chadwick organize the Boston Medical Library, was a director of the Mental Hygiene Association, advocate of the State Board of Insanity, supporter and worker for the Mass. Civic League, and organizer and administrator of the Boston Medical Library's Directory of Nurses. REFERENCES: *Boston Med. and Surg. J.*, May 7, 1914; *DAB*, 8: 275-76; Kelly and Burrage (1928), 998-99.

M. Kaufman

PUTNAM, JAMES JACKSON (October 3, 1846, Boston, Mass.-November 4, 1918, Boston). *Physician; Neurology.* Son of Dr. Charles Gideon, physician, and Mrs. Elizabeth Cabot (Jackson) Putnam, daughter of James Jackson (q.v.). Married Marian Cabot, 1886; five children. EDUCATION: 1866, A.B., Harvard College; 1870, M.D., Harvard Medical School; 1870-71, house officer, Massachusetts General Hospital; 1871-72, study at Leipzig, Germany; Vienna, Austria (with Theodor Meynert); Paris, France (with Jean Charcot); and London, England (with John Hughlings Jackson). CAREER: 1872-1912, at Harvard Medical School: 1872-74, lecturer on the application of electricity in nervous disease; 1874-75, lecturer on diseases of the nervous system; 1875-85, clinical instructor on diseases of the nervous system; 1885-93, instructor on diseases of the nervous system; and 1893-1912, professor of diseases of the nervous system; 1874-1909, neurologist and consulting physician, Massachusetts General Hospital. CONTRIBUTIONS: A founder and long-time contributor to the American Neurological Association (president, 1888). Carried out much early work on organic diseases of the nervous system. Turned attention (1890s) to functional aspects of nervous disease and psychoneurosis and did much to introduce and gain acceptance for psychoanalysis in the United States.

WRITINGS: *Studies in Neurological Diagnosis* (1902, with George A. Waterman); *Human Motives* (1915). Many of his psychoanalytic articles collected in *Addresses on Psychoanalysis* (1921). REFERENCES: *BHM* (1970-74), 145; (1975-79), 107; *Addresses on Psychoanalysis* (1921); *DAB*, 15: 282-83; Nathan Hale, ed., *James Jackson Putnam and Psychoanalysis: Letters Between Putnam and Sigmund Freud* (1971); Kelly and Burrage (1928), 999-1002; *NCAB*, 18: 36; *NUC Pre-1956 Imprints*, 476: 64-67; Edward

W. Taylor, "James Jackson Putnam," *Arch. of Neurology and Psychiatry* 3 (1928): 307-14; E. Bruce Tucker, "James Jackson Putnam: An American Perspective on the Social Uses of Psychoanalysis," *New Eng. Q.*, 51 (1978): 527-46; Russell G. Vasile, *James Jackson Putnam; From Neurology to Psychoanalysis* (1977); David S. Werman, "James Jackson Putnam: Philosophy and Psychoanalysis," *American Imago* 34 (1977): 72-85; Stephen Y. Wilkerson, "Mind Over Body: James Jackson Putnam and the Impact of Neurology on Psychotherapy in Late 19th-Century America" (Ph.D. diss., Duke University, 1978).

M. M. Sokal

Q

QUAIN, ERIC PEER (August 22, 1870, Sörsjön, Delarne, Sweden-September 11, 1962, Salem, Oreg.). *Physician; Surgeon.* Son of Per Halvor, blacksmith, farmer, and trader, and Margaret (Erickson) Quain. Married Fannie Almara Dunn (q.v.), 1903, two children; divorced, 1938; Hilda Gustafson, 1940. EDUCATION: 1898, M.D., University of Minnesota; postgraduate study, New York City, Vienna, London. CAREER: 1899-1938, physician and surgeon, Bismarck, N.Dak.; 1901-3, city health officer and coroner, Bismarck; 1903, co-founder, Quain and Ramstad Clinic (second oldest group practice in the United States); 1910, delegate from N.Dak. to the National Congress of Hygiene and Demography, Washington, D.C.; 1917, major, Medical Reserve Corps, American Expeditionary Forces; 1918, chief of surgical services, Camp Jackson, S.C.; 1918-19, chief of surgical services and director of operating teams, American Expeditionary Force hospitals, France; 1919, chief of surgical services, Fort Snelling Hospital, St. Paul, Minn.; president: 1920, Soo Line Railroad Surgical Association; 1922-23, North Dakota Medical Association; and 1924, North Dakota Officers Association; 1924, commanding officer, 379th Medical Regiment. CONTRIBUTIONS: Credited with introduction of antiseptic surgery to Bismarck area of N.Dak. Co-founded Quain and Ramstad Clinic (1903). Instrumental in founding of Bismarck Hospital (1907). Played major role in establishing Bismarck Hospital School of Nursing. Developed several surgical practices, including techniques for incisions for abdominal surgery.

WRITINGS: "A New, Quick, and Practical Surgical Knot," *Surg. Gyn. & Obst.* (Mar. 1909); "Some Observations on Cartharsis," *JAMA* 59 (1912); "The Application of the Sewing Machine Stitch in Gastric and Intestinal Anastomoses," *Surg. Gyn. & Obst.* (Oct. 1916); "Abdominal Incisions," *Arch. of Surg.* 1 (1920); "Measuring Length of Lower Extremities: A New Method," *J. of Bone and Joint Surg.* 13 (1932). Writings listed in *Quarterly Cumulated Index Medicus, 1916-1942.* REFERENCES: *Bismarck Tribune*, September 11, 1962, p. 1; Paul W. Friese, *The Story of the Quain and Ramstad Clinic* (n.d.); James Grassick, *North Dakota Medicine: Sketches and Abstracts* (1926),

129-32; Naboth Hedin, "A Pioneer Physician in North Dakota," *Am. Swedish Monthly* 49 (Apr. 1955); W. B. Hennessey, *History of North Dakota* (1910), 470; *NCAB*, 51: 428.

L. Remele

QUAIN, FANNIE ALMARA (DUNN) (February 13, 1874, Bismarck, Dak. Territory-February 2, 1950, Bismarck, N.Dak.). *Physician; Public health leader.* Daughter of John Platt III, pharmacist, and Christina Seelye (Styles) Dunn. Married Eric Peer Quain, (q.v.), 1903; divorced, 1938; two children. EDUCATION: 1898, M.D., University of Michigan. CAREER: 1898-1950, physician, Bismarck; 1909-21, secretary, North Dakota Tuberculosis Association (now the North Dakota Lung Association); 1911-12, member, Site Selection Board, North Dakota State Tuberculosis Sanitarium; 1920-40, chairperson, Nurses Training School Committee, Bismarck Evangelical Hospital (now Bismarck Hospital); 1921-28, vice-president, North Dakota Tuberculosis Association; 1923-33, member, North Dakota State Board of Health; 1928-36, president, North Dakota Tuberculosis Association; 1933-34, regional director, Medical Women's National Association; 1939-48, treasurer, North Dakota Tuberculosis Association; 1948-50, vice-president, North Dakota Tuberculosis Association. CONTRIBUTIONS: First female native of N.Dak. to enter medicine as a career. Started and worked on state campaign to eradicate tuberculosis. Developed public health awareness movements, including "baby clinics" and state sanitarium, as part of fight against tuberculosis. Contributor to development of nurse's training standards within N. Dak. REFERENCES: *American Women: III* (1939); *Bismarck Tribune*, February 2, 1950, pp. 1-2.

L. Remele

QUINLAND, WILLIAM SAMUEL (October 12, 1885, All Saints, Antigua, British West Indies-April 6, 1953, Tuskegee, Ala.). *Pathologist.* Son of William Thomas and Floretta Victoria (Williams) Quinland. Married Sadie Lee Watson, 1923; two children. EDUCATION: 1914-15, Howard University; 1918, B.S., Oskaloosa College (Ia.); 1919, M.D., Meharry Medical College; 1921, Harvard Medical School Graduate certificate in Pathology and Bacteriology; 1941-42, University of Chicago, General Education Board Fellow in Pathology. CAREER: 1919-22, Rosenwald Fellow in pathology and bacteriology, Harvard Medical School; 1921-22, assistant in pathology, Peter Bent Brigham Hospital; 1922-47, professor and head of pathology department and secretary of faculty, Meharry Medical College; at George W. Hubbard Hospital: 1922-47, pathologist; and 1931-37, associate medical director; 1947-53, pathologist and chief of laboratory service, Veterans Administration Hospital, Tuskegee, Ala. CONTRIBUTIONS: First recipient of Rosenwald Fellowship for advanced medical study (1919). First black admitted to American Association of Pathologists and Bacteriologists (1920). First black diplomate of American Board of Pathology (1937). First black elected a fellow, College of American Pathologists (1947). Directed public health clinics,

Richmond, Va.; Columbia, S.C.; and Augusta, Ga. Published widely, including several articles on pathology of Negro.

WRITINGS: Twenty-eight publications, including "Primary Carcinoma in the Negro: Anatomic Distribution of Three Hundred Cases," *Arch. Path.* 30 (1940): 393-402; "Bronchogenic Carcinoma—Report of Three Cases in Negroes," *Southern Med. J.* 35 (1942): 729-32. Writings listed in *JNMA* 45 (1953): 299-300. REFERENCES: *The Crisis* 19 (Dec. 1919): 65; obituary, *JNMA* 45 (1953): 298-300; *WWAPS* 1 (1938): 979-80.

T. L. Savitt

R

RAAB, WILHELM (January 14, 1895, Vienna, Austria-September 21, 1970, Burlington, Vt.). *Physician; Cardiologist.* Son of Richard, a civil servant, and Rosa (Gerenyi) Raab. Married Olga Palmborg, 1930, two children; Helen Hubaczek, 1970. EDUCATION: 1920, M.D., University of Vienna; 1926, M.D., German University of Prague; 1921-26, assistant to Dr. Biedl, Prague, Czechoslovakia; 1926-36, assistant to Drs. Wenckebach and Eppinger, First Medical Clinic, Vienna. CAREER: 1929-30, Rockefeller Research Fellow, Department of Physiology, Harvard; 1935-39, privatdozent, internal medicine, University of Vienna; 1936-39, physician-in-chief, Krankenhaus der Kaufmannschaft, Vienna; at University of Vermont: 1939-45, assistant professor of medicine; 1945-60, professor, experimental medicine; and 1949-70, director and attending physician, Cardiovascular Research Unit; 1957-58, Fulbright Professor, Innsbruck, Austria. CONTRIBUTIONS: Described a patient with basophilic adenoma of the pituitary (1924). Case was republished (1932) by Harvey Cushing (q.v.) with two additional ones, and the syndrome became known as Cushing's Disease. Pioneer in studies of the effects of hypoxia and brain injury on "essential" hypertension. Conducted worldwide inquiries (1932-39) into the effect of cholesterol and animal fat on arteriosclerosis and formulated the dietary rules that have held until questioned (1980). Discovered catecholamines in brain tissue (1942). Known for research in nervous and chemical mechanism in heart function. Described "loafer's heart" (the deleterious effect on the heart of lack of exercise, emotional tension, and nicotine) and worked for the mass prevention of heart disease through reconditioning. Host to symposium "The Catecholamines in Cardiovascular Pathology" (1959) and "The First International Conference on Preventive Cardiology" (1964), both at the University of Vermont.

WRITINGS: *Hormones and Metabolism* (1926); *Hormonal and Neurogenic Cardio-*

vascular Disorders (1963); *Hypokinetic Disease* (1961, with H. Kraus); *Preventive My-ocardiology* (1970). REFERENCES: *Cardiologica 45 (1964): 383-84*.

L. J. Wallman

RAMSAY, ALEXANDER (1754, Edinburgh, Scotland-November 1824, Parsonsfield, Maine). *Physician; Surgeon; Anatomist*. Never married. EDUCATION: Aberdeen University; studied medicine, London, under Matthew Baillie; Trinity College, Dublin; and Edinburgh. CAREER: Established an anatomical school and museum in Edinburgh and attracted so many pupils that authorities were forced to establish a chair of anatomy, University of Edinburgh; founded Anatomical Society, Edinburgh, which lasted until 1818; 1802, went to the United States; settled in Fryeburg, Maine, and lectured on anatomy throughout the eastern states at $30 a course, only practicing medicine occasionally; 1806, failed in an effort with others to establish a new medical school in N.Y.; 1808, hired by Dr. Nathan Smith (q.v.) to present anatomical lectures at Dartmouth Medical School. Unsuccessfully tried for years to get private and public funding for a proposed Anatomical Institution and Museum at Fryeburg. CONTRIBUTIONS: Mission in life was to "justify the ways of God to man," by means of anatomy and the allied sciences. A noted dissector and lecturer on anatomy and frequently gave a course in communities "for improvement among their medical men" as well as addressing topics such as health issues and hygiene in schools and public buildings generally. Famous for development of a fever treatment as a result of study of a yellow-fever epidemic in N.Y. (1803). Eventually published findings in *Edinburgh Medical Journal* (July 1812).

WRITINGS: Began a six-part series on anatomy but completed only one, *Anatomy of the Brain* (1812). "The Muscular System, Its Contraction from Intellectual Influence," *London Med. J.* (1814); *Prospectus of Fifteen Lectures on the Animal and Intellectual Economy of Man; Adapted to the Purpose of the Medical Practitioner, the Speculative Philosopher, the Parent, and the Young, as the Medium of that Knowledge of God and Ourselves Which Seems Connected with Health, Piety and Religion* (1816). REFERENCES: *DAB*, 8, pt. 1: 337-38; Howard Kelly, *Cyclopedia of Am. Med. Biog.*, 2: 302-4; Maine Historical Society Alexander Ramsay Collection; Maine Historical Society Collection #513, Box #2, M2, Maine Physicians compiled by James Spalding; Maine Historical Society Spalding Collection #1606; *Trans. Maine Med. Assoc.* (1883): 161-62.

B. C. Lister

RAMSAY, DAVID (April 2, 1749, Lancaster, Pa.-May 8, 1815, Charleston, S.C.). *Physician; Historian*. Son of James and Jane (Montgomery) Ramsay, Irish immigrant farmers. Married Sabrina Ellis, 1775 (d. 1776); Frances Witherspoon, 1783 (d. 1784); one son; Martha Laurens, 1787; seven surviving children. EDUCATION: 1765, A.B., College of New Jersey (Princeton); tutored for two years before entering the College of Philadelphia; College of Philadelphia: 1772, B.M., and 1774, M.D. CAREER: 1776-83, leading member, S.C. legislature (served 21 years as member of the legislature, the last seven as president of the Senate); during Revolutionary War, surgeon (captured and imprisoned for

11 months in St. Augustine, Fla.). CONTRIBUTIONS: Better known as a politician and S.C. leader than as a physician. Helped form the Medical Society of South Carolina (1789) and served as its first treasurer. Won fame as an historian.

WRITINGS: "Extracts from an Address Delivered Before the Medical Society of S.C.," *Med. Repository* 4 (1801); "Facts Concerning the Yellow Fever," *ibid.*, 4 (1801). REFERENCES: *Memoirs of the Life of Martha Laurens Ramsay* (1845); J. Carson, *History of the Medical Department of the University of Pennsylvania* (1869); *DAB*, 8, pt. 1: 338-39; L. J. Friedman, "History, Politics and Health in Early American Thought," *J. of Am. Studies* 13 (1979): 37-56; Robert Y. Hayne, "Biographical Memoir of David Ramsay, M.D.," *Analectic Mag.* (1815); J. Herring, *National Portrait Gallery of Distinguished Americans* 2 (1854); *NCAB*, 7: 285; J. I. Waring, *History of Med. in S.C., 1670-1825* (1964); C. Weeks, "David Ramsay," *Annals of Med. Hist.* 3 (1929).

J. P. Dolan

RAMSEY, WALTER REEVE (November 8, 1872, Guelph, Ontario, Canada-March 11, 1973, St. Paul, Minn.). *Pediatrician.* Son of James and Mary (Scott) Ramsey. Married Ruth A. Lusk, 1902; one child. EDUCATION: Medical studies: 1893, University of Maryland; and 1896, M.D., University of Minnesota; intern, Ancker Hospital (St. Paul City and County Hospital); Postgraduate work in pediatrics, New York, N.Y.; Boston, Mass.; Vienna, Austria; and Berlin, Germany. CAREER: 1900, began private practice; 1901, began teaching, University of Minnesota; assisted French government (under auspices of the Red Cross) for 18 months with the care of children and with refugee services following World War I. CONTRIBUTIONS: First in Minn. to specialize in pediatrics. Introduced buttermilk as an important item of infant feeding. An organizer of the Central and Northwestern Pediatric societies. Organized (1911) the Baby Clinic of St. Paul (later called the Family Nursing Service). While in France for the Red Cross, organized a children's dispensary, children's hospital, and tuberculosis preventorium (1918). Established the Children's Hospital, St. Paul, the first in the northern tier of states from Chicago, Ill., to San Francisco, Calif.

WRITINGS: *Infancy and Childhood* (1916); *Care and Feeding of Infants and Children* (1920), a textbook for nurses. REFERENCES: *J.-Lancet* (1962).

R. Rosenthal

RAMSTAD, NILES OLIVER (March 22, 1875, Meridian, Wis.-February 25, 1952, St. Petersburg, Fla.). *Physician; Surgeon.* Son of John Olaf, contractor, and Karen (Narveson) Ramstad. Married Edna Winchester, 1906; one child. EDUCATION: 1899, M.D., University of Minnesota; postgraduate study: 1902-3, University of Vienna; and 1905-8 (summers), Harvard University; 1899-1900, internship, St. Barnabas Hospital, Minneapolis, Minn. CAREER: Physician and surgeon: 1900, Appleton, Minn.; and 1900-1949, Bismarck, N.Dak.; 1903, co-founder, Quain and Ramstad Clinic (second oldest group practice in the United States); president: 1926-27, North Dakota Medical Association; and 1934-48, Bismarck Medical Club; 1938-39, governor, American College of Surgeons; 1939-49, chief of staff, Bismarck Evangelical Hospital (now Bismarck Hospital).

CONTRIBUTIONS: Nationally known surgeon who was pioneer in treatment of gallbladder diseases. Co-founder, Quain and Ramstad Clinic. Instrumental in establishment of Bismarck Evangelical Hospital (1905).

WRITINGS: "Actinomycosis," *J.-Lancet* 36 (1916); "Diagnosis and Treatment of Gall Bladder Diseases," ibid., 45 (1925); "Surgical Treatment of the Peptic Ulcer," ibid., 49 (1929); "Phytobezoar with Gastric Ulcer: Report of a Case," ibid., 58 (1938). Writings listed in *Quarterly Cumulated Index Medicus, 1916-1942*. REFERENCES: *Bismarck Tribune*, February 26, 1952, p. 1; Paul W. Friese, *The Story of the Quain and Ramstad Clinic* (n.d.); *NCAB*, 41: 232.

L. Remele

RANDALL, EDWARD (October 7, 1860, Huntsville, Tex.-August 12, 1944, Galveston, Tex.). *Physician; Educator.* Son of Samuel, physician, and Texana (Garrett) Randall. Married Laura Ballinger, April 30, 1889; two children. EDUCATION: Preparatory school, Lexington, Va.; 1879, A.B., Washington and Lee (Phi Beta Kappa); 1879-80, law clerk, Galveston; 1883, M.D., University of Pennsylvania; 1883-84, intern, Philadelphia General Hospital (Blockley); 1884-86, study in Heidelberg, Berlin, and Munich, Germany; and Vienna, Austria. CAREER: 1886-1928, practice, Galveston; professor of materia medica and therapeutics: 1888-91, Texas Medical College; and 1891-1928, University of Texas Medical Branch, Galveston; 1928-44, emeritus professor; 1909-40, president, Board of Managers, John Sealy Hospital; on University of Texas Board of Regents: 1929-40, member; and 1937-39, chairman; at Sealy and Smith Foundation: 1922-44, member; and 1938-44, chairman; in Rosenberg Library Association, Galveston: 1914-44, trustee; and 1930-44, president. CONTRIBUTIONS: Fifty years of guidance to the University of Texas Medical School, Galveston. A fourth-generation physician, devoted to teaching, public service, and marshaling resources for a progressive faculty and physical plant. Secured several million dollars of federal and private funds for more than nine major expansion projects (1930s, 1940s), including a hospital for Negroes and a research laboratory.

WRITINGS: "Planning for Outpatients in a Southern Teaching Hospital," *Modern Hosp.* 36 (Mar. 1931): 83-90; "Solving Difficult Problems for Psychiatric Department," ibid., 44 (Jun. 1935): 56-58. REFERENCES: Biography folders, Rosenberg Library, Galveston; *Bull. of John Sealy Hosp. and the School of Med., Univ. of Texas* 1 (Jan. 1939); William M. Morgan, *Trinity Protestant Episcopal Church, Galveston, Texas, 1841-1953* (1954), 359-64; *NCAB*, 35: 429; *One Hundred Faithful to the University of Texas at Austin. . .*(1976), 79; A. O. Singleton, *Handbook of Texas* 2 (1952): 436-37; *Texas Med.* 63 (1967): 112-16; *Texas State J. of Med.* 40 (Oct. 1940): 351-52; *University of Texas Medical Branch at Galveston* (1967). Randall papers are in family possession.

J. P. Morris

RANSON, STEPHEN WALTER (August 28, 1880, Dodge Center, Minn.-August 30, 1942, Chicago, Ill.). *Physician; Neurology; Anatomy.* Son of Stephen William, physician, and Mary Elizabeth (Foster) Ranson. Married Tessie Grier, 1909; three children. EDUCATION: 1902, A.B., University of Minnesota; University of Chicago: 1903, M.S.; and 1905, Ph.D.; 1907, M.D., Rush Medical College; 1907-8, intern, Cook County Hospital, Chicago; 1910-11, studied with Robert E. E. Wiedersheim, University of Freiburg. CAREER: 1908-10, practiced medicine, Chicago; 1909-24, anatomy faculty, Northwestern University Medical School; 1924-28, neuroanatomy and histology faculty, Washington University Medical School; 1928-42, neurology faculty and director, Institute of Neurology, Northwestern University Medical School; 1938-40, president, American Association of Anatomists. CONTRIBUTIONS: Wrote *Anatomy of the Nervous System* (1920), the first comprehensive treatise of the subject, which by the time of his death was in its seventh edition. Studied the processes of degeneration and regeneration of nerve fibers, the structure of the vagus nerve, vasomotor pathways, and the functional role of spinal ganglia. Developed a pyridine silver stain for differentiating nonmyelinated nerve fibers. Best known for experimental studies of the function of the hypothalamus as control center for the sympathetic nervous system. Helped edit *Archives of Neurology and Psychiatry*.

WRITINGS: "Degeneration and Regeneration of Nerve Fibres," *J. of Comparative Neurology* 22 (1912): 487; "The Structure of the Vagus Nerve of Man as Demonstrated by a Differential Axon Stain," *Anatomischer Anzeiger* 46 (1914): 522; "The Conduction within the Spinal Cord of the Afferent Impulses Producing Pain and the Vasomotor Reflexes," *Am. J. of Physiol.* 38 (1915): 128 (with C. L. von Hess); "Autonomic Responses to Electrical Stimulation of the Hypothalamus, Preoptic Region and Septum," *Arch. Neurol. Psychiat.* 33 (1935): 467 (with H. Kabat and H. W. Magoun). A bibliography is in *BMNAS. REFERENCES: BMNAS* 23 (1945): 365-97; *DAB*, Supplement 3: 619-20; *Who Was Who in Am.*, 2: 438.

S. Galishoff

RAPPLEYE, WILLARD COLE (February 11, 1892, Marinette, Wis.-August 19, 1976, New York, N.Y.). *Medical educator; Foundation president.* Son of Albert Higgins, engineer, and Elizabeth (Johnson) Rappleye. Married Elizabeth Templeton Cunningham, 1923; two children. EDUCATION: 1915, A.B., University of Illinois; 1918, M.D., Harvard University; 1918-19, medical house officer, Massachusetts General Hospital. CAREER: At University of California Medical School: 1919-20, director of clinical laboratories and biochemistry faculty; and 1920-22, director of hospitals and hospital administration faculty; 1920-22, medical adviser, California State Board of Control; and acting superintendent, Pacific Colony for the Feebleminded (Pomona); 1921-22, executive secretary, Committee on the Training of Hospital Executives (sponsored by the Rockefeller Foundation); 1922-26, superintendent, New Haven Hospital; and hospital administration faculty, Yale University School of Medicine; 1925-32, director of study, Commission on Medical Education (organized and sponsored by the Association of American Medical Colleges); 1930-31, medical economics faculty, Harvard School of Public Health; at Columbia University: 1931-58, dean, medicine faculty, College of Physicians and Surgeons; 1932-60, medical economics faculty, and 1933-45, dean, School of Dental and Oral Surgery; 1933-47, director, New

York Post-Graduate Medical School and Hospital; and 1949-58, vice-president in charge of medical affairs; at Josiah Macy, Jr., Foundation: 1933-41, member, Board of Directors; and 1941-64, president; 1940-42, commissioner of hospitals, New York City; president: *post* 1954, William J. Matheson Foundation; 1937-44, Advisory Board on Medical Specialties; 1938-39, Association of American Medical Colleges; 1939-44, Advisory Council on Medical Education; and 1962, National Health Council. CONTRIBUTIONS: Made many innovations in medical education while at Columbia University, including a program of continuing education for physicians (1931) and postdoctoral graduate education and studies leading to a Med. Sc.D. degree (1934). Consolidated teachers of medicine, dentistry, public health, and nursing into a single faculty (1945) and emphasized the unity of the entire medical curriculum. Added new facilities to the Columbia medical center, including laboratories for graduate medicine (1937), Research Cancer Hospital (1940), Institute of Administrative Medicine (1950), New York Orthopedic Dispensary and Hospital (1950), and Institute for Cancer Research (1951). Took an active interest in the development of new methods of health care delivery; in cooperation with the New York City Health Department, established the Washington Heights Health and Teaching Center (1940, now Columbia School of Public Health and Administrative Medicine); was member and chairman, Board of Directors (1947-48), Health Insurance Plan of Greater New York.

WRITINGS: *The Final Report of the Commission on Medical Education* (1932); *The Current Era of the Faculty of Medicine, Columbia University, 1910-1958* (1958). REFERENCES: H. Atkins, *The Dean; Willard C. Rappleye and the Evolution of American Medical Education* (1975); *NCAB*, J: 104-5; *N.Y. Times*, August 20, 1976.

S. Galishoff

RAUCH, JOHN HENRY (September 4, 1828, Lebanon, Pa.-March 24, 1894, Lebanon). *Physician; Public health.* Son of Bernard and Jane (Brown) Rauch. Never married. EDUCATION: 1846-47, apprentice to Dr. John W. Gloninger, Lebanon; 1849, M.D., University of Pennsylvania Medical School; 1855-56, studied with Louis Agassiz. CAREER: 1850-58, practiced medicine, Ia.; materia medica and medical botany: 1857-60, Rush Medical College; and 1859-61, Chicago College of Pharmacy; Surgeon throughout the Civil War; *post* 1866, medical practice, Chicago. CONTRIBUTIONS: Fought for improvements in medical education and regulation of medical practice. Superintended administration of Ill. Medical Practice Act with vigor. Promoted vaccination of children and physical examination of immigrants. Improved sanitation and collection of vital statistics. First president, Illinois State Board of Health (1877). A founder, Chicago College of Pharmacy (1859) and Chicago Board of Health (1867). Sanitary superintendent (1867-93). Promoted marine hospital program before U.S. Congress. Became one of the commissioners for selecting sites and assisted with planning and building at Galena, Ill., and Burlington, Ia. (both hospitals opened in 1858). An organizer, American Public Health Association (1872).

Member, Sanitary Committee for Interior Department for Centennial Exposition (1876). A founder, Sanitary Council of the Mississippi Valley (1878).

WRITINGS: *Intramural Interments in Populous Cities and Their Influence upon Health and Epidemics* (1866); *Public Parks: Their Effects upon the Moral, Physical, and Sanitary Conditions of the Inhabitants of Large Cities. With Special Reference to the City of Chicago* (1869); *Coast Defenses Against Asiatic Cholera. Report of an Inspection of the Quarantines Maintained upon the Atlantic and Gulf Coasts from the St. Lawrence to the Rio Grande* (1886); *Preliminary Report to the Illinois State Board of Health. Water Supplies of Illinois and Pollution of Its Streams* (1889); *The Smallpox Situation in the United States* (1894). REFERENCES: *DAB*, 8, pt. 1: 340-41; *NCAB*, 12: 452; F. M. Sperry, comp., *A Group of Distinguished Physicians and Surgeons of Chicago* (1904), 117-20; *Trans., Ill. State Med. Soc.* 44 (1894): 57-59.

W. K. Beatty

RAY, ISAAC (January 16, 1807, Beverly, Mass.-March 31, 1881, Philadelphia, Pa.). *Psychiatrist; Author.* Son of Isaac, shipmaster, and Lydia (Simonds) Rea. The family later changed the spelling of the name. Married Abigail May Frothingham, 1831; two children. EDUCATION: Phillips Academy, Andover, Mass.; studied at Bowdoin College; apprenticeship with Dr. George C. Shattuck (q.v.); 1827, M.D., Medical School of Maine (Bowdoin). CAREER: Practice, Portland and Eastport, Maine; superintendent: 1841-45, Maine Insane Hospital, Augusta, Maine; and 1845-66, Butler Hospital, Providence, R.I.; 1866, retired to Philadelphia, where he practiced psychiatry and served as an expert witness and a vigorous supporter of reforms in treatment of the insane. CONTRIBUTIONS: An efficient administrator and a humane physician specializing in the care and treatment of the insane. An eloquent and authoritative author and spokesman on medical-legal matters bearing on insanity. A founder (1844), Association of Medical Superintendents of American Institutions for the Insane, which became the American Psychiatric Association, and served as its president (1855-59).

WRITINGS: Known for annual reports, articles, and books. *Medical Jurisprudence of Insanity*, 6 eds. (1838); *Contributions to Mental Pathology* (1873); *Mental Hygiene* (1863). REFERENCES: *DAB*, 8, pt. 1: 404-5; Fred Jacobs, "Isaac Ray and the Profession of Psychiatry," *R.I. Hist.* 38 (1979): 99-111; Miller, *BHM*, p. 93; *Trans., R.I. Med. Soc.* 2 (1882): 391-404.

G. E. Erikson

REDMAN, JOHN (February 27, 1722, Philadelphia, Pa.-March 19, 1808, Philadelphia.). *Physician.* Son of Joseph and Sarah Redman. Grandfather of John Redman Coxe (q.v.). Married Mary Sobers; at least three children. EDUCATION: Apprenticed to John Kearsley (q.v.); 1748, M.D., University of Edinburgh; 1748-49, studied medicine, Paris and London. CAREER: Practiced medicine, Bermuda, before going to Edinburgh in 1746; *post* 1749, practiced medicine, Philadelphia; 1751-80, medical staff, Pennsylvania Hospital; trustee, College of New Jersey (now Princeton University) and College of Philadelphia (now University of Pennsylvania). CONTRIBUTIONS: Helped establish and was first president, College of Physicians of Philadelphia (1786-1804). Taught several of the founders of American medical education including John Morgan (q.v.), Benjamin Rush (q.v.), William Shippen (q.v.), and Caspar Wistar (q.v.). An ardent defender of inoculation for smallpox. Advocated the use of saline purgatives as opposed to emetics and bleeding in the treatment of yellow fever.

WRITINGS: *A Defence of Inoculation* (1760); *An Account of Yellow Fever as It Prevailed in Philadelphia in 1762* (1793). REFERENCES: Whitfield J. Bell, Jr., "John Redman, Medical Preceptor, 1722-1808," *Pa. Mag. of Hist. and Biog.* 81 (1957): 157-69; *DAB*, 15: 443; Kelly and Burrage (1928), 1018; Miller, *BHM*, p. 93; John H. Talbott, *Biographical Hist. of Med.* (1970), 265-66; *Who Was Who in Am.*, Hist. Vol.: 506.

S. Galishoff

REED, WALTER (September 13, 1851, Belroi, Va.-November 22, 1902, Washington, D.C.). *Physician; Microbiology.* Son of Lemuel Sutton, Methodist minister, and Pharaba (White) Reed. Married Emilie Lawrence, 1876; two children. EDUCATION: 1869, M.D., University of Virginia; 1870, M.D., Bellevue Hospital Medical College; 1870-72, intern, New York Infants', Kings County (Brooklyn, N.Y.), and Brooklyn City hospitals; 1890-91, studied at Johns Hopkins Medical School. CAREER: 1871-72, district physician, New York Department of Public Charities; 1873-74, sanitary inspector, Brooklyn Board of Health; 1875-1902, at Medical Corps, U.S. Army: 1876-89, assigned to garrison duty, various parts of the country; 1891-93, attending surgeon and examiner of recruits, Baltimore, Md.; 1890-91, curator, Army Medical Museum; and 1893-1902, bacteriology and clinical microscopy faculty, Army Medical School; chairman: 1898, committee to investigate typhoid fever in army camps; and 1900, Army Yellow Fever Commission; 1901-2, pathology and bacteriology faculty, Columbian University Medical School. CONTRIBUTIONS: Did earliest work on the bacteriology of erysipelas and diphtheria; helped demonstrate the contagiousness of erysipelas (1892) and was an early supporter of the use of diphtheria antitoxin and government regulation of biologic substances. Headed commission that showed that the spread of typhoid fever in military camps during the Spanish-American War was mainly attributable to flies and contact with infected fecal material. Planned a brilliant series of laboratory and field experiments that demonstrated that yellow fever was spread by the *Aedes aegypti* mosquito; with other members of the Army Yellow Fever Commission, uncovered the etiology of the disease and proved that it was caused by a filterable virus; work led to the eradication of yellow fever in Havana and the Panama Canal Zone within a few years.

WRITINGS: *The Contagiousness of Erysipelas* (1892); "Bacillus Icteroides and Bacillus Cholerae Suis," *Med. News* 74 (1899): 513-14 (with James Carroll [q.v.]); "The Specific Cause of Yellow Fever. A Reply to Dr. G. Sanarelli," ibid., 75 (1899): 321-29 (with James Carroll); "The Etiology of Yellow Fever," *Phila. Med. J.* 6 (1900): 790-96 (with J. Carroll, A. Agramonte, and J. Lazear [q.v.]); *Report on the Origin and Spread of Typhoid Fever in U.S. Military Camps During the Spanish War of 1898* (1904). A bibliography is in Howard A. Kelly [q.v.], *Walter Reed and Yellow Fever*, 3rd ed. (1923). REFERENCES: *BHM* (1964-69), 222; (1970-74), 147; (1975-79), 105; *DAB*, 15: 459-61;

DSB, 11: 345-47; Kelly and Burrage (1928), 1018-20; Miller, *BHM*, pp. 94-95; *NCAB*, 33: 143-44; *Who Was Who in Am.*, Hist. Vol.: 507.

S. Galishoff

REEVE, JAMES THEODORE (April 26, 1834, Orange County, N.Y.-November 4, 1906, Appleton, Wis.). *Physician; Surgeon; Public health.* Son of Daniel, farmer, and Mary (Valentine) Reeve. Married Laura Spofford, 1857; six children. EDUCATION: 1852, first course in medical lectures, University of Michigan, Ann Arbor, Mich.; 1854, M.D., Castleton Medical College, Vt.; 1855, M.D., Jefferson Medical College. CAREER: Practiced medicine: 1856-60, DePere, Wis.; and 1860, Green Bay, Wis.; 1861-65, U.S. Army; *post* 1865, practiced, Appleton; 1876-94, Secretary, Wisconsin State Board of Health, for its first 18 years; in Wisconsin State Medical Society: 1871-89, secretary; and 1874-75, president; 1880-90, state supervisor of inspection of illuminating oil; helped pass a law prohibiting the sale of low test fuel that was causing fatal explosions. CONTRIBUTIONS: As first secretary, Wisconsin Board of Health, pioneered in organizing local boards of health and in establishing sanitary laws in Wis. Collected vital statistics under the general direction of the secretary of state.

WRITINGS: As secretary, Wisconsin State Board of Health, wrote for and edited the annual reports. Instructed newly formed boards of health in the techniques of public health and wrote numerous pamphlets on the subject. REFERENCES: Weston A. Goodspeed, Melvin E. Bothwell, and Kenneth C. Goodspeed, *History of Outagamie County* (1911), 1022-23; *JAMA* 47 (1906): 1753; "James T. Reeve, M.D.," *The United States Biographical Dictionary and Portrait Gallery of Eminent and Self-made Men, Wisconsin Volume* (1877), 431-32; Howard A. Kelly, *Cyclopedia of Am. Med. Biog.* 2 (1912): 315-16; Kelly and Burrage (1928), 1022-23; Military Order of the Loyal Legion of the United States, *In Memoriam James Theodore Reeve* circular no. 12, series 1906, whole no. 415; Erik Timmerman, "State Historians Honor Appleton Civil War Doctor," *Appleton Post-Crescent*, July 22, 1962.

M. Van H. Jones

REICH, WILHELM (March 24, 1897, Dobrzcynica, Galicia, Austria-November 3, 1957, Federal Penitentiary, Lewisburg, Pa.). *Physician; Patent medicine.* Son of Leon, cattle rancher, and Cecilio (Roniger) Reich. Married Annie Pink, 1922, two daughters, divorced, 1933; Elsa Lindenberg, 1933 (no official marriage); Ilse Ollendorff, 1939, one son. EDUCATION: 1922, M.D., University of Vienna; Freud's first assistant, Psychoanalytic Polyclinic, Vienna. CAREER: 1922-24, postgraduate, Neurological and Psychiatric Clinic; 1924-30, conducted clinics for workers and became a member, Communist party; moved: to Berlin; back to Vienna; and 1933, to Denmark; expelled from Danish Communist party; 1934, moved to Oslo, Norway, and lived there until 1939; 1934, published *Character Analysis* and was expelled from the International Psychoanalytic Association; 1939, moved to New York City and became lecturer, New School for Social Research, until 1941; 1942, U.S. publication of *Function of the Orgasm* suggesting orgasm without inhibition as reform to reduce family rigidity (founded

Orgone Institute); 1945, left New York City for Rangeley, Maine; 1954, Federal Food and Drug Administration obtained injunction against use of orgone energy devices; defied injunction to force a test case; May 1956, held in contempt, convicted, and jailed for two-year term, Lewisburg, Pa. CONTRIBUTIONS: Early deviant from Freudian views on death instinct and masochism. Disagreed with conclusion that destructiveness is biologic instinct and that sexuality drains the individual's energy for other pursuits. Developed idea of orgone energy (also called "vegetative energy," "biopsyschic energy"). Developed Reichitis, believed that neurosis was excessive undischarged energy rooted in sexual repression; treatment involved releasing energy. Invented Orgone Energy Accumulator, a therapeutic box the size of a telephone booth designed to attract energy and help produce orgasm. Believed orgasm was the best index of a patient's mental health, and that orgone energy was a nonelectro magnetic force that permeates all of nature. Claimed that orgastic impotence was primary cause of cancer, all neurosis, cardiovascular hypertension, and anemia. Discredited through attempt to create energy-restoring devices and treatment of cancer by cosmic orgone energy (COE).

WRITINGS: *The Function of the Orgasm* (1927); *The Character Analysis* (1933); *The Mass Psychology of Fascism* (1933); *The Bions* (1938); *The Sexual Revolution* (1945); *The Cancer Biopathy* (1948); *Cosmic Superism-imposition* (1951). REFERENCES: Jerome Greenfield, *Wilhelm Reich vs. The U.S.A.* (1974); Helen Krueger, *Other Healers, Other Cures* (1974); Ilse Ollendorff Reich, *Wilhelm Reich, A Personal Biography* (1969); *World Who's Who in Sci.* (1968).

R. Edwards

REID, MONT ROGERS (April 7, 1889, near Oriskany, Va.-May 11, 1943, Cincinnati, Ohio). *Physician; Surgery.* Son of Benjamin Watson, farmer and schoolteacher, and Harriet Pendleton (Lemon) Reid. Married Elizabeth Harmon Cassatt, 1929; one child. EDUCATION: 1908, A.B., Roanoke College, Salem, Va.; Johns Hopkins University: 1912, M.D.; 1913-14, intern in pathology under Joseph C. Bloodgood (q.v.) and 1914-21, resident in surgery under William S. Halsted (q.v.). CAREER: At Johns Hopkins University: 1913-14, pathology faculty; and 1914-22, surgery faculty; during World War I, Medical Corps, U.S. Army; 1922-43, surgical faculty, University of Cincinnati; and surgical staff, Cincinnati General and Children's hospitals; 1925-26, surgery faculty, Union Medical College of Peking, China; 1926, surgeon, Asiatic expedition into Mongolia under the leadership of Roy Chapman Andrews. CONTRIBUTIONS: Made the University of Cincinnati one of the nation's outstanding training centers for surgeons. Principal scientific contributions were experimental and clinical studies of surgery of the thyroid gland and of the large blood vessels. First to demonstrate that arteriovenous aneurysms may seriously damage the heart. Also advanced the surgical treatment of angina pectoris, pigmented moles, and cancer.

WRITINGS: "The Effects of Arteriovenous Fistula upon the Heart and Blood Vessels," *Johns Hopkins Hosp. Bull.* 31 (1920): 43-50; "Sensory Disturbances Following Sympathectomy for Angina Pectoris,'' *JAMA* 83 (Jul.-Sept. 1924): 114-17 (with Gustav Eckstein); contributed the chapter on arterial surgery in *Nelson's Loose Leaf System of Surgery* (1928) and the chapter on surgery of the sympathetic nervous system in *Dean Lewis's System of Surgery* (1929); ''The Pavex (Passive Vascular Exercise) Treatment of Obliterative Arterial Diseases of the Extremities,'' *J. of Med.* 14 (Dec. 1933): 524-29 (with Louis George Herrmann). REFERENCES: *DAB*, Supplement 3: 625-26; *NCAB*, 34: 172-73; *N.Y. Times*, May 12, 1943; *Who Was Who in Am.*, 2: 442.

S. Galishoff

REID, WILLIAM WHARRY (1799, Argyle, N.Y.-December 9, 1866, drowned in Hudson River). *Physician.* 1830, married Elizabeth Manson. EDUCATION: 1825, A.B., Union College; 1826-28, studied medicine with A. G. Smith in Rochester; M.D., probably conferred on him by the Monroe County Medical Society. CAREER: Practiced medicine: 1828-64, Rochester, N.Y.; and 1864-66, New York City; president, Monroe County Medical Society (1836, 1849). CONTRIBUTIONS: Demonstrated that the existing method of treatment of dislocation of the hip requiring longitudinal traction by pulleys and brute force prevented reduction and ruptured muscles unnecessarily. Showed that hip dislocation could be reduced easily and with little pain by flexion (1844).

WRITINGS: ''Dislocation of the Femur on the Dorsum ilii, Reducible without Pulleys or any Other Mechanical Power,'' *Buffalo Med. J. and Monthly Rev.* 7 (1851-52): 129-43. REFERENCES: *DAB*, 15: 486-88; Kelly and Burrage (1928), 1026-27.

S. Galishoff

REMOND, SARAH PARKER (June 26, 1826, Salem, Mass.-after 1887, possibly in Rome, Italy). *Physician.* Daughter of John, hairdresser, caterer, merchant-trader, and Nancy (Lenox) Remond. Married ? Pintor. EDUCATION: Academy in Salem, Mass.; 1859-61, Bedford College for Ladies (London); 1866-68, medical study, Santa Maria Nuova Hospital, Florence, Italy. CAREER: Throughout life, was a champion of black rights; 1868-death, medical practice, Florence, and perhaps Rome, Italy. CONTRIBUTIONS: One of first black women trained at a medical school and teaching hospital. As an activist in black rights, successfully took Howard Athenaeum management to Boston police court for denying her a seat in theatre (1853). Participated regularly in work of the Salem Female, Essex County, and Mass. antislavery societies. Lectured throughout the North as agent for American Anti-Slavery Society (1856-58) and pursued the American antislavery and, after the Civil War, the freedmen's cause among British audiences (1859-66).

WRITINGS: ''The Negroes in the United States of America,'' reprinted in *J. of Negro Hist.* 27 (1942): 216-18; ''The Negro and Anglo-Africans as Freemen and Soldiers,'' London: Emancipation Society Tract No. 7, 1864. Writings listed in Dorothy B. Porter ''Sarah Parker Remond, Abolitionist and Physician,'' *J. of Negro Hist.* 20 (1935): 287-

93. REFERENCES: *Notable Am. Women* 3: 136-37; Dorothy B. Porter, "Sarah Parker Redmond, Abolitionist and Physician," *J. of Negro Hist.* 20 (1935): 287-93.

L. A. Falk and T. L. Savitt

REYBURN, ROBERT (August 1, 1833, Glasgow, Scotland-March 25, 1909, Washington, D.C.). *Physician; Surgery.* Son of James and Jane (Brown) Reyburn. Married Catherine White, February 5, 1854; eight children. EDUCATION: Studied medicine with Dr. Lewis D. Harlann, Philadelphia, Pa.; 1856, M.D., Philadelphia College of Medicine. CAREER: 1856-62, private practice, Philadelphia; 1862-63, acting assistant surgeon, U.S. Volunteers; moved to Washington; 1863-67, assistant surgeon and surgeon, U.S. Volunteers; 1867, assistant surgeon, U.S. Army; at Georgetown Medical School: 1866-67, professor of clinical surgery; 1873-74, professor of anatomy; 1867-75, surgeon in charge, Freedmen's Hospital; at Howard Medical School: 1868-73, professor of surgery; 1880-92, professor of physiology and clinical surgery; 1902-9, professor of preventive medicine and hygiene; 1902-9, dean. CONTRIBUTIONS: Noted for work with freed blacks. Most instrumental in establishing the Freedmen's Hospital. Fought unsuccessfully to have black physicians admitted to the Medical Society of the District of Columbia. Librarian, American Medical Association (1870). President: American Therapeutic Society, Medico-Legal Society of Washington, Washington Board of Health (1868-70). Vice-president (1891), National Microscopical Society. One of the attending surgeons to President Garfield (1881).

WRITINGS: For bibliography, see p. 39 of autobiographical sketch, *Fifty Years in the Practice of Medicine and Surgery, 1856-1906* (1907); more precise citations in *Index Catalogue*, 2nd series, 14 (1909): 518-19. *Type of Disease Among the Freed People of the United States* (1891); "Clinical History of the Case of President James A. Garfield," (1894), reprinted from *Journal of American Medical Association* 22 (1894). REFERENCES: William B. Atkinson, ed, *Physicians and Surgeons of the U.S.* (1878), 83-84; S. C. Busey, *Personal Reminiscences* (1895), 245-84, on attempts to admit blacks to the Medical Society of the District of Columbia; D. S. Lamb et al., *History of the Medical Society of the District of Columbia, 1817-1909* (1909), 281-82; *Washington Med. Annals* 8 (1909-10): 136-42; *Who Was Who in Am.*, 1: 1023.

R. A. Kondratas

RICHARDS, ALFRED NEWTON (March 22, 1876, Stamford, N.Y.-March 24, 1966, Bryn Mawr, Pa.). *Pharmacologist; Nephrology.* Son of Leonard E., Presbyterian minister, and Mary E. (Burbank) Richards. Married Lillian L. Woody, 1908; one child. EDUCATION: Yale University: 1897, B.A.; and 1899, M.A.; 1901, Ph.D., Columbia University. CAREER: At College of Physicians and Surgeons (Columbia): 1898-1904, physiological chemistry faculty; 1904-1908, pharmacology faculty; 1908-10, pharmacology faculty, Northwestern University; at University of Pennsylvania: 1910-46, pharmacology faculty; 1939-48, vice-president in charge of medical affairs; 1917-18, member, scientific staff, British Medical Research Committee; 1941-46, chairman, Committee on Medical Research, Office of Scientific Research and Development. CONTRIBUTIONS: Illuminated the field of renal physiology and directed the nation's medical research during World War II. Pioneered micropuncture and ultramicrochemical techniques of renal investigation; discovered that urine is filtered from the blood by the glomeruli of the kidneys (1915-25); developed method for measuring the rate of glomerular filtration (1930-36). With Henry H. Dale, made a definitive study of the effect of histamine on capillary contractility and shock (1917-18). Developed the first course in clinical pharmacology in the United States (1922). During World War II, headed the Committee on Medical Research, which made outstanding contributions in the fields of aviation medicine, chemotherapy, synthetic malaria drugs, blood substitutes, and insecticides; development of sulfa drugs, plasma, and especially penicillin, which was made available for use outside the laboratory for the first time, greatly altered medical practice. Played a prominent role in the revitalization of the medical school of Pennsylvania University. A founder, *Journal of Biological Chemistry*; helped edit it (1905-14).

WRITINGS: "The Vaso-Dilator Action of Histamine and of Some Other Substances," *J. of Physiol.* 52 (1918-19): 110-65 (with Sir Henry Hallett Dale); "The Nature and Mode of Regulation of Glomerular Function," *Am. J. of Med. Sci.* 170 (1925): 1-22; "Quantitative Studies of the Composition of Glomerular Urine. XIV. The Glomerular Excretion of Inulin in Frogs and Necturi," *J. Biol. Chem.* 116 (1936): 735-47 (with James P. Hendrix and B. B. Westfall). A bibliography is in *BMNAS*. REFERENCES: *Am. Phil. Soc. Yearbook* (1971), 141-53; *BHM* (1964-69), 223; (1970-74), 149; (1976), 25; *BMFRS* 13 (1967): 327-42; *BMNAS* 42 (1971): 272-318; *N.Y. Times*, March 25, 1966; *Who Was Who in Am.*, 4: 790.

S. Galishoff

RICHARDS, DICKINSON WOODRUFF (October 30, 1895, Orange, N.J.-February 23, 1973, Lakeville, Conn.). *Physician; Pulmonary and cardiac physiology.* Son of Dickinson W., lawyer, and Sally (Lambert) Richards. Married Constance B. Riley, 1931; four children. EDUCATION: 1917, B.A., Yale University; at Columbia University: 1922, M.A.; and 1923, M.D.; 1923-27, intern and resident, Presbyterian Hospital (N.Y.); 1927-28, research fellow, National Institute for Medical Research (London). CAREER: 1928-61, internal medicine faculty, College of Physicians and Surgeons (Columbia); medical staff: 1928-45, Presbyterian Hospital; and 1945-61, Bellevue Hospital. CONTRIBUTIONS: With André Cournand, developed the technique of cardiac catheterization—first pioneered by Werner Forssmann—which enabled physicians to make more precise measurements of heart and lung functions (1931-45); proved invaluable in diagnosing diseases and defects of the heart, including traumatic shock, heart failure, and congenital heart lesions; made it possible to measure cardiac output over a long period; was a major step in the development of heart surgery, for which he, Cournand, and Forssmann were awarded the 1956 Nobel Prize in medicine or physiology. With Cournand, demonstrated the superiority of whole blood in the treatment of shock (1944).

WRITINGS: ". . .Clinical Use of Concentrated Human Serum Albumin in Shock, and Comparison with Whole Blood and with Rapid Saline Infusion," *J. Clin. Invest.* 23 (1944): 491 (with A. Cournand et al.); "Measurement of Cardiac Output in Man Using the Technique of Catheterization of the Right Auricle or Ventricle," ibid., 24 (1945): 106 (with A. Cournand et al.); "The Contributions of Right Heart Catheterization to Physiology and Medicine, with Some Observations on the Physiopathology of Pulmonary Heart Disease," *Am. Heart J.* 54 (1957): 161-71; *Circulation of the Blood: Men and Ideas* (1964, editor with A. P. Fishman); *Medical Priesthoods and other Essays* (1970). A bibliography is in *Am. J. of Med.* REFERENCES: *BHM* (1970-74), 149; André F. Cournand, "Dickinson Woodruff Richards: 1895-1973. A Survey of His Contributions to the Physiology and Physiopathology of Respiration in Man," *Am. J. of Med.*, 57 (Sept. 1974): 312-28; *McGraw-Hill Modern Men of Sci.* 1 (1966): 391-92; *N.Y. Times*, February 24, 1973; *Who Was Who in Am.*, 5: 604.

S. Galishoff

RICHARDS, GEORGE GILL (September 5, 1883, Mendon, Utah-April 20, 1950, Boston, Mass.). *Physician*. Son of Stephen L., farmer, later a veterinarian, and then a physician, and Emma (Staynor) Richards. Married Florence Farnsworth, 1912; two children; Lacy Farnsworth, 1938. EDUCATION: student: 1898-1902, University of Utah; and 1903-4, University of Chicago; 1906, M.D., New York University and Bellevue Hospital Medical College; 1906, intern, Bellevue Hospital; 1910-11, 1912-13, studied in Vienna at the Allgemeines Krankenhaus and with Edmund von Neusser and Friedrich Kovacs. CAREER: 1906-50, staff, LDS Hospital; at Salt Lake Clinic: 1915, co-founder; and 1915-50, head, Department of Medicine; 1942-50, clinical professor of internal medicine, University of Utah Medical School; 1936-46, member, American Board of Internal Medicine; at American College of Physicians: 1924-34, member, Board of Governors; and 1934-37, regent; 1918-32, Captain, Medical Corps, U.S. Army Reserve; 1940, Medical Advisory Board, Selective Service. CONTRIBUTIONS: Introduced modern diagnostic methods at Latter-Day Saints (LDS) Hospital and Salt Lake Clinic.

WRITINGS: "Medical Management of Gastric Ulcers," *Annals of Internal Med.* (Feb. 1929); "The Family Doctor and Pioneer Physicians of the West," *JAMA* 98 (Jun. 11, 1932): 2035-38; "Rocky Mountain Spotted Fever," *Annals of Internal Med.* 6 (Mar. 1933): 1207-11; "Postoperative Tetany," *Rocky Mt. Med. J.* 37 (Jun. 1940): 436-40; "Are We Neglecting the Art of Physical Diagnosis?" *JAMA* (Aug. 1942). REFERENCES: *NCAB* 39 (1954): 216; Ralph T. Richards, M.D., *Of Medicine, Hospitals and Doctors* (1953), 107-9.

H. Bauman

RICHARDS, LINDA (July 27, 1841, Potsdam, N.Y.-April 16, 1930, Boston, Mass.). *Pioneer nursing educator*. Daughter of Sanford and Betsy (Sinclair) Richards. Never married. EDUCATION: 1873, Nurse Training School, New England Hospital for Women and Children; 1877, St. Thomas' School, London, under the direction of Florence Nightingale. CAREER: 1873, night superintendent,

Bellevue Training School; 1877, assisted in the development of a training school for nurses at Boston City Hospital; 1878-85, matron, Boston City Hospital; and superintendent, Training School; 1886-91, opened Japan's first training school for nurses, Doshisha Hospital, Kyoto; 1891, head, Philadelphia Visiting Nurses Society; 1892, founder, Nurse Training School, Philadelphia's Methodist Episcopal Hospital; 1893-94, 1894-95, 1895-97, strengthened and reorganized training schools, New England Hospital for Women and Children, Brooklyn Homeopathic Hospital, and Hartford (Conn.) Hospital, respectively; 1897-99, superintendent, Training School, University of Pennsylvania Hospital; 1899-1904, 1904-5, 1906-9, director, training schools at Taunton (Mass.) Insane Hospital, Worcester (Mass.) Hospital for the Insane, and Michigan Insane Asylum (Kalamazoo, Mich.), respectively; 1910-11, director, Taunton Insane Hospital. CONTRIBUTIONS: Often considered America's first trained nurse; may more accurately be described as the first American woman to receive a diploma in nursing. Developed a program (1874-77) of regular classroom instruction for nurses, Boston Training School. Success gave confidence and prestige to the entire movement for the professional training of nurses. Helped found (1877) the first Nightingale School in the United States to be established as an integral part of a hospital organization. Became the first president, American Society of Superintendents of Training Schools (1894). Purchased the first share of stock in the *American Journal of Nursing* (1900).

WRITINGS: *Reminiscences* (1911). REFERENCES: Autobiographical articles in *Am. J. of Nursing* (Nov. 1901, Jan. 1903, Dec. 1915) and biographical articles in ibid. (Oct. 1900, Nov. 1920 [by Agnes B. Joynes], Sept. 1948 [by Helen W. Munson]); R. Baker, *America's First Trained Nurse* (1959); *Notable Am. Women, 1607-1950*, 3: 148-50; (1971); *Reminiscences of Linda Richards* (1911); Alfred Worcestor, "Linda A. Richards," *New England J. of Med.* (May 29, 1930).

V. Drachman

RICHARDS, PAUL SNELGROVE (November 25, 1892, Salt Lake City, Utah-November 20, 1958, Salt Lake City). *Surgeon; Industrial medicine.* Son of Willard B., farmer and rancher, and Louise (Snelgrove) Richards. Married Ethel Bennion, 1916; three children. EDUCATION: University of Utah: 1913-16, student; and 1920, A.B.; 1920, M.D., Harvard Medical School; 1920-21, intern, Cincinnati General Hospital; 1921-22, residencies, Boston Lying-In Hospital and Free Hospital for Women, Brookline, Mass. CAREER: 1922-48, practiced, Bingham Canyon (Utah) Hospital and Clinic; 1948-53, cancer of the hands forced him to cease practicing for five years; 1953, co-founder, Memorial Medical Center, Salt Lake City; 1958, established the Richards Memorial Medical Foundation for the promotion of medical research; 1938-40, served on the Utah Medical, Labor, and Industrial Council and was a member of the committee that drafted the first occupational disease law for Utah, enacted in 1941; 1944-47, professor of industrial medicine, University of Utah Medical School; diplomate, American Board of Preventive and Occupational Medicine; member, American Board of

Industrial Medicine; 1953, received presidential citation for work with the hand-icapped. CONTRIBUTIONS: Built up the Bingham Canyon Clinic and created a 35-bed accredited hospital there. Practicing among miners and smelter workers, made innovations to prevent silicosis. Prevailed on the copper company to in-troduce safety and health features for the miners. Studied fracture rehabilitation and was one of the first to perform intervertebral disc operations. Inaugurated immunization, preventive medicine, and sex education in the community and local schools.

REFERENCES: *Memoirs of Dr. Paul*, compiled by sister Ann Barton, 1965 (typescript); *NCAB* 47 (1965): 175-76.

H. Bauman

RICHARDS, RALPH TAYLOR (September 15, 1880, Salt Lake City, Utah-June 12, 1954, Salt Lake City). *Surgeon*. Son of Joseph S., surgeon, and Louise (Taylor) Richards. Married Rhada Gibbs, 1916; two children. EDUCATION: 1903, M.D., New York University and Bellevue Hospital Medical College; 1904-5, intern, Bellevue Hospital; 1906, assistant to C. H. Mayo (q.v.) and E. S. Judd, Mayo Clinic; 1910-11, assistant to Otto Schultz in gross pathology, Cornell University Medical School; 1914, first assistant to Emil Beckman, Mayo Clinic; 1919, studied in Europe. CAREER: 1905-45, staff, Latter-Day Saints Hospital, chief of surgical services; 1915, co-founder, Salt Lake Clinic; at American College of Surgeons: 1914, diplomate, and 1935, member, Board of Governors; 1938, member, American Board of Surgery; 1941-42, active in organizing the four-year medical school, University of Utah; 1943-50, clinical professor of surgery, University of Utah Medical School. CONTRIBUTIONS: Important force in Utah for setting high surgical standards; among the first to require immediate postoperative movement and exercise.

WRITINGS: "The Goiter Problem of the Small Town," *Trans. Assoc. Resid. & ex-Resid. Physicians of the Mayo Clinic* 4 (1923): 53-58; "Utah Goiter Survey; Including Examination of 110,000 Children," *Am. J. of Surg.* 7 (Jul. 1929): 44-47; "Burns," *Rocky Mt. Med. J.* 40 (Dec. 1943): 810-15; *Of Medicine, Hospitals and Doctors* (1953), an original study of Utah medical history. REFERENCES: *Who's Important in Med.* (1952), 808-9.

H. Bauman

RICHARDSON, MAURICE HOWE (December 31, 1851, Athol, Mass.-July 31, 1912, Boston). *Surgeon*. Son of Nathan Henry and Martha Ann (Barber) Richardson. Married Margaret White Peirson, 1879; six children. EDUCATION: Graduated from Fitchburg High School; 1873, A.B., Harvard College; 1874-75, apprenticeship under Dr. Edward B. Peirson; 1876-77, attended Harvard Medical School, M.D., 1877; 1877, surgical study at the Mass. General Hospital. CAREER: 1873, taught in Salem High School while serving a medical appren-ticeship under Dr. Peirson; 1877, began medical practice in Boston; Harvard Medical School: 1877, assistant demonstrator of anatomy; 1895-1907, assistant professor of clinical surgery; 1907-12, Moseley Professor of Surgery; Mass. General Hospital: 1882-86, surgeon to out-patients; 1886-1911, visiting surgeon; 1911-12, surgeon-in-chief. CONTRIBUTIONS: Well-known surgeon and educator. Specialist in abdominal surgery. Performed the first gastrotomy for removal of a foreign body (set of false teeth) from the esophagus (1886). Became a supporter of Reginald Heber Fitz's (q.v.) operation for removal of the appendix. Wrote on the difficulties of diagnosis and surgery of the gallbladder. President, American Surgical Association, 1902.

WRITINGS: Articles in Park, *Surgery by American Authors* (1895) and in Dennis, *System of Surgery* (1896). REFERENCES: *Boston Med. and Surg. J.*, December 26, 1912; *DAB*, 8, pt. 1: 572; Kelly and Burrage (1928), 1032-34.

M. Kaufman

RICHARDSON, RODNEY HALL (November 14, 1860, Snow Hill, Md.-May 1, 1936, Reno, Nev.). *Physician.* Son of Ephraim King, merchant, and Eliza L. (Hall) Richardson. Married Penelope Rodney Plummer, 1888; one child. EDUCATION: 1881, Ph. B., Delaware College; 1884, M.D., University of Pennsylvania; intern, University of Pennsylvania hospital. CAREER: 1887-1902, physician, Pyramid Lake Indian Reservation; 1890-c.1917, practice, Ely, Nev.; 1919-26, Superintendent, Nevada Hospital for Mental Diseases, Reno, and for many years, medical staff, St. Mary's Hospital, Reno. CONTRIBUTIONS: Early Nev. physician serving the needs of the Indians on the Pyramid Lake Reservation and as a hospital administrator (1919-26). Member, Nevada State Board of Medical Examiners (1910-13). REFERENCES: Sam Davis, *History of Nevada* 2 (1913): 1234; *NCAB*, 36: 95.

J. Edwards

RICKETTS, HOWARD TAYLOR (February 9, 1871, Findley, Ohio-May 3, 1910, Mexico City, Mexico). *Physician; Pathology; Microbiology.* Son of Andrew Duncan, grain dealer, and Nancy Jane (Taylor) Ricketts. Married Myra Tubbs, 1900; two children. EDUCATION: 1894, A.B., University of Nebraska; 1897, M.D., Northwestern University Medical School; 1897-99, intern, Cook County Hospital (Chicago, Ill.); 1899-1901, fellow in pathology, Rush Medical College; 1901-2, studied in Europe. CAREER: *Post* 1902, pathology faculty, University of Chicago. CONTRIBUTIONS: Did earliest work on blastomycosis, immunology, and serums. Made pioneering studies of a group of diseases that bear his name: the rickettsial diseases; showed that Rocky Mountain spotted fever was communicable to lower animals, who kept the disease alive, and was transmitted to man by the accidental bite of an infected tick; found the organism responsible for the disease in ticks and their eggs and in the blood of humans (1906-10). Discovered the causative agent of tabardillo, or Mexican typhus fever, and proved that it was transmitted by the body louse *Pediculus vestimenti* (1910); microorganisms discovered during these investigations were later classified as members of a new genus called "Rickettsia"; work made it possible to control typhus on the Western Front during World War I.

WRITINGS: "Oidiomycosis (Blastomycosis) of the Skin and Its Fungi," *J. of Med. Research* 6 (1901): 374; *Infection, Immunity, and Serum Therapy* (1906); "The Role of the Wood Tick (Dermacentor Occidentalis) in Rocky Mountain Spotted Fever, and the Susceptibility of Local Animals to the Disease," *JAMA* 49 (1907): 24; *Y sus Trabajos sobre el Tabardillo* (1910). A bibliography is in *Contributions to Medical Science by Howard Taylor Ricketts* (1911). REFERENCES: *BHM* (1970-74), 149; *DAB*, Supplement 1: 628-29; *DSB*, 11: 442-43; Kelly and Burrage (1928), 1036; *NCAB*, 34: 543.

S. Galishoff

RIDGELY, FREDERICK (May 25, 1757, Elk Ridge, Anne Arundel County, Md.-November 21, 1824, Dayton, Ohio). *Surgeon; Teacher*. Married Eliza Short, 1797. EDUCATION: Newark Academy, Newark, Del.; 1774-76, study of medicine under Dr. Philip Thomas, Fredricktown, Md.; 1778-79, attended medical lectures, medical department, College of Philadelphia. CAREER: 1776-78, surgeon's mate, Corps of Virginia Riflemen raised in Va. and adjacent Md. counties; 1779, brief service as surgeon on privateer—escaped capture by British, returned to Philadelphia, and reentered army as surgeon, where he remained until 1784; 1784-90, practiced medicine, Anne Arundel County; 1790, moved to Lexington, Ky., and again resumed practice of medicine; 1792, also operated a drug store in Lexington with Basil Duke; 1793-95, served as surgeon, U.S. Army, under Maj. Gen. Anthony Wayne; 1795-97, practiced in partnership with James Watkins; at Transylvania University: 1799, professor of materia medica, midwifery and the practice of physic; and 1801-4, professor of medicine; 1802-4, practiced in partnership with James Fishback; 1804, retired to Woodford County, Ky. CONTRIBUTIONS: 1799, gave first medical lectures west of the Allegheny Mountains at Lexington; taught many office pupils, the most notable ones were Benjamin W. Dudley (q.v.) and Walter Brashear; May 1801, with Samuel Brown (q.v.), instituted the practice of vaccination with cowpox vaccine in Lexington. REFERENCES: Kelly and Burrage (1928), 1038; F. R. Packard, *Hist. of Med. in the U.S.* 1 (1930): 478; C. W. Short, "Obituary of Frederick Ridgely," *Transylv. J. Med.* 1 (1828).

E. H. Conner

RIIS, JACOB AUGUST (May 3, 1849, Ribe, Denmark-May 26, 1914, Barre, Mass.). *Journalist; Author; Public health*. Son of Niels Edward, teacher of Latin, and Caroline (Lundholm) Riis. Married Elizabeth Nielson, 1876, five children; Mary A. Phillips, 1907. EDUCATION: Educated by father in Denmark; apprentice to a carpenter. CAREER: 1870, went to the United States and worked at various trades until 1877; reporter: 1877-88, *New York Tribune*; and 1888-99, *New York Sun*; 1900-1914, wrote and lectured. CONTRIBUTIONS: Leading muckraker of the Progressive era, described life of the poor in N.Y.'s tenements. Exposed contamination of the N.Y. water supply, leading to purchase of the Croton Waterworks and a vast improvement of the water supply. Worked for child labor legislation. Exposures led to improvement in tenement conditions in N.Y. and elsewhere. Helped destroy the worst tenement block in N.Y. (Mulberry Bend), and replaced it with a neighborhood house named for him (1888).

WRITINGS: *How the Other Half Lives* (1890); *The Children of the Poor* (1892); *The Battle with the Slum* (1902); *Children of the Tenements* (1903). REFERENCES: *DAB* 8: 606-8; *NCAB*, 13:114; *N.Y. Times*, May 27-June 1, 1914; *Jacob A. Riis* (1903); *Who's Who in Am.*, 1914-1915.

M. Kaufman

RIPLEY, MARTHA (GEORGE) (November 30, 1843, Lowell, Vt.-April 18, 1912, Minneapolis, Minn.). *Obstetrician; Pediatrician.* Daughter of Francis Rogers and Esther Ann George. Married William Warren Ripley, 1867; three children. EDUCATION: M.D., 1883, Boston University Medical School. CAREER: Moved to Minn. after husband had an accident that forced him out of work; medical practice, Minn.; professor of children's diseases, Homeopathic School of Medicine, Minneapolis, Minn.; lectured on obstetrics and pediatrics in medical schools, Wis., Mich., and Ia. CONTRIBUTIONS: Worked on the reduction of mortality in childbirth and infant mortality. Established the Maternity Hospital for married and unmarried mothers in Minneapolis (1886), later named the Ripley Memorial Hospital. First to establish a special social service for poor and unmarried women and for homeless children born at the hospital. REFERENCES: *Notable Am. Women*, 3: 162-63; W. Solberg, in *Minnesota Hist.* 39 (1964): 1-17.

R. Rosenthal

RIVERS, THOMAS MILTON (September 3, 1888, Jonesboro, Ga.-May 12, 1962, New York, N.Y.). *Physician; Virology; Microbiology.* Son of Alonzo Burrill, cotton buyer and warehouse owner, and Mary Martha (Coleman) Rivers. Married Theresa Jacobina Riefele, 1922; no children. EDUCATION: 1909, A.B., Emory College (Oxford, Ga.); 1915, M.D., Johns Hopkins Medical School; 1915-18, intern and resident, Johns Hopkins Hospital. CAREER: 1918, Medical Corps, U.S. Army; 1919-22, bacteriology faculty, Johns Hopkins Medical School; 1920-22, pathology staff, St. Joseph's Hospital (Baltimore, Md.); 1922-55, at Rockefeller Institute for Medical Research: *post* 1927, member; 1953-55, vice-president and director; and 1937-53, director of its affiliated hospital; at National Foundation for Infantile Paralysis (later National Foundation): 1938-55, chairman, committee on virus research; 1954, chairman, Vaccine Advisory Committee; 1956-57, medical director; and *post* 1957, vice-president for medical affairs; president: 1932, American Society for Clinical Investigation; 1934, American Association of Immunologists; 1936, Society of American Bacteriologists; and 1942-43, Interurban Clinical Club. CONTRIBUTIONS: Established virology as a separate discipline in the United States. A leader in recognizing the importance of viruses as a distinct group of pathogenic organisms. Observed that viruses were obligate parasites, therefore, that they require living cells for their survival and replication (1926). Responsible for the viral research plan that culminated in the development of the Salk and Sabin vaccines against poliomyelitis. Developed an attenuated strain of vaccinia virus in tissue culture (1931); first vaccine for human use grown in cell culture; later was found to have become too attenuated to confer protection against smallpox and was discarded; however, methods used in its preparation were adopted in the development of more effective vaccines for other viral diseases, notably yellow fever. Made important discoveries about psittacosis (1929-30) and sleeping sickness, a form of encephalitis (1934). Discovered the bacillus *Hemophilu parainfluenza* and a latent virus of rabbits known as Virus III (1919-24). Edited and was a contributor to several books on viral diseases that became classics in their field. Trained many of the leading virologists of his time.

WRITINGS: *Epidemic Respiratory Disease*. . .(1921, with Eugene L. Opie [q.v.], Francis G. Blake [q.v.], and J. C. Small); "The Lesions in Rabbits Experimentally Infected by a Virus Encountered in the Attempted Transmission of Varicella," *J. of Experimental Med.* 40 (1924): 281; *Filterable Viruses* (1928, editor); "Cultivation of Vaccine Virus for Jennerian Prophylaxis in Man," *ibid.*, 54 (1931): 453; "Diagnosis of Psittacosis in Man by Means of Injection of Sputum into White Mice," *ibid.*, 61 (1935): 205-12 (with George P. Berry); *Viral and Rickettsial Infections of Man* (1948). A bibliography is in *BMNAS* 38 (1965): 263-94. REFERENCES: *BHM* (1964-69), 224; (1970-74), 149; James Bordley and A. McGehee Harvey, *Two Cent. of Am. Med.* (1976), 639-42; *Current Biog.* (1960), 336-38; *NCAB*, E: 390-91; *N.Y. Times*, May 13, 1962; *Who Was Who in Am.* 4: 796.

                                                                    S. Galishoff

ROBB, ISABEL ADAMS (HAMPTON) (1860, Welland, Ontario, Canada-April 15, 1910, Cleveland, Ohio). *Nurse.* Daughter of Samuel James, tailor, and Sarah Mary (Lay) Hampton. Married Dr. Hunter Robb, 1894; two sons. EDUCATION: Collegiate Institute, St. Catherine's, Ontario; 1883, graduated from Bellevue Hospital Training School for Nurses. CAREER: 1883-85, nurse, St. Paul's House, Rome, Italy; superintendent of nurses: 1886-89, Cook County Hospital training school; and 1889-94, Johns Hopkins Hospital; resigned to move to Cleveland with husband, who became professor of gynecology, Western Reserve University; killed in a streetcar accident at age 50. CONTRIBUTIONS: As superintendent of nursing, Johns Hopkins Hospital, introduced a systematic program that was the first graded course for nurses in America. Worked to develop a three-year course of study and an eight-hour day for nurses. Led in the organization of the American Society of Superintendents of Training Schools for Nurses, the first national nursing organization that became the National League for Nursing Education (1912). Helped organize the Nurses' Associated Alumnae (1911, became the American Nursing Association), serving as first president (1897-98).

WRITINGS: *Nursing: Its Principles and Practices* (1893); *Nursing Ethics* (1900). REFERENCES: *BHM* (1964-69), 225; (1975-79), 107; J. W. James, "Isabel Hampton and the Professionalization of Nursing in the 1890s,'' in Morris Vogel and Charles Rosenberg, *Therapeutic Revolution* (1979); *Notable Am. Women*, 3: 170-72.

M. Kaufman

ROBERTS, CARL GLENNIS (December 15, 1886, Roberts' Settlement, Hamilton County, Ind.-January 15, 1950, Chicago, Ill.). *Surgeon; Gynecologist; Medical educator.* Son of John A. and Nancy E. (Simpson) Roberts. Married Lucille E. Williams, 1908; one child. EDUCATION: 1901-5, high school, Fairmount, Ind.; 1906-11, Chicago College of Medicine and Surgery, M.D., 1911; 1911, externship, German-American Hospital, Chicago; and graduate clinical work, Illinois Post-Graduate School of Therapeutics; 1919-34, intermittent postgraduate study courses in surgery and pathology: 1919, Chicago Laboratory of Surgical Technique; 1921, Chicago Institute of Surgery; 1921-22, Illinois Post-Graduate School of Operative Surgery; 1930-33, University of Chicago Medical School; and 1933-34, Cook County Hospital Graduate School Laboratory of Surgical Pathology. CAREER: 1911-28, attending staff, Chicago General Hospital and other Chicago-area hospitals; 1912-41, closely associated with Provident Hospital, Chicago, serving as chairman, Department of Gynecology (1918-23) and Department of Surgery; 1941, activities were severely limited by a heart attack from which he never fully recovered. CONTRIBUTIONS: Involvement with Provident Hospital as leader in staff reorganizations and residency training, especially in surgery, established reputation in black medical education. Provident Hospital's surgical residency was the first in any black institution to receive official approval of American College of Surgeons and the AMA. One of first blacks to be certified by American Board of Surgery. Fought long and hard for recognition of black physicians in American organized medicine. Represented the NMA before the Senate Committee on the Wagner Bill (1940) and before the AMA House of Delegates, first time in AMA's history (1939). Served NMA as member, Board of Trustees, and as president (1925). Organized first black sanitary corps of Red Cross in Chicago during World War I and led it as commandant. REFERENCES: Charles R. Drew, ''Carl Glennis Roberts, M.D., 1886-1950,'' *JNMA* 24 (1950): 109-10; *WWCR* 1 (1915): 232; *WWICA* 7 (1950): 440-41.

T. L. Savitt

ROBERTSON, FELIX (January 11, 1781, Nashville, Tenn.-July 10, 1865, Nashville). *Physician.* Son of James, pioneer Tennessean and founder of Nashville, and Charlotte (Reeves) Robertson. Married Lydia Waters, 1808; eight children. EDUCATION: Probably attended Davidson Academy, Nashville; c. 1801, began studying medicine under Drs. Joseph Hays and Thomas A. Claiborne, Nashville; 1805, M.D., University of Pennsylvania. CAREER: 1805-65, practiced medicine, Nashville, with a special interest in children; at Cumberland College, later University of Nashville: 1809, trustee; 1850, president, Board of Trustees; and an organizer, medical department; 1825, led a group of 30 settlers to Tex. to establish the Robertson Colony and remained there about six months; in

Medical Society of Tennessee: 1830, organizer and charter member; and 1834-40, 1853-55, president; 1818, 1827-28, mayor, Nashville; friend and physician to Presidents Andrew Jackson and James K. Polk. CONTRIBUTIONS: Pioneer Tenn. physician. First native-born Tennessean to obtain an M.D. degree; sometimes referred to as Nashville's first pediatrician. M.D. thesis "Chorea Sancti Viti" (1805) was the first published medical work by a Tenn. physician. Involved in the organization of the first Nashville medical society (1821) and was its first president; served a total of eight years as president, Medical Society of Tennessee, a record that still stands. Leader in development of higher education in Nashville, mainly as a trustee, University of Nashville, and encouraged the development of the medical department. Alderman and mayor, Nashville.

WRITINGS: Eight publications have been located, mainly on clinical subjects, including valuable "Sketch of Pioneer Physicians of Nashville." Communicated the experience of father on the treatment of scalped head (1805), a major event in the history of surgery in the trans-Appalachian frontier. REFERENCES: Amos Christie, "Dr. Felix Robertson—Nashville's 'First Pediatrician,'" *J. Tenn. Med. Assoc.* 69 (1976): 469-72; T. S. Weaver, "Dr. Felix Robertson: His Life and Times," ibid., 53 (1960): 410-15.

S. R. Bruesch

ROBERTSON, WILLIAM STEPHENSON (June 5, 1831, Georgetown, Pa.-January 2, 1887, Muscatine, Ia.). *General practitioner.* Son of James M. Robertson, physician. Married Annie E. Charlton, 1856; two children. EDUCATION: Knox College (Galesburg, Ill.); 1852-54, studied medicine with his father, Columbus City, Ia.; 1856, M.D., Jefferson Medical College (Philadelphia, Pa.); 1868-69, attended lectures, Bellevue Hospital, N.Y. CAREER: 1856-68, medical practice (with father), Columbus City; 1861-63, major, Fifth Iowa Infantry; *post* 1869, medical practice, Muscatine; 1870-87, first professor of theory and practice of medicine, State University of Iowa medical department (Iowa City, Ia.); 1874, president, Iowa State Medical Society; 1878-82, Ia. state senator; 1880-87, president, Iowa State Board of Health. CONTRIBUTIONS: A member of its first faculty, was influential in the development of clinical teaching at the University of Iowa medical school; instituted Iowa's first courses in physical diagnosis and in public hygiene and "sanitary science." As the bacterial origin of infectious diseases became gradually accepted, changed his lectures accordingly, considerably in advance of other medical teachers of the time. As state senator, was the principal organizer of the Iowa State Board of Public Health. Also instrumental in founding the state institution for the "feebleminded" at Glenwood.

WRITINGS: Various papers read before the Iowa State Medical Society (for example, "Medical Inhalation"; "Thermometry in Disease"); "Over-Pressure in Schools," *Report of the Board of Health of Iowa* 3 (1885): 461. REFERENCES: W. B. Atkinson, *Biographical Dictionary of Contemporary Am. Physicians and Surgeons*, 2d ed. (1880), 94; Walter L. Bierring, *A History of the Department of Internal Medicine, State University of Iowa College of Medicine, 1870-1958* (1958), 20; David S. Fairchild, *History of Medicine in Iowa* (1923), 185-88; *Index Medicus*, 1st series; Charles H. Lothrop, *The Medical and*

Surgical Directory of the State of Iowa (1876), 217; *One Hundred Years of Iowa Medicine, 1850-1950* (1950), 125.

R. E. Rakel

ROBINS, CHARLES ARMINGTON (December 8, 1884, Defiance, Ia.-September 16, 1970, Lewiston, Idaho). *Physician.* Son of Charles M. and Rebecca J. (Burke) Robins. Married Patricia Simpson, 1939; two children. EDUCATION: 1907, A.B., William Jewell College; 1917, M.D., Rush Medical College. CAREER: 1917-18, member, U.S. Army Medical Corps; 1918, began practice, St. Maries, Idaho; 1939-46, member, Idaho Senate; 1946, elected governor, Idaho, serving a four-year term; 1950, became director, North Idaho Medical Service Bureau. CONTRIBUTIONS: As governor, worked for reforms in health and education. Although a busy physician, turned to politics and to public service. REFERENCES: *Capitol Who's Who* (1950), 178; *Daily Statesman* (Boise), September 21, 1970.

A. A. Hart

ROBINSON, G[EORGE] CANBY (November 4, 1878, Baltimore, Md.-August 31, 1960, Greenport, N.Y.). *Physician; Medical educator.* Son of Edward Ayrault, business executive, and Alice (Canby) Robinson. Married Marion Bruyette Boise, 1912; two children. EDUCATION: Johns Hopkins University: 1899, A.B.; and 1903, M.D.; 1903, assistant, Clifton Springs (N.Y.) Sanitorium; 1903-4, assistant demonstrator of anatomy, Cornell University; 1904-8, resident pathologist and resident physician, Pennsylvania Hospital (Philadelphia); 1908-9, studied physiology, Munich, with Friedrich Von Müller. CAREER: 1909, practiced medicine, Philadelphia, Pa.; 1909-10, director, pathological laboratory, Presbyterian Hospital (Philadelphia); 1910-13, resident physician, Hospital of the Rockefeller Institute for Medical Research (N.Y.), associate in medicine, Rockefeller Institute for Medical Research; at Washington University (St. Louis, Mo.): 1913-20, medicine faculty; and 1917-20, dean; 1920-28, medicine faculty and dean, Vanderbilt Medical School; 1921-22, acting professor of medicine, Johns Hopkins Medical School; 1928-35, medicine faculty, Cornell University Medical College, and director, New York Hospital and Cornell Medical College Association; 1935, medicine faculty, Peiping (China) Union Medical College; 1936-46, lecturer, medicine and preventive medicine, Johns Hopkins Medical School; 1941-45, national director, American Red Cross Blood Donor Service; *post* 1946, executive secretary, Maryland Tuberculosis Association; president: 1929-30, Harvey Society; and 1932-33, Association of American Physicians. CONTRIBUTIONS: One of the nation's leading medical educators in the period between the two world wars, reorganized and revitalized three great medical schools: Washington University (1917-20), Vanderbilt University (1920-28), and Cornell University (1928-34). At Vanderbilt University, with the help of a grant from the General Education Board, built a new hospital and medical school and recruited an outstanding faculty. At Cornell University, directed the building of the New York Hospital-Cornell Medical Center but was unable to realize all of his goals because of the Great Depression. An active medical investigator. Helped demonstrate (1906) that the causative agent in meningitis could be isolated from the blood stream. Did most important scientific work on cardiovascular disease; used electrocardiography to study cardiac arrhythmias, extended the therapeutic value of digitalis, and invented a technique for determination of the blood gases. Later work was mainly in occupational medicine and the social aspects of illness. Edited *Journal of Clinical Investigation* (from founding, 1924-30).

WRITINGS: "Bacteriological Findings in Fifteen Cases of Epidemic Cerebrospinal Meningitis," *Bull. of the Ayer Clinical Laboratory, Pennsylvania Hosp.* 1, no. 3 (1906): 27; "A Study with the Electrocardiograph of the Mode of Death of the Human Heart," *J. of Experimental Med.* 16 (1912): 291; *The Therapeutic Use of Digitalis* (1922); "The Gaseous Content of the Blood and the Output of the Heart in Normal Resting Adults," *J. of Clin. Invest.* 1 (1924): 87; *The Patient as a Person: A Study of the Social Aspects of Illness* (1939). A bibliography of his scientific writings is in *Johns Hopkins Med. J.* REFERENCES: *Adventures in Medical Education* (1957), memoirs; *DAB*, Supplement 6: 546-47; A. McGehee Harvey, "G. Canby Robinson: Peripatetic Medical Educator," *Johns Hopkins Med. J.* 143 (1978): 84-103; *NCAB*, 46: 408-10; *Who Was Who in Am.*, 4: 801.

S. Galishoff

ROBINSON, JOHN LaRUE   (1872, Keokuk, Ia.-July, 1950). *Physician; EENT*. Son of Thara and Laura Robinson. Married Mary Elizabeth Evans, June 17, 1914; two children. EDUCATION: M.D., 1898, Keokuk Medical College. CAREER: Medical practice in Nev. (licensed in Reno, Nev., 1904). CONTRIBUTIONS: Established People's Hospital, Reno (1904-5), first general hospital in Nev. Patented several instruments for eye, ear, nose, and throat treatment, including a powerful mobile magnet for drawing steel from the eye, a croup kettle, eye dropper, electric pad, and so forth. President, Nevada State Medical Society (1923).

J. Edwards

ROBINSON, PAUL TIMOTHY   (June 23, 1898, Lewisville, Ark.-February 1, 1966, Richmond, Calif.). *Surgeon*. Son of George Washington, Baptist minister, and Pearl Anna Robinson. Married Virginia Marie ? ; eight children. EDUCATION: Bishop College (Tex.): 1917, graduated from Academic and Normal Department; and 1921, B.S.; 1931, M.D., Meharry Medical College; 1931-35, turned down two-year General Education Board fellowship in pathology, Harvard University Medical School, to do internship and three-year residency in pathology, Flint-Goodridge Hospital, Tulane University, New Orleans, La. CAREER: 1917-18, student teacher, assistant librarian, laborer, Bishop College; 1918, U.S. Army; 1921-27, teacher and principal (1923-27), Northwest Industrial Normal Institute, Mansfield, La.; at Flint-Goodridge Hospital: 1935-37, clinical assistant; 1937-39, junior associate; and 1939-52, senior associate in general surgery service; 1950-58, medical director, Robinson Infirmary and Clinic (New Orleans);

1953-60s, private surgical practice, Richmond. CONTRIBUTIONS: Devoted career to serving black medical needs within the profession and among patients. Established and edited the *Journal of the New Orleans Medical, Dental, and Pharmaceutical Association* (five issues, 1938-39). Served ten years as president, New Orleans Medical Association, and one year (1940-41) as president, Louisiana State Medical Association. Led the Louisiana representatives in the NMA House of Delegates for about 15 years and served several times as secretary and as vice-speaker. Established the Robinson Infirmary and Clinic, a 40-bed private hospital (1950) to offset need for good hospital service for black patients in New Orleans during era of segregation. REFERENCES: W. Montague Cobb, "Paul Timothy Robinson, M.D., 1898-1966," *JNMA* 58 (1966): 321-23.

T. L. Savitt

ROCK, JOHN SWEAT (October 13, 1825, Salem, N.J.-December 3, 1866, Boston, Mass.). *Physician.* EDUCATION: Mid-1840s, apprentice to Drs. Sharp and Gibson, Salem; 1852 or 1853, M.D., American Medical College, Philadelphia, Pa.; 1848-49, studied dentistry under Dr. U. Harbert, Salem; 1860-61, studied law, Boston, Mass. CAREER: 1844-48, schoolteacher, Salem; 1850-53, dental practice, Philadelphia; 1853-60, medical and dental practice, Boston (gave up practice owing to poor health); 1861-66, law practice, Boston and Washington, D.C. CONTRIBUTIONS: One of the first blacks to earn a medical degree in the United States (1852 or 1853). Provided medical treatment to Boston's black population and to a number of fugitive slaves passing through to Canada. Appears to have been admitted to Massachusetts Medical Society (mid-1850s), second black to be so honored (John De Grasse was admitted in 1854), but society records do not record this event. Very active in abolitionist and black rights causes (1855-death). First black to be admitted to practice law before the bar of the U.S. Supreme Court (1865). REFERENCES: Clarence G. Contee, "John Sweat Rock, M.D., Esq., 1825-66," *JNMA* 68 (1976): 237-42; G. W. Forbes, "John S. Rock," ms., Boston Public Library, Rare Books and Manuscripts Division; Eugene P. Link, "The Civil Rights Activities of Three Great Physicians," *J. of Negro Hist.* 52 (1967): 169-84.

T. L. Savitt

RODMAN, WILLIAM LOUIS (September 5, 1858, Frankfort, Ky.-March 8, 1916, Philadelphia, Pa.). *Physician; Surgery; Medical education.* Son of John, lawyer and attorney general of Ky., and Harriet Virginia (Russell) Rodman. Married Bettie Stewart, 1882; three children. EDUCATION: 1875, M.A., Kentucky Military Institute; 1879, M.D., Jefferson Medical College; 1879-80, house surgeon, Jefferson Hospital. CAREER: 1880-82, surgeon, U.S. Army, Fort Sill, Okla. (then Indian Territory); practiced medicine: 1882-84, Abilene, Tex.; and 1884-98, Louisville, Ky.; 1885-93, demonstrator of surgery, medical department, University of Louisville; 1893-98, surgery faculty, Kentucky School of Medicine; 1898-1916, practiced medicine, Philadelphia; 1898-1916, surgery faculty, Medico-Chirurgical College of Philadelphia; 1900-1905, surgery and clinical surgery faculty, Woman's Medical College of Pennsylvania; 1900-1906, chairman, Executive Committee, North American Children's Sanitarium, Atlantic City, N.J.; president: 1902-3, Association of American Medical Colleges; and 1915, American Medical Association. CONTRIBUTIONS: Founded the National Board of Medical Examiners (1915) for the purpose of standardizing examination for medical licensure. Pioneered in the excision of the ulcer-bearing area in the treatment of gastric ulcer. An authority on the surgical treatment of mammary cancer and first to oppose the use of radium alone in cancer therapy.

WRITINGS: *Diseases of the Breast, with Special Reference to Cancer* (1908); "Pylorectomy and Partial Gastrectomy or Excision of the Ulcer-Bearing Area in the Treatment of Gastric Ulcer," *Surg. Gyn. & Obst.* 20 (Jan. 1915): 25-30. REFERENCES: Kelly and Burrage (1928), 1048-49; *NCAB*, 27: 228; *Who Was Who in Am.*, 1: 1049.

S. Galishoff

ROGERS, WILLIAM EGBERT (September 26, 1826, Hillsboro, N.C.-May 21, 1885, Memphis, Tenn.). *Physician; Medical educator; Surgery.* Son of John, physician and educator, and Margaret L. (Sheppard) Rogers. Married Elizabeth Battle, 1855; seven children. EDUCATION: Medical preceptorship under Dr. Egbert Haywood, Brownsville, Tenn.; 1848, M.D., Jefferson Medical College, Philadelphia, Pa. CAREER: 1848-58, practiced medicine, Brownsville; 1858, moved to Memphis; 1861-65, surgeon, Ninth Tennessee Infantry Regiment, Confederate States of America; 1865, resumed practice, Memphis, with emphasis on surgery; 1867, secretary, Memphis Board of Health; 1878, director, Howard Association Hospitals; attended the sick during the yellow-fever epidemics of 1867, 1873, 1878, and 1879; at Memphis Hospital Medical College: 1877, organized college; and 1880, at opening session, dean of the faculty and professor of surgery; 1883, established the Rogers' Surgical Infirmary, Memphis, assisted by son William Boddie Rogers, M.D. CONTRIBUTIONS: Founded Memphis Hospital Medical College, a very successful medical school from 1880 until its merger with the University of Tennessee in 1913. As the leading surgeon of the Memphis area, saw to it that Surgical Infirmary provided the best contemporary facilities for the latest advances in surgery.

WRITINGS: Wrote little, mainly papers about surgical topics. REFERENCES: P. M. Hamer, *Centennial Hist. of the Tenn. State Med. Assoc.* (1930), 196-97; information from family; J. M. Keating, *Hist. of Memphis* 2 (1888): 102-3.

S. R. Bruesch

ROMAN, CHARLES VICTOR (July 4, 1864, Williamsport, Pa.-August 25, 1934, Nashville, Tenn.). *Physician; Ear, Nose and Throat; (ENT); Medical Writer; Educator.* Son of James William and Anna Walker (McGuinn) Roman. Married Margaret Lee Voorhees, 1891; one child. EDUCATION: Hamilton Collegiate Institute, Ontario, Canada; 1889-90, office assistant to Dr. R. F. Boyd (q.v.), Nashville; 1890, M.D., Meharry Medical College; 1899, Post-Graduate

Medical School and Hospital of Chicago; 1904, postgraduate study, Royal Ophthalmic Hospital and Central London Ear, Nose and Throat Hospital, London, England. CAREER: Medical practice: 1890-93; and 1893-1904, Dallas Tex.; 1904-34, ENT practice, Nashville; at Meharry Medical College: 1904-31, chairman, ophthalmology and oto-laryngology; and 1931-34, professor of medical history and ethics; 1904-33, director of health, Fisk University. CONTRIBUTIONS: A founder and editor, *Journal of the National Medical Association* (1908-18). President, National Medical Association (1903-4). Founder and first head, Department of Ophthalmology and Oto-Laryngology, Meharry Medical College (1904-31). Early leader in black medical profession, as writer, specialist, teacher, and speaker and as observer of medical education at Meharry.

WRITINGS: *Meharry Medical College: A History* (1934); "Vitality of the Negroes," *JNMA* 2 (1910): 180-82; "An Appeal to Meharry Alumni," *JNMA* 3 (1911): 21-24; "Therapeutics of Pulmonary Tuberculosis," *JNMA* 4 (1912): 1-7; "The Cultural Background of Modern Medicine," *JNMA* 16 (1924): 168-70. Writings listed in *JNMA* 45 (1953): 304-5. REFERENCES: W. Montague Cobb, "Charles Victor Roman," *JNMA* 45 (1953): 301-5; Obituary, *JNMA* 26 (1934): 174-75; Charles V. Roman, *Meharry Medical College: A History* (1934); *WWCR* 1 (1915): 233; *WWICA* 3 (1930-32): 367.

T. L. Savitt

ROMAYNE, NICHOLAS (September 1756, New York, N.Y.-July 21, 1817, New York). *Physician; Medical education.* Son of John, silversmith, and Juliana (McCarty) Romeyn. Married Susan Van Dam; several children. EDUCATION: 1774, entered medical school, King's College (now Columbia University); 1780, M.D., University of Edinburgh; studied medicine: 1780-82, Paris, France; London, England; and Leyden, the Netherlands; and mid-1793, Europe; 1795, licentiate, Royal College of Physicians (London); 1800, fellow, Royal College of Physicians (Edinburgh). CAREER: *Post* 1783, practiced medicine, N.Y.; 1784-87, original member, Board of Regents, University of the State of New York; 1785-87, practice of "physic" faculty, Medical School, Columbia College; 1787-93, conducted private classes in medicine; speculated in western land; implicated in Blount Conspiracy of 1797; left United States briefly; 1806, first president, Medical Society of the City and County of New York; College of Physicians and Surgeons: 1807-11, founder, president, trustee; 1807-8, anatomy faculty; and 1808, institutes of medicine faculty; 1810, president, New York State Medical Society; 1812-16, institutes of medicine (physiology) and forensic medicine faculty, Queen's College (now Rutgers University). CONTRIBUTIONS: Established a private medical school that he associated with Queens College (1792-93). After a somewhat checkered career, *post* 1794, revived the College of Physicians and Surgeons (Columbia), dormant since 1791, and served as its president (1807).

WRITINGS: *An Address Delivered at the Commencement of the Lectures. . .*(1808). REFERENCES: *BHM* (1964-69), 227; *DAB*, 16: 127; Kelly and Burrage (1928), 1056-57;

Fred B. Rogers, "Nicholas Romayne, 1756-1817; Stormy Petrel of American Medical Education," *J. of Med. Ed.* 35 (1960): 258-63; *Who Was Who in Am.*, Hist. Vol.: 524.

S. Galishoff

ROMIG, JOSEPH HERMAN (1872, West Salem, Ill.-November 22, 1951, Colorado Springs, Colo.). *Physician; Surgeon.* Son of Moravian missionaries. Married Ellen May Ervin; Craig ? ; four children. EDUCATION: 1895, Hahnemann Medical School, Philadelphia, Pa. CAREER: 1896-1901, entered Alaska to join Bethel Moravian Mission; 1901-6, private practice, San Francisco, Calif.; 1909-19, superintendent of schools and physician, Southwest Alaska Natives; 1919-22, practice, Seward, Alaska; 1922-37, physician, Alaska Railroad. CONTRIBUTIONS: Known as "dog-sled doctor" and is reputed to have been the first to use anesthesia in the Kuskokwim River delta. Ministered to the Eskimos in the interior. Reported to have performed heroically following the devastating San Francisco earthquake. Subsequently returned to Alaska and established the first hospital in the territory west of Sitka, Alaska. Supervised the Alaska Railway Hospital, Anchorage (1930-37), and served one term as mayor, Anchorage.

WRITINGS: "Medical Practice in Western Alaska around 1900," *Anchorage Daily Times*, June 29, 1939. REFERENCES: Eva Greenslit Anderson, *Dog Team Doctor* (1940); *Times* (Anchorage), November 24, 1951, p. 1; *N.Y. Times*, January 3, 1937, II:8:5.

A.R.C. Helms

ROSE, WICKLIFFE (November 19, 1862, Saulsbury, Tenn.-September 5, 1931, Vancouver Island, Canada). *Public health and educational administrator.* Son of Kinchen Langston, clergyman, and Jeanette (Cherry) Rose. Married Ella Morio Sadler, 1891; three children. EDUCATION: University of Nashville: 1889, A.B.; and 1890, M.A. CAREER: At Peabody College and University of Nashville: 1891-92, history and mathematics faculties; 1892-1902, philosophy faculty; and 1904-7, dean; 1902-4, history and philosophy of education faculty, University of Tennessee; 1907-15, general agent, Peabody Educational Fund; 1909-23, trustee, John F. Slater Fund; 1910-15, administrative secretary, Rockefeller Sanitary Commission for the Eradication of Hookworm Disease; on Southern Education Board: 1909-15, member; and 1909-13, executive secretary; 1913-28, member, Rockefeller Foundation; with International Health Commission (later International Health Board): 1913-28, member; and 1913-23, general director; on General Education Board: 1911-28, member; and 1923-28, president; 1923-28, president, International Education Board. CONTRIBUTIONS: Planned and directed the Rockefeller Sanitary Commission's campaign to eradicate hookworm in the South; treated nearly 700,000 cases and educated the public in the need for sanitary privies and their use. Commission also provided personnel to train local health workers and offered financial assistance to state health departments to make needed improvements. Commission's successes stimulated other private philanthropies to become involved in public health. With International Health Board, directed hookworm, malaria, and yellow-fever campaigns overseas. Instrumental in getting the board to endow schools of hygiene and public health at Johns Hopkins and Harvard and overseas.

WRITINGS: *State Systems of Public Health in Twelve Southern States* (1911). REFERENCES: Mary Boccaccio, "Ground Itch and Dew Poison, The Rockefeller Sanitary Commission, 1909-1914," *J. Hist. Med.* 27 (1972): 30-53; *DAB*, Supplement 1: 639-40; John Ettling, *The Germ of Laziness* (1981); Simon Flexner, "Wickliffe Rose, 1862-1931," *Sci.* 75 (1932): 504-6; *NCAB*, 31: 478-79; *Who Was Who in Am.*, 1: 1058.

S. Galishoff

ROSENAU, MILTON JOSEPH (January 1, 1869, Philadelphia, Pa.-April 9, 1946, Chapel Hill, N.C.). *Physician; Medical educator; Public health.* Son of Nathan, merchant, and Matilda (Blitz) Rosenau. Married Myra F. Frank, 1900; Maud (Heilner) Tenner, 1935; three children by first marriage. EDUCATION: 1889, M.D., University of Pennsylvania; 1889-90, intern, Philadelphia General Hospital; studied: 1892-93, Berlin; and 1900, Paris and Vienna. CAREER: 1890-1909, with U.S. Marine Hospital Service (later U.S. Public Health Service): 1895-99, quarantine and sanitation assignments, San Francisco, Calif., Philippine Islands, and Cuba; 1899-1909, director, Hygienic Laboratory; and 1904-9, bacteriology faculty, Army and Navy Medical School; 1909-35, preventive medicine and hygiene faculty, Harvard Medical School; 1913-22, director, Harvard and Massachusetts Institute of Technology School for Health Officers; 1922-35, epidemiology faculty, Harvard School of Public Health; on Massachusetts State Board of Health: 1912-21, member; and 1914-21, chief, Division of Biologic Laboratories; and director, Antitoxin and Vaccine Laboratory; at University of North Carolina: *post* 1936, director, Division of Public Health; and epidemiology faculty, School of Medicine; and 1940-46, dean, School of Public Health; president: 1934, Society of American Bacteriologists; and 1944, American Public Health Association. CONTRIBUTIONS: Made important discoveries in preventive medicine, and through writings and work as a medical educator, helped create a corps of professionally trained public health workers. With John F. Anderson, helped elucidate the phenomenon of anaphylaxis, or sensitivity to toxin proteins; with Joseph Goldberger (q.v.), standardized the unit of diphtheria antitoxin (early 1900s). Aided the movement for a clean milk supply with studies of milk sanitation; spurred the use of pasteurization by determining that heating to 60°C for 20 minutes destroys the more harmful pathogens in milk without damaging its nutritional value. With W. T. Sedgwick (q.v.), and George C. Whipple (q.v.), established the first American school of public health at Harvard-MIT (1913). Held the first chair of preventive medicine and hygiene in an American medical school. Organized a school of public health at the University of North Carolina. Wrote an authoritative textbook, *Preventive Medicine and Hygiene* (1913), which by 1935 had run through six editions and had been translated into six languages.

WRITINGS: *The Immunity Unit for Diphtheria Antitoxin* (1905); *A Study of the Causes of Sudden Death Following the Injection of Horse Serum* (1906, with John F. Anderson); *The Standardization of Tetanus Antitoxin* (1908); *The Milk Question* (1912). REFER-

ROSS, JULIAN WALDO

ENCES: *DAB*, Supplement 4: 700-702; Miller, *BHM*, p. 97; *NCAB*, 42: 690-92; *N.Y. Times*, April 10, 1946; *Who Was Who in Am.*, 2: 459.

S. Galishoff

ROSS, JULIAN WALDO (June 10, 1884, Lee County, Ga.-April 2, 1961). *Obstetrics and gynecology*. Son of Seymour and Clara (Singleton) Ross. Married Lillian Russell Jefferson, 1910; no children. EDUCATION: 1904-5, Georgia State Industrial College (Savannah, Ga.); 1907, A.B. (magna cum laude), Lincoln University (Pa.); 1911, M.D., Howard University Medical School; 1911-12, intern, Freedmen's Hospital; 1922-35 (summers), postgraduate work, in obstetrics and gynecology, Harlem, Long Island Medical College, and Bellevue hospitals. CAREER: 1912-57, staff, Freedmen's Hospital, and Howard University Medical School: 1929-57, first chief of obstetrics and gynecology and chair of department. CONTRIBUTIONS: First black physician to receive certification in both obstetrics and gynecology by American Board of Obstetrics and Gynecology (1935). Part of Dean Numa P. G. Adams's (q.v.) program to upgrade and rebuild Howard's Medical School by serving as strong leader of obstetrics and gynecology. A model teacher, methodical surgeon, and consistent researcher. Secretary of faculty (1924-30), Howard Medical School.

WRITINGS: More than 20 publications, including "Nembutal in the Treatment of Preeclampsia and Eclampsia," *Am. J. Obstet. Gynecol.* 31 (1936): 120; "Chromic Acid for the Treatment of Chronic Infective Endocervicitis," ibid., 33 (1937): 348; "The Use of Stilbestrol in Abnormal Gynecologic Bleeding (Nonmalignant)," ibid., 56 (1938): 723-26, (with C. M. Gill); "Use of Thyroid Extract in the Treatment of Hyperplasia Endometri," *JNMA* 46 (1954): 105-6. Writings listed in *JNMA*, 52 (1960): 221-22. REFERENCES: W. Montague Cobb, "Julian Waldo Ross, M.D., 1884-," *JNMA* 48: 430; *WWAPS* (1938): 1033-34; *WWICA*, 6: 446.

T. L. Savitt

ROTCH, THOMAS MORGAN (December 9, 1849, Philadelphia, Pa.-March 9, 1914, Boston, Mass.). *Physician; Pediatrics*. Son of Rodman and Helen (Morgan) Rotch. Married Helen Rotch, 1874; one child. EDUCATION: 1870, A.B., Harvard College; 1874, M.D., Harvard Medical School; 1873-74, house officer, Massachusetts General Hospital; 1874-76, postgraduate study, Vienna, Austria; and Berlin and Heidelberg, Germany. CAREER: 1878-1914, faculty, Harvard Medical School; 1893-1914, physician-in-chief, Children's Hospital and Infants' Hospital; 1881, established West End Nursery and Infants' Hospital and became its director, 1894. CONTRIBUTIONS: Deservedly called "The Father of Pediatrics in New England;" leader in the crusade for clean milk and its appropriate modification for infants. Helped develop the Walker-Gordon Farms and milk laboratories to modify clean milk on "the percentage basis." This was his most important contribution to pediatrics, despite the fact that it was later discarded as based on concepts that were no longer considered scientific. Later used the X-ray as a means of studying the bone development of growing children.

WRITINGS: "An Historical Sketch of the Development of Percentage Feeding," *N.Y. Med. J.* 85 (1907): 532; *Pediatrics* (1895); *The Diagnosis of Diseases in Early Life by the Roentgen Method* (1910). REFERENCES: *BHM* (1970-74), 151; T. E. Cone, Jr., *History of American Pediatrics* (1979); *DAB*, 8, pt. 2: 185-86; *NCAB*, 19: 350; Fritz B. Talbot, "Thomas Morgan Rotch," *Pediatric Profiles* (1957).

T. E. Cone, Jr.

ROUS, (FRANCIS) PEYTON (October 5, 1879, Baltimore, Md.-February 16, 1970, New York, N.Y.). *Physician; Pathology; Oncology.* Son of Charles and Frances Anderson (Wood) Rous. Married Marion Eckford de Kay, 1915; three children. EDUCATION: Johns Hopkins: 1900, B.A.; 1905, M.D.; and 1905-6, resident. CAREER: 1906-8, pathology faculty, University of Michigan; 1909-45, at Rockefeller Institute for Medical Research; at National Research Council: 1918-19, vice-chairman, Division of Medicine; 1919-26, member, Executive Committee; 1957-70, member, Board of Scientific Consultants, Sloan-Kettering Institute for Cancer Research; president: 1928, Harvey Society; 1930-32, Society of Experimental Biology; and 1932, Society of Experimental Pathology. CONTRIBUTIONS: Studies of transplantation of chicken sarcoma strengthened the theory of the viral origin of cancer; passed material from a tumor through porcelain filters impermeable to cancer cells and bacteria and was then able to produce the sarcoma in other chickens by injecting them with the filtrate (1911); work had little impact until the 1930s: was believed that either the growths were not tumors or faulty laboratory techniques had allowed cancer cells to slip through the filters. With J. B. Murphy (q.v.), found that chicken sarcoma could be cultivated in embryonated chicken eggs, but here too, the importance of his discovery for viral research was not appreciated for another two decades; subsequently was awarded the 1966 Nobel Prize in medicine or physiology for work on cancer in fowls. With J. R. Turner, found a way of preserving whole blood used in transfusion; developed a solution that kept refrigerated red cells alive for weeks (1915-16); later became the mainstay of blood banks and helped save numerous lives, especially during World War II. Did important research on the physiology and pathology of the liver, the biliary system, and the human blood system (1920s, 1930s). Demonstrated that carcinogenic chemicals activated the Shope papilloma, a normally benign lesion of rabbits, and accelerated its transition to the malignant state (1930s). Discovered method for isolating the cells of solid tissues using trypsin, a proteolytic enzyme found in the pancreatic juice. For some 50 years, beginning in 1921, helped edit the *Journal of Experimental Medicine.*

WRITINGS: "A Transmissible Avian Neoplasm (Sarcoma of the Common Fowl)," *J. of Experimental Med.* 12 (1910): 696-705; 13 (1911): 397-411; "Transmission of a Malignant New Growth by Means of a Cell-Free Filtrate," ibid., 56 (1912): 198; "The Preservation of Living Red Blood Cells *in Vitro*. I. Methods of Preservation," ibid., 23 (1916): 19-48. A bibliography is in *BMNAS*. REFERENCES: *BHM* (1964-69), 229; (1970-74), 151; (1977), 29; (1980), 35; *BMNAS* 48 (1976): 275-306; *Current Biog.* (1967),

354-57; *McGraw-Hill Modern Men of Sci.*, 1 (1966): 405-7; *Who Was Who in Am.*, 5: 623.

S. Galishoff

ROUSSELOT, LOUIS MARCEL (November 3, 1902, New York, N.Y.-March 28, 1974, Puerto Rico). *Physician; Surgeon.* Son of Louis Joseph, hotelman, and Louise (Jaeck) Rousselot. Married Evelyn Hastrup, 1935; one child. EDUCATION: Columbia University: 1924, A.B.; 1927, M.D.; 1933, M.Sc. in surgery; and 1934, Med. Sci.D. in surgery; 1927-34, intern and resident, Presbyterian Hospital (later part of the Columbia-Presbyterian Medical Center); 1927-28, studied pathology, University of Vienna; 1934-35, resident surgeon, School of Tropical Medicine of Columbia University in San Juan, Puerto Rico. CAREER: Surgical staff: 1935-48, Presbyterian Hospital; and 1948-67, St. Vincent's Hospital and Medical Center; consulting surgeon to numerous other hospitals, New York City metropolitan area; 1935-48, surgery faculty, College of Physicians and Surgeons (Columbia); 1942-45, served in European Theater of Operations, U.S. Army Medical Corps; 1948-67, clinical surgery faculty, New York University School of Medicine; 1968-70, deputy assistant secretary of defense, health, and environment; 1970-71, assistant secretary of defense, health, and education; 1971-73, special assistant for graduate and postgraduate education for physicians, Bureau of Health, Manpower, Education, National Institutes of Health; 1973, director, Emergency Medical Services, National Institutes of Health. CONTRIBUTIONS: As a member of Alan Whipple's (q.v.) spleen clinic, Columbia University, began research in portal hypertension, a frequent complication of cirrhosis of the liver; established the original concepts and techniques for the measurement of portal hypertension; developed methods of portocaval shunting for the treatment of bleeding esophageal varices and cirrhotic ascites. Introduced splenoportography into the United States. Did investigative work in adjuvant chemotherapy for the surgical treatment of colorectal cancer. Created an outstanding Department of Surgery, New York University. Spent the last years of life in Washington, D.C. where he served as the nation's chief medical officer for military affairs. Presided over the initiation and upgrading of many Department of Defense medical programs. Was largely responsible for the establishment of the Uniformed Services University of the Health Sciences, providing a medical school for the armed services. Proslyetized on the value of physician assistants and other physician extenders.

WRITINGS: *Bleeding Esophageal Varices—Portal Hypertension* (1959, with H. R. Liebowitz); "A Seven-Year Experience with Side-to-Side Portocaval Shunt for Cirrhotic Ascites," *Annals of Surg.* 168 (1968): 655-68 (with Albert R. Burchell and William F. Panke); "Intraluminal Chemotherapy (5-FU) Adjuvant to Surgery for Colorectal Cancer," in *Chemotherapy of Cancer* (1969). REFERENCES: John M. Dorsey, "Louis M. Rousselot," *Trans. Am. Surg. Assoc.* 93 (1975): 87-91; *NCAB*, 58: 441-43; *N.Y. Times*, March

29, 1974; Mark M. Ravitch, *A Century of Surgery*, 2 vols. (1981); *Who Was Who in Am.*, 6: 353.

S. Galishoff

ROVENSTINE, EMERY ANDREW (July 20, 1895, Atwood, Ind.-November 9, 1960, New York, N.Y.). *Anesthesiology*. Son of Cassius Andrew, general store owner, and Lulu (Massena) Rovenstine. Married Agnes Lane, 1919; Jewel Sonya Gould, 1939. EDUCATION: 1917, A.B., Wabash College (Crawfordsville, Ind.); 1928, M.D., Indiana University; 1928-29, intern, Indianapolis Hospital; 1931-34, resident in anesthesiology under Ralph M. Waters, University of Wisconsin. CAREER: 1917-19, U.S. Army Corps of Engineers, France; 1919-23, taught mathematics and science and coached sports at high schools, Menominee, Mich. and LaPorte, Ind.; anesthesia faculty: 1929-34, University of Indiana Medical School; 1935-60, New York University Medical School; and *post* 1938, College of Dentistry, New York University; 1935-60, anesthesiology staff, Bellevue Hospital; visiting professor of anesthesiology: 1938, Radcliffe Infirmary, Oxford University; and 1939, University of Rosario, Argentina; member: 1941-46, Medical Science Division, National Research Council; and during World War II, Army Advisory Board; president: 1936, American Society of Regional Anesthesia; and 1948, American Board of Anesthesiology. CONTRIBUTIONS: Reorganized the anesthetic service at Bellevue Hospital; took it out of the hands of nurses, established a Department of Anesthesia, and encouraged young physicians to specialize in this branch of medicine. While on the Army Advisory Board during World War II, was responsible for an order to army general hospitals placing anesthesiologists in charge of operating rooms. Developed new drugs, techniques, and equipment to ease pain; conducted original research in cyclopropane anesthesia and spinal anesthesia; devised endotracheal and endobronchial anesthetic techniques and instruments. Developed a system for collecting statistical data on each patient's anesthesia and surgery. Helped found the American Board of Anesthesiology (1937).

WRITINGS: "Cyclopropane as an Anesthetic Agent: A Preliminary Clinical Report," *Current Research in Anaesthesiology and Analgesia* 13 (Mar.-Apr. 1934): 59-60 (with John Alden Stiles, W. B. Neff, and R. M.Waters); *Fundamentals of Anesthesia* (1942); "The Management of Pain in the Aged," *Geriatrics* 1 (1946): 46-53 (with Emanuel M. Papper). Wrote over 200 papers and 15 textbook chapters. REFERENCES: *DAB*, Supplement 6: 553-54; *N.Y. Times*, November 10, 1960; *Who Was Who in Am.*, 4: 814.

S. Galishoff

ROWNTREE, LEONARD GEORGE (April 10, 1883, London, Ontario, Canada-June 2, 1959, Miami Beach, Fla.). *Physician: Pharmacology; Endocrinology*. Son of George, merchant, and Phoebe Ann (Martindale) Rowntree. Married Katherine Campbell, 1914; two children. EDUCATION: 1905, M.D., Western Medical College (London, Canada); 1906, intern, Victoria Hospital (London, Canada); 1907, voluntary assistant in pharmacology and experimental therapeutics, Johns Hopkins Medical School; summers, 1910-13, postgraduate study, Europe. CAREER: 1906, practiced medicine, Camden, N.J.; at Johns Hopkins Medical School: 1909-14, pharmacology faculty; and 1914-16, medicine faculty; 1916-20, medicine faculty, University of Minnesota; 1920-32, medical staff and medicine faculty, Mayo Foundation (Graduate School of the University of Minnesota); and senior medical consultant and director of clinical research, Mayo Clinic; 1918-19, Medical Corps, U.S. Army, attached to executive office, Medical Research Board, Army Expeditionary Force, Issoudon, France; 1932-40, director, Philadelphia Institute for Medical Research; and research clinician, Philadelphia General Hospital; 1933-55, head, advisory board, Biochemistry Research Foundation, Newark, Del.; 1940-45, chief, medical division, National Headquarters, Selective Service System, Washington, D.C.; 1946-55, chairman, dean's committee, Veterans Administration Hospital, Coral Gables, Fla.; president: 1921, American Society for Clinical Investigation; and 1929, American Society of Endocrinologists. CONTRIBUTIONS: Pioneered in the field of functional tests for kidney-liver diseases; devised and introduced the phenolsulfonephthalein test for renal function (1910) and, later, the tetrachlorphthalein test for hepatic excretion. Demonstrated that a large intake of water could cause intoxication (1923); work stimulated interest in water and inorganic metabolism. Made important studies of basal metabolism. Showed the beneficial effect of cortin in Addison's disease and the role of the thymus and pineal glands in growth and development. Helped effect the standardization of digitalis. An inspiring teacher and an organizer, University of Miami Medical School (1952).

WRITINGS: "An Experimental and Clinical Study of the Functional Activity of the Kidneys by Means of Phenolsulfonephthalein," *J. of Pharmacology* 1 (Jun. 1910): 579-661 (with J. T. Geraghty); "An Experimental and Clinical Study of the Value of Phenoltetrachlorphthalein as a Test for Hepatic Function," *Johns Hopkins Hosp. Bull.* 24 (Nov. 1913): 327-42 (with S. H. Hurwitz and A. L. Bloomfield); "Pituitary Extract and Water Balance," *Med. Record* 100 (1921): 174; "The Treatment of Three Cases of Chronic Addison's Disease," *Med. Clinics North America* 7 (Jul.-Nov. 1923): 177-87; *Amid Masters of Twentieth Century Medicine* (1958). REFERENCES: A. McGehee Harvey, *Science at the Bedside* (1981), 361, 371-75; *NCAB*, 44: 546-47; *Trans., Assoc. of Am. Physicians* 73 (1960): 29-31; *Who Was Who in Am.*, 7: 494.

S. Galishoff

RUBIN, ISIDORE CLINTON (January 8, 1883, Vienna, Austria-July 10, 1958, London, England). *Physician: Gynecology.* Son of Nehemiah and Froma (Keller) Rubin. Married Sylvia Unterberg, 1914; survived by three children. EDUCATION: College of the City of New York; 1905, M.D., College of Physicians and Surgeons (Columbia); 1905-8, intern and resident, Mount Sinai Hospital; 1909, postgraduate study, Austria and Germany. CAREER: *Post* 1910, practiced medicine, New York City; 1910-46, gynecological staff, Beth Israel, Mt. Sinai, and Montefiore hospitals; 1937-47, obstetrics and gynecology faculty, College of Physicians and Surgeons (Columbia); later held a similar position at New York University and at New York Medical College; president: 1928, New York

Obstetrical Society; and 1955-56, American Gynecological Society; president: American Association of Obstetricians, Gynecologists and Abdominal Surgeons. CONTRIBUTIONS: One of the first to use X-rays in gynecology. Best known for the introduction of tubal insufflation with a gaseous medium for the diagnosis and treatment of sterility due to occlusion of the Fallopian tubes (1922), subsequently called the Rubin test. Advanced knowledge of carcinoma of the cervix, uterine endoscopy, and ectopic pregnancy. A founding fellow, American Board of Obstetrics and Gynecology and the American Academy of Obstetrics. Helped edit *International Journal of Fertility, Gynécologie Pratique, Excerpta Medica, Fertility and Sterility*, and *Journal of Obstetrics and Gynecology*.

WRITINGS: "The Nonoperative Determination of Patency of Fallopian Tubes in Sterility. Intra-Uterine Inflation with Oxygen, and Production of an Artificial Pneumoperitoneum," *JAMA* 75 (Sept. 4, 1920): 661-66; *Symptoms in Gynecology* (1923); "X-Ray Diagnosis in Gynecology with the Aid of Intra-Uterine Collargol Injection," *Surg. Gyn. Obst.* 20 (1915): 435-42; *Uterotubal Insufflation* (1947); *Integrated Gynecology*, 3 vols. (1956, with Josef Novak). Writings are in *The Collected Papers of Dr. Isidor Clinton Rubin* (1954). REFERENCES: *DAB*, Supplement 6: 554-56; Miller, *BHM*, p. 97; *N.Y. Times*, July 11, 1958; Harold Speert, "I. C. Rubin, a Gynecologic Eponym," *J. of Mount Sinai Hosp.* 25 (1958): 221-28.

S. Galishoff

RUBINOW, ISAAC MAX (April 19, 1875, Grodno, Russia-September 1, 1936, New York City). *Physician; Statistician; Social welfare.* Son of Max Simon, textile merchant, and Esther (Shereshewsky) Rubinow. Married Sophia Himowich, 1899; three children. EDUCATION: 1885-92, attended Moscow Gymnasium; migrated to America with his family in 1893; 1895, A.B., Columbia College; 1895, attended College of Physicians and Surgeons of Columbia University; 1896-98, attended University Medical College (New York University), M.D., 1898; 1900, graduate student of the social sciences, Columbia University, Ph.D., 1914. CAREER: 1898-1903, medical practice in New York City; 1904-7, U.S. Department of Agriculture analyst on economics and statistics; 1908-10, U.S. Department of Commerce and Labor, completed study of European legislation related to workmen's compensation; 1911-16, chief statistician, Ocean Accident and Guarantee Corporation; 1916, executive secretary of AMA committee on social insurance; 1919-22, in Palestine as director of a medical unit sent by the Zionist Organization of America; 1923-28, head of the Jewish Welfare Society of Philadelphia; 1927, vice president of the American Association for Old-Age Security; served as consultant and author in his later years. CONTRIBUTIONS: Advocate of social welfare legislation to uplift the poor. Report on European legislation on workmen's compensation (1911) provided the basis for state legislation passed in the U.S. from 1911 to 1920. As statistician in the insurance industry, helped systematize the premium system and wrote articles and books which were used to support various proposals for social insurance. As executive secretary of the AMA committee on social insurance, was responsible for drafting legislation which was opposed by labor, industry, insurance companies, and the AMA. Consultant to the committee which developed the old age assistance program (social security) of the New Deal. Active in Jewish and social work activities throughout his life.

WRITINGS: *Economic Condition of the Jews of Russia* (1907); *Social Insurance, with Special Reference to American Conditions* (1913); *A Standard Accident Table, as a Basis for Compensation Rates* (1915); *Standards of Health Insurance* (1916); *The Quest for Security* (1934). REFERENCES: *DAB*, Supp. 2: 585-87; *N.Y. Times*, September 3, 1936; *Who Was Who in Am.*, 1 (1942).

M. Kaufman

RUGGLES, DAVID (March 15, 1810, Norwich, Conn.-December 26, 1849, Florence, Mass.). *Hydropathic practitioner*. Son of ? and Nancy Ruggles. Never married. EDUCATION: Probably attended Sabbath School for the Poor, Norwich, Conn., and schools established by the Manumission Society in Conn.; by age 17, had ceased formal schooling; learned about hydropathy from own readings and from a German homeopathic physician, Robert Wesselhoeft, living in Cambridge, Mass., who treated Ruggles for serious ailments in the mid-1840s. CAREER: 1829-33, grocery business, New York City; 1833-42, antislavery activity, New York City; 1834-42, bookshop proprietor and jobprinter, New York City; 1843-49, hydropathic practitioner, Northampton, Mass. area. CONTRIBUTIONS: An early, famous, black hydropathist. Founded one of the first hydropathic establishments in the United States near Northampton, Mass. (1843). Treated a number of important people, including Sojourner Truth (1843) and William Lloyd Garrison (1849). An ardent abolitionist and active participant in the Underground Railroad.

WRITINGS: Numerous antislavery articles and pamphlets. Writings listed in *J. of Negro Hist.* 28 (1943): 23-50. REFERENCES: Dorothy B. Porter, "David Ruggles, An Apostle of Human Rights," *J. of Negro Hist.* 29 (1943): 23-50; idem, "David Ruggles, 1810-1849, Hydropathic Practitioner," *JNMA* 49 (1957): 67-72, 130-34.

T. L. Savitt

RUSH, BENJAMIN (January 4, 1746, Byberry, Pa.-April 19, 1813, Philadelphia, Pa.). *Physician: Chemistry; Psychiatry*. Son of John, gunsmith, and Susanna (Hall) Rush. Married Julia Stockton, 1776; eight children. EDUCATION: c. 1754-59, school of his uncle, the Rev. James Finley; 1760, A.B., College of New Jersey (later Princeton); 1760-66, apprenticed to Dr. John Redman (q.v.); 1765-66, medical courses, College of Philadelphia (later University of Pennsylvania); 1768, M.D., Edinburgh University; 1768-69, postgraduate study, London. CAREER: 1769-1813, physician; 1769-1813, medical faculty, College of Philadelphia (1776-78, interrupted by service as delegate to Continental Congress and various medical posts during the Revolution); 1783-1813, medical staff, Pennsylvania Hospital (*post* 1787, care of the insane); 1797-1813, Treasurer, U.S. Mint. CONTRIBUTIONS: 1769, first professor of chemistry in America and author of first textbook—promoted study, not experimentation. Promoted interest in psychiatry (1812); author of first book on the subject by a native American. A founder: Dickinson College, Carlisle, Pa. (1783); Philadelphia Dispensary for the Poor, first free dispensary (1786); Young Ladies Academy in Philadelphia (1787); and College of Physicians (1787). Proposed a federal university for the preparation of young men for public life and government service (1788), specifying courses and recommending languages and foreign travel. Elected to the American Philosophical Society (1767) and was successively secretary, councillor, and vice-president (1770-1801). Signed the Declaration of Independence (1776). Physician and a manager, Philadelphia Humane Society, first in United States (1780). A forceful advocate of the value of bloodletting in reducing fever—a misapprehension offset by contributions of enduring value—his recognition of the connection between decayed teeth and disease; championship of inoculation (later vaccination) in smallpox (1802); description of cholera infantum; and early advocacy of preventive medicine (1805).

WRITINGS: *An Inquiry into the Influence of Physical Causes upon the Moral Faculty*, (1786); *Medical Inquiries and Observations*, 2nd ed., 4 vols. (1805); *Medical Inquiries and Observations, upon Diseases of the Mind* (1812); *The Autobiography of Benjamin Rush* (1948, ed. G. W. Corner); *The Letters of Benjamin Rush*, 2 vols. (1951, ed. L. H. Butterfield); Writings listed in Butterfield, *Letters*, 2: 1277-79; and N. G. Goodman, *Benjamin Rush, Physician and Citizen, 1746-1813* (1934), 382-90. REFERENCES: C. Binger, *Revolutionary Doctor: Benjamin Rush, 1746-1813* (1966); E. T. Carlson and M. M. Simpson, "The Definition of Mental Illness: Benjamin Rush (1746-1813)," *Am. J. of Psychiatry* 121 (1964): 209-14; *DAB*, 9, pt. 2: 229-31; Goodman, *Benjamin Rush*; D. F. Hawke, *Benjamin Rush, Revolutionary Gadfly* (1971); W. Miles, "Benjamin Rush, Chemist," *Chymia* 4 (1953): 33-77; *NCAB*, 3: 333; R. H. Shryock, "Benjamin Rush from the Perspective of the Twentieth Century," *Trans. and Studies of the Coll. of Physicians of Phila.* 14 (1965): 121-38; idem, "The Medical Reputation of Benjamin Rush: Contrast over Two Centuries," *Bull. Hist. Med.* 45 (1971): 507-52.

E. H. Thomson

RUSSELL, FREDERICK FULLER (August 17, 1870, Auburn, N.Y.-December 29, 1960, Louisville, Ky.). *Physician; Microbiology.* Son of George Daniel and Anna Cecelia (Fuller) Russell. Married Mathilda J. W. Busse, 1899; one child. EDUCATION: 1893, M.D., College of Physicians and Surgeons (Columbia); 1897-98, studied at University of Berlin. CAREER: 1898-1920, U.S. Army Medical Corps; at Army Medical School: 1907-13, bacteriology and medical microscopy faculty; and 1913-20, bacteriology, pathology, and preventive medicine faculty; 1907-20, curator, Army Medical Museum; 1909-13, bacteriology and pathology faculty, George Washington University; 1913-14, tropical medicine faculty, New York Post Graduate Medical School; 1915-17, chief, Board of Health Laboratory, Ancon, Canal Zone; 1917-18, director, Division of Laboratories and Infectious Diseases, Surgeon-General's Office; on International Health Board, Rockefeller Foundation: 1920-23, director, Public Health Laboratory Service; and 1923-25, general director; 1924-36, member, Public

Health Council, N.Y. State; 1936-39, preventive medicine and epidemiology faculty, Harvard Medical School and Harvard School of Public Health. CON-TRIBUTIONS: Demonstrated the effectiveness of typhoid fever vaccination in the American Army (1908) and later popularized its use in the civilian population. Made numerous bacteriological discoveries including the development of a culture medium that bears his name. Did important work during army career on worm infestation, dysentery, malaria, and yellow fever.

WRITINGS: "The Control of Typhoid in the Army by Vaccination," *N.Y. State J. of Med.* 19 (1910): 535-48. "The Isolation of Typhoid Bacilli from Urine and Feces with the Description of a New Double Sugar Tube Medium," *J. of Med. Research* 25 (Sept. 1911): 217-29. REFERENCES: *Am. J. of Public Health* 26 (1936): 1148; *JAMA* 176 (1961): 237-38; *Trans. Assoc. of Am. Physicians* 74 (1961): 44-46; *Who Was Who in Am.*, 4: 820.

S. Galishoff

RUTHERFORD, FRANCES ARMSTRONG (October 8, 1842, Bath, N.Y.-May 24, 1922, Grand Rapids, Mich.). *Physician; General practice; Gynecology.* Married and divorced. EDUCATION: 1856, Elmira College (N.Y.); 1863, studied medicine with Rachel Gleason, Elmira Water Cure Institution and at New York Infirmary for Women and Children; 1868, M.D., Woman's Medical College of Pennsylvania; studied: 1873, New York Woman's Hospital; and 1882-83, Berlin and London. CAREER: 1868-1922, medical and gynecological practice, Grand Rapids; 1870, city physician, Grand Rapids; in Michigan State Medical Society: 1872, first woman member; and 1873, vice-president; 1877, second woman delegate, American Medical Association; visiting gynecologist and founder, nursing school, Union Benevolent Association Hospital, Grand Rapids; at *Medical Woman's Journal*: 1893, co-founder; and 1894-1901, associate editor. CON-TRIBUTIONS: Among the first group of women members and probably the first woman officer of a U.S. state medical society. First woman to hold office as a city physician in an American city.

WRITINGS: "New Force in Medicine and Surgery," *Med. Woman's J.* 1 (1893): 181-84; "Women Physicians in Michigan," Michigan State Med. Soc. *J.* 12 (1913): 480-85. REFERENCES: Albert Baxter, *History of Grand Rapids* (1890), 712-13; C. B. Burr, *Medical History of Michigan* 2 (1930): 370; *Grand Rapids Press*, May 25, 1922; *Med. Woman's J.* 54 (Nov. 1937): 41.

M. Pernick

S

SABIN, FLORENCE RENA (November 9, 1871, Central City, Colo.-October 3, 1953, Denver, Colo.). *Physician; Anatomist.* Daughter of George Kimball, mine superintendent, and Serena (Miner) Sabin. EDUCATION: Vermont Academy, Saxton River, Vt.; 1893, B.S., Smith College; 1900, M.D., Johns Hopkins Medical School; 1901, intern, Johns Hopkins Hospital. CAREER: At Johns Hopkins Medical School: 1902, researcher; and 1903, appointed to anatomy teaching staff and regularly promoted until 1917, when she became professor of histology; 1924, first woman elected president, American Association of Anatomists, and first female member, National Academy of Sciences; 1924, joined staff, Rockefeller Institute for Medical Research, New York City, as director of the Department of Cellular Studies; 1944, appointed chair, Interim Board of Health and Hospitals of Denver; 1948, president, American Public Health Association. CONTRIBUTIONS: Among numerous pioneering efforts, was the first woman to matriculate at and graduate from Johns Hopkins Medical School and the first woman in America to attain the rank of full professor in a medical college (1917). Research and papers were significant contributions to the limited knowledge about the origin and function of cells. Through her most important investigations, made major steps toward a better understanding of the nature of tuberculosis infection. Furthermore, civic work resulted in the passage of precedent-setting public health legislation in Colo. Although often referred to as the "little doctor," is much more accurately remembered as one of the most renowned medical scientists of her era.

WRITINGS: *An Atlas of the Medulla and the Brain* (1911); *The Origin and Development of the Lymphatic System* (1913); *Franklin Paine Mall: The Story of a Mind* (1934). REFERENCES: *BMNAS* 34 (1960): 271-369; Elinor Bluemel, *Florence Sabin: Colorado Woman of the Century* (1959); *DAB*, Supplement 5: 600-601; *DSB*, 12: 48-49; Florence Rena Sabin Papers, American Philosophical Society Library, Philadelphia, Pa.; *NCAB*, C: 288; 40: 12; *Notable Am. Women: The Modern Period* (1980); Mary K. Phelan, *Probing the Unknown* (1969); *Woman's Who's Who of Am., 1914-1915.*

F. B. Rogers

SACHS, BERNARD (January 2, 1858, Baltimore, Md.-February 8, 1944, New York, N.Y.). *Physician; Neurology.* Son of Joseph, schoolteacher, and

Sophia (Baer) Sachs. Married Bettina R. Stein, 1887; two children; Rosetta (Fechheimer) Kaskel, 1940. EDUCATION: 1878, A.B., Harvard University; 1882, M.D., University of Strassburg; 1882-84, studied medicine, Vienna, Austria, Paris, France, and London, England. CAREER: 1884-87, assistant to Isaac Adler, general practice of medicine, N.Y.; *post* 1887, established own practice, confined to mental and nervous diseases; 1885-1905, mental and nervous diseases faculty, New York Polyclinic Hospital, later, clinical neurology faculty, College of Physicians and Surgeons (Columbia); at Mount Sinai Hospital: 1893-1925, neurological staff; and 1920-23, president, medical board; 1904-20, alienist and neurologist, Bellevue Hospital; 1932-42, director, Division of Child Neurology Research Fund (Friedsam Foundation); president: 1894, 1932, American Neurological Association; and 1933-35, New York Academy of Medicine. CONTRIBUTIONS: Played a prominent role in the developing field of organic neurology. Described a new disease (1887) he called "amaurotic family idiocy," a genetically caused, arrested development of the brain that caused blindness and death in infants and young children. Since Warren Tay, a British ophthalmologist, had independently recorded the occular manifestations of the illness, it became known as Tay-Sachs disease. Had a special interest in the neurological disorders of children and published (1895) best known work, *Nervous Diseases of Children*, which was translated into Italian and German. Edited the *Journal of Nervous and Mental Disease* (1886-1911). Was instrumental in establishing international collaboration in neurology and helped organize the first International Neurological Congress, held in Bern, Switzerland (1931).

WRITINGS: "On Arrested Cerebral Development with Special Reference to Its Cortical Pathology," *J. of Nervous and Mental Disease* 14 (1887): 541-53; *Keeping Your Child Normal* (1926); *Nervous and Mental Disorders from Birth Through Adolescence* (1926, with Louis Hausman). A bibliography is in *Bernard Sachs, 1858-1914* (privately printed, 1949) and *J. of the Mount Sinai Hosp.* 9 (Dec. 1942): 262-70. REFERENCES: *DAB*, Supplement 3: 682-83; Miller, *BHM*, p. 100; *NCAB*, 34: 127; *Who Was Who in Am.*, 2: 465.

S. Galishoff

SALMON, DANIEL ELMER (July 23, 1850, Mt. Olive, N.J.-August 30, 1914, Butte, Mont.). *Veterinarian; Microbiology; Public health*. Son of Daniel Landon and Eleanor (Flock) Salmon. Married Mary Thompson Corning, 1872; Agnes Christina Dewhurst, 1904. EDUCATION: Cornell University: 1872, graduated; and 1876, D.V.M. CAREER: Practiced veterinary medicine: 1872-75, Newark, N.J.; and 1875, Asheville, N.C.; 1877, lecturer, veterinary medicine, University of Georgia; 1879, participated in N.Y. State campaign to eradicate pleuro-pneumonia of cattle; at United States Department of Agriculture: 1879-84, investigator; and 1884-1905, chief, Bureau of Animal Industry; 1906-12, director, National Veterinary School, Montevideo, Uruguay; 1912, manufactured veterinary biological products, United States; 1913, managed laboratory for the production of hog cholera serum, Butte; president: American Veterinary Medical Association (1898) and American Public Health Association. CONTRIBUTIONS: As chief of the Bureau of Animal

Industry, conducted and directed scientific investigations of animal diseases and their bearing upon the public health. Brought contagious pleuro-pneumonia and Texas fever, two serious diseases that had threatened the cattle industry, under near complete control. With Theobald Smith (q.v.), differentiated hog cholera from swine plague and found the bacillus responsible for each disease (1886-91); was later shown by others that the bacillus found in hog cholera is a secondary invader and that the disease has a viral origin. Performed one of the first experiments in immunization when he demonstrated that the injection of filtered products of the swine plague bacillus conferred immunity against the disease. Discovered a genus of bacteria most commonly associated with various types of food poisoning named after him, salmonella. Inaugurated a nationwide system of meat inspection, the quarantine of imported livestock, and the inspection of exported cattle and the ships carrying them.

WRITINGS: "The Bacterium of Swine Plague," *Am. Monthly Microscopical J.* 7 (Nov. 1886): 204-5; "On a New Method of Producing Immunity from Contagious Diseases,"*Proc. Biological Soc. of Washington* 3 (1886): 29-33 (with Theobald Smith); *Hog Cholera: Its History, Nature and Treatment* (1889, with T. Smith and F. L. Kilbourne). A list of publications is in C. W. Stiles (q.v.) and Albert Hassall, *Index-Catalogue of Medical and Veterinary Zoology*, 36 nos. (1902-12). REFERENCES: *DAB*, 16: 311-12; Kelly and Burrage (1920), 1015-16; *Who Was Who in Am.*, 1: 1074.

S. Galishoff

SANFORD, JOHN F. (April 13, 1824, Chillicothe, Ohio-1874, New York, N.Y.?). *Physician; Surgery.* EDUCATION: Studied with Dr. J. S. Prettyman; attended lectures: Medical College of Cincinnati; and 1847, Philadelphia College of Medicine (it is assumed that he received an M.D.). CAREER: 1841, began medical practice at age 17, Farmington, Ia.; 1846, elected to Ia. State Senate; 1848, professor of midwifery, Rock Island Medical School (Rock Island, Ill.); 1849, professor of surgery, College of Physicians and Surgeons of the Upper Mississippi (Davenport, Ia.); 1850-53, dean of the faculty and professor of surgery, College of Physicians and Surgeons (Keokuk, Ia.); 1850-54, editor, *Western Medico-Chirurgical Journal*; *post* 1853, lecturer, Iowa Medical School (preparatory); c. 1850-69, surgical practice, Keokuk; 1869-74, associated with a life insurance company, New York City. CONTRIBUTIONS: By all accounts, as able and excellent a teacher of medicine as could be found in the Upper Mississippi Valley. First dean, College of Physicians and Surgeons, after its move to Keokuk from Davenport until rivalry with John C. Hughes (q.v.) forced his resignation. As state senator, was instrumental in the declaration of the medical college, Keokuk, as the "medical department" of the state university (which designation it held until 1870), a degree from which automatically entitled the recipient to practice medicine in Ia. Co-founder, with S. G. Armor, and publisher of the first medical journal published west of the Mississippi and north of the Missouri. Largely responsible for the founding of the Iowa State Medical and Chirurgical Society and its first president (1850, Burlington, Ia.). REFERENCES: Walter L. Bierring, *A History of the Department of Internal Medicine, State University* *of Iowa College of Medicine 1870-1958* (1958), 13-14; Peter T. Harstad, "Health in the Upper Mississippi River Valley, 1820 to 1861" (Ph.D. diss., University of Wisconsin, 1963), chap. 10, "Medical Education"; *One Hundred Years of Iowa Medicine, 1850-1950* (1950), 110-11 (including John T. McClintock, "Medical Education in Iowa," pp. 224-309, and Charles L. Jones, "Medical Journalism in Iowa, 1850-1950," pp. 311-70).

R. E. Rakel

SANGER, MARGARET (HIGGINS) (September 14, 1879, Corning, N.Y.-September 6, 1966, Tucson, Ariz.). *Birth-control leader*. Daughter of Michael Hennessy, artist and maker of monuments, and Annie (Purcell) Higgins. Married William Sanger, 1900, three children; James Noah Henry Slee, 1922. EDUCA-TION: 1896-98, Claverack College (N.Y.); c. 1900, graduated, nurse's training school, White Plains Hospital (N.Y.); postgraduate study, Manhattan Eye and Ear Hospital; 1913-15, studied contraception methods used in Europe. CAREER: 1900-1912, housewife, Saranack (N.Y.) and New York City; 1912, did maternity nursing on Lower East Side of New York City; *post* 1912, spearheaded birth-control movement in United States and abroad; editor and publisher, *The Woman Rebel* (1914) and *Birth Control Review* (1917-28). CONTRIBUTIONS: Helped found and led the birth-control movement in the United States. Propounded the idea that control of conception was a basic human right. Coined the term "birth-control" and won support for the movement through writings, lecture tours, and organizational activities. Indicted (1915) for disseminating contraceptive information through the mails in defiance of the Comstock Law; action aroused public sympathy for her, and the case was dropped. Opened the first American birth-control clinic in Brownsville, (Brooklyn) (1916). Was arrested and convicted but won decision permitting physicians to give contraceptive advice for the "cure and prevention of disease"; liberal court interpretation of this phrase resulted in de facto repeals of most restrictions on the control of contraception. Organized (1921) the American Birth Control League (later Planned Parenthood Federation of America) and served as its first president (until 1928). Organized the first International Birth Control Conference (1927, Geneva). Spurred the creation of birth-control movements in India and elsewhere in Asia and founded the International Planned Parenthood Federation (1952, Bombay). Channeled research funds into biochemical investigations of the control of fertility. Founded (1935) the science periodical *Journal of Contraception* (later *Human Fertility*).

WRITINGS: *The Case for Birth Control* (1917); *Woman and the New Race* (1920); *The Pivot of Civilization* (1922); *My Fight for Birth Control* (1931); *Margaret Sanger: An Autobiography* (1938). REFERENCES: *BHM* (1964-69), 233; (1970-74), 154; *Current Biog.* (1944), 585-89; L. Leder and M. Meltzer, *M. Sanger. . .*(1969); *NCAB*, 52: 325-26; *N.Y. Times*, September 7, 1966; *Who Was Who in Am.*, 4: 828.

S. Galishoff

SAUGRAIN DE VIGNI, ANTOINE FRANCOIS (February 17, 1763, Paris, France-May 18, or 19, 1820, St. Louis, Mo.). *Physician*. Son of Antoine Claude, bookseller, and Marie (Brunet) Saugrain. Married Genevieve Rosalie Michau, March 20, 1793; six children. EDUCATION: Trained by brother-in-law, Dr. J. N. Guillotin; practiced surgery, Hotel-Dieu, Paris; 1783, admitted to practice of surgery, New Orleans, La. CAREER: First went to America at age 19; 1783-86, private practice, New Orleans; 1787-89, mineralogical work and medical practice, Ohio Valley; 1790-97, farmed and manufactured scientific supplies and medicines and inoculated for smallpox, Gallipolis, Ohio; 1797-99, manufactured shot and vinegar, Lexington, Ky.; 1799-1820, practiced medicine and manufactured and sold drugs, thermometers, barometers, and phosphorous matches, St. Louis, Mo. CONTRIBUTIONS: First nonmilitary physician to locate permanently in the St. Louis area and the only physician from 1800 to 1807. Introduced Jenner's cowpox vaccination technique west of the Mississippi (1809). REFERENCES: *DAB*, 16: 377-78; N. P. Dandridge, M.D., "Antoine Francois Saugrain (de Vigni)," presidential address, American Surgical Association, St. Louis, 1904 (pamphlet, Missouri Historical Society); Samuel E. Dicks, "Antoine Saugrain (1763-1820): A French Scientist on the American Frontier," *Emporia State Research Studies* 25 (1976): 5-27.

M. Hunt and
D. R. Sneddeker

SAYRE, LEWIS ALBERT (February 29, 1820, Bottle Hill, N.J.-September 21, 1900, New York, N.Y.). *Physician; Orthopedic surgeon.* Son of Archibald, farmer, and Martha (Sayer) Sayre. Married Eliza Ann Hall, 1849; four children. EDUCATION: Wantage Seminary, Deckertown, N.J.; 1839, A.B., Transylvania University; apprentice to Dr. David Green (New York City); 1842, M.D., College of Physicians and Surgeons. CAREER: 1842-52, prosector to Dr. Willard Parker (q.v.), College of Physicians and Surgeons; 1861-98, medical faculty, Bellevue Medical College; 1845-61, surgeon-general, New York Militia; 1860-66, resident physician, New York City; 1880, president, American Medical Association; medical staff, Bellevue, Charity, and St. Elizabeth's hospitals. CONTRIBUTIONS: Chief organizer, Bellevue Hospital Medical College. Occupied the first chair of orthopedic surgery in the United States and is called the father of American orthopedic surgery. Performed resection of the hip for morbus coxarius (1854), developed the Sayre method of treatment of lateral curvature, and invented numerous orthopedic instruments and devices. Improved sanitary conditions in tenements, advocated compulsory vaccination, and established quarantine regulations for the port of N.Y. to prevent the spread of cholera and other communicable diseases. Urged the AMA to publish its own journal, which resulted in the publication of the *JAMA* (1882).

WRITINGS: *Report on Morbus Coxarius* (1860); *A Practical Manual on the Treatment of Club Foot* (1869); *Lectures on Orthopedic Surgery and Diseases of the Joints* (1876); *Spinal Diseases and Spinal Curvature* (1877). REFERENCES: Theodore M. Banta, *Sayre Family* (1901), 633-36; *BHM* (1964-69), 234; *Boston Med. and Surg. J.* 143 (1900): 331; *DAB*, 8: 403-4; *N.Y. Times*, September 22, 1900; Alfred R. Shands, "Lewis Albert

Sayre, The First Professor of Orthopaedic Surgery in the United States (1820-1900),''
Current Practice in Orthopaedic Surg. 4 (1969): 22-42.

D. O. Powell

SCAMMON, RICHARD EVERINGHAM (July 9, 1883, Kansas City, Mo.-
September 15, 1952). *Anatomist; Embryologist.* Son of James and Laura (Everingham) Scammon. Married Julia Sims, 1913; two children. EDUCATION: University of Kansas: 1904, B.A.; 1906, M.A.; and 1909, Ph.D. in medical science,
Harvard University. CAREER: Taught at University of Kansas and Harvard, before
going to Minn. in 1914; 1914-30, professor of anatomy, University of Minnesota;
1931-35, dean of medical sciences; *post* 1935, distinguished service professor,
graduate school. CONTRIBUTIONS: Outstanding teacher of anatomy and embryology. Main interest was in the growth of man.

WRITINGS: Section about anatomy of the child in Isaac Abt's (q.v.) *System of Pediatrics*
(1923); *Growth of the Fetal Period* (1929, with L. A. Calkins); numerous papers about
growth and physical development of children; editor, *Am. J. of Physical Anthropology*.
REFERENCES: *Anat. Record* 116 (1953): 259-62; *Who Was Who in Am.*, 7: 504.

R. Rosenthal

SCHAMBERG, JAY FRANK (November 6, 1870, Philadelphia, Pa.-March
30, 1934, Philadelphia). *Physician; Dermatology.* Son of Gustav and Emma
(Frank) Schamberg. Married May Ida Bamberger, 1905; two children. EDU-
CATION: University of Pennsylvania: 1892, M.D.; and 1892-93, intern; 1893-
94, studied dermatology, Vienna, Paris, Berlin, Hamburg, and London. CAREER:
Post 1894, practiced medicine, Philadelphia; at University of Pennsylvania: c.
1895-1900, lecturer on infectious eruptive fevers; and 1919-34, dermatology and
syphilology faculty; 1900-18, dermatology faculty, Philadelphia Polyclinic College for Graduates in Medicine (later Pennsylvania University); dermatology and
syphilology faculty: 1910-18, Temple University; and 1918-20, Jefferson Medical College; 1912, member, Pennsylvania Vaccination Commission; 1912-20,
director, Dermatological Research Laboratories, Philadelphia Polyclinic College
for Graduates in Medicine; 1920-34, director and president, Board of Trustees,
Research Institute of Cutaneous Medicine (Philadelphia); 1925-34, special consultant in venereal diseases, U.S. Public Health Service; 1920-21, president,
American Dermatological Association. CONTRIBUTIONS: Conducted and organized research on skin diseases and syphilis. Described a progressive pigmentary
skin disease (1901) since known as Schamberg's disease. With Joseph Goldberger (q.v.), found that ''grain itch'' was caused by a small mite found in the
straw of mattresses (1909). During World War I, with John A. Kolmer and
George Raiziss, produced the first salvarsan and neosalvarsan (arsenical compounds used in the treatment of syphilis) made outside of Germany, the availability of which had been curtailed by the war; used profits from sales to endow
the Research Institute of Cutaneous Medicine, which became affiliated with
Temple University (1949) as the Institute of Public Health and Preventive Medicine; success in synthesizing these arsenical compounds provided impetus to

the development of the American pharmaceutical industry. Made important studies of psoriasis. Served on the editorial board, *Archives of Dermatology and Syphilology* (1927-34). Published several well-regarded books in his fields.

WRITINGS: *Compendium of Diseases of the Skin* (1898); *Acute Contagious Diseases* (1905, with William H. Welch [q.v.]); *Acute Infectious Diseases* (1928, with John A. Kolmer); *Treatment of Syphilis* (1932, with Carroll S. Wright). REFERENCES: *BHM* (1964-69), 234; *DAB*, 16: 418-19; Miller, *BHM*, p. 101; *NCAB*, 30: 290-91; Louis Pelner, "Jay Frank Schamberg, M.D. (1870-1934); Medical Scholar and Founder of the Independent American Pharmaceutical Industry," *Med. Times*, 97 (Dec. 1969): 95-100.

S. Galishoff

SCHICK, BELA (July 16, 1877, Boglar, Hungary-December 6, 1967, New York, N.Y.). *Physician; Pediatrics.* Son of Jacob, grain merchant, and Johanna (Pichler) Schick. Married Catherine C. Fries, 1925; no children. EDUCATION: Staats Gymnasium, Graz, Austria; 1900, M.D., Karl Franz University, Graz. CAREER: 1900-1901, captain, medical corps, Austro-Hungarian army; 1902, followed teacher Theodor Escherich to Vienna and began medical practice and research on infectious disease; at University of Vienna: 1911-18, privatdozent; and 1918-23, extraordinary professor; 1923-42, director of pediatrics, Mt. Sinai Hospital, N.Y.; 1928-42, clinical faculty, Columbia University College of Physicians and Surgeons; 1950-67, pediatrician-in-chief, Beth-El Hospital, Brooklyn, N.Y.; affiliated with several other N.Y. medical institutions; remained active until his death at age 90. CONTRIBUTIONS: In Vienna, and later as unofficial dean of American pediatricians, promoted all aspects of child welfare. Pioneered the study of immunologic and allergic phenomena; with Clemens von Pirquet, first described serum sickness and established the concept of allergy (1905). Contributed to the understanding of the pathogenesis of tuberculosis, scarlet fever, and diphtheria; advanced the study of newborn and childhood nutrition and hyperalimentation; devised the Schick test for determining susceptibility to diphtheria (1913) and subsequently played a key role in New York City's diphtheria eradication program (1920s-30s).

WRITINGS: *Serumkrankheit* (1905, with C. von Pirquet); *Scarlach* (1912, with Theodor Escherich); "Diphtheriehautreaktion als Vorprobe d. Prophylakt. Diphtherieseruminjektion," *Münch med Wchnschr* 60 (1913): 2608; *Child Care Today* (1934, with W. Rosenson). Writings listed in Antoni Gronowicz, *Bela Schick and the World of Children* (1954). REFERENCES: *BHM* (1964-69), 235; (1970-74), 155; Jerome Glaser, "Pediatric Allergy as a Specialty (Bela Schick)," *Annals of Allerg.* 30 (1972): 1-10; Gronowicz, *Schick*; Miller, *BHM*, p. 101; *NCAB*, 53: 425; E: 444; Murray M. Peshkin, "Bela Schick, Scientist, Humanitarian, Friend," *Annals of Allerg.* 26 (1968): 625-36; I. J. Wolf, *Aphorisms and Facetiae of Bela Schick* (1965).

L. P. Rubin

SCHLOSS, OSCAR MENDERSON (June 20, 1882, Cincinnati, Ohio-October 13, 1952, Southold, N.Y.). *Physician; Pediatrics.* Son of Hugo and Aurelia (Menderson) Schloss. Married Rowena Farmer, October 2, 1912; one child. EDUCATION: 1901, S.B., Alabama Polytechnic Institute (Auburn, Ala.); 1905,

M.D., Johns Hopkins University; 1905-7, house officer, King's County Hospital, Brooklyn, N.Y.; 1907-8, New York Nursery and Children's Hospital. CAREER: 1908-18, pediatric practice and teaching, Bellevue Medical College and Babies Hospital, Columbia University; and with Dr. L. Emmett Holt (q.v.), visiting physician, Willard Parker Hospital and New York Nursery and Child's Hospital; 1918-21, professor of pediatrics, Cornell Medical College; and physician-in-chief, New York Nursery and Children's Hospital; 1921-23, professor of pediatrics, Harvard Medical School; and physician-in-chief, Infants' and Children's Hospital, Boston, Mass.; 1923-33, professor of pediatrics, Cornell Medical School; and pediatrician-in-chief, New York Hospital; 1933-52, clinical professor of pediatrics, Cornell Medical College. CONTRIBUTIONS: Helped establish the study of pediatric allergy in America (1912-36). Major contributor to our understanding of the physiologic imbalance in infants with diarrheal diseases (1917-20).

WRITINGS: "A Case of Allergy to Common Foods," *Am. J. of Diseases of Children* 3 (1912): 361; "The Occurrence of Acidosis with Severe Diarrhea," ibid., 13 (1917): 218 (with R. Stetson); "Intestinal Intoxication in Infants: The Importance of Impaired Renal Function," ibid., 15 (1918): 165. REFERENCES: Harry H. Gordon, "Oscar Menderson Schloss," *Pediatric Profiles* (1957); L. Emmett Holt, Jr., "Oscar Menderson Schloss," *Arch. of Ped.* 70 (1953): 151.

T. E. Cone, Jr.

SCHUYLER, LOUISA LEE (October 26, 1837, New York, N.Y.-October 10, 1926, Highland Falls, N.Y.). *Leader in welfare work.* Daughter of George Lee Schuyler, engineer and lawyer, and Eliza (Hamilton) Schuyler. Never married. EDUCATION: Privately tutored; no formal training. CAREER: 186?, chair, Committee of Correspondence, Woman's Central Association of Relief (most important auxiliary of the U.S. Sanitary Commission during the Civil War); 1863, established a network of tributary county and village societies; 1872, formed the State Charities Aid Association, an organization of citizen groups that regularly visited public charitable institutions; 1873, helped establish a training school for nurses, Bellevue Hospital; 1884, began a massive publicity and lobbying campaign that resulted in an 1890 law turning the care of the mentally ill over to state institutions; 1907, appointed a charter trustee, Russell Sage Foundation; 1915, founded the National Committee for the Prevention of Blindness. CONTRIBUTIONS: Devoted life to founding philanthropic institutions. Active leadership role in charitable work became a model for wealthy women of her generation.

WRITINGS: *Forty-Three Years Ago*, a pamphlet published by the State Charities Aid Association (1915). REFERENCES: *NCAB*, 20: 19; *Notable Am. Women, 1607-1950*, 3: 244-46; Francis G. Peabody, *Reminiscences of Present-Day Saints*; *Louisa Lee Schuyler* (1927).

V. Drachman

SCHWEINITZ, GEORGE EDMUND de. See deSchweinitz, George Edmund

SCHWYZER, ARNOLD (May 23, 1864, Zurich, Switzerland-February 19, 1944). *Surgeon*. Son of A., businessman and officer, Swiss Army, and Katherine (Iten) Schwyzer. Married Johanna Henggeler, 1899, no children; Marguerite Mueller, 1906, three children. EDUCATION: High school, Zurich; studied basic medical science, Geneva; three years of clinical medicine, Zurich University; 1888, M.D., Zurich. CAREER: Swiss Army surgeon and then assistant, County Hospital, Glarus, Switzerland; 1891, went to United States; 1894, practice, St. Paul, Minn.; at Hamline University: 1897-1902, professor of pathology; and 1904-8, professor of clinical surgery; pathologist, City and County Hospital, St. Paul; 1927, became professor and lecturer on surgery, University of Minnesota. CONTRIBUTIONS: Did first resection of the entire transverse colon with partial resection of the pancreas and the large curvature of the stomach (1898). Introduced first set of broncho-esophogoscopes and did first removal of a foreign body from a lung (1903). Did early appendectomies and mastoidectomies. Apparently did first successful ligation (in America) of an aneurism of the innominate artery. Did early saline infusions to replace severe loss of blood. Developed a new pyeloureteral plastic for hydronephrosis (1923). Did first cystoscopy in Minn. Developed a surgical technique for the kinking of the ureter at the renal pelvis. REFERENCES: *NCAB*, 34: 411; *Who Was Who in Am.*, 2: 474.

R. Rosenthal

SCOTT, ARTHUR CARROLL (July 12, 1865, Gainsville, Tex.-October 27, 1940, Temple, Tex.). *Surgeon*. Son of Rufus F. and Martha Helen (Moran) Scott. Married Maud Sherwood, October 30, 1899; three children. EDUCATION: Apprentice to Dr. A. H. Cousan, Gainsville, Tex.; 1886, M.D., Bellevue Hospital Medical College; 1886-88, intern and resident surgeon, Western Pennsylvania Hospital, Pittsburgh, Pa. CAREER: 1888-92, practice, Gainsville; local surgeon, Santa Fe Railroad; 1892-1940, practice, Temple, and chief surgeon, Santa Fe Railroad; 1898-1904, with associate Raleigh R. White, King's Daughters Hospital, until White's death; 1904-40, senior surgeon and president, Scott and White Clinic; 1923-24, president, Texas State Medical Association; 1926-40, chairman, Texas State Medical Association Council on Scientific Work; 1927-33, Board of Governors, American College of Surgeons; 1913-25, chairman, Texas Committee of the American Society for the Control of Cancer. CONTRIBUTIONS: Founder, Scott and White Clinic, in Temple, on the Mayo model. Authority on the diagnosis and surgical treatment of cancer. Worked for penal reforms.

WRITINGS: More than 23 scientific articles. REFERENCES: *Handbook of Texas* 2 (1952): 581-82; Dayton Kelly, *With Scalpel and Scope: History of Scott and White* (1970); *NCAB*, 34: 398; Scott and White Library and archives, Temple, Tex. Articles listed in *Texas State J. of Med.* 36 (Dec. 1940): 588-90.

J. P. Morris

SCOTT, JAMES ROBERT (April 29, 1886, Hamden, N.Y.-September 14, 1956, Santa Fe, N.Mex.). *Pathologist; Public health officer*. Son of John Thompson and Ella (Fraser) Scott. Married Alice E. Simpson, 1912; two children. EDUCATION: 1908, undergraduate degree, University of California; 1912, M.D.,

Cooper Medical College (now Stanford University); 1916, Ph.D., George Washington University. CAREER: 1912-18, anatomist and microscopist, Army Medical Museum, Washington, D.C.; pathologist: 1918-19, Los Angeles County Hospital, Calif.; and 1919-20, Baker Clinic, Baker City, Oreg.; 1920-22, associate professor of pathology and bacteriology, University of South Dakota; 1922-23, pathologist, St. Joseph's Hospital, Albuquerque, N.Mex.; 1923-26, 1928-33, Bernalillo County health officer; 1935-36, District III health officer; at University of New Mexico: 1928-32, part time associate professor of health education; and 1932-40, professor of health; 1940-53, director, State Department of Public Health; 1953-56, district health officer, District IV; 1953, retired due to ill health. CONTRIBUTIONS: As scholar and teacher, as well as public health administrative officer, helped form the U.S.-Mexican Border Public Health Association, which he served as president. Sensed the need for the private citizen to become more independent and saw to it that nutrition programs emphasized better use of locally grown foods such as pinto beans. In pre-World War II, inaugurated home nursing classes to anticipate problems created by fewer doctors in the area. Directed the Santa Fe Child Guidance Center (1949-52), an agency of the State Department of Public Health. Supported dentists in their plans to induce the legislature to create a dental division within the State Department of Public Health, which reached fruition in 1953.

WRITINGS: Was writing a book when he died; completed by Myrtle Greenfield and titled *A History of Public Health in New Mexico* (1962). Several publications concerning phases of public health and disease control. REFERENCES: Myrtle Greenfield, *A History of Public Health in New Mexico* (1962); Interview with Daniel Johnson, Ph.D., formerly of the New Mexico Dept. of Public Health.

C. L. Cutter

SCUDDER, JOHN MILTON (September 8, 1829, Harrison (Hamilton County), Ohio-February 17, 1894, Daytona, Fla.). *Physician (eclectic); Educator*. Son of John, cabinet maker, and Matilda (Marvin) Scudder. Married Jane Hannah, 1849, five children; Mary Hannah James, 1861, five children. EDUCATION: Entered Miami College at age 12; apprenticeship with Dr. Milton L. Thomas; 1856, M.D., (Cincinnati) Eclectic Medical Institute. CAREER: At (Cincinnati) Eclectic Medical Institute: 1856-58, professor of general, special, and pathological anatomy; 1858-60, chair, obstetric diseases of women and children; 1860-87, chair, principles and practices of medicine; 1887-94, continued to lecture in hygiene, physical diagnosis, and specific diagnosis; *post* 1862, dean, treasurer, and president; 1856-62, maintained a very successful practice, until he closed practice to devote entire time to the college; 1868-94, editor, *Eclectic Medical Journal*. CONTRIBUTIONS: Foremost eclectic physician of his time. Organizational abilities enabled the Cincinnati Eclectic Medical Institute to become the strongest eclectic college west of the Alleghenies. Developed the theory of specific diagnosis, specific medication, and specific medicines.

WRITINGS: *Eclectic Practice of Medicine* (1864); *Principles of Medicine* (1867); *Specific Medication* (1871); *Specific Diagnosis* (1874); *A Practical Treatise on the Diseases*

of Women (1858); *Materia Medica and Therapeutics* (1860, with L. E. Jones). REFER-
ENCES: *DAB*, 8, pt. 2: 524; Harvey Wickes Felter, *Biographies of John King, M.D.,
Andrew Jackson Howe, A.B., M.D., and John Milton Scudder, M.D.* (1912); Miller,
BHM, p. 102; *NCAB*, 28: 419; Cecil Striker, ed., *Medical Portraits* (1963).

G. P. *Jenkins*

SEAMAN, VALENTINE (April 2, 1770, North Hempstead, N.Y.-July 3,
1817, New York, N.Y.). *Physician; Surgeon.* Son of Willet, merchant, and
Martha (Valentine) Seaman. Married Anne Ferris, 1794; nine children. EDU-
CATION: Apprentice to Dr. Nicholas Romayne (q.v.); resident physician, New
York City Almshouse; 1792, M.D., University of Pennsylvania Medical School.
CAREER: 1792-1817, private practice, New York City; 1796-1817, medical staff,
New York Hospital; 1811-16, medical faculty, Medical Institution of the State
of New York, Queens College. CONTRIBUTIONS: Argued that yellow fever was
not contagious. Introduced vaccination for smallpox in New York City (1800).
Delivered systematic lectures to midwives (1799) and the first clinical lectures
on surgery, New York Hospital (1811). Published the first book on midwifery
in the United States (1800).

WRITINGS: *An Account of Epidemic Yellow Fever. . .1795* (1796); *The Midwives
Moniter, and Mothers Mirror. . .*(1800); *An Account of the Introduction of Vaccination
or Kine-Pock Inoculation in New York* (1802). REFERENCES: Kelly and Burrage (1928),
1088; James M. Phalen, "Dr. Valentine Seaman: Pioneer Surgical Case Report," *Mil.
Surg.* 86 (1940): 594-95; Mary T. Seaman, *The Seaman Family* (?), 127-28; Glenn
Sonnedecker, "Earliest Formulary for a Civilian Hospital, U.S.A. Seaman's *Pharma-
coepia Chirurgica* of 1811," *Drug Intelligence and Clinical Pharmacy* 6 (1972): 425-
34; Stephen W. Williams, *Am. Med. Biog.* (1845), 509-12.

D. O. *Powell*

SEDGWICK, WILLIAM THOMPSON (December 29, 1855, West Hartford, Conn.-January 26, 1921, Boston, Mass.). *Biologist; Educator; Epidemiology; Sanitary engineering.* Son of William and Anne Louise (Thompson)
Sedgwick. Married Mary Katrine Rice, 1881; no children. EDUCATION: 1877,
Ph.B., Sheffield Scientific School (Yale); 1881, Ph.D., Johns Hopkins University. CAREER: 1879-83, physiological chemistry faculty, Johns Hopkins University; 1883-1921, biology faculty (*post* 1911, biology and public health),
Massachusetts Institute of Technology; 1888-1921, consulting biologist, Massachusetts State Board of Health; *post* 1902, member, advisory board, Hygienic
Laboratory, U.S. Public Health Service; 1913-22, chairman, administrative board,
Harvard-Massachusetts Institute of Technology School for Health Officers; member, International Health Board, Rockefeller Foundation; president: 1900, Society of American Bacteriologists; and 1914-15, American Public Health
Association. CONTRIBUTIONS: Helped establish the profession of sanitary engineering in the United States and pioneered in the application of bacteriology to
sanitary science. Using the facilities of the Lawrence Experiment Station (Massachusetts State Board of Health), made important studies of sewage disposal.
With Hiram F. Mills (q.v.), demonstrated that a severe typhoid epidemic that

swept the Merrimac valley (1890) was caused by pollution of the Merrimac River, from which the cities along its banks obtained their water supply; published findings in influential book *Principles of Sanitary Science and the Public Health* (1902). Demonstrated how chlorine could be used to disinfect water and sewage. Developed one of the first courses in sanitation and public health and trained many of the leading public health workers of his time. Took an active role in the founding and early development of the Harvard-Massachusetts Institute of Technology School for Health Officers, the nation's first school of public health.

WRITINGS: *General Biology* (1886, with E. B. Wilson); *A Report of the Biological Work of the Lawrence Experiment Station. Experimental Investigation by the State Board of Health of Massachusetts upon Sewage, etc.* (1890); *The Human Mechanism: Its Physiology and Hygiene and the Sanitation of its Surroundings* (1906, with Theodore Hough). A bibliography is in E. O. Jordan, G. C. Whipple, and C.-E.A. Winslow, *A Pioneer of Public Health, William Thompson Sedgwick* (1924). REFERENCES: *DAB*, 16: 552-53; Miller, *BHM*, p. 102; *NCAB*, 13: 290-91; *Who Was Who in Am.*, 1:1101.

S. Galishoff

SEGUIN, EDOUARD (January 20, 1812, Clamecy, France-October 28, 1880, New York, N.Y.). *Psychiatrist; Neurologist; Special education.* Son of T.O. Seguin. Married ?, one child; married Elsie M. Mead, 1880; no children. EDUCATION: College of Auxerre; Lycee St. Louis, Paris; Parisian medical schools; 1861, M.D., University of the City of New York. CAREER: c. 1830-1840, worked with Dr. Esquirol on problems of idiot children, Paris; 1839-50?, founded and conducted a school for idiots in France; 1850, emigrated to the United States; 1851-54, general medical practice, Cleveland, Ohio; 1854-57, taught at New York State School for Idiots (Syracuse), and traveled around the country helping establish similar schools; 1857-60, returned to France; 1860-63, medical practice, Mt. Vernon, New York; 1863-80, practiced at Randall's Island (New York City) idiot asylum, and operated Seguin Physiologic School (Orange, N.J.). CONTRIBUTIONS: Developed theory that idiocy was not result of deficiency or malformation of brain, but rather an arrest of mental development before or at birth, which could, with training, be at least partially overcome. Technique involved physiological training of the senses. Ideas were studied by the French Academy of Sciences and disseminated worldwide through his book receiving instant acceptance and adoption. Schools for idiots were established in many countries, based on Seguin's system of education. Aided in establishment of several schools for idiots in America after his arrival. Taught his method of training idiots to many students, and educated many children labeled mentally defective. Helped popularize the clinical thermometer in America through several publications (1870s).

WRITINGS: *Traitement Moral, Hygiène et Éducation des Idiots* (1846); *Idiocy and Its Treatment by the Physiological Method* (1866); many articles on his physiological method and on clinical thermometry. Writings listed in *NCAB*, 15: 151-52; *Annals of Medical History* 6 (1924): 478-79. REFERENCES: *NCAB*, 15: 151-52; *DAB*, 16: 559-60; *Appleton's*

CAB, 2: 454; Kelly and Burrage (1928), 1089-90; I. Kraft, "Edouard Seguin and 19th Century Moral Treatment of Idiots," *Bulletin Hist. Med.*, 35 (1961): 393-418.

T. L. Savitt

SEGUIN, EDWARD CONSTANT (1843, Paris, France-February 19, 1898). *Neurologist.* Son of Edouard Seguin (physician) (q.v.). Married Margaret Amidon; three children; married a second time. EDUCATION: 1864, M.D., College of Physicians and Surgeons, New York; 1865-67, intern, New York Hospital; 1869-70, studied neurology with Brown-Sequard, Charcot, and Ranvier, Paris. CAREER: 1862-65, medical cadet, then acting assistant surgeon, Union army; 1867-69, post surgeon at forts Craig and Selden, New Mexico; 1869-84, taught diseases of the nervous system at College of Physicians and Surgeons, New York; 1870-94, neurology practice, New York, N.Y. CONTRIBUTIONS: Helped popularize thermometer through publication of first fever chart in pioneer article on medical thermometry (1866). Studies and papers on aphasia, infantile paralysis, and especially on localization of brain lesions, stimulated the study of neurology in America. With Silas Weir Mitchell and William A. Hammond, one of the leading neurologists in the United States. Edited *American Clinical Lectures* (1876-78), and *Archives of Medicine* (1879-84). A founder, American Neurological Association and New York Neurological Society.

WRITINGS: Collected all his writings into *Opera Minora* (1884); "The use of the Thermometer in Clinical Medicine," *Chicago Med. Journal* (May 1866). REFERENCES: *DAB*, 16: 560-61; Kelly and Burrage (1928), 1088-89; *Who Was Who in Am.*, Hist. Vol.: 473.

T. L. Savitt

SELLARDS, ANDREW WATSON (1884, Scranton, Kans.-December 1, 1942). *Physician; Microbiology.* Never married. EDUCATION: University of Kansas: 1903, A.B.; and 1904, M.A.; 1909, M.D., Johns Hopkins Medical School. CAREER: 1909-11, worked in the Philippines as an instructor, Philippine General Hospital, and as an assistant, Bureau of Science, Manila; 1911-14, medicine faculty, Johns Hopkins Medical School; and medical staff, Johns Hopkins Hospital; 1914-42, tropical medicine faculty, Harvard University; 1917-18, Medical Corps, U.S. Army; during and after World War I, member, American Red Cross committee on typhus; 1926-27, studied yellow fever in Brazil and Africa under the auspices of the Rockefeller Foundation. CONTRIBUTIONS: Demonstrated that the early administration of alkalies prevented death from uremia in cases of Asiatic cholera (1909-11). Showed that the symptoms of uremia, whether occurring in Asiatic cholera or in chronic renal disease, were not caused by the presence of a toxin, as was commonly believed then, but by a deficiency of alkali in the blood. With E. L. Walker, determined the incubation period of amoebic dysentery and demonstrated that *E. histolytica* was almost always the cause; further showed that it survived outside the body in cysts in the stool of patients and carriers (1913, 1923). Helped prove that Weil's disease and yellow fever were separate entitites. Isolated a virus strain from a case of yellow fever

(1927) and developed a technique for preserving its virulence for at least 12 days by freezing; subsequently attenuated the virus by passage from brain to brain of mice until it no longer caused yellow fever in monkeys, at which time he injected his mouse brain virus into man and showed that it conferred immunity (1931); helped prepare the way for Max Theiler's (q.v.) development of a safe and effective yellow-fever vaccine.

WRITINGS: "Indications of Acid Intoxication in Asiatic Cholera," *Philippine J. of Sci.* 6 (1911): 53 (with A. O. Shaklee); "The Determination of the Equilibrium in the Human Body between Acids and Bases with Especial Reference to Acidosis and Nephropathies," *Johns Hopkins Hosp. Bull.* 23 (1912): 289; Experimental and Amoebic Dysentery," *Philippine J. of Sci.* 8 (1913): 253; "A Clinical Method for Studying Titratable Alkalinity of the Blood and Its Application to Acidosis," *Johns Hopkins Hosp. Bull.* 25 (1914): 101; "The Behavior of the Virus of Yellow Fever in Monkeys and Mice," *Proc., Nat. Acad. of Sci.* 17 (1931): 339. REFERENCES: A. McGehee Harvey, *Research and Discovery in Medicine; Contributions from Johns Hopkins* (1981), 306-16.

S. Galishoff

SENN, NICHOLAS (October 31, 1844, Buchs, Switzerland-January 2, 1908, Chicago, Ill.). *Surgeon; Teacher; Military surgery.* Son of John and Magdelena Senn. Married Amelia S. Muehlhauser, 1869; two children. EDUCATION: 1864, Fond du Lac (Wis.) High School; 1864-66, apprentice to Dr. Emanuel Munk, Fond du Lac; 1868, M.D., Chicago Medical College; 1868-69, intern, Cook County Hospital; 1878, M.D., University of Munich; 1887, Ph.D., University of Wisconsin. CAREER: Practiced medicine: 1869-74, Elmore, Wis.; 1874-91, Milwaukee, Wis.; and 1893-1908, Chicago, Ill.; 1884-88, surgery, College of Physicians and Surgeons, Chicago; 1890-1908, surgery and pathology, Rush Medical College; surgeon-general: 1882-91, National Guard of Wis.; and 1893-1908, National Guard of Ill.; 1898, served in Cuba during Spanish-American War. CONTRIBUTIONS: Did pioneer experimental and clinical work in abdominal surgery, surgical management of tuberculosis, and plastic surgery. Promoted use of antiseptic methods and clinical microscopy. Developed use of rectal insufflation of hydrogen to diagnose visceral injury (1888). One of first to investigate gastrointestinal anastomosis experimentally (1893). Did major experimental and clinical surgery on the pancreas (1886). Proponent of conservative surgical treatment for gunshot wounds. Opposed traction in treatment of inflamed joints (1878). Developed widely used operative procedures for fractures of the neck of the femur (1883). Improved military surgery and medicine by work with National Guards of Wis. and Ill., by founding (1891) and guiding of Association of Military Surgeons (of the National Guard) of the United States, by active service in the Spanish-American War, and by writings. Early used Roentgen rays in treatment of leukemia (1903). Collected one of the best private medical and surgical libraries in the United States (given to Newberry Library, later transferred to John Crerar Library).

WRITINGS: "Rectal Insufflation of Hydrogen Gas an Infallible Test in the Diagnosis of Visceral Injury of the Gastrointestinal Canal in Penetrating Wounds of the Abdomen," *JAMA* 10 (1888): 767-77; "Enterorrhaphy; Its History, Technique and Present Status,"

JAMA 21 (1893): 215-35; "The Surgery of the Pancreas, as Based Upon Experiments and Clinical Researches," *Trans., Am. Surg. Assoc.* 4 (1886): 99-232; *Experimental Surgery* (1889); *Intestinal Surgery* (1889); *Surgical Bacteriology* (1889; 2nd ed., 1891). Writings listed in Ella Maude Salmonsen, "Nicholas Senn, M.D., Ph.D., LL.D. (1844-1908). Master Surgeon, Pathologist, and Teacher. Biographical Sketch, with a Complete Bibliography of His Writings," *Bull. of the Soc. of Med. Hist., Chicago* 4 (1928-35): 268-94. REFERENCES: Arthur Dean Bevan, "Nicholas Senn's Work in Experimental Surgery and Surgical Pathology, and Its Influence on the Surgery of His Time," *Surg. Gyn. & Ob.* 61 (1935): 414-16; *BHM* (1975-79), 116; (1980), 37; *DAB*, 8, pt. 2: 584-85; Miller, *BHM*, p. 102; *NCAB*, 6: 371; *Q. Bull. Northwestern Univ. Med. School* 9 (1907-8): 360-73; Salmonsen, "Nicholas Senn," pp. 268-94; F. M. Sperry, comp., *A Group of Distinguished Physicians and Surgeons of Chicago* (1904), 15-31; Samuel Cecil Stanton, "Editorial Expression: Vale, Nicholas Senn," *Mil. Surg.* 22 (1908): 144-51.

W. K. Beatty

SEWALL, HENRY (May 25, 1855, Winchester, Va.-July 8, 1936, Denver, Colo.). *Physician; Physiologist.* Son of Thomas and Julia Elizabeth (Waters) Sewall. Married Isabel Josephine Vickers, 1887; no children. EDUCATION: 1876, B.S., Wesleyan University; 1879, Ph.D., Johns Hopkins University; 1889, M.D., University of Denver; 1879-80, studied in Europe with Willy Kühne, Carl Ludwig, and Michael Foster. CAREER: 1882-88, professor of physiology, University of Michigan; 1889, resident physician, Adirondack Cottage Sanitarium; 1890-1908, professor of physiology, University of Denver and Denver & Gross Medical College; 1911-20, professor of medicine, University of Colorado; 1891-93, assistant health commissioner, Denver; 1893-99, secretary, Colorado State Board of Health; president: 1915, American Climatological Association; 1916, Denver Medical Society; 1915-16, American Association of Physicians; 1924, Colorado Medical Society; and 1926, National Tuberculosis Association; 1917-36, editorial staff, *American Review of Tuberculosis.* CONTRIBUTIONS: Showed that a stimulus not of itself strong enough to cause a reaction nevertheless modifies the reaction to a succeeding stimulus (1879). Described sensory functions of the heart that affect changes in blood pressure, foreshadowing subsequent studies on the carotid sinus (1885). Demonstrated the immunization of an animal to a foreign protein and the principle of antitoxin production (injection of rattlesnake venom in pigeons, 1887). Described the form and staining characteristics of various strains of tubercle bacilli and experimented with tuberculo-proteins as sensitizing agents (1915-18). Contributed studies on climatological aspects of tuberculosis therapy, and a critique of artificial pneumothorax (1928). REFERENCES: *NCAB*, A: 199; 26: 323; Florence R. Sabin, "The Contributions of. . .Henry Sewall to Medicine," *Sci.* 86 (1937): 357-64; Gerald B. Webb and Desmond Powell, *Henry Sewall, Physiologist and Physician* (1946), contains bibliography of 150 items (pp. 175-86), by F. R. Sabin.

F. B. Rogers

SHADD, FURMAN JEREMIAH (October 24, 1852, Washington, D.C.-June 24, 1908, Washington, D.C.). *Physician; Medical education.* Son of Absalom, free black restauranteur, and Eliza Brockett Shadd. Married Alice Parke, 1882; three children. EDUCATION: Howard University: *post* 1867, preparatory course; 1875, A.B.; 1878, A.M.; and 1881, M.D. CAREER: At Howard University Normal Department: 1875-83, teacher; and 1878-81, principal; 1881-95, assistant surgeon and resident physician, Freedmen's Hospital; 1886-1908, faculty member, 1896-1908, secretary-treasurer, Howard University Medical School; taught various subjects during his career at Howard. CONTRIBUTIONS: Third black appointed to Howard's medical faculty; highly respected teacher and efficient secretary-treasurer of medical school. Rejection (1891) from the all-white Medical Society of the District of Columbia created reaction that, combined with other incidents, resulted in revival of the black Medico-Chirurgical Society of the District of Columbia (1895).

WRITINGS: Presented several papers (1898-1905) at regional conferences on black mortality and sanitary conditions. Writings listed in *JNMA* 72 (1980): 152. REFERENCES: Rayford W. Logan, *Howard University, 1867-1967* (1969), 94, 160, 165; Henry S. Robinson, "Furman Jeremiah Shadd, M.D., 1852-1908," *JNMA* 72 (1980): 151-53.

T. L. Savitt

SHAFFER, PHILIP ANDERSON (September 20, 1881, Martinsburg, W.Va.-December 4, 1960, St. Louis, Mo.). *Biochemistry*. Son of Joseph, businessman, and Hannah (Anderson) Shaffer. Married Nan Jefferson Evans, June 1904; three children. EDUCATION: 1900, B.A., University of West Virginia; 1904, Ph.D., Harvard University; 1900-1903, research biological chemist, McLean Hospital, Waverly, Mass. CAREER: 1904-10, instructor in chemical pathology, Loomis Laboratory, Cornell Medical College; 1910-46, professor and head, Department of Biological Chemistry, Washington University School of Medicine, St. Louis; at Washington University School of Medicine: 1915-19, 1937-46, dean; 1946-52, distinguished service professor of biological chemistry; and 1952-60, professor emeritus. CONTRIBUTIONS: Initial reputation came from his development, with Dr. Warren Coleman, of a high-calorie, high-protein diet for typhoid-fever patients to prevent weight loss during the illness. For most of the remainder of his career, dealt with questions related to diabetes. Developed methods for determining ketones, and with A. F. Hartmann (q.v.), developed a widely used test for blood sugar (1921). Was working independently on insulin when its discovery was announced, and his preparation of it for use in the pediatrics department led to a workable means of producing and purifying insulin on a large scale. Work also established that insulin was a protein. As dean, Washington University School of Medicine, was instrumental in introducing full-time clinical departments in his first term and resolved long-standing organizational conflicts between the medical school and its teaching hospitals in second term.

WRITINGS: "A Method for the Quantitative Determination of B-oxybutyric Acid in Urine," *J. Biol. Chem.* 5 (1908): 211-22; "Protein Metabolism in Typhoid Fever," *Arch. of Int. Med.* 4 (1909): 538-600 (with W. Coleman); "The Determination of Oxybutyric Acid," *J. Biol. Chem.* 16 (1913): 265-80 (with W. McKim Marriott); "The Iodometric Determination of Copper and Its Use in Sugar Analysis 1. Equilibria in the Reaction

Between Copper Sulphate and Potassium Iodine," *ibid.*, 45 (1921): 349-64 (with A. F. Hartmann); "On the Preparation of Insulin," *ibid.*, 60 (1924): 31-58 (with M. Somogyi and E. A. Doisy). Writings listed in *BMNAS*. REFERENCES: *BMNAS* 40 (1969): 321-36.

D. R. Sneddeker

SHAKESPEARE, EDWARD ORAM (May 19, 1846, Rosemont, Pa.-June 1, 1900, Philadelphia, Pa.). *Physician; Ophthalmalogy; Epidemiology.* Son of William McIntire and Catherine (Haman) Shakespeare. Married Mary Louise Baird, 1889; two children. EDUCATION: 1864, B.A., Dickinson College; 1869, M.D., University of Pennsylvania; 1883, 1885, 1891, studied bacteriology in Germany and Switzerland. CAREER: 1869-74, practiced medicine with Dr. Isaac Jurup, Dover, Del.; 1874-1900, practiced medicine, Philadelphia, specializing in ophthalmalogy; pathology staff and bacteriology and hygiene staff, Philadelphia Hospital; ophthalmic surgery faculty, University of Pennsylvania; chairman: 1881, committee to make pathological examination of the brain of Guiteau, the assassin of President Garfield; and 1888, committee to investigate hog cholera, U.S. secretary of agriculture; 1885, U.S. representative to Spain to investigate cholera; 1898, member, U.S. commission to investigate typhoid fever in American army camps during the war against Spain. CONTRIBUTIONS: Best known to his contemporaries for work in ophthalmalogy, is better remembered today for epidemiological investigations of typhoid fever. Invented an improved ophthalmoscope and ophthalmometer (1876). Was asked by the mayor, Philadelphia, to report upon an epidemic of typhoid fever, Plymouth, Pa. (1885), which, because of its severity and the town's previous immunity to the disease, was attracting nationwide attention. Confirmed the conclusion reached by a local investigator that the epidemic had been caused by the accidental contamination of the town's water supply by the excreta of a single typhoid fever victim; demonstrated that even the purest water supply could become dangerously contaminated upon occasion; incident speeded up research on methods of water treatment, which resulted in the development of the first successful sand filters eight years later. Member, Spanish-American War typhoid fever commission, which revealed the role of the human carrier and the common housefly in transmitting the disease.

WRITINGS: "Description of a New Ophthalmoscope and Ophthalmometer, Devised for Clinical Use and for Physiological and Therapeutic Investigation on Men and Animals," *Am. J. of Med. Sci.* 71 (1876): 45-61. A partial bibliography is in Irving A. Watson, *Physicians and Surgeons of Am.* (1896). REFERENCES: *JAMA* 34 (Jan.-Jun. 1900): 1504; Kelly and Burrage (1928), 1097; R. F. Stone, *Biog. of Eminent Am. Physicians and Surgeons* (1894), 462; Watson, *Physicians and Surgeons of Am.*, 163-64.

S. Galishoff

SHATTUCK, GEORGE CHEYNE (July 17, 1783, Templeton, Mass.-March 18, 1854, Boston, Mass.). *Physician.* Son of Dr. Benjamin and Mrs. Lucy (Barron) Shattuck. Married Eliza Cheever Davis, 1811, only one surviving child, Dr. George C. Shattuck, Jr. (q.v.); Amelia Bigelow, 1835. EDUCATION: 1803,

A.B., Dartmouth College, 1806, M.B., Dartmouth; studied at Harvard Medical School and the University of Pennsylvania; 1807, M.D., University of Pennsylvania. CAREER: 1807 to death, medical practice, Boston. CONTRIBUTIONS: One of the busiest and most successful physicians in Boston. Although not connected with any medical college, always had private students in his office and had a dissecting room in the back of his house. Known for philanthropy: charged as little in 1840 as he did in 1808, and an indigent Harvard or Andover student would receive a prescription for free medication and a note to a tailor to furnish the bearer with a suit "appropriate to his status." President, Massachusetts Medical Society (1836-40). Consulting physician, Boston. Donated money to Dartmouth for the College Observatory, gave Harvard more than $26,000, and established the Shattuck Professorship of Pathological Anatomy, Harvard Medical School. A co-founder, *New England Journal of Medicine and Surgery* and Massachusetts Dispensary. REFERENCES: *DAB*, 9: 31-32; *NCAB*, 12: 197; notebooks and ledgers in the Countway Library, Harvard, Boston, Mass.; Lemuel Shattuck, *Shattuck Genealogy* (1855).

                                                                                            G. C. Sanchez

SHATTUCK, GEORGE CHEYNE, JR. (July 22, 1813, Boston, Mass.-March 22, 1893, Boston). *Physician, Educator*. Son of Dr. George C. (q.v.) and Eliza Cheever (Davis) Shattuck. Married Anne Henrietta Brune, 1840; three children. EDUCATION: Boston Latin School; Round Hill School, Northampton, Mass.; 1831, A.B., Harvard College; studied one year, Harvard Law School; 1835, M.D., Harvard Medical School; postgraduate study, Europe. CAREER: 1839, returned to Boston and founded a private clinic, where he taught private medical students; 1849, succeeded Oliver Wendell Holmes (q.v.) as visiting physician, Massachusetts General Hospital; at Harvard: 1855-59, professor of clinical medicine; 1859-73, professor of theory and practice of medicine; and 1864, dean. CONTRIBUTIONS: Came under the influence of Pierre Louis when he studied in Paris after graduation from Harvard Medical School. Credited with the introduction in the United States of the case method of teaching medicine. Helped found the Boston Society of Medical Observation. A founder, St. Paul's School, Concord, N.H. (1855), as well as the Shattuck School of Fairbault, Minn., a missionary school for Indians.

WRITINGS: *On Fever* (1838); "On the Continued Fever of Great Britain," *Medical Examiner* (1840); *Yellow Fever*, by Pierre Louis (1839, translation). REFERENCES: Caleb Bradlee, *Brief Sketch of the Life of Dr. George Shattuck* (1894); *DAB*, 9: 32-33; Journals in the Countway Library, Boston; Dale Smith, "The Emergence of Organized Clinical Instruction in the Nineteenth Century American Cities of Boston, New York, and Philadelphia" (Doctoral thesis, University of Minnesota, 1979); Alfred Stillé, *Notice of the Life and Character of George Cheyne Shattuck, M.D.* (1893).

                                                                                            G. C. Sanchez

SHATTUCK, LEMUEL (October 15, 1793, Ashby, Mass.-January 17, 1859, Boston, Mass.). *Public health innovator; Vital statistics*. Son of John, farmer, and Betsey (Miles) Shattuck. Married Clarissa Baxter, 1825; five children. ED-

UCATION: Almost entirely self-taught. CAREER: 1817-22, schoolteacher, Troy and Albany, N.Y., and Detroit, Mich.; 1823-33, merchant, Concord, Mass.; 1834, bookseller, Cambridge, Mass.; 1834-59, self-employed bookseller, publisher, genealogist, public health writer, and statistician, Boston; 1840-50, intermittently a legislator for Boston and Mass. CONTRIBUTIONS: Provided impetus to expansion and institutionalization of public health work at local and state levels; his Sanitary Report of 1850 constituted a model for eventual establishment of state boards of health, first in Mass. (1869) and then elsewhere in the United States. A principal promoter and organizer of statistics in mid nineteenth-century America; initiated the establishment of the American Statistical Association (1839); stimulated and shaped reform of state vital statistics provisions in Mass. (1840-50), thus providing a prototype and standard for other states; instituted major improvements in and expansion of census work through census of Boston (1845) and suggestions for the federal census (1850). Played an important role in the improvement and standardization of the nomenclature of the causes of death (1842-50), particularly through work on Mass. vital statistics registration but also through work for AMA committees. Stimulated studies of heredity through contributions to improvement of genealogical records and local history sources (1830-55). Introduced important measures for systematization and organization of local and state government in Massachusetts.

WRITINGS: *History of the Town of Concord. . .*(1835); *Census of Boston for the Year 1845* (1846); *Report. . .Relating to a Sanitary Survey of the State* [of Mass.] (1850); *Memorials of the Descendants of William Shattuck* (1855). Writings listed in *DAB; Who Was Who in Am.; Appleton's CAB*. REFERENCES: John B. Blake, "Lemuel Shattuck and the Boston Water Supply," *Bull. Hist. Med.* 29 (1955): 554-62; James H. Cassedy, "The Roots of American Sanitary Reform, 1843-47: Seven Letters from John H. Griscom to Lemuel Shattuck," *J. Hist. Med.* 30 (Apr. 1975): 136-47; *DAB*, 9, pt. 1: 33-34; Charles Hudson, "Memoir of Lemuel Shattuck," *Proc., Mass. Hist. Soc.* 18 (Jun. 1880): 155-65; W. G. Smillie et al., "Lemuel Shattuck—Still a Prophet," *Am. J. of Public Health* 39, no. 2 (Feb. 1949): 135-62; Walter F. Willcox, "Lemuel Shattuck, Statist, Founder of the American Statistical Association," *J. Amer. Stat. Assoc.* 35 (1940): 224-35.

J. H. Cassedy

SHEW, JOEL (November 13, 1816, Providence, N.Y.-October 6, 1855, Oyster Bay, N.Y.). *Hydropath*. Married Marie Louise Shew. EDUCATION: c. 1842, M.D. CAREER: 1843-55, operator of hydropathic institutions, N.Y. and Vt. CONTRIBUTIONS: Introduced water-cure system of Vincent Priessnitz to the United States, opening the first hydropathic establishment in America in New York City (1843). Edited *Water Cure Journal* (1845-48). A leader of American Vegetarian Society (1850-55).

WRITINGS: *Hydropathy, or the Water-Cure* (1844); *Cholera Treated by Water* (1848); *Children: Their Hydropathic Management* (1852); *The Hydropathic Family Physician* (1854). REFERENCES: *Appleton's CAB* 5 (1888): 508-9; Russell Trall, "Death of Dr.

Shew," *Water Cure J.* 20 (1855): 104-5; Harry Weiss and Howard Kemble, *The Great American Water-Cure Craze* (1967), 69-70.

J. C. Whorton

SHIPP, ELLIS REYNOLDS (January 20, 1847, Davis County, Ia.-January 31, 1939, Salt Lake City, Utah). *Obstetrics; Health education.* Daughter of William F., farmer, and Anna (Hawley) Reynolds. Married Milford Bard Shipp, 1866; ten children. EDUCATION: 1878, M.D., Woman's Medical College of Pennsylvania. CAREER: 1878-1935, taught classes in obstetric nursing, Salt Lake City; after two terms of six months each, students were examined and certified by the Salt Lake City Board of Health; during this period, also taught classes of three months duration in midwifery and obstetric nursing in outlying Mormon settlements over a broad western territory, from Mexico to Alberta, Canada, and from Colo. to Nev.; 1882-90, on the staff of Deseret Hospital, which was established by the Relief Society of the Mormon Church mainly for accouchement, and where the first nurses' training school in Utah Territory was established; active in the women's rights movement, was a delegate to the National Council of Women; 1938, elected to Utah's Hall of Famous Women. CONTRIBUTIONS: By her systematic and thorough training of about 2,000 midwives and obstetrical nurses, writings on hygiene, and public lectures on hygiene and nutrition, contributed to the elevation of public health, the decline of infant mortality and maternal deaths, and the welfare of women.

WRITINGS: "Hygiene of Beds," *Salt Lake Sanitarian* 1 (May 1888): 32-34; "Mothers' Methods," pt. 1, *ibid.*, 1 (Jun. 1888): 67-68; pt. 2 (Jul. 1888): 85-86; pt. 3 (Aug. 1888): 109-12; pt. 4 (Sept. 1888): 143-46; pt. 5 (Oct. 1888): 170-72; pt. 6 (Nov. 1888): 181-83; "Poisons and their Antidotes," *ibid.*, 2 (Jun. 1889): 68-71. REFERENCES: Claire Noall, "Ellis Reynolds Shipp," in *Guardians of the Hearth. Utah's Pioneer Midwives and Women Doctors* (1974), 115-30; Ralph T. Richards, M.D., *Of Medicine, Hospitals and Doctors* (1953), 233-34.

H. Bauman

SHIPPEN, WILLIAM (October 21, 1736, Philadelphia, Pa.-July 11, 1808, Germantown, Pa.). *Physician; Surgeon; Educator.* Son of William, physician, and Susannah (Harrison) Shippen. Married Alice Lee, 1760; only son died in 1798. EDUCATION: Reverend Finley's Nottingham Academy; 1754, A.B., Princeton College; 1754-57, medical student of his father, William Shippen; studied in London and Edinburgh; 1761, M.D., University of Edinburgh; 1761-62, studied in France. CAREER: 1762, returned to America; 1762, began teaching anatomy at his father's house, using anatomy pictures given to the Pennsylvania Hospital by Dr. John Fothergill; 1765, elected professor of anatomy and surgery, College of Philadelphia; 1776, chief physician and director-general of hospitals, Continental Army, N.J.; 1776, director-general of all hospitals west of the Hudson River; 1777-81, chief physician and director-general, Medical Corps, Continental Army; 1779, only faculty member, College of Philadelphia, to accept a post at the newly created University of Pennsylvania; 1783, professor in both the university and the college medical schools; 1791, when schools merged, held chair of anatomy, surgery, and midwifery; 1778-79, 1791-1802, physician, Pennsylvania Hospital. CONTRIBUTIONS: A founding medical educator in America, teaching in the early years of the College of Philadelphia, the first American medical school. A founder, College of Physicians of Philadelphia. Created a quarrel with John Morgan (q.v.) and took over his post during the Revolutionary War. Was court-martialed (1780) but vindicated. REFERENCES: B. C. Corner, *William Shippen, Jr.* (1951); *DAB*, 9: 117-18; F. P. Henry, *Standard History of the Med. Profession in Phila.* (1897); Kelly and Burrage (1928), 1104-6; T. C. Morton and F. Woodbury, *History of the Pennsylvania Hosp.* (1895); *NCAB*, 10: 384.

D. I. Lansing

SHOPE, RICHARD EDWIN (December 25, 1901, Des Moines, Ia.-October 2, 1966, New York, N.Y.). *Animal pathologist; Virology.* Son of Charles Cornelius, physician, and Mary (Hast) Shope. Married Helen Madden Ellis, 1925; four children. EDUCATION: 1924, M.D., State University of Iowa. CAREER: 1924-25, pharmacology and materia medica faculty, State University of Iowa; at Rockefeller Institute for Medical Research (later Rockefeller University): 1925-49, researcher in animal pathology, Princeton campus; and 1952-66, member and animal pathology faculty, N.Y. campus; 1942-44, director, War Disease Control Station, Grosse Isle, Quebec, Canada; 1949-52, associate director, Merck Institute for Therapeutic Research, Rahway, N.J.; served on numerous scientific committees. CONTRIBUTIONS: A leading investigator of animal viral disease. With Paul A. Lewis, uncovered the etiology of swine influenza (1931); showed that serious illness resulted from the concerted action of a bacterium, *Pfeiffer bacillus*, and a virus; argued on the basis of the similarity of the disease to the Spanish flu of 1918-19 that the same viral agent was involved in both illnesses. Described a method of animal vaccination against influenza that laid the basis for the development of a human flu vaccine. Explained the survival of hog influenza in nature by demonstrating that the swine lungworm provided a reservoir of infection. Showed that the "mad itch" of cattle is caused by a pseudorabies virus for which pigs act as an intermediate host (early 1930s). Demonstrated that infectious papillomatosis and infectious fibromatosis of cottontail rabbits are viral diseases (early 1930s); work was extended by Peyton Rous (q.v.), who proved that the Shope papilloma virus could cause malignancies in domestic rabbits, thereby lending support to the concept of a virus etiology of cancer. Developed a vaccine against rinderpest, a serious epidemic disease of cattle (1942-44).

WRITINGS: "Swine Influenza: Hemophilic Bacillus from Respiratory Tract of Infected Swine," *J. of Experimental Med.* 54 (1931): 361-71 (with Paul A. Lewis); "A Transmissible Tumor-Like Condition in Rabbits," ibid., 56 (Dec. 1932): 793-803; "Infectious Papillomatosis of Rabbits, with Note on Histopathology," ibid., 58 (1933): 607-24 (with E. W. Hurst). REFERENCES: *Am. Philosophical. Soc. Yearbook* (1971), 179-84; *Am. Veterinary Med. Assoc. J.* 131 (Nov. 1957): 486-87; *Current Biog.* (1963), 384-86; Greer Williams, *Virus Hunters* (1959), 200-209; *N.Y. Times*, October 3, 1966; *Trans. Assoc. Am. Physicians* 84 (1971): 36-38; *Who Was Who in Am.*, 4: 860.

S. Galishoff

SHORE, CLARENCE ALBERT (November 26, 1873, Salem, N.C.-February 10, 1933, Raleigh, N.C.). *Physician; Pathologist.* Son of Henry Washington and Lavinia Elizabeth (Boyer) Shore. Married Ellen Dortch, 1914. EDUCATION: 1901, B.S., University of North Carolina; 1907, M.D., Johns Hopkins; 1902, M.S., University of North Carolina. CAREER: 1901-4, instructor in biology, University of North Carolina; 1908-33, director, State Laboratory of Hygiene. CONTRIBUTIONS: Organized (1908) and directed (1908-33) the State Laboratory of Hygiene, providing the only free service in the state for histopathology, surgical pathology, and other standard laboratory diagnostic tests. The service provided was vital for the state as there were never more than three professional pathologists in N.C. during Shore's 25 years of work at the State Laboratory. REFERENCES: Dorothy Long, ed. *Medicine in North Carolina* (1972), 112, 114, 129-30, 590, 600; *Who Was Who in Am.*, 1 :1121..

T. L. Savitt

SHOULDERS, HARRISON H. (February 27, 1886, Whitleyville, Jackson County, Tenn.-November 17, 1963, Nashville, Tenn.). *Physician; Surgeon.* Son of Leonard H. and Belle M. (Clark) Shoulders. Married Virginia Swiggert, 1922; three children. EDUCATION: Potter Bible College, Bowling Green, Ky.; 1909, M.D., University of Nashville; 1909-10, intern, St. Thomas Hospital, Nashville; 1910-12, house surgeon, Forts Infirmary, Nashville; 1920, resident surgeon, St. Luke's Hospital, New York City; 1921, house surgeon, Hospital for Ruptured and Crippled, New York City. CAREER: 1912-17, assistant director, Tennessee Department of Health; 1917-19, captain, U.S. Army Medical Corps, mostly overseas; 1922-55, private practice of surgery, Nashville; 1927-45, secretary, Tennessee State Medical Association, and editor of its journal; 1946-47, 100th president, American Medical Association; 1930-55, associate clinical professor of surgery, Vanderbilt; organizer and first president, Nashville Surgical Society; certified (1940, Founders Group), American Board of Surgery. CONTRIBUTIONS: Devised several new surgical procedures and contributed extensively to surgical literature. Aided the advancement of surgery through his leadership skills. Contributed to organized medicine through service in local, state, and national medical and surgical organizations, culminating in the presidency of the American Medical Association.

WRITINGS: Published extensively in surgical journals. REFERENCES: Morris Fishbein, ed., *History of the American Medical Association* (1947), 827-28; *NCAB*, 51: 175.

S. R. Bruesch

SHRADY, GEORGE FREDERICK (January 14, 1837, New York, N.Y.-November 30, 1907, New York City). *Physician; Surgeon; Editor.* Son of John and Margaret (Beinhauer) Shrady. Married Mary Lewis, 1860; Hester Ellen Cantine, 1888; five children. EDUCATION: Free Academy, New York City; 1858, M.D., College of Physicians and Surgeons; 1857-58, resident surgeon, New York Hospital. CAREER: Assistant Surgeon, U.S. Army; medical staff, St. Francis, Columbus, N.Y., and Red Cross hospitals; editor: 1860-64, *American Med-*

ical Times; and 1866-1904, *Medical Record*; medical editor, N.Y. *Herald*. CON-
TRIBUTIONS: Founded the *Medical Record* and crusaded for the reform of medical
education and public health and against medical charlatans. A pioneer in plastic
surgery.

WRITINGS: *Surgical and Pathological Reflections on President Garfield's Wound* (1881);
The College of Physicians and Surgeons (1903); *General Grant's Last Days* (1908).
REFERENCES: *DAB*, 9: 132; *Herald* (N.Y.), December 1, 1907; *JAMA* 49 (1907): 1938;
Kelly and Burrage (1928), 1108-9; *NCAB*, 7: 271; *N.Y. Times*, December 1, 1907.

D. O. Powell

SHRYOCK, RICHARD HARRISON (March 29, 1893, Philadelphia, Pa.-
January 30, 1972, Fort Lauderdale, Fla.). *Educator; Medical history.* Son of
George Augustus and Mary Harrison (Chipman) Shryock. Married Rheva Ott,
1921; two children. EDUCATION: University of Pennsylvania: 1917, B.S. in
education; and 1924, Ph.D. CAREER: 1913-16, teacher, public schools, Philadelphia; 1917-18, Field Ambulance Corps, U.S. Army; 1918, student, U.S.
Army Medical School; history faculty: 1921-24, Ohio State University; 1924-
25, 1938-49, 1958-63, University of Pennsylvania; and 1925-38, Duke University; 1935-36, fellowship secretary, Social Science Research Council, N.Y.;
1944-49, medical history faculty, Woman's Medical College of Pennsylvania;
1946-47, acting director, American Council of Learned Societies; 1949-58, director, Institute of the History of Medicine, Johns Hopkins University; 1950-
53, member, National Historical Publications Committee; 1958-65, librarian,
American Philosophical Society; 1956-65, member of board, Russell Sage Foundation; 1959, member, History of Medicine Study Section, National Institutes
of Health; president: 1941-42, History of Science Society; 1946-47, American
Association for the History of Medicine; 1950, American Association of University Professors; and 1958, International Association of University Professors;
primarily a medical historian but also wrote about other aspects of American
history. CONTRIBUTIONS: Leading interpreter of modern medical history, being
the first to emphasize the interplay of social and scientific factors in medicine.
Most distinguished work was *The Development of Modern Medicine. . .*(1936),
which was translated into German, Japanese, and French. Edited *Pennsylvania
Magazine of History and Biography* (1940-46).

WRITINGS: *American Medical Research; Past and Present* (1947); *The National Tuberculosis Association, 1904-1954* (1957); *The History of Nursing. . .*(1959); *Medicine
and Society in America, 1660-1860* (1960); *Medicine in America; Historical Essays*
(1966). A bibliography is in Lloyd G. Stevenson, "A Salute to Richard Shryock," *J.
Hist. Med. & Allied Sci.* 23 (Jan. 1968): 1-15. REFERENCES: Whitfield J. Bell, Jr.,
"Richard H. Shryock: Life and Work of a Historian," *J. Hist. Med. & Allied Sci.* 29
(Jan. 1974): 15-31; *BHM* (1970-74), 159; *Who Was Who in Am.*, 5: 660.

S. Galishoff

SIBLEY, JOHN (May 19, 1757, Sutton, Mass.-April 8, 1837, Natchitoches,
La.). *Physician.* Son of Timothy and Anne (Waite) Sibley. Married Elizabeth
Hopkins, 1780; Mary White Winslow, 1791; Eudalie Malique, 1813; one

son. EDUCATION: Apprentice to Dr. John Wilson, Hopkinton, Mass. CAREER: Surgeon's mate, American Revolution; practice, Great Barrington, Mass., moving next to Fayetteville, N.C.; 1802, moved to New Orleans, La.; became contract surgeon, U.S. Army; 1805-14, Indian agent, Orleans Territory; judge, member of the legislature, officer in the state militia, serving in the 1819 raid on Tex.; owned a cotton plantation. CONTRIBUTIONS: An early physician, Louisiana Territory and in La. Reports to Thomas Jefferson are an important source of information on the Louisiana Territory shortly after its purchase from France.

WRITINGS: Reports in *American State Papers: Indian Affairs* (1832). REFERENCES: *DAB* 9: 146-47; John Duffy, *History of Medicine in Louisiana* 1 (1958); Miller, *BHM*, p. 103.

                                                                            M. Kaufman

SIGERIST, HENRY ERNEST (April 7, 1891, Paris, France-March 17, 1957, Pura, Ticino, Switzerland). *Medical historian.* Son of Ernst Heinrich, businessman, and Emma (Wiskemann) Sigerist. Married Emmy M. Escher, 1916; two daughters. EDUCATION: 1910, Literargymnasium, Zurich; 1910-11, student of oriental philology, University of Zurich and University College, London; 1917, M.D., University of Zurich (summer 1914, University of Munich); 1912-22, Periodic service, Medical Corps, Swiss army; 1919, student of Karl Sudhoff, University of Leipzig. CAREER: At University of Zurich: 1921-25, privatdozent of history of medicine; and 1924, titular-professor; 1925-32, professor of history of medicine and director of institute of the history of medicine, University of Leipzig; at Johns Hopkins University: 1932-47, William H. Welch Professor of History of Medicine and director of the institute of the history of medicine; and 1942-45, acting librarian, William H. Welch Medical Library; 1947-57, research associate in the history of medicine, Yale University. CONTRIBUTIONS: Leading medical historian of his generation. Introduced graduate studies in medical history in United States. Promoted the social history of medicine and sought to make medical history an integral part of American medical education. Founded the *Bulletin of the History of Medicine* and reorganized the American Association for the History of Medicine.

WRITINGS: *Great Doctors* (1933); *American Medicine* (1934); *Socialized Medicine in the Soviet Union* (1937); *Civilization and Disease* (1943); *A History of Medicine* (Vol. 1. *Primitive and Archaic Medicine*, 1951; Vol. 2. *Early Greek, Hindu and Persian Medicine*, 1961). Writings listed in Genevieve Miller, *A Bibliography of the Writings of Henry E. Sigerist* (1966). REFERENCES: Elisabeth Berg-Schorn, *Henry E. Sigerist (1891-1957), Medizinhistoriker in Leipzig und Baltimore: Standpunkt und Wirkung* (1978); *DAB*, Supplement 6: 580-81; "Henry E. Sigerist Issue," *J. Hist. Med. & Allied Sci.* 13 (1958): 125-250; "Henry E. Sigerist Valedictory Number," *Bull. Hist. Med.* 22 (1948): 1-93; *NCAB*, 46: 436; M. Terris, "The Contributions of Henry E. Sigerist to Health Service Organization," *Milbank Mem. Fund Q.* 53 (1975): 489-530; F. G. Vescia, "Henry E. Sigerist: the Years in America," *Medizinhist. J.* 14 (1979): 218-232.

                                                                            G. Miller

SILLIMAN, BENJAMIN (August 8, 1779, North Stratford, now Trumbull, Conn.-November 24, 1864, New Haven, Conn.). *Scientist; Educator.* Son of

Gold Selleck, lawyer and farmer, and Mary (Fish) Silliman. Married Harriet Trumbull, 1809, nine children; Sarah Isabella (McClellan) Webb, 1851. EDUCATION: Prepared for college by Rev. Andrew Eliot; 1796, A.B., Yale College; 1798, studied law under Simeon Baldwin, New Haven, Conn., and was admitted to the bar, March 1802; 1802-4, medical school, University of Pennsylvania. CAREER: 1797-98, taught in a private school, Wethersfield, Conn.; at Yale College: 1799, appointed tutor; 1801, appointed first professor of chemistry and natural history; and 1813-53, professor of chemistry, medical institute. CONTRIBUTIONS: Instrumental in the appointment of Dr. Nathan Smith (q.v.) and others to the first faculty of the Medical School. Taught chemistry and pharmacy to the medical students at Yale for nearly 40 years, during which time the Medical School flourished. Founded the *American Journal of Science and the Arts* (1818) and edited it for the next 20 years. Made a member, American Philosophical Society (1805). First president, Association of American Geologists (1840). Original member, National Academy of Sciences (1863).

WRITINGS: Edited *The Elements of Experimental Chemistry*, 2 vols. (1814); and Robert Bakewell's *An Introduction to Geology* (1829). Published his own *Elements of Chemistry*, 2 vols. (1830-31) in addition to works on his travels, eulogies, and reports listed in F. B. Dexter, *Biographical Sketches of the Graduates of Yale College* 5 (1885): 224-27. REFERENCES: F. B. Dexter, *Biographical Sketches of the Graduates of Yale College* (1885); *DAB*, 9, pt. 1: 160-63; John F. Fulton and Elizabeth H. Thomson, *Benjamin Silliman, 1779-1864, Pathfinder in American Science* (1947); *NCAB*, 2: 386; Leonard G. Wilson, ed., *Benjamin Silliman and His Circle* (1979).

J. W. Ifkovic

SIMMONS, GEORGE HENRY (January 2, 1852, Moreton, England-September 1, 1937, Chicago, Ill.). *Physician; Medical editor.* Son of George, farmer, and Sarah Louise (Clifford) Simmons. Married Kate Vedder Monell (second marriage); no children. Went to the United States in 1870. EDUCATION: 1871-72, Tabor College, Ia.; 1872-76, University of Nebraska; 1882, M.D., Hahnemann Medical College, Chicago; 1883-84, studied in Europe; 1892, M.D., Rush Medical College. CAREER: 1884-99, practiced medicine, Lincoln, Nebr.; 1896-99, founder and editor, *Western Medical Review*; 1899-1911, general secretary, American Medical Association; at *Journal of American Medical Association*: 1899-1924, editor; and *post* 1901, general manager; 1921, president, Institute of Medicine, Chicago. CONTRIBUTIONS: Initiated the movement for reorganization of the American Medical Association that culminated (1901) with the acceptance of the plan proposed by Joseph N. McCormack (q.v.). Undertook the publication of several periodicals devoted to medical specialties, including *American Journal of Diseases of Children* and the various *Archives*: of *Internal Medicine, Neurology and Psychiatry, Dermatology and Syphilology,* and *Surgery*. Began publication of *Hygeia*, a popular health journal, and *American Medical Directory*. Inaugurated a cumulative quarterly index of medical publications that made available to physicians the latest scientific advances reported in the periodical literature; was later combined with *Index Medicus* to become

Quarterly Cumulative Index Medicus. Helped bring about the elimination of inferior medical colleges by publishing the results of state examinations for licensure together with the medical schools from which the applicants had graduated; published similar statistics regarding appointments to hospitals, internships, and residencies. Established within the AMA committees and councils for matters such as medical education, medical ethics, health and public instruction, and pharmacy and chemistry, which greatly broadened the association's influence. Was especially active in combatting fraud and quackery.

WRITINGS: Most of what little he wrote appeared anonymously in *JAMA* and is briefly described in his obituary in that journal. REFERENCES: *DAB*, Supplement 2: 612-13; *JAMA* 109 (Sept. 1937): 807-8; *N.Y. Times*, September 2, 1937; *Who Was Who in Am.*, 1: 1126-27.

S. Galishoff

SIMPSON, JOHN (March 19, 1869, Mason, W.Va.-November 23, 1947, Morgantown, W.Va.). *Medical educator*. Son of Mason and Phoebia (Kennedy) Simpson. EDUCATION: 1893, B.A., University of Nashville; 1902, M.D., Johns Hopkins Medical School; study in Vienna and Paris for three summers. CAREER: At West Virginia University School of Medicine: 1902-12, head of the faculty; and 1917-35, dean. CONTRIBUTIONS: Organized the first two years of medical curriculum (1903-4). Policies enabled West Virginia University Medical School to survive the Flexner Report. REFERENCES: Edward J. Van Liere and Gideon S. Dodds, *History of Medical Education in West Virginia (1965)*.

K. Nodyne and R. Murphy

SIMS, J[AMES] MARION (January 25, 1813, Lancaster, S.C.-November 13, 1883, New York, N.Y.). *Physician; Surgeon; Gynecology*. Son of John and Mahala (Mackey) Sims. Married Eliza Theresa Jones, 1836; five surviving children. EDUCATION: 1832, graduate of South Carolina College; 1833, entered Charleston Medical College; 1834, enrolled in Jefferson Medical School, Philadelphia, Pa.; 1835, M.D., Jefferson Medical College. CAREER: Began practice, Lancaster, S.C., where his first two patients died; moved: to Mount Meigs, Ala.; 1840, Montgomery, Ala.; 1853, New York City, for practice of surgery; and 1861, Europe; 1868, returned to N.Y.; 1870, returned to France for two years; 1872, returned to N.Y.; and member, Board of Surgeons, Women's Hospital; president: 1876, American Medical Association; and 1880, American Gynecological Society. CONTRIBUTIONS: Established Women's Hospital (1854), N.Y., for the instruction of students and physicians in gynecological surgery. Performed the celebrated operations for vesico-vaginal fistula. Experimented with silver sutures. Leading gynecologist of his time.

WRITINGS: "The Treatment of Epiethelioma of the Cervix Uterine," *Am. J. of Obstet.* (1879); "Remarks on the Treatment of Gunshot Wounds of the Abdomen in Relation to Modern Peritonal Surgery," *British Med. J.* (1881); "The Surgical Treatment of President Garfield," *North Am. Rev.* (1881). REFERENCES: I. Abell, "J. Marion Sims: An Appreciation," *Southern Med. J.* (1933); *BHM* (1964-69), 246; (1970-74), 160; (1975-79), 118; E. B. Carmichael, "J. Marion Sims: Inventor, Physician, Surgeon," *J. of the*

International Coll. of Surgeons 33 (1960); *DAB*, 9, pt. 1: 186-88; Seale Harris, *Woman's Surgeon* (1950); Miller, *BHM*, pp. 105-6; *NCAB*, 2: 356; J. Marion Sims, *The Story of My Life* (1968); G. G. Ward, "The Contribution and the Origin of Modern Gynecology," *Bull. of the N.Y. Acad. of Med.* 12 (1936); J. I. Waring, *Hist. of Med. in S.C., 1825-1900* (1967).

J. P. Dolan

SKENE, ALEXANDER JOHNSTON CHALMERS (June 17, 1837, Fyvie, Scotland-July 4, 1900, Brooklyn, N.Y.). *Gynecologist.* Son of Johnston and Jean (McConachie) Skene. Married Annette Wilhelmine Lillian Van der Wegen; one adopted child. EDUCATION: Studied medicine in King's College, Scotland; migrated to America in 1857; 1860, studied medicine in Toronto, Canada; 1861-62, attended University of Michigan medical department; 1863, M.D., Long Island College Hospital Medical School. CAREER: 1864, medical practice in Brooklyn; 1864-65, served in U. S. Army medical corps as assistant surgeon; 1865-99, practiced medicine and surgery in Brooklyn; 1883-86, professor of gynecology, New York Post-Graduate Medical School; Long Island College Hospital, 1868-93, professor, also dean and president (1886-1893); 1884, opened private sanitarium in Brooklyn; 1899, operated Skene's Hospital for Self-Supporting Women. CONTRIBUTIONS: Pioneering gynecologist. Wrote on the urethral glands (1880). Was conservative in his outlook as indicated by his failure to succumb to "the epidemic of vaginal hysterectomy" when virtually every surgeon tried to eliminate pelvic pain by removing the ovaries. A founder of the American Gynecological Society and its president (1886-87). A founder of the International Congress of Gynecology and Obstetrics (honorary president at the Geneva Congress of 1896). Associate editor of the *Archives of Medicine* (1883-84), the *American Medical Digest* (1884-89), and the *New York Gynecological and Obstetrical Journal* (1891-1900). Discovered Skene's urethral glands (1880).

WRITINGS: *Diseases of the Bladder and Urethra in Women* (1878); *Treatise on the Diseases of Women* (1888); *Education and Culture as Related to the Health and Diseases of Women* (1889); *Electro-haemostasis in Operative Surgery* (1889); *Medical Gynecology* (1895). REFERENCES: Kelly and Burrage (1928), 1117-18; *Trans. of the Am. Gynecological Soc.*, 26 (1901); *DAB*, 9, pt. 1: 194-95.

M. Kaufman

SLEYSTER, ROCK (June 14, 1879, Waupun, Wis.-March 7, 1942, Wauwatosa, Wis.). *Physician; Psychiatry.* Son of William, grain merchant, and Addie (Butts) Sleyster. Married Clara Sarah Swift, 1903; no children. EDUCATION: 1902, M.D., University of Illinois. CAREER: Private practice: 1902-7, Appleton, Wis.; and 1907-19, Waupun, Wis.; 1907-19, prison physician, Wisconsin State Prison, Waupun; medical director: 1907-19, Central State Hospital for the Criminal Insane, Waupun; and 1919-42, Milwaukee Sanitarium, Wauwatosa; in Wisconsin State Medical Society: 1914-24, secretary; 1924-25, president; and 1926-39, treasurer; 1918-23, editor, *Wisconsin Medical Journal*; in American Medical Association: 1926-37, trustee; 1935-37, chairman of the board; and 1939-40, president; 1916-20, chief, Bureau of Postgraduate Medical Instruction, University of Wisconsin Extension Division. CONTRIBUTIONS: Following 26 years of service to the AMA, assumed its presidency (1939), the first Wis. resident to do so. Fame rests as much on institutional contributions as on research. Appointment as physician, Wisconsin State Prison (1909), led to specialization in psychiatry, especially the psychological basis of crime. Became medical director, Milwaukee Sanitarium (1919), a model institution devoted to the care of mental patients. At the time of his death was known as one of the nation's leading psychiatrists.

WRITINGS: "The Criminal Physique: A Preliminary Report on the Physical Examination of One Thousand, Five Hundred and Twenty-One Prisoners at the Wisconsin State Prison," *JAMA* 60 (1913): 1351-53; "The Physical Basis of Crime as Observed by a Prison Physician," *Bull. of the Am. Acad. of Med.* 14 (1913): 396-407; "Some Data Gathered in a Study of 269 Murderers," *Ill. Med. J.* 25 (1914): 236-39; "Mind of Man and His Security," *JAMA* 112 (May 20, 1939): 2003-6. Writings listed in *Index Medicus*. REFERENCES: Morris Fishbein, *History of the American Medical Association, 1847 to 1947* (1947), 808-9; *NCAB*, 33: 91; Arthur J. Patek, "Dr. Rock Sleyster," *Annals of Internal Med.* 16 (Apr. 1942): 806-7; *Wisconsin Med. J.* 41 (Apr. 1942): 339-40.

                                                                                                    R. B. Schoepflin

SMILLIE, WILSON GEORGE (November 2, 1886, Eaton, Colo.-August 4, 1971, Newfane, Vt.). *Physician and educator; Public health.* Son of John Wilson, rancher, and Christina (Trenholme) Smillie. Married Faye Anderson, 1914; Octavia Hall, 1923; two children by each marriage. EDUCATION: 1908, A.B., Colorado College; Harvard University: 1912, M.D.; and 1916, D.P.H.; 1912-14, intern and resident, Peter Bent Brigham Hospital. CAREER: 1914-16, preventive medicine faculty, Harvard Medical School; 1917-27, scientific staff, International Health Division, Rockefeller Foundation; 1919-21, director, Institute of Hygiene, Sao Paulo, Brazil; 1927-37, public health administration faculty, Harvard School of Public Health; 1937-55, public health and preventive medicine faculty, Cornell University Medical College; 1955-58, director, New York State Charities Aid Association. CONTRIBUTIONS: Influenced the development of American public health, especially epidemiology, through teachings and writings. Authored two textbooks that were widely used in medical colleges and schools of public health; wrote the first comprehensive history of American public health. Established the first school of public health in South America, the Institute of Hygiene, in Sao Paulo (1919-21).

WRITINGS: *Public Health Administration in the United States* (1935); *Preventive Medicine and Public Health* (1946); *Public Health, Its Promise for the Future: A Chronicle of the Development of Public Health in the United States, 1607-1914* (1955). REFERENCES: *N.Y. Times*, August 6, 1971; George Rosen, "Some Recollections of Wilson G. Smillie, M.D. (1886-1971)," *Am. J. of Public Health* 62 (Mar. 1972): 431-34; *Who Was Who in Am.*, 5: 669.

                                                                                                    S. Galishoff

SMITH, ALBAN GILPIN (March 22, 1795, probably in New Castle County, Del.-1876, New York, N.Y.). *Surgeon; Medical educator.* Son of Samuel and

Lydia (Gilpin) Smith. Married Taliaferro Middleton, 1817, seven children; Ann Higby, 1845. Changed name to Goldsmith by an act of legislature of state of N.Y., April 20, 1839. EDUCATION: Before December 1809, apprenticed to Ephraim McDowell (q.v.), Danville, Ky.; 1821-22, private medical lectures of Dr. Joseph Parrish (q.v.), Philadelphia, Pa.; 1829, in Paris to study Jean Civiale's technique of lithotripsy. CAREER: Practiced: until 1817, Danville, with his preceptor; and 1817-21, Port Tobacco, Md.; 1822-26, returned to Danville from Philadelphia and became a partner of E. McDowell; until 1831, remained in Danville, when he moved to Louisville, Ky. CONTRIBUTIONS: While a partner of E. McDowell, performed the third successful ovariotomy (May 1823). A bold innovative surgeon, performed the first documented laminectomy for relief of paralysis secondary to fracture of a vertebra (1829). First in the United States to perform lithotripsy for bladder stone using Civiale's instruments and technique (1831). Obtained first charter for the Louisville Medical Institute (1833) but was unable to assemble a faculty. Appointed professor of surgery, Medical College of Ohio (fall 1833) but was not reappointed four years later when faculty was reorganized. Accepted the chair of surgery, University of State of New York (1837), but resigned after only two years. Remained in practice, New York City, the rest of his life.

WRITINGS: *Lithotripsy* (1843); *Diseases of the Genito Urinary Organs* (1857). REFERENCES: E. H. Conner, "Alban Gilpin Smith (Alban Goldsmith), M.D." in Dorothy M. Schullian, ed., "Notes & Events," *J. Hist. Med. & Alled Sci.* 32 (1977): 205-10; J. E. Gilpin, *Genealogy of the Family of Gideon Gilpin* (1897).

E. H. Conner

SMITH, ALBERT HOLMES (July 19, 1835, Philadelphia, Pa.-December 14, 1885, Philadelphia). *Obstetrician; Gynecologist.* Son of Dr. Moses and Mrs. Rachel (Coate) Smith. Married Emily Kaighn, 1860; seven children. EDUCATION: Westtown Quaker Boarding School; Gregory's Classical School; 1853, B.S., University of Pennsylvania; apprentice to Dr. George B. Wood (q.v.); 1856, M.D., University of Pennsylvania; 1856-59, intern, Frankford Asylum and Pennsylvania Hospital. CAREER: 1859, obstetrical practice, Philadelphia; at Philadelphia Lying-In Charity: 1859-62, assistant physician; and 1862 to his death, attending physician; 1867, became consulting physician, Woman's Hospital of Philadelphia; 1863-71, a manager, Wills Ophthalmic Hospital. CONTRIBUTIONS: A leading obstetrician, championed the rights of women in the medical profession. Founder, Obstetrical Society of Philadelphia (June 1868, in his own office), and president (1874-76). Founder, American Gynecological Society, and president (1884). Inventor of medical instruments, especially a pessary still in occasional use.

WRITINGS: *An Improved Speculum* (1869); *Retarded Dilation of Os Uteri in Labor* (1877); *Pendulum Leverage of the Obstetrical Forceps* (1878); *The Present Aspect of Puerperal Diseases* (1884). REFERENCES: *Am. J. of Obst.* (1886); *American Gynecological Society, 1876-1900* (1901); *DAB*, 9: 234-35; Kelly and Burrage (1920), 1063; *Med. News* (1885); *NCAB*, 25: 62; Kaighn Smith (grandson), presidential address, Obstetrical Society of Philadelphia, May 1981 (to be published in *Trans.* of the Society); *Trans., Am. Gyn. Soc.* 11 (1886): 422; *Proc. of the Am. Philosophical Soc.* (1886); *Trans., Coll. of Physicians of Phila.* (1887).

D. I. Lansing

SMITH, ALONZO de GRATE (July 29, 1890, East Orange, N.J.-October 26, 1970, Washington, D.C.). *Pediatrician.* Son of Greene, blacksmith, and Mary (Baker) Smith. Married Marie Wright, 1928; one child. EDUCATION: 1914-15, Howard University; 1923, B.S., College of the City of New York; 1919, M.D., Long Island Medical College (now Downstate Medical School); 1919-20, intern, Kansas City General Hospital #2; 1932, M.S., Columbia University, (biochemistry); 1935-40, completed classroom requirements for an M.A. in child psychology, Catholic University of America. CAREER: 1920-32, private pediatrics practice, New York City; 1922-32, served for varying periods on pediatrics staffs, Vanderbilt Clinic, Mt. Sinai Hospital, and Harlem Hospital, all in New York City; 1932-56, faculty, Howard University Medical School: 1932-45, associate professor and chief, Division of Pediatrics, Department of Medicine; 1945-56, clinical associate professor of pediatrics; and 1953, clinical professor of pediatrics; 1932-45, pediatrician, Freedmen's Hospital; 1956-70, emeritus associate professor of pediatrics, Howard University College of Medicine. CONTRIBUTIONS: First black, full-time clinician on an American medical faculty (Howard University, 1932). Worked for very low salary at Howard in order to build the school and train black physicians. Started pediatrics residency program at Howard (1935). Started research program in pediatrics at Howard (mid-1930s). Often viewed as the "dean" of black American pediatricians. First black to become diplomate, American Board of Pediatrics (1934). During N.Y. years, was physician to preschool clinic, Association for Improving the Condition of the Poor. Wrote weekly health columns, *New Amsterdam News* (1925-27), *New York Age* (1928-30), and *Afro-American* (1945-47).

WRITINGS: "Rheumatism in Children Under Five Years of Age," *Arch. Ped.* 39 (1922): 799-810; "Incidence of Physical Defects in Negro Children," *J. Negro Ed.* 5 (1937): 393; "Treatment of Rickets with Minimal Viosterol Dosage," *J. Pediat.* 16 (1940): 76. Writings listed in *JNMA* 61 (1969): 358-60. REFERENCES: W. Montague Cobb, "Alonzo de Grate Smith, M.S., M.D., 1890-," *JNMA* 61 (1969): 358-60; *NCAB*, 56: 182-83.

T. L. Savitt

SMITH, ANDREW C. (July 14, 1856, Richland County, Wis.-April 12, 1943, Portland, Oreg.). *Physician; Surgeon.* Son of Patrick C., farmer and ship captain, and Elizabeth (Tully) Smith. Married Anna B. McDonald, 1907; no children. EDUCATION: 1877, M.D., Pacific Medical College; 1888-89, postgraduate study, New York Polyclinic and hospitals: Vienna, Austria; Glasgow, Scotland; Berlin, Germany; and London, England. CAREER: 1877-79, surgeon, U.S. Navy; practice: 1880-87, Amador City, Calif.; and 1890-1943, Portland; 1891-98, county physician, Multnomah County, Oreg.; member: 1901-3, 1915-17, Oreg. legislature; and 1903-27, Oregon State Board of Health. CONTRIBUTIONS: Practiced in several fields of surgery; performed first subtotal thyroidectomy on the Pacific Coast (1896). By 1900, was the outstanding surgeon in Portland if not in the Pacific Northwest. Helped organize the Coffey Hospital, Multnomah County Hospital, and Portland Open Air Sanitarium. One of the first to use X-ray equipment in Oreg. Elected to state senate (1901). Prepared a bill to create a state board of health and county boards of health and succeeded in getting legislature to adopt it (1903). Elected first president of this board and served as a member for 24 years. Under his presidency, board took measures to control smallpox, typhoid fever, and tuberculosis; urged creation of better water supply systems for towns; and took the lead in creating Oregon State Health Association (1906). Urged State Board of Medical Examiners to tighten its standards. Organized financing and construction of Medical Arts Building in Portland (1925).

REFERENCES: *Encyclopedia of Northwest Biog.* (1943), 260-62; H. K. Hines, *An Illustrated History of the State of Oregon* (1893); O. Larsell, *The Doctor in Oregon* (1947).

G. B. Dodds

SMITH, ANDREW HEERMANCE (August 27, 1837, Charlton, N.Y.-April 8, 1910, New York, N.Y.). *Physician; Industrial hygiene.* Son of Archibald and Cornelia Heermance Smith. Married Jane T. Sheldon, 1884. EDUCATION: Undergraduate education, Ballston Spa Institute and Union College; 1858, M.D., College of Physicians and Surgeons (Columbia); postgraduate study, universities of Göttingen and Berlin, Germany. CAREER: 1859-61, practiced medicine, N.Y.; 1861-67, surgeon, U.S. Army; *post* 1868, practiced medicine, N.Y.; medical staff, St. Luke's and Presbyterian hospitals; surgical staff, Manhattan Eye, Ear and Throat Hospital; 1895-1910, vice-president, New York Post Graduate Medical School and Hospital. CONTRIBUTIONS: Discovered the cause of caisson disease and how to prevent it; showed that underwater workers who went from their caissons to the surface without first undergoing decompression developed nitrogen narcosis as a result of moving from an atmosphere of high air pressure to air of ordinary pressure. Did significant research on the therapeutic benefits and dangers of oxygen and compressed air.

WRITINGS: *The Physiological, Pathological and Therapeutical Effects of Compressed Air* (1886); *The Effects of High Atmospheric Pressure, Including the Caisson Disease* (1873). Several of more important writings are listed in Kelly and Burrage. REFERENCES: *JAMA* 14 (Jan.-Jun. 1910): 1396; Kelly and Burrage (1928), 1123; *N.Y. Times*, April 9, 1910; *Who Was Who in Am.*, 1: 1137.

S. Galishoff

SMITH, ASHBEL (August 13, 1805, Hartford, Conn.-January 21, 1886, Galveston Bay, Tex.). *Physician; Public servant.* Son of Moses and Phoebe (Adams) Smith. Never married. EDUCATION: 1824, A.B., Yale, with honors in Greek and Latin; 1824-27, read law and taught high school, Salisbury, N.C.; 1828, M.D., Yale. CAREER: 1828-31, practiced medicine, Salisbury, N.C.; 1831-32, staff, Neckar Hospital, Paris; 1832-37, practice, Salisbury (also newspaper editor);

1837-38, surgeon-general, Tex.; 1839-42, medical practice, Galveston, Tex.; 1842-44, Texas chargé d'affairs to England and France; 1844-45, Tex. secretary of state; and negotiated independence from Mexico; brief service in Mexican War; 1855, elected to Tex. legislature; 1861-65, Civil War, colonel, Confederate Army; 1866, 1878, elected to Tex. legislature; 1881-86, regent, University of Texas, and president, Board of Regents; 1881-82, president, Texas Medical Association (although retired from practice). CONTRIBUTIONS: Pushed for improved sanitation, education, transportation, and fiscal restraint. Short in stature but a giant in service to Tex. Began the process of creating a university for Texans.

WRITINGS: Wrote about cholera in Paris (1832); yellow fever in Galveston (1839); reminiscences of the Tex. Republic (1876); many speeches and treatises, plus active correspondence in the Smith papers, Barker History Center, University of Texas, Austin, Tex. REFERENCES: *BHM* (1964-69), 247; *Biographical Encyclopedia of Texas* (1880); *DAB*, 9, pt. 1: 239-40; *Handbook of Texas* 2 (1952): 620-21; C. D. Leake, in *Yale J. of Biol. and Med.* 20 (Jan. 1948): 225-32; Miller, *BHM*, p. 106; *NCAB*, 10: 160; *Encyclopedia of Southern Hist.* (1979), 1119; S. C. Red, *Biographical Sketch of Ashbel Smith* (1929); writings about Tex. medicine by Pat I. Nixon (q.v.).

J. Morris

SMITH, CLARENCE AUSTIN (January 24, 1861, Derby, Conn.-September 10, 1953). *Physician; Physical therapy; Editor.* Son of Ell Stone and Eliza (Holbrook) Smith. Married Susan Selden Chichester, 1890; four children. EDUCATION: 1882, B.A., Yale University; 1887, M.D., College of Physicians and Surgeons, Columbia University. CAREER: Medical practice, Seattle, Washington; 1897-1898, city health officer, Seattle; 1903-38, editor, *Northwest Medicine*; 1915-25, physician and surgeon, Seattle City Hospital; 1925-31, chief, physical therapy, Seattle City Hospital; *post* 1925, chief, physical therapy, King County Hospital. CONTRIBUTIONS: Editor of *Northwest Medicine* (1903–38). Served as president, King County Medical Society (1898), and Washington State Medical Association (1909).

REFERENCES: *WWAPS* (1938): 1121; *Who's Who in the State of Washington, 1939-40*, 170.

T. L. Savitt

SMITH, FRED M. (May 31, 1888, Yale, Ill.-February 23, 1946, Iowa City, Ia.). *Physician; Internal medicine.* Son of John Alfred and Sarah Ellen (Newlin) Smith. Married Helen Louise Bushee, 1917; three children. EDUCATION; 1914, B.S., University of Chicago; 1914, M.D., Rush Medical College; 1914-16, intern, Presbyterian Hospital, Chicago, Ill.; Rush Medical College: 1916-18, assistant in internal medicine; and 1918-20, associate in internal medicine; 1927, postgraduate study, University of Vienna. CAREER: 1918-19, 1st lieutenant, Medical Corps; 1916-24, medical staff, Presbyterian Hospital, Chicago; 1920-24, faculty, Rush Medical College; 1923-24, medical staff, Evanston Hospital, Evanston, Ill.; 1924-46, professor and head, Department of Theory and Practice of Medicine, State University of Iowa College of Medicine; 1924-46, physician-in-chief, University Hospital, Iowa City; 1937-41, secretary and chairman, Section on Internal Medicine, AMA; 1939-46, editor, *American Heart Journal*; 1942-45, member, Committee on Medicine, Division of Medical Sciences, National Research Council. CONTRIBUTIONS: Conducted important experimental studies in obstruction of the coronary arteries and electrocardiographic research (especially 1918, with James B. Herrick [q.v.], Chicago); played a major role in clinical research in the treatment of coronary artery disease; studied functional disorders of the digestive tract, particularly during the Depression, when there was widespread financial anxiety. Throughout tenure as head of internal medicine at Iowa, actively encouraged faculty interest in clinical research and publishing.

WRITINGS: Among numerous articles and chapters are "The Ligation of Coronary Arteries with Electrocardiographic Study," *Arch. Int. Med.* 22 (1918): 8; "Concerning the Anatomy of the Coronary Arteries," *Am. J. of Med. Sci.* 156 (1918): 706; "Diseases of the Heart and Pericardium," in John Herr Musser, ed., *Internal Medicine, Its Theory and Practice* (1932); "Theophylline in the Treatment of Diseases of Coronary Arteries," *Arch. Int. Med.* 56 (1935): 1250. REFERENCES: Walter L. Bierring, *A History of the Department of Internal Medicine, State University of Iowa College of Medicine, 1870-1958* (1958); *Who Was Who in Am.*, 2: 1943-50; *Who's Important in Med.* (1945); *Who's Who in Am. Med., 1925*; *WWAPS* 1 (1938).

R. E. Rakel

SMITH, HARRY PRATT (February 18, 1895, West Branch, Ia.-April 11, 1972, Columbia, Mo.). *Physician; Pathology*. Son of Walter Z. and Estella M. (Pratt) Smith. Never married. EDUCATION: 1916, A.B., University of California (Berkeley, Calif.); University of California: 1917-19, George Williams Hooper Foundation Fellow; 1918, M.S.; and 1921, M.D.; 1921-23, assistant and instructor in pathology, Johns Hopkins University; 1923-24, National Research Council Fellow in Chemistry, Columbia University and Europe. CAREER: 1924-30, assistant and associate professor, pathology, University of Rochester; 1930-45, professor and head, pathology, State University of Iowa College of Medicine; 1941, received Ward Burdick Award, American Society of Clinical Pathologists; 1945-60, Delafield Professor and head, pathology, College of Physicians and Surgeons, Columbia University; 1945-60, director, pathology service, Presbyterian Hospital, N.Y.; 1960-69, reference librarian and archivist, American Society of Clinical Pathologists, Chicago, Ill.; 1970-72, lecturer and consultant, pathology, University of Missouri; president: 1948, American Society for Experimental Pathology; and 1949, Federation of the American Societies for Experimental Biology and Medicine. CONTRIBUTIONS: As a young man, research in the determination of blood volume at high altitude firmly established that erythrocyte mass is the main contributor to the expanded blood volume (1925) and is still regarded as an important precursor of erythropoietin studies. Other research involved plasma proteins, blood substitutes, bile salt metabolism, vital staining, fibrinogen and thrombin, vitamin K and prothrombin, and hepatic injury. Introduced the basic concept of quantitation in work on blood coagulation and the plasma procoagulants. Work on vitamin K and the correction of the bleeding defect in obstructive jaundice, with related studies in blood coagulation, was recognized by the Burdick Award. Also wrote on the history and clinical practice of pathology and was widely recognized as an outstanding teacher and administrator who believed strongly in multidisciplined research. During "retirement," was an oft-consulted expert on the organizational and "legislative" operation of the AMA. A pioneer in computer applications in clinical pathology.

WRITINGS: Published over 100 professional articles, including "Blood Volume Changes at High Altitudes," *Am. J. of Physiol.* 71 (1925): 395 (with A. E. Belt and H. R. Arnold); "The Titration of Prothrombin in Certain Plasmas," *Arch. Pathol.* 18 (1934): 587 (with E. D. Warner and K. M. Brinkhous); "A Quantitative Study on Blood Clotting: Prothrombin Fluctuations under Experimental Conditions," *Am. J. of Physiol.* 114 (1936): 667 (with E. D. Warner and K. M. Brinkhous); "Bleeding Tendency and Prothrombin Deficiency in Bile Fistula Dogs: Effects of Feeding Bile and Vitamin K," *J. of Experimental Med.* 67 (1938): 911 (with E. D. Warner and K. M. Brinkhous); "Prothrombin Deficiency and the Bleeding Tendency in Obstructive Jaundice and Biliary Fistula. Effect of Feeding Bile and Alfalfa (Vitamin K)," *Am. J. of Med. Sci.* 196 (1938): 50 (with E. D. Warner and K. M. Brinkhous). REFERENCES: *Am. Men of Med.* (1961); Kenneth M. Brinkhous, "Harry P. Smith (1895-1972): Pathologist, Teacher, Investigator, Administrator," *Am. J. Clin. Pathol.* 63 (1975): 605; *JAMA* 221 (Sept. 11, 1972); University of Iowa Archives, Iowa City, Ia.; *WWAPS* 1 (1938); *Who's Important in Med.* (1945).

R. E. Rakel

SMITH, HOMER WILLIAM (January 2, 1895, Denver, Colo.-March 25, 1962, New York, N.Y.). *Physiologist; Renal physiology.* Son of Albert Charles and Margaret E. (Jones) Smith. Married Carlotta Smith, 1921; Margaret Wilson, 1949, one child. EDUCATION: 1917, A.B., University of Denver; 1921, D.Sc., Johns Hopkins University; 1923-25, research fellow in physiology, Harvard Medical School; 1928, 1930, Guggenheim Fellow in Physiology, Africa and Southeast Asia. CAREER: 1917-18, Chemical Warfare Station, American University, Washington, D.C.; 1919, research pharmacologist, Hygienic Laboratory, U.S. Public Health Service, Washington, D.C.; 1921-23, research chemist, Eli Lilly and Company, Indianapolis, Ind.; 1925-28, physiology faculty, University of Virginia; 1928-61, physiology faculty and director, physiological laboratories, New York University College of Medicine; during World War II, member, Chemistry Division, National Defense Research Committee; 1948-51, chairman, National Research Council-Atomic Energy Commission Postdoctoral Fellowship Board in Medical Sciences; associated with: 1930-38, American Museum of Natural History; 1938-62, New York Zoological Society; 1926-62, Mt. Desert Island Biological Laboratory; and 1938-62, Bermuda Biological Station for Research; achieved distinction as a philosophical novelist and evolutionary biologist. CONTRIBUTIONS: One of the leading authorities of his time on renal physiology. Independently of A. N. Richards (q.v.), who was working on the same problem, discovered (1930s) that inulin could be used to measure glomerular filtration rate; led to advances in medical and surgical treatment of kidney and heart diseases. Illuminated functional alterations in renal disease and helped explain how the kidney "clears" creatine, urea, mannitol, sodium, and inulin. Made important studies of differential blood flow in both normal and diseased kidneys and explored the role of the kidneys in hypertension.

WRITINGS: *The Physiology of the Kidney* (1937); "The Measurement of the Tubular Excretory Mass, Effective Blood Flow and Filtration Rate in the Normal Human Kidney," *J. Clin. Invest.* 17 (May 1938): 263-78 (with W. Goldring and H. Chasis); *The Kidney: Structure and Function in Health and Disease* (1951); *Principles of Renal Physiology* (1956). A bibliography is in *BMNAS*. REFERENCES: *BMNAS* 39 (1967): 445-70; H. Chasis and W. Goldring, eds., *Homer William Smith, Sc.D.: His Scientific and Literary Achievements* (1965); *DSB*, 12: 470-71; *NCAB*, 52: 321-22; *N.Y. Times*, March 26, 1962; *Who Was Who in Am.*, 1: 876.

S. Galishoff

SMITH, JAMES McCUNE (April 18, 1813, New York, N.Y.-November 17, 1865, Williamsburg, L.I., N.Y.). *Physician.* Son of a slave freed by N.Y. Emancipation Act and a self-emancipated bondswoman. Married; five children. EDUCATION: African Free School, New York City; University of Glasgow, Scotland: 1835, B.A.; 1836, M.A.; and 1837, M.D.; 1837, studied at Paris Hospital clinics. CAREER: 1838-63, medical practice, New York City. CONTRIBUTIONS: First black with a medical degree to practice in United States. In addition to practicing medicine, lectured and wrote in support of abolition of slavery and black equality. Answered John C. Calhoun's and others' attacks on black health and insanity, especially after 1840 census report of supposed high rate of black lunacy. Showed this data to be false and misleading. Attacked arguments about small size and weight of Negro brain with information based on his knowledge of medicine. First black to operate a pharmacy in United States (New York City, 1838). Served for 20 years on medical staff of Free Negro Orphan Asylum, New York City.

WRITINGS: "On the Haitian Revolution with a Sketch of the Character of Toussaint L'Overture" (1841), 28 pp., available in Henry P. Slaughter Collection, Atlanta University Library, Atlanta, Ga.; "On the Influence of Opium upon the Catamenial Functions," *N.Y. J. of Med.* 2 (1844): 57-58; "The Influence of Climate on Longevity: With Special Reference to Life Insurance," *Hunt's Merchants' Magazine* 14 (1846): 319-29, 402-19; "Lay Puffery of Homeopathy," *The Annalist* 2 (1847-48): 348-51; "Facts Concerning Free Negroes" [The Memorial of 1844 to the United Senate], in Herbert Aptheker, *Documentary History of the Negro People in the U.S.* 1 (1951): 238-43. Many writings are listed in *DAB*, 9: 288-89. REFERENCES: Benjamin G. Brawley, *The Negro Genius* (1937), 44-46; W. Montague Cobb, "James M. Smith," *JNMA* 44 (1952): 160; *DAB*, 9: 288-89; Guido Furman, M.D., "Obituary of James McCune Smith," *The Medical Register of the City of New York for the Year Commencing June 1, 1866*, pp. 201-4; Arthur A. Schomburg, "James McCune Smith," *Negro Hist. Bull.* 9 (1945): 41-42.

L. A. Falk and T. L. Savitt

SMITH, JOB LEWIS (October 15, 1827, Onondaga County, N.Y. (near Syracuse, N.Y.)-June 9, 1897, New York, N.Y.). *Physician; Pediatrics.* Son of Lewis, a farmer active in the political life of Onondaga County, and Chloe (Benson) Smith. Married Mary Anne (Hannah) Smith, 1858; eight children.

EDUCATION: 1849, B.A., Yale College; 1849-50, entered medical apprenticeship; 1853, M.D., College of Physicians and Surgeons (New York City); 1853, curator, Nursery and Child's Hospital; CAREER: 1853-97, private practice; 1858, established a children's clinic, Northwestern Dispensary; 1860, attending physician in charge of infants and sick children, Charity Hospitals of New York; 1861, lecturer in morbid anatomy, Bellevue Hospital Medical College; 1869, appointed attending physician, Infant Asylum of New York; 1871-72, professor of morbid anatomy, Bellevue Medical College; 1876-96, clinical professor of diseases of children, Bellevue; in American Pediatric Society: 1888, founder; 1889, elected second president. CONTRIBUTIONS: Helped establish the study of the diseases of infants and children in America. A staunch advocate of preventive medicine in pediatrics. Incorporated own observations and experiences in a textbook, *A Treatise on the Diseases of Infancy and Childhood* (1869), which passed through eight editions in the next 27 years. Clinical and teaching skills led to recognition as one of America's leading pediatricians, a position he shared with Abraham Jacobi (q.v.). Served on the staffs of eight major New York City hospitals.

WRITINGS: *A Treatise on the Diseases of Infants and Children* (1869); "Scarlatinal Nephritis," *Trans., Am. Pediat. Soc.* 3 (1892): 201-14; "The Etiology of Tetanus Neonatorum,"*ibid.*, 6 (1894): 143-48. REFERENCES: *DAB*, 9, pt. 1: 293-94; Eliot Ellsworth, "Memorial to Job Lewis Smith," *N.Y. Acad. of Med., Trans.*, 2nd series, 13 (1897): 220; S. X. Radbill, "Job Lewis Smith: New York Pioneer of Pediatrics," *Episteme* 8 (1974): 339-58; J. Shrady, "Memoir of J. Lewis Smith," *Trans., N.Y. State Med. Assoc.* 14 (1897): 524.

                                                                                      T. E. Cone, Jr.

SMITH, LYNDON ARNOLD (November 11, 1795, Haverhill, N.H.-December 15, 1865, Newark, N.J.). *Physician.* Son of Ethan, minister, and Bathsheba (Sanford) Smith. Married Frances Louisa Griffin, 1823; six children. EDUCATION: Common schools, Hopkinton, N.H.; Phillips Exeter Academy; 1817, A.B., Dartmouth College; 1822, M.D., Dartmouth Medical School. CAREER: Private practice: 1822-27, Williamstown, Mass.; and 1827-65, Newark. CONTRIBUTIONS: As the president of the Medical Society of New Jersey (1837), provided the stimulus and was largely responsible (in cooperation with Dorothea Dix [q.v.]) for the state legislature establishing (1845) the State Hospital at Trenton, the first mental hospital in N.J. REFERENCES: J. Q. Bittinger, *History of Haverhill, N.H.* (1888), 223; J. Henry Clark, *The Medical Men of New Jersey, in Essex District, from 1666 to 1866* (1867), 61-62; *Daily Advertiser* (Newark), December 15, 16, 19, 20, 1865; "The New Jersey Lunatic Asylum," *N.J. Med. Rep.* 1 (1848): 111-16, 504; "New Jersey Lunatic Asylum," *ibid.*, 2 (1849): 128-30; "Our State Institutions," *J. of the Med. Soc. of New Jersey.* 13 (1916): 303-4; Fred B. Rogers, "Lyndon A. Smith: Prime Mover for Mental Hospitals," *ibid.*, 63 (1966): 29-30.

                                                                                          W. Barlow

SMITH, MARGARET G. (February 10, 1896, Carnegie, Pa.-May 1, 1970, St. Louis, Mo.) *Pathologist.* Daughter of William Smith, machine shop foreman.

EDUCATION: 1918, A.B., Mount Holyoke College; 1922, M.D., Johns Hopkins. CAREER: At Johns Hopkins Medical School: 1922-23, assistant in pathology; 1923-26, instructor in pathology; and 1926-29, associate in pathology; at Washington University School of Medicine: 1929-43, assistant professor in pathology; 1953-57, associate professor of pathology; 1957-64, professor of pathology; and 1964-70, professor emeritus and lecturer in pathology. CONTRIBUTIONS: Prominent in infectious disease pathology, was best known for work in isolating the St. Louis encephalitis and salivary gland viruses. First to propagate the herpes simplex virus in a mouse and first to discover the cytomegetic inclusion disease virus.

WRITINGS: "Tumors of Islands of Langerhans and Hypoglycemia," *Am. J. of Path.* 7 (1931): 723-39 (with M. G. Seibel); "Isolation of St. Louis Encephalitis Virus During Inter and Epidemic Periods," *Proc. Soc. for Experimental Biol. Med.* 37 (1937): 288-90 (with H. McCordock and E. Moore); "Isolation of the Virus of Herpes Simplex and the Demonstration of Intranuclear Inclusions in a Case of Acute Encephalitis," *Am. J. of Path.* 17 (1941): 55-68 (with E. Lennette and H. Reames); M. G. Smith, "Propagation in Tissue Cultures of a Cytopathogenic Virus from Human Salivary Gland Virus Disease," *Proc., Soc. for Experimental Biol. & Med.* 92 (1956): 424-30. REFERENCES: *JAMA* 214 (1970): 159.

M. Hunt

SMITH, MORGAN (March 8, 1868, Union County, Ark.-September 14, 1935, Little Rock, Ark.). *Physician; Pediatrics.* Son of James Monroe, farmer, and Mary Josephine (Morgan) Smith. Married Mrs. Henri Ellen Schulenberger, 1891; two stepdaughters. EDUCATION: 1889, M.D., Department of Medicine of Arkansas Industrial University; 1904, postgraduate study, Tulane University medical department. CAREER: Private practice: 1889-96, Hillsboro, Ark.; 1896-1904, Eldorado, Ark.; and 1904-35, Little Rock, Ark.; at University of Arkansas Department of Medicine: 1904-35, pediatrics faculty; and 1912-23, 1924-27, dean; 1909-11, state director, Rockefeller Commission for the Eradication of Hookworm Disease; 1913-14, State Health Officer. CONTRIBUTIONS: Supported higher standards of medical practice and education as editor, *Monthly Bulletin of the Arkansas Medical Society* (1907-9), the society's secretary (1907-11), and its president (1911-12). Drafted an amendment to a medical practice act adopted in 1907 to require graduation from a recognized medical school as a prerequisite to examination by the state licensing board. Served in the Arkansas House of Representatives (1929-34), where he amended and maneuvered a bill to successful passage that required a preliminary examination in all basic sciences for licensure of applicants in all fields of medical practice, including osteopathy and chiropractic. Wrote the health code embodied in the 1913 act creating a State Board of Health for Ark. As first state health officer, established the operational procedures for the State Board of Health, including a Bureau of Vital Statistics. As dean, University of Arkansas Department of Medicine, raised the premedical requirements to two years of college and persuaded the University of Arkansas to establish a premedical program, obtained use of several Little Rock hospitals for clinical experience, extended the school term to nine months, promoted greater reliance on faculty committees, and obtained an A rating from the AMA Council on Medical Education. Successfully promoted the establishment of the Arkansas State Pediatric Society as last major accomplishment (1935). REFERENCES: W. David Baird, *Medical Education in Arkansas* (1979), 89-90, 105-11; Dallas T. Herndon, *Centennial History of Arkansas* 3 (1922): 1023; *NCAB*, 27: 378.

D. Konold

SMITH, NATHAN (September 30, 1762, Rehoboth, Mass.-January 26, 1829, New Haven, Conn.). *Physician; Surgeon.* Son of John, farmer, and Elizabeth (Ide, Hills) Smith. Married Elizabeth Chase, 1791, and Sarah Hall Chase, 1794; ten children. EDUCATION: District schools, Chester, Vt.; 1783, studied Latin and Greek with Rev. Whiting, Rockingham, Vt.; 1784-87, apprenticed to Dr. Joshua Goodhue, Putney, Vt.; 1790, B.M., Harvard College; 1796-97, studied medicine, Edinburgh and Glasgow, Scotland; and London, England. CAREER: 1787-89, 1790-96, practiced medicine, Cornish, N.H.; 1797-1813, professor of anatomy, surgery, and chemistry, Dartmouth College, and carried on a practice as physician, surgeon, and consultant, central New England; 1813-28, professor of surgery and obstetrics, Yale Medical School. CONTRIBUTIONS: Founder, Dartmouth College Medical School. Devised a plan for a professorship of medicine and studied in England and Scotland for a year to fit himself for the post (1797). At Dartmouth, was the entire medical faculty, occasionally assisted by Lyman Spalding (q.v.) and Cyrus Perkins. President, New Hampshire State Medical Society (1811). When the Yale Medical School was established (1813), was appointed professor of surgery and obstetrics after he "renounced" his religious "infidelity." Largely instrumental in the school obtaining a $200,000 appropriation from the Conn. legislature. Performed the second ovariotomy in the United States (1821). Found time to assist in the founding of the medical school, Bowdoin College (1821), and to lecture there each summer until 1826, and at the University of Vermont, where his son Nathan Ryno (q.v.) was developing a department of medicine.

WRITINGS: *Practical Essay on Typhus Fever* (1824). *Medical and Surgical Memoirs* (1831). Co-editor of the *American Medical Review* (1824-26). REFERENCES: *BHM*, (1964-69), 247; (1975-79), 119; *DAB*, 9, pt. 1: 324-27; Samuel C. Harvey, "The Education of Nathan Smith," *Yale J. of Bio. and Med.* 1 (May 1929): 259-68; idem, "Surgery of the Past in Connecticut," in Herbert Thoms, ed., *Heritage of Connecticut Medicine* (1942), 172-80; Oliver S. Hayward, M.D., "Dr. Nathan Smith (1762-1829), American Pioneer," *New England J. of Med.* 261 (Sept. 3, 1959): 489-94; idem, "A Search for the Real Nathan Smith," *J. Hist. Med.* 15 (Jul. 1960): 268-81; idem, "Nathan Smith (1762-1829), Politician," *New England J. of Med.* 263, nos. 24, 25 (Dec. 15, 22, 1960): 1235-42, 1288-91; Kelly and Burrage (1920); Gustaf E. Linskog, M.D., "Yale's First Professor of Surgery: Nathan Smith, M.D. (1762-1829)," *Surgery* 64, no. 2 (Aug. 1968): 524-28; Miller, *BHM*, p. 107; *NCAB*, 3: 153.

J. W. Ifkovic

SMITH, NATHAN RYNO (May 21, 1797, Cornish, N.H.-July 3, 1877, Baltimore, Md.). *Surgeon; Teacher.* Son of Nathan (q.v.), physician, and Sarah

Hall (Chase) Smith. Married Juliette Octavia Penniman, 1824; eight children. EDUCATION: First educated by tutors and then went to Dartmouth; Yale: 1817, A.B.; and 1823, M.D. (where he studied under his father); winters of 1825 and 1826, postgraduate work, University of Pennsylvania Medical School. CAREER: 1817-19, tutor, Fauquier County, Va., for the Thomas Turner family; 1824, began practice of surgery, Burlington, Vt.; 1825, professor of surgery and anatomy, medical department, University of Vermont; 1825-26, co-editor, *The American Medical Review* (Philadelphia, Pa.); 1825-27, professor of anatomy, Jefferson Medical College (Philadelphia); 1827-28, editor, *Philadelphia Monthly Journal of Medicine and Surgery*; at University of Maryland: 1827-38, 1841-70, surgery faculty; 1828-29, 1841, dean; and 1870-72, president, medical and chirurgical faculty; 1830-31, editor, *Baltimore Monthly Journal of Medicine and Surgery*; 1832, co-editor, *New York Medical Journal*; 1838-41, professor of the practice of medicine, Transylvania University, Lexington, Ky. CONTRIBUTIONS: A founder, medical department, University of Vermont (1824). With Dr. George McClellan (q.v.), helped establish Jefferson Medical College, Philadelphia (c. 1826). Founded *Philadelphia Monthly Journal of Medicine and Surgery* (1827), which merged (1828) with *American Journal of the Medical Sciences*. Began *Baltimore Monthly Journal of Medicine and Surgery* (1830). Invented the lithotome, an instrument used to perform vesical lithotomy (news of the apparatus was first published in *Medical and Surgical Memoirs*, 1831). Early innovator in surgical removal of the thyroid gland (did first thyroidectomy, 1835). Invented the anterior suspensory apparatus or anterior splint for thigh and leg fractures.

WRITINGS: *Medical and Surgical Memoirs* [of Nathan Smith including Nathan R. Smith's own memoirs] (1831); *Surgical Anatomy of the Arteries* (1832; 2d ed., 1835); *Treatment of Fractures of the Lower Extremity, by the Use of the Anterior Suspensory Apparatus* (1867); writings listed in *Kelly's Encyclopedia of Medical Sources*, p. 380; E. F. Cordell, *The Medical Annals of Maryland* (1903), 573-74; and *Index Catalogue*, 1st series, 13: 217. REFERENCES: George H. Callcott, *A History of the University of Maryland* (1982), 117; Samuel Clagett Chew, "Essays Commemorative of Professor Nathan Ryno Smith. . .," *Maryland Med. J.* 3 (Sept. 1878): 407-30; E. F. Cordell, *Historical Sketch of the University of Maryland School of Medicine & The Medical Annals of Maryland* (1891), 573-74; *DAB*, 9: 327-29; S. D. Gross, *Autobiography* 1 (1887): 385-87; Oliver S. Hayward, "Three American Anatomy Letters (1817-1830)," *Bull. Hist. Med.* 38, no. 4 (Jul.-Aug. 1964): 377-78; Kelly and Burrage (1928), 1135-37; Richard A. Leonardo, *Lives of Master Surgeons* (1948), 402-3; Alexius McGlannan, "The Surgical and Anatomical Works of Nathan Ryno Smith," *U. of Md. Bull. of the School of Med.* 9 (Apr. 1925); *NCAB*, 3: 154; E. A. Smith, *The Life and Letters of Nathan Smith (1914)*; *Who Was Who in Am.*, Hist. Vol.: 563.

C. Donegan

SMITH, PETER (February 6, 1753, probably N.J.-December 31, 1816, Donnel's Creek, Ohio.). *Itinerant preacher; Farmer; "Indian doctor."* Son of Hezekiah, "Indian doctor," and Sarah Smith. Married Catherine Stout, 1776; 12 children. EDUCATION: Reported to have studied medicine under his father; purported attendance at and graduation from the College of New Jersey (Princeton).

CAREER: Itinerant preacher and practitioner of medicine; c. 1780, left N.J. and claimed to have learned much in travels from German physicians and other practitioners of medicine; evidence of some familiarity with Culpeper, Tissot, Rush, and Brown; first settled in Ga. and then in Ohio, which he reached about 1794, and where he continued to preach and practice medicine. CONTRIBUTIONS: As an "Indian doctor," relied mainly on herbs, roots, and other remedies known to the Indians. *Indian Doctor's Dispensatory* is said to be the first medical book published west of the Alleghenies and is one of the leading examples of American folk medicine that found its way into print. Used common and local names for his botanicals, and many cannot be identified with certainty. The book has a claim to scientific fame in that Rafinesque cited it.

WRITINGS: *The Indian Doctor's Dispensatory, Being Father Smith's Advice Respecting Diseases and Their Cure* (1813). REFERENCES: O. Juettner, "Peter Smith, The Indian Doctor: An Historical Sketch," *Ohio State Med. J.* 11 (1915): 90-99; J. U. Lloyd, "Biography of Peter Smith," in P. Smith, *The Indian Doctor's Dispensatory*, in *Lloyd Lib., Bull. No. 2* (1901), reproduction series, no. 2; P. Smith's "Preface," in his *The Indian Doctor's Dispensatory* (1813); S. S. Smith, "Peter Smith of Jamaica, Long Island, and Some of His Descendants," *N.Y. Genealogical and Biographical Record* 85 (1954): 92, 95, 156; S. S. Smith, "Some Connections of Hezekiah Smith of Newton, Hanover and Piscataway," *Genealogical Mag. N.J.* 22 (1947): 73-78.

D. L. Cowen

SMITH, PHILIP EDWARD (January 1, 1884, DeSmet, S.D.-December 8, 1970, Florence, Mass.). *Anatomist; Endocrinology.* Son of John E., Congregational minister, and Lydia Elmina (Stratton) Smith. Married Irene Patchett, 1913; two children. EDUCATION: 1908, B.S., Pomona College; Cornell University: 1910, M.S.; and 1912, Ph.D. (anatomy). CAREER: 1908-9, employed as entomologist, southern Calif.; anatomy faculty: 1910-12, Cornell University; 1912-26, University of California (Berkeley, Calif.); 1926-27, Stanford University; and 1927-52, College of Physicians and Surgeons (Columbia); 1956-63, research associate, Stanford University; president: 1937-38, Society for Experimental Biology and Medicine; 1938-40, Harvey Society; 1939-40, Association for Study of Endocrine Glands; 1940-42, American Association of Anatomists. CONTRIBUTIONS: Developed a surgical procedure for the removal of the hypophysis (pituitary gland) without causing brain damage. Demonstrated that hypophysectomy in mammals caused cessation of growth; loss of weight; and atrophy of the reproductive system, thyroid gland, and adrenal cortex. Showed that symptoms could be reversed by daily implants of material derived from anterior pituitary extracts.

WRITINGS: "The Pigmentary Growth and Endocrine Disturbances Induced in the Anuran Tadpole by the Early Ablation of the Pars Buccalis of the Hypophysis," *Am. Anatomical Memoirs* 11 (1920): 1-151; "The Induction of Precocious Sexual Maturity by Pituitary Homotransplants," *Am. J. of Physiol.* 80 (1927): 114-25; "Experimental Evidence Regarding the Role of the Anterior Pituitary in the Development and Regulation of the Genital System," *Am. J. of Anatomy* 40 (1927): 159-217 (with E. T. Engle); "Hypophysectomy and Replacement Therapy in the Rat," ibid., 45 (1930): 205-73. A compilation of most important writings is in *DSB*. REFERENCES: *DSB*, 12: 472-77; *N.Y. Times*, December 9, 1970; *Who Was Who in Am.*, 5: 674.

S. Galishoff

SMITH, RELLIFORD STILLMON (November 30, 1889, Americus, Ga.-June 28, 1965, Washington, D.C.). *Physician; Venereal disease; Obstetrics-gynecology.* Son of Dennis and Mollie (Daniels) Smith. Married Gertrude Savage, 1920 (d. 1946), some children; Cynthiabelle Blacke Gordon, 1947, no children. EDUCATION: c. 1910, B.S., Shaw University; 1910-14, Leonard Medical College; 1914, M.D., University of West Tennessee Medical College (Memphis); 1916, M.D., Meharry Medical College; postgraduate courses: 17 years, Medical College of Georgia; 1931-32, Grady Hospital (Emory University Medical School); 1935-41, Gynecology and Venereal Disease courses, University of Georgia; 1938, three-month venereal disease course, Howard University; 1939, two-month course in surgery and treatment of neurosyphilis, Mayo Clinic. CAREER: 1916-18, private medical practice, Americus (passed state licensing exams in Ga., S.C., Md., D.C.); 1918-19, assistant regimental surgeon, U.S. Army Medical Corps, Camp Wheeler, Macon, Ga.; 1919-65, private practice, Macon. CONTRIBUTIONS: Pioneer black physician of Ga. who continued medical education throughout career despite racial and financial barriers. Owing to perseverance and hard labor, gained local, state, and national recognition as a medical practitioner and efficient civil rights worker for physicians. Obtained funds from U.S. Public Health Service to allow southern black physicians to attend postgraduate venereal disease courses at Howard (1938). Organized and directed for eight years Venereal Disease Clinic at Macon-Bibb County Hospital. Active in NMA: president (1958-59); vice-president, Board of Trustees (six years); chair, Budget Committee (three years); Judicial Council (six years); House of Delegates (24 years). Considered one of NMA's best presidents owing to excellent sense of organization and numerous innovations and hard work. Served as president, Macon Academy of Medicine, Dentistry and Pharmacy and Georgia State Medical Association of Physicians and Pharmacists. Constantly supported efforts to break down racial barriers in the South. Was immediately admitted to Bibb County Medical Society when changed rules permitted integration (1965). REFERENCES: W. Montague Cobb, "Relliford Stillmon Smith, M.D., 1889-1965," *JNMA* 58 (1966): 145-47; *WWICA* 7 (1950): 477-78.

T. L. Savitt

SMITH, STEPHEN (February 19, 1823, Skaneateles, N.Y.-August 26, 1922, Montour Falls, N.Y.). *Surgeon; Sanitary reformer.* Son of Lewis, farmer and member, N.Y. State Assembly, and Chloe Benson Smith. Married Lucie Culver, 1858; nine children. EDUCATION: Cortland Academy, Homer, N.Y.; Geneva Medical College; Buffalo Medical College; College of Physicians and Surgeons, N.Y., M.D., 1850; 1850-52, house officer, Bellevue Hospital. CAREER: 1854-96, attending surgeon, Bellevue Hospital; at *New York Journal of Medicine*: 1853-57, assistant editor; and 1857-60, editor; 1860-64, editor, *American Med-*

ical Times; at Bellevue Hospital Medical College: 1861-65, professor of principles of surgery; and 1865-72, professor of anatomy; member: 1868-75, Metropolitan Board of Health, N.Y.; 1879-83, National Board of Health; and 1881-82, 1888-1918, New York State Board of Charities; 1882-88, state commissioner in lunacy, N.Y.; 1894, delegate, International Sanitary Conference, Paris. CONTRIBUTIONS: Extensive writing and editing and long surgical teaching career made him a leading late nineteenth-century American surgeon. Active in promulgating the doctrine of antisepsis in surgery (1870s) and developed an improved technique for amputation of the leg. Organized efforts for passage of the Metropolitan Health Bill in New York City (1866). Later an active member of the board. Principal founder, American Public Health Association (1872), and its first president (1872-74). As commissioner in lunacy, N.Y., introduced training schools for hospital attendants and was responsible for the State Care Act of 1890 that removed responsibility for the mentally ill to state hospitals and out of county almshouses. Actively supported the founding of the Nursing School, Bellevue Hospital (1873). President, New York Medical Association (1892). An authority on hospitals—designed the Roosevelt Hospital in New York City (1866), actively promoted Bellevue Hospital improvements, and was one of five authorities invited to submit plans for the Johns Hopkins Hospital (1875).

WRITINGS: Published several score articles in medical journals (1851-1917). Pocket-size *Handbook of Surgical Operations* (1862) was widely used by the Union Forces. *Doctor in Medicine* (1872) was a collection of his editorials from the *American Medical Times*. Published a large text (1879), *Manual of the Principles and Practice of Operative Surgery*, revised and enlarged (1887). *The City That Was* (1911) described long efforts to improve the health conditions of New York City, and *Who is Insane* described work in the care of the mentally ill. REFERENCES: Gert H. Brieger, "Sanitary Reform in New York City: Stephen Smith and the Passage of the Metropolitan Health Bill," *Bull. Hist. Med.* 40 (Sept.-Oct. 1966): 407-29; John Duffy, *History of Public Health in New York City* (1968-74). Biographical sketches appear in most biographical dictionaries.

G. H. Brieger

SMITH, THEOBALD (July 31, 1859, Albany, N.Y.-December 10, 1934, New York, N.Y.). *Physician; Microbiology; Comparative pathology; Immunology.* Son of Philip, tailor, and Theresa (Kexel) Smith. Married Lillian Hillyer Egleston, 1888; three children. EDUCATION: 1881, Ph.B., Cornell University; 1883, M.D., Albany Medical College. CAREER: 1884-95, director, pathology laboratory, Bureau of Animal Industry, Department of Agriculture; 1886-95, bacteriology faculty, Columbian (later George Washington) University; 1895-1915, director, antitoxin laboratory, Massachusetts State Board of Health; at Harvard University: 1895-96, applied zoology faculty; and 1896-1915, comparative pathology faculty; at Rockefeller Institute for Medical Research (later Rockefeller University): *post* 1901, member, Board of Scientific Directors; 1924-33, vice-president; 1933-34, president; and 1914-29, director, Department of Animal Pathology; president: 1903, Society of American Bacteriologists; 1925, National Tuberculosis Association; and 1928, Congress of American Physicians and Surgeons. CONTRIBUTIONS: Determined the etiology of numerous diseases of man and animals and is considered by many to have been America's greatest bacteriologist. Established one of the first departments of bacteriology in an American medical school at Columbian University (1886). With Daniel E. Salmon (q.v.), differentiated hog cholera from swine plague and found the bacillus responsible for each disease (1889-91); was later shown by others that the bacillus found in hog cholera is a secondary invader and that the disease has a viral origin. Demonstrated that the injection of heat-killed cholera bacilli conferred immunity against the disease, thereby preparing the way for the preparation of other dead vaccines. In most important work, showed that Tex. cattle fever was spread by ticks; was first proof of the role of insects in transmitting disease (1888-93); led to the identification of mosquito and other anthropod vectors of human disease. Differentiated between human and bovine tubercle bacilli and convinced adversaries, notably Robert Koch, that bovine tuberculosis was communicable to man (1896-98). Observed anaphylaxsis in guinea pigs that had received a second injection of antitoxin that, for many years, was referred to as the "Theobald Smith phenomenon" (1904). Made important studies of parasitology in animals; proved that "blackhead" in turkeys was caused by a protozoa transmitted by an intestinal worm parasite and did the first work on coccidiosis in cattle. In addition, did important immunological research, improved the production of smallpox vaccine and antitoxins for diphtheria and tetanus, developed methods of culturing bacteria, and established techniques for the bacteriological examination of milk, water, and sewage.

WRITINGS: *Hog Cholera; Its History, Nature and Treatment* (1889, with D. E. Salmon and F. L. Kilborne); *Special Report on the Cause and Prevention of Swine Plague* (1891); *Investigations into the Nature, Causation, and Prevention of Texas or Southern Cattle Fever* (1893, with F. L. Kilborne); "The Relation between Bovine and Human Tuberculosis," *Med. News* 80 (1902): 343-46; *Parasitism and Disease* (1934). Bibliography is in *BMNAS* 17 (1936): 261-303. REFERENCES: *BHM* (1970-74), 161; P. F. Clark, "T. Smith. . ." *J. Hist. Med.* 14: 490-514; *DAB*, Supplement 1: 665-67; *DSB*, 12: 480-86; Miller, *BHM*, p. 107; *NCAB*, 35: 5-6; *Who Was Who in Am.*, 1: 1149.

S. Galishoff

SMITH, THOMAS JEFFERSON (April 21, 1841, Mannington, N.J. June 14, 1932, Bridgeton, N.J.). *Physician*. Son of Peter, farmer, and Elizabeth (Ellett) Smith. Married Mary G. Glover, 1871; no children. EDUCATION: Salem (N.J.) Academy; Williams College: 1862, A.B.; and 1865, M.A.; apprentice to Dr. Quinton Gibbon and Dr. H. Lenox Hodge (Philadelphia, Pa.); 1866, M.D., University of Pennsylvania Medical School; did postgraduate work in obstetrics under Dr. Edward A. Spooner (Philadelphia). CAREER: Private practice: 1867-69, Camden, N.J.; 1869-1930s, Bridgeton; medical staff, Bridgeton Hospital; 1883-91, editor, *Transactions of the Medical Society of New Jersey*; 1896, president, Medical Society of New Jersey; member, Board of Directors, New Jersey Training School for Feeble Minded Children; medical director, Cumberland County (N.J.) Hospital for the Insane; member, Board of Managers, New

Jersey State Village for Epileptics. CONTRIBUTIONS: Largely responsible for the N.J. State legislature establishing (1898) the New Jersey State Village for Epileptics. REFERENCES: *J. of the Med. Soc. of New Jersey* 29 (1932): 616; Francis Bazley Lee, ed., *Genealogical and Memorial History of the State of New Jersey* 3 (1910): 850-51; "New Jersey State Village for Epileptics, Skillman, N.J.," *J. of the Med. Soc. of New Jersey* 13 (1916): 310; Irving A. Watson, *Physicians and Surgeons of Am.* (1896), 802-3.

W. Barlow

SMITH, WARREN GEORGE (December 29, 1883, Tully, Onandaga County, N.Y.-December 1, 1954, Carlsbad, N.Mex.). *General practitioner*. Son of Norman Murphy, teacher, and Ida Elizabeth (Morrison) Smith, a music teacher. Married Alma Elizabeth Arnold, R.N., 1915; five children. EDUCATION: 1905, M.D., Cornell University Medical School; 1906, internship, St. Elizabeth's Hospital, Newark, N.J. CAREER: 1906, went to N.Mex. to recover from tuberculosis; practiced in the N.Mex. mining areas of Santa Fe, Pecos, Las Vegas, Mora, and Terrado; 1925-40, company doctor, American Metals (mining) Company; 1940 to death, practiced, potash mining area of Carlsbad, N.Mex.; was known as the medical practitioner who traveled by buckboard. CONTRIBUTIONS: As medical career was spent in the mining areas, became involved in treatment of work-related ailments such as black lung and other respiratory pulmonary diseases. They were problems from which he, himself, also suffered. Tended to the accident victims of the mining industry. Also delivered babies, did minor surgery, and performed other "routine" medical services demanded of rural doctors who had to be jacks-of-all-trades. With a Dr. Milne, worked on legislation that eventually required mandatory inoculation against prevalent smallpox and diphtheria, as well as tetanus and pertussis. Served as the elected representative from the northern counties of N.Mex. in the state legislature (1926-28), thereby representing in the political arena the people whom he knew intimately as patients in his practice. REFERENCES: Interviews with son, Daniel F. Smith, M.D., and daughter-in-law, Jean Smith.

C. L. Cutter

SNOW, EDWIN MILLER (May 8, 1820, Pomfret, Vt.-December 22, 1888, Providence, R.I.). *Physician; Public health*. Son of Nathan and Rhoda (Miller) Snow. Married Anna E. W. Pike, 1850; five children. EDUCATION: Brown University: 1845, graduated; and 1848, A.M.; 1849, M.D., College of Physicians and Surgeons (Columbia). CAREER: 1849, practiced medicine, Holyoke, Mass.; in Providence: *post* 1850, practiced medicine; 1855-88, city registrar; and 1856-88, superintendent of health; member for 26 years, [R.I.] State Registration Committee; Civil War, special inspector, Union Army General Hospitals; 1872, U.S. delegate, International Statistical Congress, St. Petersburg, Russia; 1876, president, American Public Health Association; on State Board of Charities and Correction: state prison inspector, quarantine officer, and member. CONTRIBUTIONS: America's first professional public health officer. Inaugurated an extensive program of sanitary reform in Providence. One of the nation's foremost authorities on the collection and use of vital statistics; city and state registration reports set a standard of excellence for American reformers. A leader and early president, American Public Health Association.

WRITINGS: *Statistics and Causes of Asiatic Cholera. . .*(1855). Most important writings are in *Annual Reports of the Superintendent of Health of Providence* (1856-88). REFERENCES: William B. Atkinson, *Physicians and Surgeons of the U.S.* (1878), 375; James H. Cassedy, "Edwin Miller Snow: An Important American Public Health Pioneer," *Bull. Hist. Med.* 35 (Mar.-Apr. 1961): 156-62; *NCAB*, 13: 285.

S. Galishoff

SNOW, WILLIAM FREEMAN (July 13, 1874, Quincy, Ill.-June 12, 1950, Bangor, Maine). *Physician; Public health administrator.* Son of William, grocery store owner, and Emily M. (Streeter) Snow. Married Blanche Malvina Boring, 1899; two children. EDUCATION: Stanford University: 1896, B.A.; and 1897, M.A.; 1900, M.D., Cooper Medical College (later part of Stanford University); 1901-2, studied ophthalmology, Johns Hopkins. CAREER: *Post* 1903, practiced medicine, Palo Alto, Calif.; at Stanford University: 1902-9, hygiene faculty; and 1909-19, hygiene and public health faculty; early 1900s, deputy county health officer and voluntary epidemiologist, State Board of Health; 1909-14, secretary and executive officer, California State Board of Health; in American Social Hygiene Association: *post* 1914, general secretary (later general director); 1940, chairman, Executive Committee; and 1944, chairman, Board of Directors; 1917-19, secretary, general medical board, Council of National Defense; chairman: 1918, Committee on Civilian Cooperation in Combatting Venereal Diseases, Council of National Defense; and 1918-22, Executive Committee, U.S. Interdepartmental Social Hygiene Board; 1920-26, lecturer in hygiene, Johns Hopkins School of Hygiene and Public Health; 1924-28, chairman, League of Nations Committee to Study Traffic in Women and Children; 1927-34, president, National Health Council; 1928-40, lecturer in health education, Columbia University; 1930-36, lecturer in preventive medicine, New York University; *post* 1936, special consultant, U.S. Public Health Service; president: 1912-13, Association of State and Provincial Boards of Health; and 1946-50, International Union against the Venereal Diseases. CONTRIBUTIONS: Directed the social hygiene movement from just before World War I to the late 1930s. Sought to change American attitudes toward venereal disease from a hidden sin to a serious public health problem to be dealt with openly and scientifically. Believed that both medical science and moral persuasion were needed in dealing with the problem. Devoted efforts to educate the public and to coordinate the work of voluntary public health organizations, especially the American Social Hygiene Association and government agencies established to combat venereal disease. During World War I, persuaded the armed forces to attempt to prevent the spread of gonorrhea and syphilis by forbidding prostitution in and around army camps and by providing moral education and wholesome recreational activities for servicemen.

WRITINGS: *The Venereal Diseases: Their Medical, Nursing, and Community Aspects* (1924). REFERENCES: *DAB*, Supplement 4, 758-59; Miller, *BHM*, p. 107; *NCAB*, 39: 262-63; *Who Was Who in Am.*, 3: 802.

S. Galishoff

SOLIS-COHEN, JACOB DaSILVA (February 28, 1838, New York, N.Y.- December 22, 1927, Philadelphia, Pa.). *Physician; Laryngology.* Son of Myer David and Judith Simiah (DaSilva Solis) Cohen. Married Miriam Binswanger, 1875; nine children. EDUCATION: 1860, M.D., University of Pennsylvania; 1860-61, intern, Philadelphia Hospital. CAREER: Medical Corps: 1861-64, U.S. Navy; and 1864-65, U.S. Army; *post* 1866, practiced medicine, Philadelphia; at Jefferson Medical College: 1867-69, electro-therapeutics faculty; and *post* 1869, diseases of the throat and chest faculty; 1880-82, president, American Laryngological Association; *post* 1883, diseases of the throat and chest faculty, Philadelphia Polyclinic and College for Graduates in Medicine; consulting or visiting physician, several Philadelphia hospitals; acoustics faculty, Stevens Institute of Technology. CONTRIBUTIONS: Through publications and teaching, helped establish laryngology as a medical specialty in the United States. One of the first Americans to study the use of the laryngoscope. Performed the first successful operation for laryngeal cancer (1867) but generally opposed the operation because of its high risks. Wrote *Diseases of the Throat* (1872), a widely used textbook that for many years was the only comprehensive English-language work in its field. Trained many of the leading laryngologists of his time. A founder, American Laryngological Association and Philadelphia Polyclinic (1883). Helped edit *Archives of Laryngology* for several years.

WRITINGS: *Inhalation; Its Therapeutics and Practice* (1867); *Croup in Its Relations to Tracheotomy* (1874); "Does Excision of the Larynx Tend to the Prolongation of Life," *Med. News* 43 (1883): 20-22. REFERENCES: *BHM* (1970-74), 162; Louis H. Clerf, "Jacob DaSilva Solis-Cohen, M.D., Pioneer Laryngologist," *Annals of Otology, Rhinology, and Laryngology* 81 (Aug. 1972): 599-602; *DAB*, 4: 275; *NCAB*, 10: 92; *N.Y. Times*, December 23, 1927.

S. Galishoff

SOLIS-COHEN, SOLOMON (September 1, 1857, Philadelphia, Pa.-July 12, 1948, Philadelphia). *Physician; Medical writer.* Son of Myer David Cohen and Judith Simiah (da Silva Solis) Cohen. Married Emily Grace da Silva Solis, 1885; four children. EDUCATION: Central High School, Philadelphia: 1872, A.B.; and 1877, A.M.; 1883, M.D., Jefferson Medical College. CAREER: 1888-1927, lecturer and professor (*post* 1902), clinical medicine, Jefferson Medical College; 1887-1902, professor, clinical medicine and therapeutics, Philadelphia Polyclinic; 1890-92, lecturer, therapeutics, Dartmouth College; 1887-1927, physician, Philadelphia General, Jefferson, and Jewish hospitals; active in Philadelphia Jewish affairs entire life. CONTRIBUTIONS: Developed standard diagnostic and therapeutic techniques, including physical, physiological, and pharmacological therapies; influenced hundreds of physicians through his texts.

WRITINGS: *Essentials of Diagnosis, Arranged in the Form of Questions and Answers, Prepared Especially for Students of Medicine* (1892; 2nd ed., 1900; with Augustus A. Eshner); *A System of Physiologic Therapeutics: A Practical Exposition of the Methods Other Than Drug Giving, Useful in the Treatment of the Sick*, 11 vols. (1901-5, editor); *Pharmacotherapeutics, Materia Medica and Drug Action* (1928, with Thomas Stotesbury Githens); *Judaism and Science, with Other Addresses and Papers, from the Writings of Solomon Solis-Cohen* (1940). REFERENCES: bibliography, *Judaism and Science*; *JAMA* 138 (1948): 375; *NUC Pre-1956 Imprints*, 555; 450-55; *N.Y. Times*, July 13, 1948, p. 27.

M. M. Sokal

SOLLMANN, TORALD HERMANN (February 10, 1874, Coburg, Germany-February 11, 1965, Cleveland, Ohio). *Medical educator; Pharmacology.* Son of August and Adelheid (Eckardt) Sollmann. Married Alice M. Sersall, 1902; one child. EDUCATION: 1884-87, Gymnasium, Coburg, Germany; 1896, M.D., Western Reserve University ; 1899, special studies, Strassburg, France. CAREER: At Western Reserve University School of Medicine: 1896-98, demonstrator in physiology and histology; 1898-99, lecturer in pharmacology and demonstrator in physiology; 1899-1901, lecturer in pharmacology; 1901-3, assistant professor in pharmacology and materia medica; 1903-4, associate professor; 1904-44, professor of pharmacology; 1928-44, dean; and 1944, emeritus professor. CONTRIBUTIONS: Called the "Father of American Pharmacology," wrote the first comprehensive textbook on pharmacology in the English language. Established new techniques for determining the actions of many drugs and the reactions of tissues. Pioneered in organizing the Society for Pharmacology and Experimental Therapeutics and Council of Pharmacy and Chemistry of the American Medical Association. Trained many leaders of pharmacology in laboratory at Western Reserve University and guided the Medical School successfully through the depression and World War II.

WRITINGS: *Textbook of Pharmacology with Some Allied Sciences* (1901, with R. A. Hatcher); *The Action of Drugs: A Course of Elementary Lectures for Students of Pharmacy* (1917); *Manual of Pharmacology* (1917); *An Introduction to Experimental Pharmacology* (1928, with Paul J. Hanzlik); many journal articles. REFERENCES: Adelaide B. Curtiss, "Doctor Torald Sollmann," *Western Reserve Univ. School of Med. Alumni Bull.* 22 (first quarter, 1958). 3-6, Miller, *BHM*, p. 107; *Sollmann Bibliographies* (1957, a compilation of the bibliographies appearing in *Manual of Pharmacology* throughout its many editions; Carl J. Wiggers, "Torald Sollmann—the Professor and Dean," *Clin. Bull. of the School of Med. of Western Reserve Univ. and Its Associated Hospitals* 8 (Nov. 1944): 82-84.

G. P. Jenkins

SOLLY, S[AMUEL] EDWIN (May 5, 1845, London, England-November 18, 1906, Asheville, N.C. *Laryngologist; Climatologist.* Son of Samuel, senior surgeon, St. Thomas Hospital, and Jane (Barrett) Solly. Married Alma Helena Sandwell, 1872 (d. 1875), two children; Mrs. Elizabeth Mellor Evans, 1887. EDUCATION: Rugby School; St. Thomas Hospital; 1867, graduated, Royal College of Surgeons; 1869, Society of Apothecaries. CAREER: 1874, immigrated to

Colorado Springs, Colo.; president: 1888, Colorado Medical Society; and 1895, American Climatological Association; 1897, a founder and several times president, El Paso County Medical Society; 1899, president, American Laryngological, Rhinological, and Otological Society. CONTRIBUTIONS: An early advocate of the climatological therapy of tuberculosis. Founder, planner, and first director, Cragmor Sanitarium, Colorado Springs (1905-6).

WRITINGS: *Manitou, Colorado, U.S.A., Its Mineral Waters and Climate* (1875); *Health Resorts of Colorado Springs and Manitou* (1883); *Handbook of Medical Climatology* (1897). Contributed chapter "Climate" to H. A. Hare's *System of Practical Therapeutics* 1 (1891): 385-451. Wrote chapter "Diseases of the Nose and Nasopharynx; Diseases of the Larynx" in A. E. Loomis's *System of Practical Medicine* 2 (1897): 19-83. REFERENCES: P. F. Gildea, "Solly, Samuel Edwin," *Colorado Med.* 3 (1906): 332-33; James A. Hart, "Samuel Edwin Solly, M.D., M.R.C.S.," *Trans., Am. Climatological Assoc.* 23 (1907): xxv-xxvii; Kelly and Burrage (1928), 1141-42; obituary, *British Med. J.* 2 (Dec. 1, 1906): 1611-12; Horace G. Wetherill, "Samuel Edwin Solly," *J. of the Outdoor Life* (Summer 1932): 347-48.

                                                                                            F. B. Rogers

SOUCHON, EDMUND (December 1, 1841, Opelousas, La.-August 5, 1924, New Orleans, La.). *Surgeon.* Son of Eugene, dentist, and Caroline (Pettit) Souchon. Married Corinne LaVie, 1869; three children. EDUCATION: Studied in Paris; intern, Charité Hospital (Paris); 1867, M.D., University of Louisiana; while in Paris, served as interpreter and assistant to J. Marion Sims (q.v.) while he was demonstrating his operations in Europe. CAREER: 1867, began medical and surgical practice, New Orleans; at University of Louisiana: 1873-76, demonstrator of anatomy; and 1885-1908, professor of anatomy and clinical surgery; 1898-1908, president, Louisiana State Board of Health. CONTRIBUTIONS: As a surgeon and anatomist, studied aneurysms and shoulder dislocations, developed museum of anatomical specimens, using a technique of injecting specimens with a colored formula that made the structure more readily understandable. Overhauled the Louisiana State Board of Health, preparing a complete sanitary code embodying all health laws of the state (1898) and participated with other southern health officers in establishing quarantine regulations to protect the region from yellow fever. Declared war on the stegomyia mosquito (1903), to reduce disease in his state. Encouraged development of local health boards in La. Designed and superintended the Richardson Building of the Tulane Medical School.

WRITINGS: "Aneurysms of the Arch of the Aorta," *New Orleans Med. and Surg. J.* (1867). REFERENCES: *BHM* (1964-69), 249; *DAB* 9: 402-3; John Duffy, *History of Medicine in Louisiana* 2 (1962); *JAMA* (Aug. 16, 1924); *NCAB* 9: 132; Irving A. Watson, *Physicians and Surgeons of the U.S.* (1896).

                                                                                            M. Kaufman

SOUTH, LILLIAN HERRELD (January 31, 1879, near Bowling Green, Ky.-September 14, 1966, PeeWee Valley, Ky.). *Physician; Bacteriologist; Epidemologist.* Daughter of J. F., physician, and Martha Bell (More) South. Married Judge H. H. Tye, July 8, 1926. EDUCATION: 1897, B.A., E.B. Potter College,

Bowling Green; Paterson General Hospital, Paterson, N.J.: 1897-99, School of Nursing; and 1899, R.N., School of Nursing; 1900-1904, Women's Medical College of Pennsylvania, Philadelphia, Pa., M.D., 1904; 1910, laboratory training under William H. Park (q.v.) and at the Rockefeller Institute, Mayo Clinic, and Pasteur Institute (Paris); M.S., School of Public Health, Johns Hopkins University. CAREER: 1906-10, general practice of medicine, Bowling Green, in partnership with Drs. J. N. and A. T. McCormack (q.v.); 1908, with associates, established St. Joseph's Hospital (42 beds), Bowling Green; at Kentucky State Department of Health: 1910, became director, newly created Bureau of Bacteriology; and 1910-50, director, Bureau of Bacteriology and Epidemiology; 1913, elected third vice-president (first woman vice-president), American Medical Association; 1920-c. 1926, lecturer in bacteriology, School of Public Health, University of Louisville; 1930, director, School for Laboratory Technicians, School of Public Health, University of Louisville. CONTRIBUTIONS: Established and became director, first Bacteriology Laboratory, Kentucky State Health Department (1910) and continued to improve its capabilities until retirement. Made a survey of hookworm infestation in Ky. (1912), and the State Department of Health received a $20,000 grant from the Rockefeller Foundation to eradicate the disease in Ky. Business manager, *Journal of Kentucky Medical Association* (1907-c. 1943). Continued to render valuable services to the *Journal* until 1951. REFERENCES: *JAMA* 199 (1967): 352; *J. Ky. Med. Assoc.* 64 (1966): 890; *Who Was Who in Am.*, 6: 384.

E. H. Conner

SOUTHARD, ELMER ERNEST (July 28, 1876, Boston, Mass.-February 8, 1920, New York, N.Y.). *Physician; Neuropathology; Psychiatry*. Son of Martin, mill superintendent, and Olive Wentworth (Knowles) Southard. Married Mabel Fletcher Austin, 1906; three children. EDUCATION: Harvard University: 1897, A.B.; 1901, M.D.; and 1902, M.A.; 1901-3, intern and assistant in pathology, Boston City Hospital; 1902, studied at Senckenberg Institute, Frankfort, Germany, and University of Heidelberg. CAREER: 1904-20, neuropathology faculty, Harvard Medical School; 1906-9, medical and pathology staffs, Danvers State Hospital [for the insane]; 1909-20, pathology staff, Massachusetts State Board of Insanity (later, Commission on Mental Diseases); 1912-20, director, Boston Psychopathic Hospital (later, Massachusetts Psychiatric Institute); member, Board of Scientific Directors, Bedford Hills Laboratory, Bureau of Social Hygiene, N.Y.; director, Eugenics Record Office, Cold Spring Harbor, N.Y.; president, American Medico-Psychological Association (1919). CONTRIBUTIONS: Pioneered in the fields of neuropsychiatry and psychotherapy. An early advocate of social work in hospitals. While at Boston Psychopathic Hospital, established an outpatient clinic for psychiatric treatment. With Mary Jarrett, introduced the term "psychiatric social work" and established (1918) the first professional school in this field at Smith College. Developed the concept of orderly exclusion in psychiatric diagnosis. Made important contributions to the neuropsychiatry of syphilis and shell shock. A leading figure in the American eugenics movement.

Helped edit *Journal of Nervous and Mental Diseases, Psychiatric Bulletin*, and *Journal of Clinical and Laboratory Medicine*.

WRITINGS: *Outlines of Neuropathology* (1906); *Neurosyphilis* (1917, with H. C. Solomon); *The Brains of the Feeble Minded* (1918, with Walter E. Fernald); *Shell Shock and Neuropsychiatry* (1919). REFERENCES: Leland B. Alford, "Dr. E. E. Southard's Scientific Contributions to Psychiatry." *Am. J. of Psychiatry* 92 (1935): 675-93; *DAB*, 17: 410-11; Kelly and Burrage (1928), 1143-44; *NCAB*, 19: 113-14; *N.Y.Times*, February 9, 1920; *Who Was Who in Am.*, 1: 1157-58.

                                                                                          S. Galishoff

SPAFFORD, FREDERICK ANGIER (October 13, 1855, Ludlow, Vt.-March 3, 1922, Flandreau, S.Dak.) *Physician; Surgery.* Son of Alva M., contractor, and Mary (Angier) Spafford. Married Hattie Davis, 1881; one child. EDUCATION: Black River Academy, Ludlow; 1879, M.D., Dartmouth College; postgraduate work, Edinburgh and Berlin. CAREER: 1881-84, professor of anatomy, Leonard Medical College, Raleigh, N.C.; 1884, opened practice, Flandreau. CONTRIBUTIONS: Prominent figure in the development of education and medical care in S. Dak. Served twice as president, State Medical Association (1898, 1913), and as secretary (1919-22). First vice-president, State Board of Health (1887). Served on the Territorial Board of Health and as physician, Flandreau Indian School. Member, South Dakota Board of Regents and president, Flandreau School Board, for a great many years. During World War I, helped mobilize the medical doctors of the state. Associate editor, *Journal-Lancet*. REFERENCES: Lowe Barlett, *Heroes and Hero Tales of South Dakota*, ed. N. E. State (1931), 129; George W. Kingsbury, *History of Dakota Territory* (1915); *Memorial and Biographical Record-The Black Hills Region* (1899), 616, 619; George Martin Smith, *South Dakota, Its History and Its People: Biographical* 4 (1915): 94.

                                                                      D. W. Boilard and P. W. Brennen

SPALDING, JAMES ALFRED (August 20, 1846, Portsmouth, N.H.-February 27, 1938, Portland, Maine). *Physician; Ophthalmologist; Aural surgeon.* Son of Lyman Dyer and Susan (Parker Parrott) Spalding. Married Sarah Chase Shepley, 1882; no children. EDUCATION: 1866, A.B., Dartmouth College; entered Harvard Medical School; deafness was becoming more pronounced and Dr. O. W. Holmes (q.v.) advised him upon graduation to go abroad and study diseases of the eye and ear; 1870 , M.D., Harvard Medical School; study in Moorefield's Ophthalmic Hospital, London, and in Vienna. CAREER: 1872, returned to Portsmouth but moved to Portland, 1873; 1881-1914, on Maine General Hospital staff as ophthalmologist and aural surgeon. CONTRIBUTIONS: Established Eye and Ear clinics in Portland, Augusta, and Bangor, Maine, and helped establish young specialists in his field throughout the state; Necrologist, Maine Medical Association (1908-36). Man most responsible for the *Journal of the Maine Medical Association* becoming a monthly publication replacing the *Transactions*. Early advocate of a state eye and ear hospital and an institute for the deaf.

WRITINGS: Prolific writer, with works including two books, *Life of Dr. Lyman Spalding* (1917) and *Maine Physicians of 1820* (1929). A complete list is in the Maine Historical

Society's Spalding Collection #1606. REFERENCES: *J. of the Maine Med. Assoc.*, 18, no. 8 (Aug. 1927): 149-53; Maine Historical Society, "Maine's Hall of Fame," vol. 2, pp. 14-15; Maine Historical Society, Portland Obituary Scrapbook, vol. 18, pp. 133-34; Maine Historical Society, Spalding Collection #1606; *Maine Med. J.*, 21, no. 8 (Aug. 1930): 133-38; 22, no. 10 (Oct. 1931): 192-96; 29, no. 3 (Mar. 1938): 60-61.

B. C. Lister

SPALDING, LYMAN (June 5, 1775, Cornish, N.H.-October 21, 1821, Portsmouth, N.H. *Physician; Surgeon.* Son of Col. Dyer and Elizabeth Cady (Parkhurst) Spalding. Married Elizabeth Coues, 1802; five children. EDUCATION: Charleston, N.H., Academy; 1797, M.B., Harvard; winter 1809-10, attended medical lectures, Philadelphia, Pa. CAREER: 1797-1800, first lecturer on chemistry at the new Dartmouth Medical School; practiced: 1799-1813, Portsmouth, N.H.; and 1813 until death, New York City; at College of Physicians and Surgeons of the Western District of New York, Fairfield: 1810-17, professor of anatomy, physiology, and surgery; and 1813-17, president; although successful as a medical educator, and famous as an operator, resigned positions at Fairfield when the school became a political pawn and could not pay his salary; unsuccessful in obtaining other academic appointments; proposals for publishing an American edition of Robert Willan's pioneering work on skin disease and his own "Institutes of Medicine" were never realized. CONTRIBUTIONS: Worked actively with lifelong friend Nathan Smith (q.v.) during the establishment of new medical school, Dartmouth. While at Portsmouth, published annual bills of mortality for the town, partly because of his interest in the incidence of consumption and partly for their actuarial value. Bills, distinguished for their wealth of detail, became the basis for annuity calculations for at least one insurance company. Introduced inoculation with cowpox matter to N.H. as a participant in Benjamin Waterhouse's (q.v.) short-lived "Vaccination Trust" and conducted public tests of the new method's efficacy (1801, 1802). Chief contribution to medicine began with proposal (1817), as secretary, New York County Medical Society, for a national pharmacopoeia that would insure the uniform preparation of drugs with proven efficacy throughout the country. First pharmacopoeia to be developed through a process of nationwide professional consensus, the *United States Pharmacopoeia*, appeared (December 1820) under Spalding's guidance.

WRITINGS: *Inaugural Dissertation on the Production of Animal Heat* (1797); *Bills of Mortality for Portsmouth, N.H.* [11 broadsides] (1802-12); *Reflections on Fever* (1817); *Reflections on Yellow Fever Periods* (1819); *United States Pharmacopoeia* (1820, editor-in-chief). REFERENCES: *BHM* (1975-79), 120; *DAB*, 9, pt. 1: 423-24; J. Worth Estes, *Hall Jackson and the Purple Foxglove* (1979), 87-139; Morris C. Leikind, "An Episode in the History of Smallpox Vaccination in New Hampshire," *Bull. Hist. Med.* 7 (1939): 671-86; *NCAB*, 2: 199; James Alfred Spalding, *Dr. Lyman Spalding* (1916).

J. W. Estes

SPITZKA, EDWARD CHARLES (November 10, 1852, New York City-January 13, 1914, New York City). *Psychiatrist, Neurologist.* Son of Charles Anthony, clockmaker, and Johanna (Tag) Spitzka. Married Catherine Watzek, 1875; one child. EDUCATION: Attended City College of New York; 1873, M.D., University of the City of New York (NYU); 1873-76, postgraduate study in Leipzig and Vienna, Austria. CAREER: 1876, began medical practice in New York City, 1879, began to specialize in nervous and mental illness; professor of anatomy and physiology, Columbia Veterinary College; 1882-87, professor of anatomy and physiology of the nervous system and medical jurisprudence, New York Post-Graduate Medical School. CONTRIBUTIONS: Pioneering neurologist. Work on the pathology of insanity (1882) won an award from the British Medico-Psychological Association. A well-known consultant and medico-legal expert; most famous case that of Charles Guiteau, the assassin of President James Garfield, in which he was the only expert who testified to the defendent's insanity. Editor (1881-84) of the *American Journal of Neurology and Psychiatry*. President of the New York Neurological Society (1883-84), and of the American Neurological Association (1890).

WRITINGS: *The Somatic Etiology of Insanity* (1882); *Insanity, Its Classification, Diagnosis, and Treatment* (1883); Bibliography in *J. of Nervous and Mental Disease*, 41 (1914). REFERENCES: *DAB*, 9, pt. 1: 461-62; Kelly and Burrage (1928), 1148-49; *N.Y. Times*, September 6, 1922.

M. Kaufman

SPIVAK, CHARLES DAVID (December 25, 1861, Krementchug, Russia-October 16, 1927, Denver, Colo.). *Physician; Medical bibliographer*. Son of Samuel David and Deborah (Dorfman) Spivakowsky. Immigrated to the United States in 1882. Married Jennie Charsky, 1893; three children. EDUCATION: 1890, M.D., Jefferson Medical College; 1891-92, postgraduate studies, University of Berlin. CAREER: 1896, went to Denver; 1896-1902, on faculty, University of Denver, as associate professor of anatomy, lecturer on diseases of the gastrointestinal tract, and associate professor of medicine; 1902-7, clinical professor of medicine, Denver & Gross Medical College. CONTRIBUTIONS: A founder (1903), of the Jewish Consumptives' Relief Society (JCRS), of which he was secretary until his death. Became administrator of the new JCRS Sanatorium (1904), which he had planned and organized. Compiled (1897) a catalog of all medical books in the personal libraries of Denver physicians. Editor and publisher (1898-1902), *Medical Libraries* (five vols), a monthly journal that became the official organ of the Association of Medical Libraries, founded with his encouragement (1898). With Henry Sewall (q.v.), was a leading spirit in the Colorado Medical Library Association and its president (1902). Librarian of the short-lived Denver Academy of Medicine.

WRITINGS: Compiled a 50-year bibliography of the writings of Colo. physicians that was published in *Medical Coloradoana* (1922), 22-142. Contributed articles on medicine in the Bible and rabbinic literature to the *Jewish Encyclopedia* and was co-author (with Solomon Bloomgarden) of a *Yiddish Dictionary* (1911). REFERENCES: *BHM* (1970-74), 163; (1980), 38; *DAB*, 17: 462-63; A. Levinson, "Charles D. Spivak's Contribution to

Medicine," *Med. Life* 35 (1928): 46-54, contains a partial bibliography of Spivak's writings (pp. 52-54).

F. B. *Rogers*

SPRAGUE, EDWARD WHARTON (April 6, 1880, Centerville, N.Y.-February 21, 1974, Newark, N.J.). *Physician; Surgeon.* Son of Wharton Edward and Sarah (Allen) Sprague, teacher. Married Harriet Thorne Newman, 1906, two children; Mae Stone, 1949, no children. EDUCATION: Tutored privately; public schools, Sandy Creek, Kasoag, Pulaski, N.Y.; apprentice to Dr. Francis Low (Pulaski); 1903, M.D., College of Physicians and Surgeons of Baltimore; 1903-5, intern, Newark City Hospital. CAREER: 1905-72, private practice, Newark; senior surgeon: St. James Hospital, Newark; Presbyterian Hospital, Newark; and Newark City Hospital; consulting surgeon; Mountainside Hospital, Montclair, N.J.; St. Barnabas Hospital, Livingston, N.J.; and Clara Maass Hospital, Belleville, N.J.; although he "laid down his own scalpel on his 90th birthday," he "stood in" at operations until death six years later. CONTRIBUTIONS: Performed with Dr. E. Zeh Hawkes the first blood transfusion (1908) and the first total gastrectomy (1929) in N.J. Helped found (1929) Presbyterian Hospital, Newark. Played preeminent role in the establishment (1942) of the Medical-Surgical Plan of New Jersey and served as a member, original Board of Trustees.

WRITINGS: Writings listed in Morris H. Saffron, "Edward Wharton Sprague, M.D., F.A.C.S.," Studies in the Medical History of New Jersey Dedicated to Edward Wharton Sprague, *Acad. of Med. of N.J. Bull.* 16 (1970): 11. REFERENCES: Irving P. Borsher, "Dr. Sprague's Role in the Early History of MSD," *J. Med. Soc. of New Jersey* 63 (1966): 498-501; "Dr. Edward W. Sprague," *ibid.*, 71 (1974): 326; "Dr. Edward W. Sprague Honored By National Blue Cross Association," *ibid.*, 65 (1968): 469; "Dr. Edward W. Sprague Receives the Edward J. Ill Award," *ibid.*, 42 (1945): 181-84; *JAMA* 228 (1974): 1597; *News* (Newark), May 3, 1945; December 18, 1970; Saffron, "Edward Wharton Sprague," pp. 3-11; *Who Was Who in Am.*, 6: 387.

W. *Barlow*

SPRAY, ROBB SPALDING (February 19, 1890, Omaha, Nebr.-May 14, 1966, Cumberland, Wis.). *Bacteriology.* EDUCATION: 1914, B.S., Purdue; 1917, M.S., Penn State; University of Chicago: 1920-21, Logan Fellow; and 1923, Ph.D. CAREER: 1915-18, instructor of botany, Penn State University; 1918-20, assistant professor of animal pathology, Purdue University; at West Virginia University: 1921-25, associate professor of hygiene and bacteriology; 1926-46, professor; and 1946-66, professor emeritus; 1958-66, bacteriologist, Cumberland Memorial Hospital. CONTRIBUTIONS: Pioneer research investigator in the field of anaerobic bacteria. One of the first to work in the field. First to grow organisms that require low oxygen pressure, such as the tetanus bacillus.

WRITINGS: "An Outbreak of Food Poisoning Probably Due to Rat Virus," *JAMA* 86 (1926): 109; "Heated Blood Derivatives for Cultivation of the Hemo-globinophilic Organisms," *J. Lab. and Clin. Med.* 16 (1930): 166; "Sporadic Typhoid Fever, with Discovery of a Carrier," *West Virginia Med. J.* 26 (1930): 553; "Further Application of Semi-Solid Media in Cultivation and Identification of the Sporulating Anaerobes," *J.*

of Bacteriology 29 (1935): 18; 32 (1936): 135. REFERENCES: Interview with Dr. Clark
Sleeth, Morgantown, W. Va.; records of the Medical School of West Virginia University,
Morgantown, W. Va.; St. Paul *Sunday Pioneer Press*, December 14, 1957.

K. Nodyne and R. Murphy

SQUIBB, EDWARD ROBINSON (July 5, 1819, Wilmington, Del.-October
25, 1900, Brooklyn, N.Y.) *Physician; Pharmacist; Pharmaceutical manufacturer.* Son of James R. and Catherine H. (Bonsall) Squibb. Married Caroline
Lownds Cook, 1852; four children. EDUCATION: Private tutor, Wilmington; 1837-
42, apprenticed to Warder Morris and Morris and Sprague, pharmacists, Philadelphia, Pa.; 1845, M.D., Jefferson Medical College. CAREER: 1845-47, medical practitioner, Philadelphia; U.S. Navy: 1847-52, assistant surgeon; and 1852-
57, assistant director and director, Pharmaceutical Laboratory; 1857, partner,
Thomas E. Jenkins & Co., Louisville, Ky.; 1858, founder, "Edward R. Squibb,
M.D." Laboratory, Brooklyn, predecessor of E. R. Squibb & Sons (1886);
1869-71, professor of pharmacy, College of Pharmacy of the City of New York;
1858, vice-president, American Pharmaceutical Association; 1860, chairman,
Special Committee, American Medical Association, on the Drug Adulteration
Act. CONTRIBUTIONS: A pioneer in the manufacture of pharmaceuticals and
chemicals in the United States, developed and perfected processes for the manufacture of ether, chloroform, fluid extracts, bismuth salts, calcium chloride,
phosphoric acid, and ergot preparations, among others. Emphasized the purity
and integrity of product, rejected secrecy, and based operations on scientific and
technical foundations. Contributed prolifically to the literature of the scientific
and technical aspects of practical pharmacy. Invented numerous devices (e.g.,
a burette and a specific gravity apparatus). Participated actively in and advocated
vociferously the reform of the Pharmacopoeia of the United States (1870, 1880).
Sponsored pure food and drug legislation. Credited with the authorship of the
N.Y. and N.J. statutes. Advocated a universal pharmacopoeia.

WRITINGS: *The American Medical Association and the Pharmacopoeia of the United
States of America* (1877). Contributor to many journals, especially the *Transactions of
the Medical Society of New York, American Journal of Pharmacy*, and *Proceedings of
the American Pharmaceutical Association*. In the last two, contributed over 100 items.
List of writings in the *American Journal of Pharmacy* and *Proceedings of the American
Pharmaceutical Association* is in J. P. Remington, "Edward Robinson Squibb, M.D.,"
Am. J. Pharm. 73 (1901). Issued and distributed on request, sporadically: *An Ephemeris
of the Materia Medica*, which disseminated useful and practical drug information. "A
Universal Pharmacopoeia," *Trans. of the Internat. Med. Cong.* (1876). REFERENCES:
L. G. Blockman, *Doctor Squibb: The Life and Times of a Rugged Idealist* (1958); *DAB*,
9, pt. 1: 487-88; *The Journal of Edward Robinson Squibb*, 2 vols. (1930); Miller, *BHM*,
p. 108; *NCAB*, 19: 56; Remington, "Edward Robinson Squibb," pp. 419-31; G. Sonnedecker, *Kremers and Urdang's History of Pharmacy*, 4th ed. (1976).

D. L. Cowen

STANLEY, WENDELL MEREDITH (August 16, 1904, Ridgeville, Ind.-
June 15, 1971, Salamanca, Spain). *Biochemist; Virology.* Son of James G.,

newspaper publisher, and Claire (Plessinger) Stanley. Married Marian Staples Jay, 1929; four children. EDUCATION: 1926, B.S., Earlham College; University of Illinois: 1927, M.S.; and 1929, Ph. D.; 1930-31, National Research Fellow, Munich, Germany. CAREER: 1931-48, scientific staff, Rockefeller Institute for Medical Research; University of California: 1940, Hitchcock professor; 1948-69, biochemistry faculty; 1948-69, director, virus laboratory; 1958-69, virology faculty; served on numerous scientific committees. CONTRIBUTIONS: Awarded a share of the 1946 Nobel Prize in chemistry for isolation and crystallization of the tobacco mosaic virus. Influenced by the work of James B. Sumner and John H. Northrup, co-recipients of the prize, who had purified and crystallized several enzymes and showed them to be proteins (1920s). Demonstrated that the tobacco mosaic virus was a chemical substance that had the ability to replicate itself when placed on the leaf of a tobacco plant and that could be transmitted to other plants (1932-35); work refuted the commonly held belief that viruses were living submicroscopic organisms; showed instead that viruses provided a link between living and nonliving matter; research opened the way for the development of new vaccines against viral diseases and other scientific advances. During World War II, developed a centrifuge-purified influenza vaccine that was more effective than previous vaccines. Developed the virus laboratory at the University of California into one of the world's leading centers for work in molecular biology and biochemistry.

WRITINGS: "Isolation and Properties of Tobacco Mosaic and other Virus Proteins;" Harvey Lecture, *Bull., N.Y. Acad. of Med.*, 14 (1938): 398-428; "The Preparation and Properties of Influenza Virus Vaccines Concentrated and Purified by Differential Centrifugation," *J. of Experimental Med.*, 81 (1945): 193-218; *Viruses and the Nature of Life* (1961, with Evans Valens). Writings are briefly described in *NCAB*. REFERENCES: *Am. Philos. Soc. Yearbook* (1971), 184-90; *Current Biog.* (1947), 604-7; Greer Williams, *Virus Hunters* (1959), 88-107; *McGraw-Hill Modern Men of Sci.* 1 (1966): 440-41; *NCAB*, 57: 161-63; *N.Y.Times*, June 16, 1971; *Who Was Who in Am.*, 5: 686.

S. Galishoff

STASTNY, OLGA FRANCES (September 13, 1878, Wilber, Nebr.-August 21, 1952, Omaha, Nebr.). *Physician; Surgeon*. Daughter of Frank John, public official, and Teresa (Jurka) Sadilek. Married Charles Jan Stastny, dentist, October 25, 1895; two children. EDUCATION: 1895, Wilber High School; 1913, M.D., University of Nebraska College of Medicine; postgraduate study, College of Medicine of New York City; and Mary Thompson Hospital, Chicago, Ill.; postgraduate work, Prague, Czechoslovakia; and Berlin, Germany; 1913-14, intern, New England Hospital for Women and Children, Boston, Mass. CAREER: 1913-16, practice of medicine, Omaha; 1918-19, anesthetist, American Women's Hospital, France, receiving the French Government's Medallie de la Reconnaissance; 1919-20, faculty (hygiene), School of Social Service, Prague; 1919-22, director, International YMCA, Department of Health, Czechoslovakia; 1923-24, supervisor, Macronissi quarantine station for refugees of Greece and Asia Minor; at University of Nebraska College of Medicine: 1925-29, clinical assistant in medicine; 1929-31, assistant instructor in obstetrics and gynecology; 1931-48, instructor in obstetrics and gynecology; and 1948-52, instructor, emeritus. Entered Government Medical Reserve and served with American Women's Hospital in France; thence to Czechoslovakia and Greece. CONTRIBUTIONS: Considered "Dean" of women physicians in Nebr.

WRITINGS: "Dyspituitarism," *Nebraska State Med. J.* 3 (February 1918): 60; "Diathermy in Pelvic Disease," *Med. Woman's J.* 36 (December 1929): 318-20; "Trichomonas Vaginalia," *Nebraska State Med. J.* 20 (March 1938): 105-8; "Clinical Use of Estrogenic Compounds," ibid., 27 (Aug. 1942): 286-87. REFERENCES: Archives, University of Nebraska Medical Center Library of Medicine, Omaha; E. P. Lovejoy, *Women Doctors of the World* (1957), 199, 340-41; *Who's Who in Nebraska* (1940), 389.

B. M. Hetzner

STEELE, HENRY KING (April 1, 1825, Dayton, Ohio-January 20, 1893, Denver, Colo.). *Physician; Public health administrator.* Son of Dr. John and Cornelia (King) Steele. Married Frances Dunlevy, 1855; three children. EDUCATION: 1844, B.A., Centre College; 1848, M.D., University of the City of New York. CAREER: 1848-70, practiced medicine with father in Dayton; 1861-64, surgeon, 44th Ohio Infantry and 8th Ohio Cavalry; 1870, moved to Denver; surgeon, Kansas Pacific Railroad and Denver & South Park Railroad; president: 1873, Denver Medical Society; 1875, Colorado Territorial Medical Society; 1877, Denver School Board; and 1879-84, Colorado State Board of Health; 1882-87, professor of surgery and dean, University of Denver medical department; 1887, retired from active practice; 1887-90, traveled and studied in Europe. CONTRIBUTIONS: As Denver health commissioner (1891-92), systematically inventoried and tackled the problems of his office and made great improvements in the sanitary conditions of the city. Insisted on serving without pay, diverting salary to two assistants of his own choosing (Drs. Henry Sewall [q.v.] and Wm. P. Munn). REFERENCE: Henry Sewall, "Memoir of Dr. Henry King Steele," *Denver Med. Times* 22 (1902): 598-602.

F. B. Rogers

STEELE, WILLIAM L. (February 17, 1833, Pendleton, S.C.-May 16, 1909, Butte, Mont.). *Physician; Surgeon; Public health.* One of 16 children. Married Agnes Forbis, 1865; three children. EDUCATION: Private tutoring and Kennedy Thalian Institute, S.C.; clerkship under Dr. Poosher, Greenville, S.C.; 1857, M.D., South Carolina Medical College in Charleston. CAREER: 1859-63, physician on mining frontier, Central City, Colo.; 1863, moved to Bannock in Mont. Territory and practiced medicine and mined; practiced, Virginia City, Mont., and also maintained several businesses; elected miner's president in Alder Gulch and served as local judge; 1866, moved to Prickly Pear Canyon; 1869, elected sheriff of Lewis and Clark County; 1872 until death, practiced medicine, Helena, Mont., area; army surgeon after Battle of Big Hole (Nez Perce War, 1877); served as county coroner (ten years); mayor of Helena two terms, county treasurer one term, and member of state legislature (1896); physician-surgeon, Northwest

Mounted Police; served native American Indian community. CONTRIBUTIONS: Worked to improve public health and hygiene and to improve Indian-white relations. Much in demand as surgeon during period of Indian wars. Helped organize first Montana Medical Association and provided standards for practice of medicine.

WRITINGS: Only surviving documents are interview (1907) and contemporary historical collections. REFERENCES: *Helena Daily Independent*, January 2, 1907 (interview), p. 8; *Helena Independent*, May 16, 1909, p. 1; Michael A. Leeson, ed., *History of Montana, 1739-1885* (1885), 1254; *Progressive Men of the State of Montana* (1902), 1248; Helen F. Sanders, *A History of Montana* 2 (1913): 898.

P. C. Mullen

STEENBOCK, HARRY (August 16, 1886, Charlestown, Wis.-December 25, 1967, Madison, Wis.). *Biochemist.* Son of Henry and Christine (Oesan) Steenbock, farmers. Married Evelyn Carol Van Donk, March 6, 1948; no children. EDUCATION: University of Wisconsin, 1908, B.A.; 1910, M.S.; 1916, Ph.D.; 1912, graduate study, Yale University; 1913, studied, University of Berlin. CAREER: At University of Wisconsin: 1908-38, agricultural chemistry faculty; 1938-56, professor of biochemistry; and 1956-67, emeritus professor and researcher. CONTRIBUTIONS: Studied animal and human nutrition, specifically the role of fat-soluble vitamins, minerals, and the biological action of ultraviolet radiation. Discovered the relationship between vitamin D and ultraviolet light and their essential role in body growth and bone calcification (1923). Showed (1925) that irradiation of sterol-containing foodstuffs would concentrate vitamin D and prevent rickets. The commercial application of this discovery, the Steenbock Process, led to the elimination of rickets in young children in the United States. Subsequently discovered vitamin A activity in carotene and other yellow pigments and the need for vitamin E in the diet.

WRITINGS: "Calcium and Phorphorous Supply of Farm Feeds and Their Relation to Animals Requirements," *Wis. Agricultural Experiment Station Research Bull.*, no. 30 (1911): 1-28, (with E. B. Hart and J. G. Fuller); "Fat Soluble Vitamins: Light in Its Relation to Ophthalmia and Growth," *J. Biol. Chem.* 56 (1923): 355 (with E. M. Nelson); "The Antirachitic Property of Milk and Its Increase by Direct Radiation and by Irradiation of the Animal," ibid., 66 (1925): 441 (with E. B. Hart, C. A. Hopoert, and Archie Black); "Fat Soluble Vitamins; The Induction of Growth Promoting and Calcifying Properties in Fats and their Unsaponifiable Constituents by Exposure to Light," ibid., 64 (1925): 263 (with Archie Black); "The Quantitative Determination of Vitamin A," ibid., 72 (1927): 59 (with K. H. Coward). Writings listed in *Science Citations Index*. REFERENCES: *BHM* (1970-74), 164; *NCAB*, 54: 357-8; E. N. Todhunter, "Biographical Notes from the History of Nutrition," *J. Am. Diet. Assoc.* 54 (1969): 432.

C. G. Borst

STEINDLER, ARTHUR (June 22, 1878, Graslitz, Bohemia-July 21, 1959, Iowa City, Ia.). *Physician; Orthopedic surgery.* Son of Leopold and Caroline (Goldberg) Steindler. Married Louise Junk, March 1, 1914. EDUCATION: 1896-

98, University of Prague; 1902, M.D., University of Vienna, Austria. CAREER: 1902-7, studied with Edward Albert, Adolph Lorenz, and Carl Friedlander, Vienna; 1907, went to United States; 1907-10, associate to Dr. John Ridlon, St. Luke's Hospital, Chicago, Ill.; and orthopedic surgeon, Home for Crippled Children; 1910-15, professor, orthopedic surgery, Drake Medical School, Des Moines, Ia.; and orthopedic surgeon, Iowa Methodist and Iowa Lutheran hospitals, Des Moines; 1914, became naturalized citizen of United States; 1915-48, professor and head, orthopedic surgery, State University of Iowa College of Medicine, Iowa City; 1918, contract surgeon; lieutenant colonel, U.S. Army Medical Reserve Corps; *post* 1947, Board of Directors, Iowa Society for Crippled Children and the Disabled; 1949-59, chief of orthopedic surgery, Mercy Hospital, Iowa City; 1932-33, president, American Orthopedic Association. CONTRIBU-TIONS: A world-famous orthopedic surgeon and teacher, trained more than 250 others from all over the world. Knowledge of Latin and modern European languages was vast; made European orthopedic developments accessible to American medicine. Pioneer treatment of scoliosis by the compensatory method, as well as pioneer treatment of other spinal deformities and pes cavus. Developed a number of important orthopedic operations, including reconstructive surgery of the upper extremity, and was a pioneer in the development of occupational therapy. Kinesiology and the biophysics of locomotion occupied his attention from the mid-1920s. From late 1930s, concerned with the differential diagnosis of orthopedic pain. Interests spanned all of orthopedics, and combined a well-grounded knowledge of basic principles with sound surgical inventiveness and careful evaluation of long-term results.

WRITINGS: For a bibliography, see Ignacio V. Ponseti, "Arthur Steindler (1878-1959)," *Clin. Orthopedics* 19 (1961): 1. Steindler authored more than 100 scientific articles and nine books, including *Reconstructive Surgery of the Upper Extremity* (1923); *Operative Orthopedics* (1925); *Diseases and Deformities of the Spine and Thorax* (1929); *The Mechanics of Normal and Pathological Locomotion of Man* (1935); *Kinesiology of the Human Body* (1955). REFERENCES: *JAMA* 171, no. 6 (Oct. 10, 1959): 854; Solomon R. Kagan, *Jewish Contributions to Medicine in America* (1939); Ignacio V. Ponseti, "Arthur Steindler (1878-1959)," *Clin. Orthopedics* 19 (1961): 1; University of Iowa Archives, Iowa City; *Who Was Who in Am.* 3 (1951-60); *Who's Who in Am. Med.* (1925); *Who's Who in the Midwest* (1952); *WWAPS* 1 (1938).

R. E. Rakel

STERNBERG, GEORGE MILLER (June 8, 1838, Hartwick Seminary, Ostego County, N.Y.-November 3, 1915, Washington, D.C.). *Physician; Army officer; Microbiology.* Son of Levi, Lutheran clergyman, and Margaret Levering (Miller) Sternberg. Married Louisa Russell, 1865; Martha L. Pattison, 1869; no children. EDUCATION:1860, M.D., College of Physicians and Surgeons (Columbia). CAREER: 1860-61, practiced medicine, Elizabeth, N.J.; 1861-1902, with Medical Corps, U.S. Army (rising in rank from assistant surgeon to brigadier general); 1861-65, field and hospital duties, Civil War; 1865-79, Indian campaigns and cholera and yellow fever epidemics, various army posts; 1879, member and secretary, Havana Yellow Fever Commission, National Board of Health; 1898, in command of medical service, war with Spain; 1885, president, American Public Health Association. CONTRIBUTIONS: Introduced Americans to the work of Louis Pasteur and Robert Koch and made pioneering bacteriological investigations of his own. Almost simultaneously with Pasteur, announced the discovery of pneumococcus (1881). First American researcher to demonstrate the protozoan responsible for malaria (1885) and the bacilli of tuberculosis and typhoid fever (1886). With Koch, began the scientific study of disinfection. Advanced the technique of photomicrography. Opened the Army Medical School (1893). Organized the army's nurse and dental corps. Established the Typhoid Fever Board (1898), which revealed the importance of flies and contact infection in the spread of typhoid. Organized the Yellow Fever Commission (1900), which proved that yellow fever was transmitted by the *Aëdes aegypti* mosquito. One of the first to show that viruses in people could be tracked by the antibodies they produced.

WRITINGS: "A Fatal Form of Septicemia in the Rabbit, Produced by the Subcutaneous Injection of Human Saliva," *Reports of the National Board of Health, No. 3* (1881): 87-92; *Photomicrographs and How to Make Them* (1883); "Disinfection and Individual Prophylaxsis Against Infectious Diseases," *The Lomb Prize Essays* (1886), 99-136; *A Manual of Bacteriology* (1892). Bibliography is in John M. Gibson, *Soldier in White: The Life of General George Miller Sternberg* (1958). REFERENCES: *DAB*, 17: 590-92; Gibson, *Soldier in White*; Miller, *BHM* p. 109; *NCAB*, 4: 388; *N.Y. Times*, November, 4, 1915; *Who Was Who in Am.*, 1: 1179.

S. Galishoff

STEUART, RICHARD SPRIGG (November 1, 1797, Baltimore, Md.-July 13, 1876, Anne Arundel County?, Md.). *Physician; Psychiatrist.* Son of Dr. James and Mrs. Rebecca (Sprigg) Steuart. Married Juliette O. Penniman, 1824; at least one son. EDUCATION: St. Mary's College, Baltimore; 1817-18, studied law under General Winder; 1822, M.D., University of Maryland. CAREER: 1822-40, shared private medical practice, Baltimore, with Dr. William Donaldson and took over the practice when Donaldson died; 1828-76, superintendent and president, Board of Visitors, Old Maryland Hospital for the Insane (Baltimore), and, after it was moved, New Hospital for the Insane, Spring Grove, Md. (was active as superintendent primarily from 1828 to 1842 and 1869 to 1876); 1843, although he never lectured, was appointed professor of the practice of medicine, University of Maryland; 1848-49, 1850-51, president, Medical and Chirurgical Faculty of Maryland; 1849, vice-president, American Medical Association; 1857, chairman, Board of Commissioners, Maryland Lunatic Asylum. CONTRIBUTIONS: Pressured the state legislature to reclaim the old City Hospital then leased to two private physicians (1828-34). Established a board of visitors that regularly inspected the hospital that the state recovered (1834). Helped bring Dorothea Dix (q.v.) to speak in behalf of the insane to the state legislature (1852), Annapolis, Md.; report, as chairman, Board of Commissioners, Maryland State Lunatic Asylum, was submitted (1858) to the legislature asking for funds to construct what became the new Spring Grove State Hospital near Catonsville, Md.

WRITINGS: *Letter to John L. Carey, on the Subject of Slavery* (1845); [Md.] Commissioners to Construct a State Hospital for Insane, *Report of the Commissioners of the Maryland State Lunatic Asylum, to the General Assembly of Maryland* (Jan. 1858). Writings listed in J. R. Quinan, *Medical Annals of Baltimore*. . . (1884), 163. REFERENCES: E. F. Cordell, *Medical Annals of Maryland*. . .(1891), 581; J. Gilman, "Richard Steuart Sprigg," *TAMA* 28 (1877): 618-20; Kelly and Burrage (1928), 1160-61; Quinan, *Medical Annals of Baltimore*, pp. 163-64.

C. Donegan

STEVENSON, SARAH ANN HACKETT (February 2, 1841, Buffalo Grove, Ill.-August 14, 1901, Chicago, Ill.). *Physician.* Daughter of John Davis, merchant, and Sarah T. (Hackett) Stevenson. Never married. EDUCATION: 1863, State Normal University, Normal, Ill.; one year of study, South Kensington Science School, London, England; 1874, M.D., Woman's Hospital Medical College of Chicago (valedictorian); postgraduate studies abroad, visiting hospitals and clinics. CAREER: 1875, opened practice, Chicago; 1876, delegate, American Medical Association Convention, Philadelphia, Pa.; at Woman's Hospital Medical College: 1875-80, professor of physiology and histology; and 1880-94, professor of obstetrics; 1881, appointed to staff, Cook County Hospital, Chicago (first woman); consulting physician, Woman's and Provident hospitals; and attending physician, Mary Thompson Hospital; 1893, first woman appointed to the Illinois State Board of Health. CONTRIBUTIONS: First female member, American Medical Association (1875). Leader in the founding of the Illinois Training School for Nurses (1880). One of the most widely known women physicians of Ill. and the Midwest. In addition to medical career, devoted to reform movements—participated in the Woman's Christian Temperance Union (WCTU), serving as first superintendent (1881-82), National Department of Hygiene, and as president of the staff, National Temperance Hospital, organized by the Chicago WCTU (1886).

WRITINGS: *Boys and Girls in Biology* (1875); *The Physiology of Woman* (1880). REFERENCES: Phoebe A. Hanaford, *Daughters of America* (1883), 543-46; *History of Medicine and Surgery, and Physicians and Surgeons of Chicago* (1922); *Notable Am. Women, 1607-1950*, 3: 374-76.

V. Drachman

STICKNEY, VICTOR HUGO (April 13, 1855, Plymouth, Vt.-July 26, 1927, Dickinson, N.Dak.). *Physician; Surgeon.* Son of John W., farmer, and Anna (Pinney) Stickney. Married Margaret Hayes, 1885; two children. EDUCATION: 1881, B.S., New Hampshire College; 1883, M.D., Dartmouth University. CAREER: 1883-1914, physician and surgeon, Dickinson, Dakota Territory, and N. Dak.; 1883-1914, surgeon, Northern Pacific Railway; 1915-16, president, North Dakota Medical Association; 1917, lieutenant, Medical Corps, American Expeditionary Force; and chairperson, Medical Section, Council of National Defense for North Dakota; 1917-19, captain, Medical Corps, American Expeditionary Force. CONTRIBUTIONS: For more than a decade, the only doctor for southwestern N.Dak., an area of more than 50,000 square miles. Personified the physician to thousands of western N.Dak. pioneers.

WRITINGS: "The Pioneer Doctor," *J.-Lancet* 21 (1921). REFERENCES: *Dickinson*

Press, July 29, 1927, pp. 1,2; James Grassick, *North Dakota Medicine: Sketches and Abstracts* (1926), 118-20.

L. Remele

STILES, CHARLES WARDELL (May 15, 1867, Spring Valley, N.Y.-January 24, 1941, Baltimore, Md.). *Zoologist; Medical zoology; Public health.* Son of Samuel Martin, Methodist minister, and Elizabeth (White) Stiles. Married Virginia Baker, 1897; two children. EDUCATION: 1885-86, studied at Wesleyan University; 1886-89, studied at the Sorbonne, Collège de France, and universities of Göttingen, Berlin, and Leipzig; 1890, Ph.D., University of Leipzig; 1890-91, studied in Berlin, Germany; Trieste, Italy; and Paris, France. CAREER: 1891-1904, zoologist, Bureau of Animal Industry, U.S. Department of Agriculture; 1892-1906, medical zoology faculty, Georgetown University; zoology faculty: 1894-1902, Army Medical School; and 1897-1937, Johns Hopkins University; 1898-99, agricultural and scientific attaché, U.S. Embassy, Berlin; 1902-10, zoology faculty, Navy Medical School; 1902-32, chief, Division of Zoology, U.S. Public Health Service; 1909-14, scientific secretary, Rockefeller Sanitary Commission; secretary: *post* 1894, Advisory Committee, Smithsonian Table at Naples Zoological Station; 1898-1936, International Commission on Zoological Nomenclature; and 1910-27, International Commission on Medical Zoology; 1931-38, zoology faculty, Rollins College (winter faculty). CONTRIBUTIONS: Investigated several parasitic diseases of animals that were doing great harm to the American economy, including trichinosis in pork and the internal parasites of the fur seal. Found a new type of hookworm indigenous to the western hemisphere (1902). Showed that the alleged laziness of poor whites in the rural South was largely attributable to widespread anemia caused by hookworm infestation. Sought support for a movement to eradicate hookworm in the South, which led to the establishment of the Rockefeller Sanitary Commission. As medical director of the commission, directed a highly successful five-year campaign against hookworm disease relying heavily upon rural sanitation and education (1909-14). Uncovered many new species of parasitic worms and helped develop a systematic zoology in the United States. With Albert Hassall, prepared *Index-Catalogue of Medical and Veterinary Zoology*, an ongoing work spanning several decades (*post* 1902). Publication was said to be comparable in scope and importance to the *Index Catalogue*.

WRITINGS: *Trichinosis in Germany* (1901); "A New Species of Hookworm (Uncinaria Americana) Parasitic in Man," *American Medicine* 3 (1902): 777-78; *Report on Hookworm Disease* (Uncinariasis) *in the United States* (1903); *Studies on Intestinal Parasites* (Especially Amoebae) *in Man* (1923). REFERENCES: *BHM* (1970-74), 110; (1975-79), 122; J. H. Cassedy, "The Germ of Laziness," *Bull. Hist. Med.* 45 (1971): 159-69; *DAB*, Supplement 3: 737-39; *DSB*, 13: 62-63; J. Ettling, *The Germ of Laziness* (1981); *NCAB*, D: 62-63; *N.Y. Times*, January 25, 1941; *Who Was Who in Am.*, 1: 1187.

S. Galishoff

STILL, ANDREW TAYLOR (August 6, 1828, Jonesville or Jonesboro, Va.-December 12, 1917, Kirksville, Mo.). *Physician; Osteopath.* Son of Abraham,

Methodist minister and missionary among the Shawnee Indians, and Martha Poage (Moore) Still. Married Mary Margaret Vaughan, June 29, 1849 (d. 1859), five children; Mary E. Turner, November 15, 1860 (d. 1910), seven children. EDUCATION: No formal schooling; attended occasional classes in Kansas School of Physicians and Surgeons; became an eclectic physician in Kansas City, Mo. CAREER: 1849-53, practiced medicine in Adair and Macon counties, Mo.; 1853, moved family to Kans.; active antislave advocate; October 1857, elected Free Soil Candidate to the first Kans. legislature; during the Civil War, major, 21st Kansas Volunteers; 1865, lost three children to spinal meningitis; *post* 1874, practiced, Kirksville; 1892, incorporated the American School of Osteopathy, Kirksville (charter granted the right to confer the M.D. degree; however, the D.O. degree was chosen; 16 men and three women graduated in the first class of 1894). CONTRIBUTIONS: With the loss of his children, centered interests in the spinal cord and illnesses caused by spinal irritation or dislocation from falls or strains, treating them by manipulation. Theory was that disease is a failure of nerves to conduct the fluids of life properly. All remedies necessary to health exist in the human body. Disease stems from tissues slipping out of place creating local damage; through manipulation tissues can be placed in their normal location. Developed a system of manipulation intended to realign functional deviations and abnormalities; only necessary to manipulate the spine or twist the neck.

WRITINGS: *Autobiography of A. T. Still* (1897; rev., 1908); *Philosophy of Osteopathy* (1899); *The Philosophy on Mechanical Principles of Osteopathy* (1902); *Osteopathy, Practice and Research* (1910). REFERENCES: *BHM* (1970-74), 164; (1975-79), 122; (1980), 38; *DAB*, 9, pt.2: 21-22; Geoffrey Marks and William Beatty, *The Story of Med. in Am.* (1973), 189-93; *NCAB*, 26: 245; Francis Schiller, "Spinal Irritation and Osteopathy," *Bull. Hist. Med.* 45 (1971): 250-66.

R. Edwards

STILL, JAMES (April 9, 1812, Indian Mill, Burlington County, N.J.-1885, Mt. Holly, N.J.). *Self-taught practitioner*. Son of Levin and Charity Still. Married Angelina Willow, 1835 (d. 1838); one child; Henrietta Thomas, 1839; one child. EDUCATION: No formal education beyond three months of training in the three "R's"; self-taught. CAREER: 1833-34, worker in glue factory, Philadelphia, Pa.; 1834-43, farmer, southern N.J.; 1843-85, medical practice, Mount Holly, N.J. area. CONTRIBUTIONS: Early, highly successful black practitioner in South Jersey. Treated both black and white patients, primarily with botanic remedies.

WRITINGS: *Early Recollections and Life of Dr. James Still* (1877). REFERENCES: W. Montague Cobb, " 'Dr.' James Still-New Jersey Pioneer," *JNMA* 55 (1963): 196-99; Margery Cridland, "Historical Sketch," pp. v-ix of introduction to 1971 reprint of Still's autobiography; *Early Recollections and Life of Dr. James Still* (1877).

T. L. Savitt

STILLÉ, ALFRED (October 30, 1813, Philadelphia, Pa.-September 24, 1900, Philadelphia). *Physician; Pathology*. Son of John and Maria (Wagner) Stillé. Married Caroline Barnett, 1841, three children; Katharine A. Blackiston, 1899. EDUCATION: Yale College; University of Pennsylania: 1832, A.B., 1835, A.M.;

and 1836, M.D.; 1850, M.A., Yale College; 1836-38, study in Europe, where he was influenced by Pierre Louis. CAREER: 1836, house physician, Blockley (Philadelphia General Hospital); 1839-41, resident physician, Pennsylvania Hospital; 1841, began private practice, Philadelphia; 1849-77, visiting physician, St. Joseph's Hospital; 1845-51, lecturer on pathology and practice of medicine, Philadelphia Association for Medical Instruction; 1854-59, professor of medicine, Pennsylvania Medical College; 1864-83, professor of the theory and practice of medicine, University of Pennsylvania. CONTRIBUTIONS: A leading American physician of his time. A founder, American Medical Association, its first secretary and president (1871). A founder, Philadelphia Pathological Society and its president (1859-62). President, College of Physicians of Philadelphia (1883). Author of textbooks in pathology and therapeutics and materia medica.

WRITINGS: *Elements of General Pathology* (1848); *Therapeutics and Materia Medica* (1860); *Epidemic Meningitis . . .* (1867). Collaborated on the production of the *National Dispensatory* (1878). REFERENCES: *DAB*, 9: 23-24; *NCAB*, 9: 358; *Trans., Coll. of Physicians of Phila.* (1902).

M. Kaufman

STOKES, JOSEPH, JR. (February 22, 1896, Moorestown, N.J.-March 9, 1972, Chestnut Hill, Pa.). *Physician; Pediatrics.* Son of Joseph, Sr., physician, and Mary (Emlen) Stokes. Married Frances Eikitnon, 1921; four children. EDUCATION: 1916, B.S., Haverford College; 1920, M.D., University of Pennsylvania; 1920-22, intern and resident, Massachusetts General Hospital; 1922-24, resident, Pennsylvania Hospital and Children's Hospital of Philadelphia. CAREER: At University of Pennsylvania Medical School: 1923-28, instructor, pediatrics; 1928-31, associate in pediatrics; 1931-36, assistant professor, pediatrics; 1936-38, associate professor, pediatrics; 1939-62, William H. Bennett, Professor of pediatrics; and 1962-72, professor emeritus; at Children's Hospital of Philadelphia: 1936-38, associate physician-in-chief; and 1939-63, physician-in-chief; 1930-39, director, Pediatric Services, Abington Hospital; 1939-62, chief, Pediatric Service, Hospital of the University of Pennsylvania; 1958-59, president, American Pediatric Society. CONTRIBUTIONS: Discovered the value of gamma globulin as a method for the prevention of epidemic hepatitis (1944). Actively involved in field trials for a number of new vaccines, including those for rubella and mumps. Also responsible for introducing the first diagnostic virus laboratory into any clinical department in the United States (1939).

WRITINGS: "Prevention and Attenuation of Infectious Hepatitis by Gamma Globulin, Preliminary Note," *JAMA* 127 (1945): 144-45 (with J. R. Neefe); "Methods of Protection Against Homologous Serum Hepatitis," *JAMA* 138 (1948): 336-41 (with others); "Measles Vaccines: Assured Safety," *Sci.* 157 (1967): 626-28; "Trivalent Combined Measles Mumps Rubella Vaccine," *JAMA* 218 (1971): 57-61 (with others). REFERENCES: Alfred M. Bongiovanni, "Obituary—Joseph Stokes, Jr.," *Pediatrics* 50 (1972): 163-64; Horace L. Hode, "Presentation of the John Howland Medal and Award to Dr. Joseph Stokes, Jr.," *Am. J. of Diseases of Children 104* (1962): 440-42.

N. Gevitz

STONE, WARREN (February 3, 1808, St. Albans, Vt.-December 6, 1872, New Orleans, La.). *Surgeon.* Son of Peter, farmer, and Jerusha (Snow) Stone.

Married Malvina Dunreith Johnson, 1843; three children. EDUCATION: Apprentice to Dr. Amos Twitchell (q.v.), Keene, N.H.; 1831, M.D., Berkshire Medical Institution (Pittsfield, Mass.). CAREER: 1832, began practice, Troy, N.Y.; December 1832, moved to New Orleans; 1832-72, practice, New Orleans; 1834-72, staff, Charity Hospital; 1839, with Dr. W. E. Kennedy, founded the Maison de Santé, an early private hospital, New Orleans; 1834-72, University of Louisiana (later Tulane University) as professor of surgery (1839-72); during Civil War, surgeon-general, La., and imprisoned by federal authorities; 1857-68, co-editor, *New Orleans Medical and Surgical Journal.* CONTRIBUTIONS: A leading surgeon, first to resect part of a rib to secure drainage in empyema. First successful case of traumatic vertebral aneurism by open incision and packing (1850). First use of silver wire to ligate the external iliac. Claimed to be the first to use quinine in yellow-fever cases. Discovered (1832) that cold water, used internally and externally, was of benefit to cholera patients.

WRITINGS: *Clinical Memoranda* (1868); *Notes from the Lectures of Dr. Warren Stone* (1868). REFERENCES: *DAB*, 9: 85-86; John Duffy, *History of Medicine in Louisiana* 2 (1962); Miller, *BHM*, p. 110; *NCAB*, 5: 22; Kelly and Burrage (1920); R. F. Stone, *Biog. of Eminent Am. Physicians & Surgeons* (1894).

M. Kaufman

STORER, DAVID HUMPHREYS (March 26, 1804, Portland, Maine-September 10, 1891, Boston, Mass.). *Physician; Naturalist; Obstetrics.* Son of Woodbury and Margaret (Boyd) Storer. Married Abby Jane Brewer, 1829; five children. EDUCATION: 1822, A.B., Bowdoin College, Brunswick, Maine; 1825, M.D., Harvard Medical School; 1825, apprentice to Dr. John Collins Warren (q.v.), Boston. CAREER: 1837, a founder of and taught at Tremont Street Medical School, Boston; 1854-68, professor of obstetrics and medical jurisprudence, Harvard Medical School; and obstetrician, Boston Lying-in Hospital; 1855-64, dean, Harvard Medical School. CONTRIBUTIONS: Popular Boston teacher of obstetrics, contributed to medical education. Founder, Obstetrical Society of Boston (1861) and American Gynecological Society (1876). Made important contributions to ichthyology, conchology, and natural history, describing many original species.

WRITINGS: *Report on the Fishes and Reptiles of Massachusetts* (1839); *A Synopsis of the Fishes of North America* (1846); *A History of the Fishes of Massachusetts* (1867). Writings listed in *Bowdoin College Library Bull.* no. 2 (Aug. 1892): 72-78. REFERENCES: *DAB*, 9: 93-94; George E. Gifford, Jr., "The Ichthyologist Dean," *Harvard Med. Alumni Bull.* 39 (1964): 22-27; Frederick C. Irving, "Father and Son," in *Safe Deliverance* (1942), 104-19; *NCAB*, 11: 336; Samuel H. Scudder, "Biographical Notice of David Humphreys Storer," *Proc., Am. Acad. of Arts and Sci.* 27 (1893): 388-91.

L. D. Longo

STORER, HORATIO ROBINSON (February 27, 1830, Boston, Mass.-September 18, 1922, Newport, R.I.). *Physician; Obstetrics and gynecology.* Son of David Humphreys (q.v.), physician, and Abby Jane (Brewer) Storer. Married Elvira Gilmore, 1853, four children; Augusta Caroline Gilmore, 1872, one child; Frances S. Mackenzie, 1876. EDUCATION: Boston Latin School; 1850, A.B.,

Harvard College; 1853, M.D., Harvard Medical School; 1853-55, studied in Paris, London, and Edinburgh; 1868, LL.B., Harvard Law School. CAREER: 1855-62, practiced, Boston; 1862-72, specialized in gynecology; 1865-67, professor of obstetrics and medical jurisprudence, Berkshire Medical Institution, Pittsfield, Mass. CONTRIBUTIONS: Respected gynecologist, advocate of chloroform for obstetrical anesthesia, and one of first to perform caesarean-hysterectomy. Founder and president, Boston Gynecological Society. Amassed remarkable collection of more than 2,000 medals (the Storer Memorial Collection of Medical Medals), which he gave to the Boston Medical Library.

WRITINGS: "Eutokia: A Word to Physicians and Women upon the Employment of Anesthetics in Childbirth" (1863); *Criminal Abortion, Its Nature, Its Evidence, Its Law* (1868), edited, with F. F. Heard; *Why Not! A Book for Every Woman . . .* (1868); *Is It I—A Book for Every Man* (1869); *The Causation, Course and Treatment of Reflex Insanity in Women* (1871). REFERENCES: *DAB*, 9: 95-96; John W. Farlow, *The History of the Boston Medical Library* (1918), 58, 141-47; *NCAB*, 11: 337.

L. D. Longo

STRAUS, NATHAN (January 31, 1848, Otterberg, Rhenish Bavaria-January 11, 1931, New York, N.Y.). *Merchant; Public health philanthropist.* Son of Lazarus, merchant, and Sara (Straus) Straus. Went to the United States with family in 1854. Married Lina Gutherz, 1875; three children. EDUCATION: Graduated from Packard's Business College. CAREER: 1866, entered father's pottery and glassware importing business; later was associated with Abraham and Straus and R. H. Macy and Company; 1914, retired to devote full time to philanthropic activities; 1898, president, New York City Board of Health; 1911, 1912, U.S. delegate, International Health Congress. CONTRIBUTIONS: Established hundreds of milk stations in American and foreign cities, where pasteurized milk was sold to the poor at or below cost; maintained stations at own expense until they were provided for by government; demonstrated that there were far fewer deaths among babies given pasteurized milk than those fed raw milk; led to a gradual acceptance of pasteurization, which helped bring about a sharp reduction in the high infant mortality rates of the early twentieth century. Established the first tuberculosis preventorium for children in Lakewood, N.J. (1909). Provided some of the first modern health facilities in Palestine, including a health bureau to fight malaria and trachoma, a Pasteur Institute, child-health welfare stations, and the Nathan and Lina Straus Health Centers in Jerusalem and Tel Aviv (1912-27).

WRITINGS: Author of pamphlets on pasteurization and various social problems. REFERENCES: *Am. J. of Public Health* 21 (1931): 233; *Biog. Index*, 8: 656; 9: 681; *DAB*, 18: 129-30; *N.Y. Times*, January 12, 1931; *Who Was Who in Am.*, 1: 1197.

S. Galishoff

STREETER, GEORGE LINIUS (January 12, 1873, Johnstown, N.Y.-July 27, 1948, Gloversville, N.Y.). *Physician; Embryology.* Son of George Austin, glove manufacturer, and Hannah Green (Anthony) Streeter. Married Julia Allen Smith, 1910; three children. EDUCATION: 1895, B.A., Union College; 1899,

M.D., A.M., College of Physicians and Surgeons (Columbia); 1899-1900, intern, Roosevelt Hospital, New York City; 1902-3, studied anatomy and embryology, Germany. CAREER: 1900-1902, assistant to Henry Hun, neurologist, Albany, N.Y.; anatomy faculty: 1901-2, Albany Medical College; 1904-6, Johns Hopkins Medical School; 1906-7, Wistar Institute of Anatomy and Biology, Philadelphia, Pa.; and 1907-14, University of Michigan; at Carnegie Institution of Washington, located at the Johns Hopkins Medical School: 1914-17, research associate; 1917-40, director, Department of Embryology; 1935-40, chairman, Division of Animal Biology; and *post* 1940, research associate; 1926-28, president, American Association of Anatomists. CONTRIBUTIONS: A brilliant descriptive embryologist, principal researches were in the development of the human brain, nerves, and auditory system. Chapter on the development of the major structures of the brain in Franz Keibel and Franklin P. Mall's (q.v.) *Manual of Human Embryology* (1912) has not been superseded. Described (1918) the development of the labyrinth of the human ear. Published charts and data (1920s) showing the size and weight of human embryos and fetuses at successive stages of development. At the Carnegie Institution, encouraged both morphological and experimental work that made his department preeminent in embryological research. Directed the publication of 22 volumes (viii-xxix) of the *Contributions to Embryology of the Carnegie Institution*. Encouraged John Rock and Arthur T. Hertig, Boston, Mass., in their important study of the first days of human development. After retirement (1940), wrote a series of papers entitled "Developmental Horizons in Human Development" (1942-51), a descriptive and pictorial account of the stages of embryonic development to about the 48th day of gestation. Argued that morbid processes in the fetus are largely due to genetic causes rather than defective uterine environment.

WRITINGS: "On the Development of the Membranous Labyrinth and the Acoustic and Facial Nerves in the Human Embryo," *Am. J. of Anatomy* 6 (1907): 139-65; "The Developmental Alterations in the Vascular System of the Brain of the Human Embryo," *Contributions to Embryology* 8 (1918): 5-38; "The Histogenesis and Growth of the Otic Capsule and Its Contained Periotic Tissue-Spaces in the Human Embryo," *ibid.*, 7 (1918): 5-55; "Weight, Sitting Height, Head Size, Foot Length, and Menstrual Age of the Human Embryo," *ibid.*, 11 (1920): 143-70; "The Significance of Morbid Processes in the Fetus," *Harvey Lectures* 29 (1934): 204-19. A bibliography is in *BMNAS*. REFERENCES: *BMNAS* 28 (1954): 261-87; *DAB*, Supplement 4: 800-802; *DSB*, 13: 96-97; *NCAB*, 37: 356-57.

S. Galishoff

STUBBS, FREDERICK DOUGLASS (1906, Wilmington, Del.-February 9, 1947, died on train from Philadelphia, Pa., to New York, N.Y.). *Surgeon*. Son of J. Bacon, physician, and Blanche (Williams) Stubbs. Married Marion V. Turner, 1934; two children. EDUCATION: 1927, A.B., Dartmouth College (magna cum laude); 1927, Rufus Choate Scholar for summer study, Marine Biology Lab, Woods Hole, Mass.; 1931, M.D., Harvard Medical School (cum laude); 1931-33, intern, Cleveland City Hospital (first black)—studied general and thoracic surgery; 1933-34, resident in surgery, Douglass Memorial Hospital, Philadelphia; 1937-38, resident in thoracic surgery, Sea View Hospital, N.Y. (tuberculosis); while a Harvard Medical School student, spent one summer at an informal clinical course in medicine, Freedmen's Hospital, Washington, D.C., and another summer studying experimental surgery, Long Island Biological Lab., Cold Spring Harbor, Long Island, N.Y. CAREER: 1934-37, 1938-47, surgical practice, Philadelphia: surgical staff, Philadelphia General Hospital (first black); administrator, Philadelphia Health Center, Philadelphia Department of Health; chief of surgery, Douglass Hospital, Philadelphia; Mercy Hospital, Philadelphia; acting chief, Division of Tuberculosis, Philadelphia General Hospital (first black), 1947, named chief, Tuberculosis Division, Jefferson Medical School, but died before assuming duties. CONTRIBUTIONS: First formally trained black thoracic surgeon (1938), the pioneer black surgeon in Philadelphia, and leading black medical figure in Philadelphia at time of his death. President, Pennsylvania Medical, Dental, and Pharmaceutical Association. Vice-president, NMA. Contributing editor, *Journal of the National Medical Association*. Member, various tuberculosis committees and commissions.

WRITINGS: Wrote several articles, primarily on lung diseases, for example, "Acute Silicosis," *Arch. Path.* 24 (1939): 274; "The Fundamental Physiologic Concepts Underlying Major Surgery of the Chest," *JNMA* 35 (1943): 1. Writings listed in *JNMA* 40 (1948): 26. REFERENCES: W. Montague Cobb, "Frederick Douglass Stubbs, 1906-1947, An Appreciation," *JNMA* 40 (1948): 24-26; *N.Y. Times,* February 10, 1947, p. 29.

T. L. Savitt

SULLIVAN, HARRY STACK (February 21, 1892, Norwich, N.Y.-January 14, 1949, Paris, France). *Physician; Psychiatry.* Son of Timothy J. and Ella M. (Stack) Sullivan. Never married. In 1927, adopted informally a patient, James Inscoe, as James I. Sullivan. EDUCATION: Cornell University: 1908, entered; and 1909, suspended; 1911-17, Chicago College of Medicine and Surgery (later part of Loyola University), M.D., 1917; psychoanalysis (in Chicago, Ill., 1916-17; in Baltimore, Md., and New York, N.Y., with Clara M. Thompson). CAREER: 1917, industrial surgeon, Chicago; 1917-18, 1st lieutenant, U.S. Medical Corps; 1919-22, assistant medical officer, Rehabilitation Division, Federal Board for Vocational Education; 1922-23, veterans' liaison officer, St. Elizabeth's Hospital, Washington, D.C.; 1923-30, director of clinical research, Sheppard and Enoch Pratt Hospital, Baltimore, 1930-39, private practice of psychiatry, N.Y.; 1939-49, private practice and consulting, Washington, D.C. CONTRIBUTIONS: Established (1938) William Alanson White Psychiatric Foundation (named for superintendent of St. Elizabeth's Hospital), which supported Washington School of Psychiatry and *Psychiatry* (which Sullivan edited). With assistance from anthropologists and sociologists, developed psychiatric system that stressed social forces as determinants of personality traits and psychological disorders. Looked upon "interpersonal event" as unit of psychological study. Attempted to apply psychiatry to study of social problems— took part in the 1948 UNESCO study of "tensions that cause wars." Consultant in establishing psychiatric examinations for recruits for the Selective Service System (1940).

WRITINGS: *Conceptions of Modern Psychiatry* (1940; rep. with additions, 1947,

1953); *Personal Psychopathology* (1972; privately circulated in typescript, 1932). After death, published and unpublished essays were collected by Helen Swick Perry and published in five volumes: *The Interpersonal Theory of Psychiatry* (1953); *The Psychiatric Interview* (1954); *Clinical Studies in Psychiatry* (1956); *Schizophrenia as a Human Process* (1962); *The Fusion of Psychiatry and Social Science* (1972).REFERENCES: Arthur H. Chapman, *Harry Stack Sullivan: His Life and Work* (1976); Kenneth L. Chatelaine, *"Harry Stack Sullivan—The Formative Years"* (Ph.D. diss., University of Maryland, 1978); *Current Biog.* (1942); *DAB*, Supplement 4: 805-8; David Elkind, " 'Good Me' or 'Bad Me'—The Sullivan Approach to Personality," *N.Y. Times Magazine*, September 24, 1972, pp. 18-19 ff.; Leslie Farber, "Harry Stack Sullivan and the American Dream," *Times Literary Supplement*, April 1, 1977, pp. 386-88 (cf. letter by Ralph M. Crowley, *Times Literary Supplement*, April 29, 1977); Patrick Mullahy, *The Beginnings of Modern American Psychiatry: The Ideas of Harry Stack Sullivan* (1973); *NUC Pre-1956 Imprints*, 576: 141-42; *N.Y. Times*, January 16, 1949, p. 68. Two bibliographies are Ralph M. Crowley, "Harry Stack Sullivan: The Complete Bibliography," in *Interpersonal Approach to Psychoanalysis: Contemporary View of Harry Stack Sullivan*, ed. Gerard Chrzanowski (1977), 219-34; and *Psychiatry* 3 (1940): 172-73.

                                                                                                M. M. Sokal

SULLIVAN, JOHN JEROME (January 23, 1877, Virginia City, Nev.-December 14, 1951, Reno, Nev.). *Physician*. Married Maude Hobart, November 16, 1910; two children. EDUCATION: 1898, premedical studies, University of Nevada; 1901, M.A., St. Francis Xavier College (New York City); 1902, M.D., Columbia College. CAREER: Medical practice, Reno, Nev.; 1915-18, superintendent, Nevada State Hospital; 1908-12, member, Nevada State Board of Health. CONTRIBUTIONS: Native Nevadan who went east for medical degree and training and returned to Nev. for lifetime of practice. Chief of staff, St. Mary's Hospital (Reno), and member, Nevada Board of Medical Examiners. Appointed regent, University of Nevada (1909-11, 1914-24).

                                                                                                J. Edwards

SUMMERS, JOHN EDWARD, JR. (January 2, 1858, Fort Kearney, Neb.-February 7, 1935, Omaha, Neb.). *Physician*; *Surgeon*. Son of Brigadier Gen. John Edward, U.S. Army medical department, and Mrs. Carolyn Jane (Stewart) Summers. Married Laura Marian Hoagland, August 24, 1895; two children. EDUCATION: West Point Military Academy; 1881, M.D., College of Physicians and Surgeons, N.Y.; 1883-85, studied in Vienna and British Isles. CAREER: 1881-83, U.S. Army acting assistant surgeon, frontier posts in northern Wyo.; chief surgeon: 1885-1935, Bishop Clarkson Memorial Hospital, Omaha; and 1891-1931, Douglas County Hospital, Immanuel Hospital, and Wise Memorial Hospital; at Omaha Medical College: 1887-1902, professor of surgery; 1890-1901, member, Board of Trustees; 1891, secretary; and 1897, president of the faculty; 1913-35, professor of clinical surgery, University of Nebraska College of Medicine; charter member, fellow, and governor, American College of Surgeons; fellow, American Medical Association; president: 1895-96, Nebraska State Medical Association; and 1895-96, Western Surgical Association; continued in active practice, Omaha, until death due to a heart attack. CONTRIBUTIONS: Made the first wide-open incision for contracture of cervical muscles and the first nephropexy in Neb. (1889). Other pioneering procedures included removal of gangrenous appendix in a child of less than two years old (1891); first nephrectomy for tuberculosis of the kidney in Neb. (1893); surgery for tubal pregnancy; internal esophagostomy; first reported case (1900) in America of *choled ocho enterostomy*; and an early advocate of jejunostomy. Did the first cardiolysis (1913) in America and reported (1928, 1929) on duodenojejunostomy followed by investigation (1930) of the use of Normet's solution as an emergency substitute for blood transfusion. In the vanguard of those American surgeons to use spinal anesthesia. Well known for successful treatment for puncture wound of the heart.

WRITINGS: *Modern Treatment of Wounds* (1899); 207 publications listed in *Nebraska State Med. J.* 17 no. 4 (Apr. 1932): 135-45. REFERENCES: Archives, University of Nebraska Medical Center Library of Medicine, Omaha; *NCAB*, 28: 406-7; *Nebraska State Med. J.* 17, no. 4 (Apr. 1932): 135-45; H. W. Orr, *History of Medicine in Nebraska* (1952), 21, 77; A. T. Tyler, and E. F. Auerbach, *History of Medicine in Nebraska* (1977, enlarged by B. M. Hetzner), 153-54.

B. M. Hetzner

SUTHERLAND, EARL WILBUR, JR. (November 19, 1915, Burlingame, Kans.-March 9, 1974, Miami, Fla.). *Physician; Endocrinology; Physiology; Biochemistry*. Son of Earl Wilbur and Edith (Hartshorn) Sutherland. Married Mildred Rice, 1937, three children; Claudia S. Smith, 1963. EDUCATION: 1937, B.S., Washburn College; 1942, M.D., Washington University (St. Louis, Mo.); 1942-43, intern, Barnes Hospital, St. Louis; 1940-42, assistant in pharmacology, Washington University. CAREER: At Washington University: 1945-46, instructor in pharmacology; 1946-50, instructor; 1950-52, assistant professor; and 1952-53, associate professor, biochemistry; 1953-63, professor of pharmacology, Case-Western Reserve University School of Medicine; 1963-73, professor of physiology, Vanderbilt University School of Medicine; 1973-74, distinguished professor of biochemistry, University of Miami School of Medicine. CONTRIBUTIONS: Made first major discovery (1955) of hormonal aspects of carbohydrate metabolism; showed the method by which adrenaline regulates the breakdown of carbohydrates stored in the liver; demonstrated that it activates the enzyme phosphorylase, which in turn stimulates the release of glucose from glycogen in the liver. A few years later, isolated a previously unknown chemical, cyclic adenosine 3'5'-monophosphate, or cyclic AMP, which functions in an intermediate role in many hormonal processes; proved that hormones do not directly activate their target organs but rather trigger production of cyclic AMP, which stimulates or inhibits cellular activity. Proposed a unifying concept for the molecular basis of hormone action in which cyclic AMP acts as a "second messenger" and hormones as "first messengers"; was awarded the 1979 Nobel prize in medicine or physiology for this work.

WRITINGS: "The Biological Role of Adenosine 3'5'-Phosphate," *Harvey Lecture Series* 57 (1962): 17-33. A bibliography is in *BMNAS*. REFERENCES: *Am. Men and Women of Sci.* (1973); *BMNAS* 49 (1978): 319-50; *British Med. J.* 4 (1971): 188; *JAMA*

228 (1974): 970; R. H. Kampmeier, in *Southern Med. J.* 64: 1413-14; *N.Y. Times*, March 10, 1974; *Sci.* 174 (1971): 392-93; *Time Magazine*, October 25, 1971; *Who Was Who in Am.*, 6: 399.

S. R. Bruesch

SUTTON, WILLIAM LOFTUS (May 21, 1797, near Georgetown, Scott County, Ky.-July 20, 1862, Georgetown). *Physician; Vital statistician.* Son of John, Jr., farmer, and Mary (Coleman) Sutton. Married Mary Belle Catlett, May 14, 1820, three children; Nancy Cooper, 1836, two children; Mrs. Ann Tibbs Webb, August 20, 1843, three children. EDUCATION: Early schooling, Rittenhouse Academy, Georgetown; and Bourbon Academy, Paris, Ky.; 1815-17, apprentice, in medicine, of Richard B. Ferguson (q.v.), Louisville, Ky.; 1817-18, Transylvania University Medical Department, Lexington, Ky.; 1818, M.D., Transylvania University; 1818-19, Medical College of Maryland (University of Maryland medical department), Baltimore, Md.; 1819, M.D., Medical College of Maryland. CAREER: 1814, taught school, Louisville; December 10, 1818, licensed to practice medicine by Medical and Chirurgical Society of Maryland; practiced: 1818 (summer), 1819-20, Catlettsburg, Ky.; 1820 (February)-33, Morganfield, Union County, Ky.; and 1833-62, Georgetown; 1851, president (first), Kentucky State Medical Society. CONTRIBUTIONS: Spent professional lifetime in efforts to raise the standards of medical education; to institute public health laws, especially the registration of births, marriages, and deaths; to improve obstetric care and the reporting of communicable (epidemic) diseases. As chairman, Kentucky State Medical Society, Committee on Registration of Births, Marriages and Deaths (1851-52), campaigned for the adoption of the proposed law and demonstrated its need and usefulness. First Vital Statistics Law in Ky. (1852) passed with Sutton's guidance and the efforts of the Kentucky State Medical Society. Was in effect the registrar of vital statistics (1853-59), since he prepared the annual reports of registration of births, marriages, and deaths for the state legislature and for publication. Proposed new registration form patterned after R.I. form (1857). Obtained an amended Kentucky Registration of Vital Statistics Law (1859) providing for a state registrar. (The laws concerning registry of vital statistics were repealed [1862] and not reinstituted in Ky. until 1910.) Chairman, Committee on Epidemics of American Medical Association (1851-55) and contributed to the study of the influence of weather, geology, and topography on the etiology and spread of epidemic disease. Chairman, American Medical Association Committee on a Uniform Plan for Registration Reports of Births, Marriages and Deaths (1858). Report also included a list of the causes of death, an early effort at achieving a standard nomenclature.

WRITINGS: "Facts and Conjectures on the Trembles and Milk Sickness" *Western J. of Med. & Sci.* 6 (1842): 181-85; *A History of the Diseases Usually Called Typhoid Fever. . .*(1850); "Report on the Medical Topography and the Epidemic Diseases of Kentucky," *TAMA* 11 (1858); "Report on a Uniform Plan for Registration Reports of Births, Marriages and Deaths," ibid., 12 (1859): 137-82. A bibliography of 57 publications is in Goldsborough and Fisher, *William Loftus Sutton, M.D., 1797-1862* (1948), pp. 168-73. REFERENCES: C. T. Goldsborough and A. G. Fisher, *William Loftus Sutton,*

M.D., 1797-1862 (1948); *Papers Presented Before the Ephraim McDowell Memorial Meeting Centennial of the Kentucky State Medical Association* (1952), p. xxx.

E. H. Conner

SWAIN, CLARA (July 18, 1834, Elmira, N.Y.-December 25, 1910, Castile, N.Y.). *Physician; Medical missionary.* Daughter of John and Clarissa (Seavey) Swain. Never married. EDUCATION: 1869, M.D., Woman's Medical College of Pennsylvania; 1865, 1867-69, worked at the Castile Sanitarium with Dr. Cordelia Green. CAREER: 1869, sailed with Isabella Thoburn, another Methodist missionary, to Bareilly, India; there, under the auspices of the Woman's Foreign Missionary Society of the Methodist Episcopal Church, provided medical care to Indian women; 1870, began lectures in anatomy, physiology, materia medica, and diseases of women and children for Indian women, Bareilly; 1874, opened the first hospital for women in India (Bareilly); 1885, became palace physician for the Rani of Khetri and Rajah of Rajputana (Khetri). CONTRIBUTIONS: First woman medical missionary in Asia. As a woman physician, was able to provide health care for Indian women who otherwise could not receive medical attention because of the religious customs that secluded women in Zenanas and forbade a woman being looked upon by any male other than her relative.

WRITINGS: "A Doctor Lady's Story," in Ross C. Houghton, *Women of the Orient* (1877); *A Glimpse of India* (1909). REFERENCES: Archives and Special Collections on Women in Medicine, the Medical College of Pennsylvania (alumnae files and Dr. Marion S. Fay Collection); Margaret I. Balfour and Ruth Young, *The Work of Medical Women in India* (1929); *DAB*, 9, pt. 2: 221-30; *Notable Am. Women, 1607-1950*, 3: 411-13; Mary Sparkes Wheeler, *First Decade of the Woman's Foreign Missionary Society of the Methodist Episcopal Church, with Sketches of Its Missionaries* (1881); Dorothy Clarke Wilson, *Palace of Healing: The Story of Dr. Clara Swain* (1968).

S. L. Chaff

SWIFT, HOMER FORDYCE (May 5, 1881, Paines Hollow, N.Y.-September 24, 1953, New York, N.Y.). *Physician; Internal medicine.* Son of Charles Fayette, Baptist clergyman, and Nancy Maria (Fordyce) Swift. Married Emma Fordyce MacRae, 1922; no children. EDUCATION: 1902, Ph.B., Western Reserve University; 1906, M.D., New York University and Bellevue Hospital Medical College; 1906-8, intern, Presbyterian Hospital (N.Y.). CAREER: 1908-10, pathology and dermatology faculties, New York University and Bellevue Hospital Medical College; 1910-14, medical staff, Hospital of the Rockefeller Institute for Medical Research (later Rockefeller University); medicine faculty: 1914-17, Columbia University; and 1917-19, Cornell Medical College; 1917-19, U.S. Marine Medical Corps; 1917-18, member, American Red Cross Trench Fever Commission; 1919-46, at Rockefeller Institute for Medical Research; 1923-48, member, Board of Directors, Russell Sage Institute of Pathology; 1942-47, consultant, secretary of war; president: 1928, American Society for Clinical Investigation; and 1925-26, Harvey Society. CONTRIBUTIONS: Collaborated in a study of trench fever sponsored by the American Red Cross, which for many years was the definitive source in its field (1918). With Arthur W. M. Ellis, introduced the Swift-Ellis treatment of syphilis of the central nervous system, which was used widely until it was superseded by other treatments. Made valuable studies of rheumatic fever, rheumatic heart disease, and streptococcal infections.

WRITINGS: "The Intestinal Treatment of Syphilis," *JAMA* 59 (Oct. 5, 1912): 1251-54; *Trench Fever* (1918, with others). Was a contributor to Frederich Forchheimer, *Therapeusis of Internal Diseases* (1914); John H. Musser and Howard A. Kelly, *Practical Treatment* (1917); Nelson, *Loose-Leaf Medicine* (1920); *A Textbook of Medicine by American Authors* (1927); *Oxford Loose-Leaf Medicine* (1938); and René Dubos, *Bacterial and Mycotic Infections of Man* (1948). REFERENCES: *NCAB*, 40: 69; *N.Y. Times*, September 25, 1953; *Who Was Who in Am.*, 3: 838.

S. Galishoff

SYDENSTRICKER, EDGAR (July 15, 1881, Shanghai, China-March 19, 1936, New York, N.Y.). *Public health statistician and investigator*. Son of Rev. Absalom, missionary, and Mrs. Caroline (Stulting) Sydenstricker. Married Alice May Ringer, 1908, two children; Phyllis Perrott, 1932, no children. EDUCATION: 1896, returned to America from China; 1900, B.A., Fredericksburg College, Va.; 1902, M.A., Washington and Lee University; 1907-8, postgraduate education, University of Chicago. CAREER: 1902-5, principal, Onancock High School, Va.; 1905-7, editor, *Lynchburg Daily Advocate*; 1907-11, special investigator, U.S. Commission on Immigration; 1914-15, staff, U.S. Commission on Industrial Relations; 1915, became statistician, U.S. Public Health Service; 1920-28, chief, Office of Statistical Investigations; 1923, while on leave, served as the first chief, statistical and epidemiological service, League of Nations; 1926-35, consultant, director of research, administrative head, Milbank Fund. CONTRIBUTIONS: A leading investigator of public health conditions and the impact of economics on health. With the U.S. Public Health Service, worked with Dr. Joseph Goldberger (q.v.) on causes of pellagra in the South (1916-20); with Dr. Wade H. Frost (q.v.) on influenza epidemics in America. Studied morbidity in a representative community (1921, Hagerstown Morbidity Studies, published 1926-29). Member, Committee on the Costs of Medical Care (1927-32), working to analyze statistical information. During beginning of the Great Depression, served President Hoover to evaluate impact of depression on public health.

WRITINGS: *Conditions of Labor in American Industries* (1917); *Health and Environment* (1933). REFERENCES: *BHM* (1975-79), 124; *DAB*, Supplement 2: 645-47; *NCAB*, 27: 203; *N.Y. Times*, March 21, 1936; *Who Was Who in Am.* 1 (1942).

M. Kaufman

T

TAIT, F. DUDLEY (1862, San Francisco, Calif.-February 26, 1918, San Francisco). *Physician; Surgeon.* Son of George Tait, college professor. EDU-CATION: 1886, M.D., Bellevue Hospital Medical College; 1889, M.D., University of Paris. CAREER: 1889 to death, practiced, San Francisco; surgeon-in-chief, French Hospital, and attending surgeon, Woman's Hospital; 1901-9, California Board of Medical Examiners and thereafter connected with the Experimental Surgical Laboratory, University of California. CONTRIBUTIONS: Although a skillful operator and contributor to experimental medicine, was best known in his time as a forceful advocate of higher educational standards and a revised college curriculum based largely upon the French model.

WRITINGS: "Experimental and Clinical Notes on the Subarachnoid Space," *JAMA* 35 (1900): 6-10 (with G. Caglieri); "Eversion of the Tunica Vaginalis as a Remedy for Hydrocele," *Annals of Surg.* 33 (1901): 305-10; "Electric Sleep: An Experimental and Clinical Study," *JAMA* 53 (1909): 1611-14 (with R. Russ); "Mistakes in Medical Education," *Calif. State J. of Med.* 9 (1911): 413-25; "Fibrous Atrophy of the Parotid Gland with Especial Reference to the Treatment of the Salivary Fistula," *Surg. Gyn. & Obst.* 14 (1912): 456-62. REFERENCES: Henry Harris, *California Medical Story* (1932), 206-7; "Obituary: F. Dudley Tait," *Calif. State J. of Med.* 16 (1918): 272.

N. Gevitz

TAKAMINE, JOKICHI (November 3, 1854, Kanazawa, Japan-July 22, 1922, New York, N.Y.). *Biochemist.* Son of Seiichi, physician, and Yukiko Takamine. Married Caroline Hitch, 1885; two children. EDUCATION: 1880, graduate of College of Science and Engineering, Tokyo; 1880-83, graduate study, Anderson's College, Glasgow, and at Glasgow University. CAREER: 1883, Department of Agriculture and Commerce (Japan); 1884, Japanese commissioner, World's Industrial and Cotton Centennial Exposition, New Orleans, La.; 1884, chief, Division of Chemistry, Department of Agriculture and Commerce (Japan); 1886, acting chief, Patent Bureau (Japan); 1887-90, developer and manager, Tokyo

Artificial Fertilizer Co.; c. 1887-90, private laboratory, Tokyo; 1890, founder, Takamine Ferment Co., Chicago, Ill.; *post* 1895, consultant, Parke, Davis & Co.; 1905, founder, Sankyo & Co., Ltd., Tokyo; founder and president: 1906, International Takamine Ferment Co., N.Y.; and 1914, Takamine Laboratory, Inc., Clifton, N.J.; c. 1913, founder, Rikagaku Kenkiujo (Research Institute in Chemistry and Physics, Japan). CONTRIBUTIONS: Developed, in Japan, Taka-diastase, a starch-digesting enzyme, which, after it failed to get the interest of the distilling industry in Ill., was successfully introduced (1895) into medicine through Parke, Davis & Co. as a digestive product useful for the relief of starch intolerance. Isolated the powerful and dramatic vasopressor, adrenalin, from the adrenal glands of animals, in a stable and definitive form (1900), the first hormone to be isolated (Abel's "epinephrine" isolated earlier, contained a benzoyl radical).

WRITINGS: "The Production of Diastase by Microscopical Plants," *N.E. Med. Month* (1898); "Production of Digestive Ferments by Microscopical Plants," *Virginia Med. Semi-Month*, 3 (1898-99): 41-43; "The Blood-Pressure Raising Principles of the Su-prarenal Glands," *Therap. Gaz.*, 3rd series, 16 (1901): 221-24; "Enzymes of Aspergillus Oryzae and the Application of Its Amyloclastic Enzyme to the Fermentation Industry," *J. Ind. Eng.* 6 (1914): 824-28. REFERENCES: *DAB*, 9, pt. 2: 275-76; H. George III, "Homage to Takamine," *Coronet* (Sept. 1937): 168-70; K. K. Kawakami, *Jokichi Tak-amine: A Record of His Achievements* (1928); W. Miles, *American Chemists and Chemical Engineers* (1976), 468-69; *NCAB* 40 (1955): 64-65; *N.Y. Times*, July 23, 1922.

                                                                                      D. L. Cowen

TATUM, EDWARD LAWRIE (December 14, 1909, Boulder, Colo.-November 5, 1975, New York, N.Y.). *Geneticist; Biochemist.* Son of Arthur Lawrie, physiologist and pharmacologist, and Mabel (Webb) Tatum. Married June Alton, 1934, two children; Viola Kantor, 1956; Elsie Bergland. EDUCATION: University of Wisconsin: 1931, A.B.; 1932, M.S.; 1934, Ph.D.; and 1934-35, research assistant in agricultural chemistry and agricultural bacteriology; 1936-37, General Education Board Fellow in Bacteriological Chemistry, University of Utrecht, Holland. CAREER: At Stanford University: 1937-41, research associate; 1942-45, 1948-56, biology faculty; and 1956-57, biochemistry faculty; at Yale University: 1945-46, botany faculty; and 1946-48, microbiology faculty; 1957-75, member, Rockefeller Institute for Medical Research (later Rockefeller University); served on many scientific committees. CONTRIBUTIONS: With George W. Beadle, studied the nutritional requirements and metabolic activity of the pink bread mold *Neurospora crassa*, whose use in genetic research they pioneered (early 1940s); irradiated the mold to induce mutations and produced one mutant that would grow if it was given vitamin B-6; allowed them to conclude that the gene that had been altered by X-ray bombardment was the one that specified the makeup of the enzyme protein needed to promote the making of vitamin B-6; further demonstrated that when normal and mutated molds were mated, the offspring requiring dietary supplement appeared in correct Mendelian ratio; proved that genes functioned through the control of specific enzymes, the one gene-one enzyme concept; knowledge was used to accelerate the production of penicillin during World War II and since then has been used in methods for assaying vitamins and amino acids in foods and tissues. With Joshua Lederberg, extended research (1946) to the common intestinal bacterium, *Escherichia coli*, an organism that until then had not been used much in genetic research; showed that exchange of genetic material between different strains of *E. coli*, a process known as genetic recombination, led to progeny with biparental inheritance; led to experiments with recombinant DNA, currently the object of intense examination, since it enables man to create new forms of life.

WRITINGS: "Genetic Control of Biochemical Reactions in Neurospora," *Proc., Nat. Acad. of Sci.* 27 (1941): 499-506 (with George W. Beadle); "Neurospora II. Methods of Producing and Detecting Mutations Concerned with Nutritional Requirements," *Am. J. of Botany* 32 (1945): 678-86 (with George W. Beadle); "Gene Recombination in the Bacterium Escherichia Coli," *J. of Bacteriology* 53 (1947): 673-93 (with Joshua Lederberg). REFERENCES: *Am. Philos. Soc. Yearbook* (1977), 97-101; *Current Biog.* (1959), 437-39; *McGraw-Hill Modern Men of Sci.*, 1: 464-65; *Nature* 179 (1957): 290-91; *NCAB* J: 475-76; *N.Y. Times*, November 7, 1975; *Who Was Who in Am.*, 6: 402.

S. Galishoff

TAUSSIG, FREDERICK JOSEPH (October 26, 1872, Brooklyn, N.Y.-August 21, 1943, Bar Harbor, Maine). *Physician; Gynecology; Public health.* Son of Joseph S., banker, and Mary L. (Cuno) Taussig. Married Florence Gottschalk, 1907; two children. EDUCATION: 1893, A.B., Harvard University; 1898, M.D., Washington University Medical School; 1898-1900, intern and assistant superintendent, St. Louis Female Hospital; 1901, gynecologic training in Berlin and Vienna. CAREER: *Post* 1902, practiced medicine, St. Louis; 1902-43, clinical obstetrics and gynecology faculty, Washington University Medical School; gynecological staff, Barnard Free Skin and Cancer, Jewish, and St. Louis City hospitals; 1936-37, president, American Gynecological Society; 1938, director, American Society for the Control of Cancer. CONTRIBUTIONS: Prosyletized physicians and the public on the need to regard abortion as a vital factor in preventive medicine and maternal health. In book *Abortion, Spontaneous and Induced: Medical and Social Aspects* (1936), cited statistics indicating that 25 percent of puerperal deaths resulted from butchied abortions. Argued that the law should be liberalized to permit physicians to perform an abortion "to preserve the health of the mother and the integrity and well-being of the family." Further argued that the best way to prevent the need for abortion was to disseminate contraceptives among the poor. Other major interest was the prevention and proper treatment of vulvar cancer. Believed that untreated leucoplakia of the vulva inevitably led to cancer, a view that has since been sharply modified by new research; strenuously urged surgical excision of the vulva as a method of treatment.

WRITINGS: *The Prevention and Treatment of Abortion* (1910); *Diseases of the Vulva* (1923); "Iliaclymphadectomy with Irridation in the Treatment of Cancer of the Cervix,"

Am. J. Obstet. Gynecol. 28 (Nov. 1934): 650-67. REFERENCES: *DAB*, Supplement 3: 763-64; *N.Y. Times*, August 23, 1943; *Who Was Who in Am.*, 2: 524.

S. Galishoff

TAYLOR, CHARLES FAYETTE (April 25, 1827, Williston, Vt.-January 25, 1899, Los Angeles, Calif.). *Orthopedic surgeon.* Son of Brimage, farmer, and Miriam (Taplin) Taylor. Married Martha Skinner, 1850; Mary Salina Skinner, 1854; four children by second marriage. EDUCATION: 1855, attended New York Medical College; 1856, M.D., University of Vermont; 1856-57, studied the "Swedish movement" system, kinesipathy, of Per Henrik Ling with Dr. Mathias Roth in London. CAREER: 1857-82, practiced medicine in New York City; surgeon-in-chief for eight years, New York Orthopedic Dispensary and Hospital; *post* 1882, his health declined and after traveling widely abroad he settled in southern California. CONTRIBUTIONS: Introduced the so-called "Swedish movements" (therapeutic exercises) into the United States and invented many machines which increased their effectiveness. Invented braces and other orthopedic devices for chronic bone, joint, and muscle lesions. Greatest achievement was a method for relieving and eventually curing Pott's disease (tuberculosis of the spine). Was instrumental in establishing the New York Orthopedic Dispensary, from which developed the New York Orthopedic Dispensary and Hospital.

WRITINGS: *The Theory and Practice of the Movement Cure* (1861); *Mechanical Treatment of Angular Curvature or Pott's Disease of the Spine* (1863); *Spinal Irritation or the Causes of Backache among American Women* (1864); *Infantile Paralysis* (1867); *Mechanical Treatment of Diseases of the Hip* (1873). REFERENCES: *DAB*, 18: 317-18; Kelly and Burrage (1928), 1186-87; *NCAB*, 9: 362; A. R. Shands, "Charles Fayette Taylor and His Times—1827 to 1899," *Surg. Gyn. & Obst.*, 143, No. 5 (Nov. 1976): 811-18; *Who Was Who in Am.*, 1: 1371.

S. Galishoff

TAYLOR, EUGENE TIVOLI (September 7, 1882, LaVernia, Tex.-April 11, 1975, St. Louis, Mo.). *Physician.* Son of Tucker, farmer, and Betty Taylor. EDUCATION: Graduated from Guadalupe Normal School, Seguin, Tex.; 1911, A.B., Leland College (New Orleans, La.); 1915, M.D., Meharry Medical College. CAREER: 1915-75, private practice, St. Louis; taught obstetrics and gynecology, Homer G. Phillips Hospital (formerly City Hospital No. 2), St. Louis, for 30 years. CONTRIBUTIONS: Served as physician to black St. Louis community for 60 years. Treasurer, NMA, for 33 years (1936-69). Involved in St. Louis community affairs. REFERENCES: W. Montague Cobb, "Eugene Tivoli Taylor, M.D., 1882-," *JNMA* 66 (1974): 525-26; *JAMA* 233 (1975): 1219 (brief obituary).

T. L. Savitt

TENNENT, JOHN (c. 1700, England-c. 1760). *Physician; Medical author.* Married Dorothy Paul, 1730; Mrs. Carey, c. 1739. CAREER: C. 1725, probably settled first in Spotsylvania County, Va.; 1735, in Williamsburg; after failing to gain acceptance from the Va. colonists for use of rattlesnake-root for the treatment of pleurisy and peripneumony, returned to London; subsequent career was both unhappy and scandalous; c. 1740, may have traveled to Jamaica to find a more hospitable environment. CONTRIBUTIONS: Best known for medical writings; most famous work, *Every Man His Own Doctor*, became a popular medical guide for laymen. Wrote about the epidemic diseases of America, constitutional effects of climate, and therapeutic uses of rattlesnake-root. Wrote several works on own problems to win acceptance and to clear reputation.

WRITINGS: *Every Man His Own Doctor*, 2nd ed. (1724); *An Epistle to Dr. Richard Mead, Concerning the Epidemical Diseases of Virginia, Particularly a Pleurisy and Peripneumony* (1738); *Physical Enquires* (1742); *Detection of a Conspiracy to Suppress a General Good in Physics. . .* (1743); *Physical Disquisitions* (1745). REFERENCES: Wyndham Blanton, *Medicine in Virginia in the Eighteenth Century* (1931); *DAB* 9, pt. 2: 369; Howard A. Kelly, *Cyclopedia of Am. Med. Biog.* (1912); letter from John Tennent to Sir Hans Sloane, *William and Mary Q.* 3 (1923): 211.

P. Addis

THACHER, JAMES (February 14, 1754, Barnstable, Mass.-May 23, 1844, Plymouth, Mass.). *Physician; Surgeon*. Son of John T. and Content (Norton) Thacher. Married Susannah Hayward, 1785; six children. EDUCATION: 1771-75, pupil of Dr. Abner Hersey, Barnstable; 1808, M.A. (hon.), Harvard; 1810, M.D. (hon.), Harvard and Dartmouth. CAREER: 1775-82, surgeon, Revolutionary War, Boston, Mass.; Ticonderoga and Albany, N.Y.; and Yorktown, Va.; 1784 until death, practiced, Plymouth. CONTRIBUTIONS: One of the most influential, but least flamboyant, physicians of his time. Books were widely regarded as reflecting the best available medical information of the early nineteenth century. They are still remarkable for their clarity of organization and style and well document early American medical practices. *Dispensatory* (1810) delineates with great precision current concepts of drug action and efficacy and still provides a detailed guide to eighteenth-century therapeutic concepts. *American Modern Practice* (1817) was the first native production of its kind published in this country. Both books reflect his wide reading in all of the available medical literature of his day. Attacked quackery in minor works *Hydrophobia* (1812) and *Demonology* (1831). *Military Journal* (1823) is still a major source of information about the Revolution, although it is not much concerned with medicine. *History of Plymouth* (1835) was the first local history of a Mass. town, and *American Medical Biography* (1828) was the progenitor of the works of Stephen West Williams (1844), Samuel D. Gross (1861), William B. Atkinson (1878), R. F. Stone (1894), Irving A. Watson (1896), and Howard A. Kelly and Walter Burrage (1920, 1928), as well as of the present volume.

WRITINGS: *The American New Dispensatory* (1810, 1813, 1817, 1821); *Observations on Hydrophobia* (1812); *American Modern Practice* (1817, 1826); *An Essay on Demonology* (1831); *History of the Town of Plymouth* (1832, 1835). REFERENCES: *BHM* (1964-69), 257; James Bartlett Brewster, *James Thacher of Plymouth, Mass.* (1891); *DAB*, 9. pt. 2: 387-88; J. Worth Estes, "Therapeutic Practice in Colonial New England," in Philip

Cash, Eric H. Cristianson, and J. Worth Estes, eds., *Medicine in Colonial Massachusetts, 1620-1820* (1980), 289-383; Miller, *BHM*, pp. 111-12; *NCAB*, 7: 401; Walter R. Steiner, "Dr. James Thacher of Plymouth, Massachusetts, an Erudite Physician of Prerevolutionary and Post-Revolutionary Fame," *Bull. Hist. Med.* 1 (1933): 157-73; Betsey Hayward Thacher, sketch of Dr. Thacher's life, c. 1843-44, Boston Medical Library, Boston, Mass.; Henry R. Viets, "James Thacher and His Influence on American Medicine," *Virginia Med. Monthly* 76 (1949): 384-99.

J. W. Estes

THACHER, THOMAS (May 1, 1620, England-October 15, 1678, Boston, Mass.). *Cleric; Physician.* Son of Rev. Peter Thacher. Married twice; five children. EDUCATION: Student for the ministry and read medicine under Charles Chauncy, who became the second president of Harvard College; 1644, ordained. CAREER: Practiced, Weymouth, Mass., for 23 years before moving to Boston in 1667; 1670, became the first minister of the Old South Church. CONTRIBUTIONS: Authored a broadside on smallpox (1678), the first publication on a medical subject in America, wherein he explained the nature of the disease, gave directions for its control, described its course, offered rules of treatment, and put forward a theory of its cause, all of which was based upon the work of Thomas Sydenham (1624-89).

WRITINGS: *Brief Rules to Guide the Common People of New England How to Order Themselves and Theirs in the Small Pocks or Measles* (1678). REFERENCES: Harry Bloch, "Rev. Thomas Thacher, First Colonial Medical Pamphleteer," *N.Y. State J. of Med.* 73 (1973): 700-702; Kelly and Burrage (1928), 1197-98.

N. Gevitz

THAYER, SAMUEL WHITE (May 21, 1817, Braintree, Vt.-November 14, 1882, Burlington, Vt.). *Physician; Surgeon.* Son of Dr. Samuel W. and Mrs. Ruth (Packard) Thayer. Married Sarah Louise Pratt, 1841; one son. EDUCATION: 1832, Thetford (Vt.) Academy; 1835, studied in his father's office and attended lectures, Dartmouth; 1838, M.D., Vermont Medical College (Woodstock, Vt.). CAREER: 1837-41, demonstrator of anatomy, Woodstock; 1841-50, medical practice, Northfield, Vt.; 1854-82, practice, primarily surgical, Burlington; at University of Vermont: 1854-72, professor, dean, and secretary of faculty of medicine; 1872-82, emeritus professor of anatomy; and 1879-82, dean; 1865-66, first health officer, Burlington; 1870, Vt. commissioner of the insane; 1879, president, Vermont State Medical Society; early in career, became consultant to the Vermont Central Railroad; 1870, as medical director, Northern Pacific Railroad, organized its medical services and in the course of duties, made a collection of botanical specimens of the American West that was exhibited at the World's Fair in Vienna and made part of its permanent collection. CONTRIBUTIONS: Prime mover in the reestablishment (1854) of the College of Medicine, University of Vermont (which had lapsed for 20 years). Donated personal museum to the college for teaching of medical students. During the Civil War, was medical examiner for recruiting medical officers; surgeon-general, Vt.; and as assistant surgeon, U.S. Army, established military hospitals in three parts of the state; served at the front for short periods. REFERENCES: *Burlington Free Press*, November 15, 1882; *History of Chittenden County* (1886); *Proc., Vermont State Med. Soc.* (1883), 77-81.

L. J. Wallman

THAYER, WILLIAM SYDNEY (June 23, 1864, Milton, Mass.-December 10, 1932, Washington, D.C.). *Physician; Internal medicine*. Son of James Bradley, law professor, and Sophia Bradford (Ripley) Thayer. Married Susan Chisolm Read, 1901; one child. EDUCATION: Harvard University: 1885, A.B.; and 1889, M.D.; 1889, intern, Massachusetts General Hospital; 1889-90, studied in Berlin and Vienna. CAREER: 1890-1921, medical staff, Johns Hopkins Hospital; 1896-1921, medicine faculty, Johns Hopkins Medical School; 1917-18, deputy commissioner, American Red Cross Mission to Russia; 1918-19, director of general medicine, American Expeditionary Force; president: 1910, American Society of Tropical Medicine; 1913, American Society for Clinical Investigation; 1915, Congress of American Physicians and Surgeons; 1921, Association of American Physicians; and 1928, American Medical Association. CONTRIBUTIONS: An outstanding medical investigator and teacher in the tradition of William Osler (q.v.), under whom he worked at Johns Hopkins. Investigated the condition of the blood in several diseases, including leukemia (1891), typhoid (1895), and malaria (1893-1900). Used the new techniques of tissue staining he had learned in Germany to study malaria; with John Hewetson, published *The Malarial Fevers of Baltimore* (1895), in which he showed that the different species of malaria parasites were characterized by distinct fever cycles. Advanced knowledge of cardiology with his studies of heart block, angina pectoris, arteriosclerosis, bacterial endocarditis, heart murmurs, and the third heart sound. Trained many of the nation's future leaders in internal medicine.

WRITINGS: *Lectures on Malarial Fevers* (1897); "Ulcerative Endocarditis Due to the Gonococcus; Gonorrheal Endocarditis," *Johns Hopkins Hosp. Bull.* 7 (1896): 57-63; "On the Early Diastolic Heart Sound (the So-Called Third Heart Sound)," *Boston Med. and Surg. J.* 158 (May 7, 1908): 713-26; *Studies on Bacterial Endocarditis* (1925); *Osler and Other Papers* (1931). REFERENCES: *BHM* (1970-74), 168; *DAB*, 18: 414-15; *DSB*, 13: 300-301; *NCAB*, 24: 409-10; *Who Was Who in Am.*, 1: 1227.

S. Galishoff

THEILER, MAX (January 30, 1899, Pretoria, South Africa-August 11, 1972, New Haven, Conn.). *Physician; Virology*. Son of Arnold, veterinary scientist, and Emma (Jegge) Theiler. Married Lillian Graham, 1928; one child. EDUCATION: 1916-18, student, University of Capetown; 1922, licentiate, Royal College of Physicians (London); and D.T.M. and H., London School of Tropical Medicine. CAREER: 1922, went to the United States; 1922-30, tropical medicine faculty, Harvard Medical School; at Rockefeller Foundation: 1930-64, scientific staff, International Health Division; and 1951-64, director, Division of Medicine and Public Health Laboratories; 1964-67, epidemiology and microbiology faculty, Yale University. CONTRIBUTIONS: With others, showed that yellow fever was caused by a filterable virus and not a bacterium as theorized by Hideyo Noguchi (q.v.). Demonstrated that the disease could be transmitted to mice, thereby freeing yellow-fever investigators of their dependence on expensive rhesus monkeys. Experimented with two strains of the virus, a neurotropic strain discovered by French investigators, and a viscerotropic strain; developed a vaccine from the French strain by cycling the virus through the brains of mice; was used by France in its African territories but was found to cause encephalitis in some persons (early 1930s). Turned next to the viscerotropic (Asibi) strain and produced a vaccine that to prevent kidney damage was combined with serum from the blood of persons who had recovered from yellow fever; appeared to be effective but could not be tested on a large scale because of the difficulty of obtaining human-immune serum; led Theiler to experiment with tissue-culture methods to produce attenuated yellow-fever virus suitable for vaccination; using chicken embryo tissue, succeeded (1937) in producing a standardized vaccine (17 D) that was used to inoculate 8 million American servicemen during World War II. For this work, was awarded the 1951 Nobel Prize in physiology or medicine.

WRITINGS: "Studies on the Action of Yellow Fever Virus in Mice," *Annals of Tropical Med. and Parasitology* 24 (1930): 249-72; "Vaccination Against Yellow Fever with Immune Serum and Virus Fixed for Mice," *J. of Experimental Med.* 55 (1932): 945-69 (with S. F. Kitchen and W.D.M. Lloyd); "The Use of Yellow Fever Virus Modified in Vitro Cultivation for Human Immunization," *ibid.*, 65 (1937): 787-800. REFERENCES: *Current Biog.* (1952); *McGraw-Hill Modern Men of Sci.* 1 (1966): 473-74; *Who Was Who in Am.*, 5: 717.

S. Galishoff

THOMAS, MARY FRAME (MYERS) (October 28, 1816, Bucks County, Md.-August 19, 1888, Richmond, Ind.). *Physician; Woman's rights advocate.* Daughter of Samuel and Mary (Frame) Myers. Married Dr. Owen Thomas, 1839; three children. EDUCATION: Medical study under the tutelage of her husband; 1853-56, Pennsylvania Medical University for Women; 1853-54, Western Reserve Medical College; 1854, M.D. CAREER: 1854-56, practiced medicine with husband, Fort Wayne, Ind.; 1856, moved to Richmond, where she practiced with husband for the rest of her life. CONTRIBUTIONS: An early and tireless worker for woman's rights, particularly in medicine. Accepted into the Wayne County Medical Society, thereby becoming the first female member of the Indiana State Medical Society. Was primarily responsible for female physicians in Ind. gaining acceptance as staff members to institutions serving female patients. A prime mover in the establishment of a woman's prison and girls' reformatory in the state. Editor and publisher, *The Lilly*, devoted to woman's rights.

WRITINGS: Writings are limited to material in the *Trans., Indiana State Med. Soc.* Little has been written about this tireless worker, whose achievements can only be appreciated from the perspective of the late twentieth century. REFERENCES: *Notable Am. Women*, 3: 450-51.

C. A. Bonsett

THOMAS, T[HEODORE] GAILLARD (November 21, 1831, Edisto Island, Charleston, S.C.-February 28, 1903, Thomasville, Ga.). *Physician; Gynecology.* Son of Edward, minister, and Jane Marshall (Gaillard) Thomas. Married Mary Gillard; Mary T. Willard, 1862; five children. EDUCATION: Charleston College, Charleston, S.C.; 1852, M.D., Medical College of the State of South Carolina; 1852-53, intern, Bellevue Hospital, New York City; 1853-55, studied in Paris and Dublin. CAREER: 1855, commenced practice, N.Y.; 1855-63, professor of obstetrics, University of the City of New York; at College of Physicians and Surgeons, N.Y.: 1863-79, professor of obstetrics; and 1879-90, professor of gynecology; 1872-87, attending surgeon, Woman's Hospital, N.Y. CONTRIBU-TIONS: Prominent gynecologist, prolific writer, had wide influence in both Amer-ica and Europe. First described oophorectomy per vaginum; championed gastro-elytomy as a substitute for caesarean section.

WRITINGS: *A Practical Treatise on the Diseases of Women* (1868), 6 eds.; *The History of Nine Cases of Ovariotomy* (1869); "Vaginal Ovariotomy," *Am. J. of Med. Sci.*, n.s, 59 (1870): 387-90; *Abortion and Its Treatment, from the Stand-point of Practical Ex-perience. . .from Notes by P. Brynberg Porter, M.D.* (1890). REFERENCES: *DAB*, 9: 446-47; "In Memoriam—Theodore Gaillard Thomas," *Trans., Am. Gyn. Soc.* (1903 or 1904); *NCAB*, 26: 49.

L. D. Longo

THOMAS, WILLIAM McKINLEY (May 5, 1903, Bryan, Tex.-March 5, 1958, San Francisco, Calif.). *Surgeon.* Son of Edmund W. and Laura Harriett (Forrester) Thomas. Married Hortense E. McClanahan, 1932; two children. EDUCATION: 1926, A.B., Wiley College (Marshall, Tex.); 1930, M.D., Meharry Medical College; 1930-31, intern, Kansas City General Hospital No. 2, Kansas City, Mo.; postgraduate study: 1941-42, Harvard School of Public Health; 1943, Army Medical Inspectors School; and 1950, Stanford University Medical School. CAREER: 1931-41, medical practice, Leavenworth, Kans.; 1942-45, U.S. Army Medical Corps; 1945-58, surgical practice, San Francisco, Calif. CONTRIBU-TIONS: Became first black physician named to a standing External Advisory Group of Public Health Service when he was appointed to five-year term on National Advisory Mental Health Council (1954). Served NMA as Board of Trustees member (1934-41), youngest chair of board (1935-41), chair of NMA-AMA Liaison Committee (1953), chair of Committee on Distinguished Service Award (1953-58). Proposed idea of NMA Distinguished Service Award. In-volved in city affairs—first black to serve on city commission, San Francisco. REFERENCES: Obituary, *JNMA* 50 (1958): 221; *WWICA* 7 (1950): 504.

T. L. Savitt

THOMPSON, MARY HARRIS (April 15, 1829, Fort Ann, N.Y.-May 21, 1895, Chicago, Ill.). *Surgeon; Teacher.* Daughter of John Harris, partner in an

iron mine, and Calista (Corbin) Thompson. Never married. EDUCATION: 1862-
63, intern, New York Infirmary for Women and Children; 1863, M.D., New
England Female Medical College, Boston, Mass.; 1870, M.D., Chicago Medical
College. CAREER: 1865-95, head physician and surgeon, Hospital for Women
and Children, Chicago; 1870-95, hygiene, obstetrics, and gynecology, Woman's
Medical College. CONTRIBUTIONS: Founder, Hospital for Women and Children,
Chicago (1865), renamed Mary Thompson Hospital of Chicago, and Woman's
Hospital Medical College (1870). First woman to perform major surgery in
Chicago. Devised widely used abdominal needle for surgery.

WRITINGS: "A Case of Prolonged Gestation and Unusual Labor," *Med. & Surg.*
Reporter (Philadelphia, Pa.) 44, no. 21 (May 21, 1881): 561-65; "Two Interesting Cases
of Ovariotomy," *Am. J. of Obstetrics* 17, no. 10 (Oct. 1884): 1040-46; "Why Diseases
of Children Should Be Made a Special Study," *JAMA* 7, no. 15 (Oct. 9, 1886): 399-
402. REFERENCES: Emilia J. Giryotas, *J. of the Am. Med. Women's Assoc.* 5 (1950):
236-38; *NCAB*, 13: 550; *Notable Am. Women*, 3 (1971): 455-56; F. M. Sperry, comp.,
A Group of Distinguished Physicians and Surgeons of Chicago (1904), 57-62.

W. K. Beatty

THOMPSON, SOLOMON HENRY (August 10, 1870, Charleston, W. Va.-
December 11, 1950, Kansas City, Kans.). *Physician.* Son of Jasper and Dolly
A. Thompson. Married Belle Jane Armstrong, 1898; four children. EDUCATION:
1886, B.A., Storer College, Harper's Ferry, W.Va.; 1892, M.D., Howard University; 1892, intern, Freedmen's Hospital, Washington, D.C. CAREER: 1892-
1946, private practice, Kansas City, Kans.; 1899-1946, first chief of staff, Douglass Hospital, Kansas City. CONTRIBUTIONS: Founded, with Dr. T. C. Unthank,
Douglass Hospital, Kansas City (1899), first Negro hospital established west of
the Mississippi River, and training school for nurses. Strong supporter and
motivating force of Douglass Hospital for many years. REFERENCES: W. Montague
Cobb, "Solomon Henry Thompson, M.D., 1870-1950," *JNMA* 49 (1957): 274-78; *WWICA*
6 (1941-44): 514.

T. L. Savitt

THOMPSON, WILLIAM GILMAN (December 25, 1856, New York, N.Y.-
October 27, 1927, New York). *Physician; Industrial and rehabilitative medicine.*
Son of Joseph Parrish, minister, and Elizabeth Coit (Gilman) Thompson. Married
Harriet Howard Pomeroy, 1887. EDUCATION: 1877, Ph.B., Sheffield Scientific
School (Yale); 1881, M.D., College of Physicians and Surgeons (Columbia);
1881-83, intern, New York Hospital. CAREER: *post* 1883, practiced medicine,
N.Y.; at New York University Medical College: 1887-96, physiology faculty;
and 1896-98, therapeutics and materia medica faculty; visiting physician: 1887-
94, New York Hospital; and 1887-1912, Presbyterian Hospital; *post* 1888, director, Loomis Laboratory; 1898-1916, medicine faculty, Cornell University
Medical College; consulting physician, Bellevue and Reconstruction hospitals;
chairman for many years, industrial hygiene division, New York Labor Department. CONTRIBUTIONS: As director of the Loomis Laboratory, the first in-

stitute of experimental medicine in the United States, vigorously supported the development of clinical research along with laboratory investigation as the basis of scientific medical discovery. Wrote books on dietetics and practical therapeutics. Conducted research and wrote on industrial hygiene and sanitation. Organized a reeducational clinic during World War I, which led to his founding of Reconstruction Hospital. Pioneered reeducation in connection with war and industrial diseases.

WRITINGS: *Practical Dietetics* (1895); *Textbook of Practical Medicine* (1900); *Occupational Diseases* (1914). REFERENCES: *DAB*, 18: 477-78; "Industrial Medicine's Hall of Fame: William Gilman Thompson, M.D., 1856-1927," *Industrial Med.* 28 (1959): 524-27; *Trans., Assoc. of Am. Physicians* 43 (1928): 7-8; *Who Was Who in Am.*, 1: 1235.

S. Galishoff

THOMS, ADAH B. (SAMUELS) (January 12, 1863, Va.-February 21, 1943, New York, N.Y.). *Nurse*. Daughter of Harry and Melvina Samuels. Married Mr. Thoms, very early in life; Henry Smith, 1923; no children. EDUCATION: 1900, graduate of Woman's Infirmary and School of Therapeutics and Massage, New York City; 1903-5, School of Nursing, Lincoln Hospital, New York City; 1905, graduate nurse. CAREER: 1900-1903, nurse, New York City; and head nurse, St. Agnes Hospital, Raleigh, N.C.; 1905-6, operating room nurse, Lincoln Hospital, New York City; 1906-23, assistant director of nursing, Lincoln Hospital; 1923, retired. CONTRIBUTIONS: Pioneer black registered nurse. Helped found the National Association of Colored Graduate Nurses (1908), serving as treasurer and president (1916-23). Opposed a proposed merger with the National Medical Association and preferred to work toward eventual merger with the American Nurses' Association (which finally occurred in 1951, after her death). Unsuccessfully tried to convince the U.S. Surgeon General to allow black nurses to work with the Red Cross in World War I, after gaining approval of Jane A. Delano (q.v.).

WRITINGS: *Pathfinders; A History of the Progress of Colored Graduate Nurses* (1929). REFERENCES: *Notable Am. Women*, 3: 455-57; M. K. Staupers, *No Time for Prejudice* (1961); Adah B. Thoms, *Pathfinders*.

M. Kaufman

THOMSON, SAMUEL (February 9, 1769, Alstead, N.H.-October 4, 1843, Boston, Mass.). *Botanical medicine*. Son of John and Hannah (Cobb) Thomson. Married Susan Allen, July 7, 1790; eight children. EDUCATION: Self-taught. CAREER: Farmer, became a botanical practitioner, first in rural N.H., then as an itinerant healer, and finally as founder of a medical sect based on botanical medicine and his primitive medical ideas. CONTRIBUTIONS: Founder, Thomsonian medical sect. Developed theory that to cure, it was important to increase body heat. Postulated that the stomach acted as a furnace of the body, maintaining heat and life. When it is clogged, therefore, it must be cleansed, by natural herbs rather than by mineral drugs administered by orthodox physicians. Steamed a patient to raise external heat and promote free perspiration: followers became known popularly as "steamers." Rallying cry was "Every man his own physician." After successfully defending himself in manslaughter case (1809), received government patent on his system of medical practice, wrote a two-volume set of books describing his theory and practice, and sold the books for $20 a set to anyone wishing to be his own physician; actually sold "family rights" authorizing the purchaser to practice Thomsonian medicine upon his family. Engaged in constant controversy with his followers.

WRITINGS: *A Brief Sketch of the Causes and Treatment of Diseases* (1821); *The New Guide to Health* (1822); *New Guide to Health Prefixed by Narrative of the Life and Medical Discoveries of the Author* (1825). REFERENCES: Alex Berman, "The Thomsonian Movement and Its Relation to American Pharmacy and Medicine," *Bull. Hist. Med.* 25 (1951), 520-28; *BHM* (1975-79), 125; (1980), 39; *DAB*, 9, pt. 2: 488-89; *NCAB*, 6: 70; F. Packard, *Hist. of Med. in the U.S.* (1931), 1233-34; W. G. Rothstein, *Am. Physicians in the 19th Century* (1972), 128-51.

R. Edwards

THORNTON, MATTHEW (1714, Londonderry, Ireland-June 24, 1803, Newburyport, Mass.). *Physician.* Son of James, farmer, and Elizabeth (Jenkins?) Thornton. Married Hannah Jack, 1760; five children. EDUCATION: c. 1740, apprenticed to Dr. (Rev.) Thomas Green, Leicester, Mass. CAREER: 1743-75, practiced, Londonderry, N.H., when he began to devote most of time to public life; became involved in local and state politics: 1758-62, provincial legislator; 1770, selectman; 1771-76, town moderator; 1771-75, justice of the Court of Common Pleas and justice of the peace; 1776-82, Superior Court justice; 1775-76, Provincial Congress delegate; 1775, chairman, N.H. Committee of Safety; 1776, speaker, N.H. House of Representatives; 1776-77, member, state's Council, and delegate, Continental Congress; and 1777-87, N.H. state representative; 1789, retired from public life. CONTRIBUTIONS: Virtually nothing is known of his medical practice. Remembered today chiefly because he was one of the two N.H. physicians who signed the Declaration of Independence. REFERENCES: Charles Thornton Adams, *Matthew Thornton of New Hampshire* (1903); *BHM* (1975-79), 125; *DAB*, 9, pt. 2: 503-4; J. Worth Estes, "Honest Dr. Thornton: The Path to Rebellion," in George E. Gifford, Jr., ed., *Physician Signers of the Declaration of Independence* (1976), 70-98; *NCAB*, 11: 540.

J. W. Estes

TIBBALS, FRANK BURR (October 14, 1864, Salem, Mich.-April 25, 1931, Detroit, Mich.). *Surgeon; Medical jurisprudence.* Son of Henry Elliott, farmer, and Mary Babbitt (Burr) Tibbals. Married Laura Adelaide West, 1893; two children. EDUCATION: Fairfield Academy (Conn.); 1888, A.B., Yale University; 1891, M.D., University of Michigan. CAREER: 1891-98, surgical practice (with Donald Maclean), Detroit; 1902, president, Wayne County Medical Society; 1909-31, founding chairman, Medical Defense Committee, Michigan State Medical Society; 1914-29, associate professor and then professor of medical juris-prudence, Detroit College of Medicine. CONTRIBUTIONS: Launched a nationwide movement for the creation of "medical defense" committees by state medical societies; as outlined in his remarkably candid article for the *Medical History of Michigan*, the purpose of these committees was to pressure doctors against testifying for plaintiffs in malpractice cases, as well as to defend all accused physicians.

WRITINGS: "Medical Defense," in C. B. Burr, *Medical History of Michigan* 2 (1930): 133-44. REFERENCES: Burr, *Medical History of Michigan*, 2: 146, 474; Michigan State Med. Soc., *J*. 30 (1929): 472; *NCAB*, 22:65.

M. S. Pernick

TILDON, TOUSSAINT TOURGEE (April 5, 1893, Waxahachie, Tex.-July 22, 1964, Tuskegee, Ala.). *Physician; Psychiatry and general medicine*. Son of John Wesley, physician, and Margaret (Hilburn) Tildon. Married Margaret Cecelia Greene, 1924; four children. EDUCATION: 1912, A.B., Lincoln University (Pa.); 1912-13, prelaw course, Harvard University; first year of medical school, Meharry; 1923, M.D., Harvard University; 1923, special training program in psychiatry and neurology at Boston University for new Veteran's Bureau Hospital, Tuskegee, Ala. CAREER: At Veteran's Administration Hospital, Tuskegee: 1923-58, began as junior medical officer, first in psychiatry and then in medicine; rose to clinical director; *post*, 1946, director. CONTRIBUTIONS: Pioneered (1920-58) in establishing black physicians in government medical positions and in setting up fully accredited residency programs for black medical and dental graduates at the Tuskegee Veteran's Administration Hospital, where black physicians were first hired on a large scale to staff a government hospital.

WRITINGS: "Residua of Encephalitis Lethargica Among Negro Veterans," *U.S. Veterans' Bureau Med. Bull*. 3 (1927): 214-17; "Syphilis of the Intrathoracic Vessels," ibid., 5 (1929): 752-59; "Heart Disease in Pulmonary Tuberculosis," ibid., 7 (1931): 833-38. Writings listed in *JNMA* 56 (1964): 567. REFERENCES: Samuel L. Younge, "Toussaint Tourgee Tildon, Sr., M.D., 1893-1964," *JNMA* 56 (1964): 565-67.

T. L. Savitt

TILLETT, WILLIAM SMITH (July 10, 1892, Charlotte, N.C.-April 4, 1974, Chester, Conn.). *Physician; Microbiology*. Son of Charles Walter and Carolyn (Patterson) Tillett. Married Dorothy Stockbridge, 1928; one child. EDUCATION: 1913, A.B., University of North Carolina; 1917, M.D., Johns Hopkins Medical School; 1920-22, intern and resident, Hospital of Rockefeller Institute. CAREER: 1922-30, medical staff, Hospital of Rockefeller Institute; 1930-37, medicine faculty, Johns Hopkins Medical School; at New York University College of Medicine: 1937-38, bacteriology faculty; and 1938-58, medicine faculty; 1938-58, medical staff and member, Executive Committee (secretary, *post* 1941), Bellevue Hospital; 1958-74, director, research trainee grant program, U.S. Public Health Service. CONTRIBUTIONS: With Thomas Francis, Jr. (q.v.), found that minute doses of the capsular polysaccharides of pneumococci are antigenic in humans (1920s); until then it was believed that only proteins were antigenic. With Francis, discovered a new protein, C-reactive protein, in the blood of patients with a wide variety of inflammatory diseases; discovery was used in clinical medicine to measure inflammation and other pathological processes (1920s). With L. R. Christensen and Sol Sherry, isolated and partially purified the enzymes streptokinase and streptodornase from the streptococcus organism and demonstrated their usefulness as liquefying agents in dissolving the products of chronic infections; showed that streptokinase, especially, could be used to dissolve accumulations of pus and fibrin clots; combined with penicillin therapy, enabled physicians to treat many ailments, notably pyemia, without surgery (late 1930s, early 1940s).

WRITINGS: "Cutaneous Reactions in Pneumonia: The Development of Antibodies Following the Intradermal Injection of Type-Specific Polysaccharide," *J. of Experimental Med.* 52 (1930): 573-85 (with Thomas Francis, Jr.); "The Fibrinolytic Activity of Hemolytic Streptococci," ibid., 58 (1933): 485-502 (with R. L. Garner). REFERENCES: *J. of Infectious Diseases* 130 (1974): 311-12; *McGraw-Hill Modern Men of Sci.* 2 (1966): 546-47; *N.Y. Times*, April 5, 1974; *Who Was Who in Am.*, 6: 408.

S. Galishoff

TILTON, JAMES (June 1, 1745, Kent County, Del.-May 14, 1822, Wilmington, Del.). *Surgeon.* Never married. EDUCATION: Nottingham Academy, Nottingham, Md.; apprentice to Dr. Charles Ridgely, Dover, Del.; College of Philadelphia: 1768, B.M.; and 1771, M.D. CAREER: 1771-76, private practice, Dover, Del.; 1776-77, surgeon, Delaware Regiment; 1777-80, in charge of Continental Army hospital, Princeton, Trenton, and New Windsor, Md.; 1780-83, senior hospital physician and surgeon, Continental Army; 1781, refused offer of the chair of materia medica, University of Pennsylvania School of Medicine; 1783-1802, private practice, Dover; 1802-13, gave up medical practice and farmed in New Castle County, near Wilmington; 1813-15, physician and surgeon-general, U.S. Army; 1815-22, retired to farm outside of Wilmington. CONTRIBUTIONS: During the American Revolution, became deeply concerned with unhygienic conditions in army hospitals and the resultant hospital fevers. As an alternative to the large, open army hospital ward, designed the "Tilton Hut," a small, well-ventilated log building, partitioned into three sections. A great decrease in army hospital mortality from contagious disease followed in areas that adopted this innovation. Remembered as an early pioneer in army sanitation and the prevention of the spread of contagious disease. The publication of well-known *Economical Observations on Military Hospitals, etc.* (1813) brought him to the attention of President Madison and led to appointment as physician and surgeon-general. For the first time, duties of army medical officers and other personnel were spelled out. In medical practice, was a close follower of the teachings of Benjamin Rush (q.v.) and bled, purged, and frequently prescribed mercurial ointments to cure patients. First president, Medical Society of Delaware

(1789-1822). Member, Continental Congress (1783-85), for several years in the Del. House of Representatives and as government commissioner of loans for Del. (1785-1801).

WRITINGS: *The Biographical History of Dionysius, Tyrant of Delaware*, by Timoleon (1788); *Economical Observations on Military Hospitals and the Prevention and Cure of Diseases Incident to an Army* (1813). REFERENCES: *BHM* (1975-79), 126; *DAB*, 9, pt. 2: 550-51; *Delaware Gazette* (Wilmington), May 17, 1822; Kelly and Burrage (1928), 1214; Miller, *BHM*, p. 112; *NCAB*, 3: 515; Alfred Shands, "James Tilton, M.D.: Delaware's Greatest Physician," *Delaware Med. J.* (Jan. 1974); James Thacher, *Am. Med. Biog.* 2 (1828).

W. H. Williams

TIMBERLAKE, GIDEON (March 6, 1876, Charlottesville, Va.-March 1, 1951, St. Petersburg, Fla.). *Physician; Urology*. Son of Crawford Goodman, merchant and farmer, and Sarah Jane (Garland) Timberlake. Married a woman from Charleston, W.Va., sometime between 1904 and 1907; Sallie Virginia Helms, 1922, two children. EDUCATION: 1902, M.D., University of Virginia; 1903, intern, Lying-In, Bellevue, and Marine hospitals, N.Y.; c. 1907, studied urology under Hugh Young (q.v.), Johns Hopkins University. CAREER: Practiced medicine: 1904-7, Charleston, W. Va.; and 1907-26, Baltimore, Md.; 1910-26, urology faculty, University of Maryland School of Medicine; c. 1909, assistant demonstrator in bacteriology, Johns Hopkins University; 1910-26, urological staff, Johns Hopkins, St. Agnes, and Franklin Square hospitals; 1918, organizer, director, Army School of Urology, Fort Oglethorpe, Ga.; 1918-c. 1926, urological staff, Walter Reed Hospital, Washington, D.C.; practiced medicine: 1926-28, Greenville, S.C.; and *post* 1928, St. Petersburg, Fla. CONTRIBUTIONS: Developed new urological techniques and instruments, including an obturator for resectoscope sheath, a declotting canula for urinary bladder, and electrolysis in transurethral resections. Helped found the American Board of Urology (1935).

WRITINGS: "Electrocoagulation of Vesicle Neoplasms under Water with Adjustable Electrode," *J. of Urology* 19, no. 5 (May 1928): 629-33; "Aids to Control of Post-Operative Hemorrhage in Transurethral Resection," ibid., 61, no. 3 (Sept. 1948); "A Device for Removing Clots from the Bladder; A New Irrigating Nozzle," ibid., 62, no. 3 (Sept. 1949): 394-95. REFERENCES: *DAB*, Supplement 5: 688-89; *NCAB*, 40: 151-52; *N.Y. Times*, March 2, 1951; *Who Was Who in Am.*, 3: 855.

S. Galishoff

TIMME, WALTER (February 24, 1874, New York, N.Y.-February 12, 1956, St. Petersburg, Fla.). *Physician; Neurology; Endocrinology*. Son of Frederick J. E., Lutheran minister, and Emma (Wirth) Timme. Married Ida Helen Haar, 1901; Anne Cecil Auwell, 1951. EDUCATION: 1893, B.S., City College of New York; 1897, M.D., College of Physicians and Surgeons (Columbia); 1912-13, postgraduate study, University of Berlin. CAREER: *Post* 1897, practiced medicine, N.Y.; 1898-1901, 1913-16, neurological staff, Vanderbilt Clinic; at Neurological Institute of New York: 1910-16, neurological staff; 1917-18, military director, in charge of training medical officers in neuropsychiatry; and 1918-37, neuro-endocrine staff; 1929-37, clinical neurology faculty, Columbia University; president: 1920-25, 1928-29, Association for Research in Nervous and Mental Diseases; and 1924, American Society for the Study of Internal Secretions. CONTRIBUTIONS: An early leader in endocrinology. Played an active role in the Association for the Study of Internal Secretions and was associate editor of its journal *Endocrinology*. Major work was on pluriglandular endocrinologic disturbances; described ovarian and adrenal insufficiency leading to compensatory hypopituitarism, now known as "Timme's syndrome." Founded and served as first president (1920), Association for Research in Nervous and Mental Diseases. Advocated the sterilization of the feebleminded (1920s) because of belief that endocrinopathic inheritance of hypoplastic body characteristics correlated directly with subsequent criminal activity.

WRITINGS: "A New Pluriglandular Compensatory Syndrome," *Endocrinology* 2 (Jul.-Sept. 1918): 209-40; *Lectures in Endocrinology* (1928). REFERENCES: *DAB*, Supplement 6: 634-35; *NCAB*, C: 141; *N.Y. Times*, February 13, 1956; *Who Was Who in Am.*, 3: 855.

S. Galishoff

TINKHAM, HENRY CRAIN (December 7, 1856, Brownington, Vt.-December 6, 1925, Burlington, Vt.). *Surgeon; Educator.* Son of Samuel Stone and Clarissa (Richmond) Tinkham. Married Clara E. Day, 1886. EDUCATION: Derby Academy, Vt.; 1883, M.D., University of Vermont. CAREER: 1883-1925, practice, Burlington; 1884-92, instructor of anatomy, University of Vermont; at University of Vermont College of Medicine: 1892-94, adjunct professor of anatomy; 1894-1925, professor of anatomy; and 1898-1925, dean. CONTRIBUTIONS: As dean, University of Vermont College of Medicine, worked to preserve the institution in the face of the devastating Flexner Report recommendation that the school be closed. Marshaled Vt. physicians and legislators in defense of the school; managed to improve standards in line with current trends and developments, gained state financial support, and ultimately gained complete approval by the AMA Council on Medical Education and the Association of American Medical Colleges. Defended the need for rural medical schools and the continuing role of the general practitioner rather than the scientifically trained Johns Hopkins-type physician advocated by the Flexner Report. REFERENCES: Martin Kaufman, *University of Vermont College of Medicine* (1979); ms. material, University of Vermont Archives, Burlington; *Who Was Who in Am.*, 1:1242.

M. Kaufman

TODD, ELI (July 22, 1769, New Haven, Conn.-November 17, 1833, Hartford, Conn.). *Physician; Psychiatry.* Son of Michael, wealthy merchant who died insane when Eli was 5, and Mary (Rowe) Todd. Lived with his great-uncle Rev. Jonathan Todd of Guilford, Conn. Married Rhoda Hill, 1796; her sister, Catherine Hill, 1828. EDUCATION: Tutored by Rev. Elizur Goodrich of Durham,

Conn.; 1783-87, attended Yale College, A.B., 1787; studied medicine by apprenticing to Dr. Ebenezer Beardsley of New Haven. CAREER: 1790-1812, 1816-20, practice of medicine in Farmington, Conn.; 1812-16, medical practice in New York City; 1820-24, practiced medicine in Hartford; 1824-33, superintendent of the Hartford Retreat (mental hospital). CONTRIBUTIONS: Had an interest in the treatment of the insane because father and a sister had suffered from mental illness. Appointed to the Connecticut Medical Society committee on the condition of the mentally ill (1812). Helped to organize (1821 and 1824) the Society for the Relief of the Insane and led the drive to raise funds for the construction of the Connecticut Retreat for the Insane at Hartford. Its first superintendent (1824). Influenced by the reforms William Tuke had instituted in England's York Retreat, instituted humane treatment at the Hartford Retreat. The Hartford Retreat became known as the best hospital for the insane in America. REFERENCES: *Boston Med. and Surg. J.*, April 20, 1836; *DAB, 9*, pt. 2: 570-71; L. Eaton, "Eli Todd and the Hartford Retreat," *New England Q.* 26 (1953): 435-53; Kelly and Burrage (1928), 1215.

M. Kaufman

TODD, THOMAS WINGATE (January 15, 1885, Sheffield, England-December 28 or 29, 1938, Cleveland, Ohio). *Physician; Anatomy.* Son of James, Methodist minister, and Katharine (Wingate) Todd. Married Eleanor Pearson, 1912; three children. EDUCATION: 1907, M.B., Ch. B., Manchester University; 1907, intern, London Hospital. CAREER: 1907-8, demonstrator in anatomy, Manchester University; 1909-10, house surgeon, Manchester Royal Infirmary; 1910-12, lecturer in anatomy, Manchester University; 1912, appointed Henry Willson Payne Professor of Anatomy, Western Reserve University; director: 1920, Hamann Museum of Comparative Anatomy; and 1928, Brush Foundation; captain, Canadian Army Medical Corps. CONTRIBUTIONS: Built, with Carl Hamann, the Hamann Museum of Comparative Anatomy, which contained 2,400 skeletons, one-eighth of all skeletal material available for study in the world. Established scientific criterion for determining the effects of age, sex, and race on the development of the human skeleton and the age of any skeleton with virtual certainty. Explored the influence of mental states on the motility of the alimentary tract (Beaumont Lecture, 1930). Studied the development of the bones of children by making quarterly radiographic examinations of 800 children to determine normal ossification at different ages. Developed the head spanner for measuring the skull.

WRITINGS: *The Clinical Anatomy of the Gastro-Intestinal Tract* (1915); "The Estimation of Cranial Capacity," *Am. J. Phys. Anthro.* 13 (1925): 251-59; "Skeletal Adjustment in Jaw Growth," *Dental Cosmos* 17 (Dec. 1926); *Behavior Patterns of the Alimentary Tract* (1930); *Atlas of Skeletal Maturation* (1937). Author of an enormous literature on the subjects of anthropometry, anthroposcopy, demography, dentition, skin, skeletal systems, skeletal age changes, muscular systems, nervous systems, gastrointestinal systems, and so on. REFERENCES: Montague Cobb, "Thomas Wingate Todd: A Biography," *JNMA* 51 (May 1959): 233-46, 223-25 (includes an excellent bibliography);

DAB, Supplement 2: 665-66; Arthur Keith, "In Memoriam: Thomas Wingate Todd, 1885-1938," *J. of Anat.* 73 (1939): 350-53; *NCAB*, 38: 639; *Who Was Who in Am.*, 1: 1244.

G. P. Jenkins

TOLAND, HUGH HUGER (April 16, 1806, Guilder's Creek, S.C.-February 27, 1880, San Francisco, Calif.). *Surgeon; Medical educator.* Son of John, planter and banker, and Mary (Boyd) Toland. Married Mary Goodwin, no children; Mary Avery, 1844, two daughters; Mrs. Mary B. (Morrison) Gridley, 1860, one adopted son. EDUCATION: Read medicine with Dr. George Ross; 1827, M.D., Transylvania University (at head of class). CAREER: 1828-30, practice, Pageville, S. C.; 1833, established successful surgical practice, Columbia, S.C.; 1852, went to San Francisco, where he practiced medicine and surgery for 28 years. CONTRIBUTIONS: Founded the Toland Medical College (1864) in San Francisco, serving as faculty president and professor of surgery until death. This school was transferred to the University of California (1873) and established as its Department of Medicine. REFERENCES: *DAB*, 9, pt. 2: 575-76; F. T. Gardner, "The Little Acorn . . . ," *Bull. Hist. Med.* 24 (1950): 61-69; Henry Harris, *California's Medical Story* (1932), 360-65.

Y. V. O'Neill

TONER, JOSEPH MEREDITH (April 30, 1825, Pittsburgh, Pa.-July 30, 1896, Cresson, Pa.). *Physician; Historian; Collector.* Son of Meredith and Ann (Layton) Toner. Never married. EDUCATION: Western University of Pennsylvania (now University of Pittsburgh) and Mt. St. Mary's College, Emmitsburg, Md.; studied medicine with Dr. John Lowman, Johnstown, Pa.; 1850, M.D., Vermont Medical College; 1853, M.D., Jefferson Medical College. CAREER: Practiced: Summit, Pa.; Pittsburgh, Pa.; Harper's Ferry, Va.; and *post* 1855, Washington, D.C.; attending physician, Providence Hospital and St. Joseph's, St. Vincent's, and St. Anne's Orphan asylums, Washington, D.C.; Board of Directors, Garfield, Columbia, and St. Elizabeth's hospitals, Washington, D.C.; president: 1873, American Medical Association; and 1874, American Public Health Association. CONTRIBUTIONS: Undertook but did not complete a biographical dictionary of American physicians. Opened personal library (more than 27,000 volumes when given to Library of Congress, 1882) to physicians and others. Compiled subject index of contents of American medical journals before 1870. Wrote on public health problems, vital statistics, vaccination, tuberculosis, yellow fever.

WRITINGS: *Contributions to the Annals of Medical Progress and Medical Education in the United States Before and During the War of Independence* (1874); *Medical Men of the Revolution* (1876); other historical addresses and monographs. Edited several writings of George Washington. REFERENCES: *Bull. Hist. Med.* 47 (1973): 1-24; *DAB*, 9, pt. 2: 586-87; Medical Society of the District of Columbia, *Trans.*, n.s., 1 (1897):

135-58; Philosophical Society of Washington, *Bull.* 13 (1895-99): 426-30; Smithsonian Institution, *Annual Report* (1896), 637-43.

W. Bell, Jr.

TOOMEY, JOHN AUGUSTUS (May 25, 1889, Cleveland, Ohio-January 1, 1950, Cleveland). *Physician; Pediatrician.* Married Mary Louise Bagot, 1918, four children; Helen Katharine, 1949. EDUCATION: St. Ignatius College (now John Carroll University): 1910, A.B.; and 1912, A.M.; 1913, LL.B., Cleveland Law School; 1919, M.D., Western Reserve University School of Medicine; City Hospital, Cleveland: 1919-20, intern; and 1920-22, resident. CAREER: At Western Reserve University: 1920-22, demonstrator in anatomy; 1921-22, demonstrator in medicine; 1922-24, instructor, pediatrics; 1924-28, senior instructor in contagious diseases; 1928-33, assistant professor; 1933-40, associate professor in pediatrics; and 1940-50, professor of pediatrics and contagious diseases; at City Hospital, Cleveland: 1922, appointed physician-in-charge, Division of Contagious Diseases; and 1945, acting head of pediatrics. CONTRIBUTIONS: Produced poliomyelitis in monkeys by injecting virus into lumen of the intestine; first to suggest that the entry of the polio virus was through the intestinal tract, possibly from contaminated food and water. Advocated heat, massage, stimulation, exercise, and balanced gait for treatment of acute polio, which later became the common method of treatment.

WRITINGS: "Spread of Poliomyelitis from Gastrointestinal Tract," *Proc., Soc. for Experimental Biol. & Med.* 31 (Mar. 1934): 680; "Explanation of Mechanism of Infantile Paralysis Production in Human Being," *Annals of Internal Med.* 8 (Jan. 1935): 854; "Observation on Treatment of Infantile Paralysis in Acute Stage," *Trans. and Studies of the Coll. of Physicians of Phila.* 12 (Apr. 1944): 14. Contributed about 300 articles to medical journals. REFERENCES: *Am. J. of Diseases of Children* 79 (1950): 714-15; *Annals of Internal Med.* 32 (1950): 1011-12; Morris Fishbein et al., ed., *A Bibliography of Infantile Paralysis, 1789-1949*, 2nd ed. (1951).

G. P. Jenkins

TOWNE, SOLON RODNEY (December 20, 1846, Stowe, Vt.-January 27, 1932, Omaha, Nebr.). *Physician; Surgeon.* Son of Jess, shoe manufacturer, and Salome Esther (Seabury) Towne. Married Harriet Christina Somers, July 23, 1873; four children. EDUCATION: 1868, People's Academy of Morrisville, Vt.; 1872, A.B., 1875, M.D., Dartmouth College. CAREER: Medical practice: 1875, Brookfield, Vt.; 1876-88, Enfield, Mass.; and 1888-1925, Omaha; professor of public health: 1894-1900, Creighton University, Omaha; and 1900-1915, Omaha Medical College and its successor, University of Nebraska College of Medicine; 1891-97, commissioner, Omaha City Health Department; 1898-1905, state health inspector, Nebraska Board of Health; 1892-98, inspector of contagious diseases, Omaha; 1897-1905, physician, Nebraska School for the Deaf; 1907-10, Executive Committee, 1910-28, president, Nebraska TB Association; author, quarantine law for Nebr. CONTRIBUTIONS: Recognized as Nebr.'s authority in public health (1890-1932). Promoted advances in medicine and public health in relation to obligations of various agencies—local, state, federal and professional. Traveled throughout the state diagnosing and quarantining for communicable diseases. Active supporter of health legislation—local, state, and federal. Devoted great effort toward education of the public in matters of preventive medicine, sanitation, nutrition, and immunization.

WRITINGS: "School Hygiene," *Western Med. Rev.* 2 (Nov. 15, 1897): 331-33; "Considerations of Etiology of Croupous Pneumonia," *Omaha Clinic* 2, no. 5 (Aug. 1889): 109-16; "A Few Notes on Recent Epidemic of Smallpox," *Western Med. Rev.* 6 (Aug. 15, 1901): 232-34; "Care in Vaccination," *ibid.*, 7 (Sept. 15, 1902): 282-84; "Medical Inspection of Schools," *Trans., Nebraska State Med. Soc.* 35 (1903): 33-36. REFERENCES: S. M. Baldwin and R. M. Baldwin, *Nebraskana* (1932), 1203; Alice T. Deweese and Alice Horsfall, "Two Doctors Come to Omaha," MS., University of Nebraska Medical Center Library of Medicine, Omaha; *Nebraska State Med. J.* 17, no. 3 (Mar. 1932): 130.

B. M. Hetzner

TRACY, MARTHA (April 10, 1876, Plainfield, N.J.-March 22, 1942, Philadelphia, Pa.). *Physician; Medical administrator; Oncology; Public health.* Daughter of Jeremiah Evarts, lawyer, and Martha Sherman (Greene) Tracy. Never married. EDUCATION: 1898, A.B., Bryn Mawr College; 1904, M.D., Woman's Medical College of Pennsylvania; 1911, studied physiological chemistry, Sheffield Scientific School (Yale); 1917, D.P.H., University of Pennsylvania. CAREER: 1904-7, assistant, research department of experimental pathology, Cornell University Medical School; 1907, assistant to Meningitis Committee, New York City Board of Health; 1907-9, researcher, Huntington Fund for Cancer Research (N.Y.); at Woman's Medical College of Pennsylvania: 1907-13, chemistry faculty; 1913-23, physiological chemistry faculty; 1923-31, preventive medicine faculty; and 1917-40, dean; at Philadelphia Board of Health: 1936-40, member; and 1940-42, assistant director; 1920-21, president, Medical Women's National Association. CONTRIBUTIONS: Helped William B. Coley (q.v.) develop "Coley's Fluid," (erysipelas and prodigiosus toxins), a long-used treatment for inoperable sarcomas. Believing that co-educational schools did not provide adequate opportunities for women in medicine, fought for many years to keep Woman's Medical College of Pennsylvania, the only American medical school controlled by women, independent and healthy. With Sarah Logan Wistar Starr (Mrs. James Starr, Jr.), staved off bankruptcy and checked faculty dissension that threatened to destroy the institution; also, raised entrance requirements, modernized the curriculum, and built a modern plant in a better part of town.

WRITINGS: "The Treatment of Experimental Tumors with Bacterial Toxins," *JAMA* 49 (1907): 1493-98 (with S. P. Beebe); "The Woman's Medical College of Pennsylvania; Its Relation to All Women in Medicine," *Women's Med. J.* 29 (1919): 202-8 (with E. C. Potter). Bibliography is in a memoir written by Catharine Macfarlane in *Trans. and Studies of the Coll. of Physicians of Phila.*, 4th series, no. 10 (1942-43): 179-81. REFERENCES: *DAB* 3: 474-75; *NCAB*, 31: 205-6; *N.Y. Times*, March 23, 1942; Fred B.

Rogers, "Martha Tracy (1876-1942): Exceptional Woman of Public Health," *Arch. of Environmental Health* 9 (1964): 819-21; *Who Was Who in Am.*, 2: 537.

S. Galishoff

TRALL, RUSSELL THACHER (August 5, 1812, Vernon, Conn.-September 23, 1877, Florence, N.J.). *Hydropath; Health reformer.* Married Rebecca L. Trall; one child. EDUCATION: Mid-1830s, Albany Medical College. CAREER: 1844-77, manager, hydropathic institutions, N.Y. and N.J., and prolific writer on popular hygiene. CONTRIBUTIONS: Opened second water-cure establishment in the United States, in New York City (1844). Edited *Water Cure Journal* (1849-61) and *Herald of Health* (1863-66). Directed several hydropathic schools, including the Hygeio-Therapeutic College, Florence Heights, N.J. (1867-77).

WRITINGS: *Hydropathic Encyclopedia* (1852); *The Complete Gymnasium* (1857); *The True Temperance Platform* (1864-66); *Sexual Physiology* (1866); *Water-Cure for the Million* (1867). REFERENCES: "Death of Dr. Trall," *Herald Health* 30 (1877): 251-52; "Imperishable Truths From Our Fathers and Mothers," *J. of Hygeio-Therapy* 1 (1877): 2-6; Ronald Numbers, "Health Reform on the Delaware," *N.J. Hist.* 92 (1974): 5-12; obituary, *N.Y. Times*, September 26, 1877, p. 4; "Russell T. Trall. Portrait, Character, and Biography," *Herald Health* 4 (1864): 2-4.

J. C. Whorton

TRASK, JAMES DOWLING (August 21, 1890, Astoria, N.Y.-May 24, 1942, Chicago, Ill.). *Physician; Microbiology; Pediatrics.* Son of James Dowling, physician, and Julia Norton (Hartshorne) Trask. Married Phyllis Hayden Randall, 1921; one child. EDUCATION: 1913, Ph.B., Sheffield Scientific School (Yale University); 1917, M.D., Cornell Medical College; 1917-18, intern, Bellevue Hospital (N.Y.). CAREER: 1918-19, Medical Corps, U.S. Army; 1919-21, at Rockefeller Institute for Medical Research; at Yale University: 1921-27, medicine faculty; and 1927-42, pediatrics faculty; 1921-42, medical staff, New Haven Hospital and Dispensary; member: *post* 1931, Yale Poliomyelitis Commission; 1939-42, New Haven Board of Health; and 1941-42, Army Epidemiological Board. CONTRIBUTIONS: With Francis G. Blake (q.v.), proved that measles was a viral disease (1919-21). With Blake and others, investigated hemolytic streptococci and developed a serum treatment for scarlet fever (early 1920s). With John R. Paul (q.v.) did important research on poliomyelitis (1930s); demonstrated that asymptomatic cases were common in families or neighborhoods where the disease was present; detected the virus in sewage and in parts of the body other than the throat; developed a method for spotting hidden outbreaks of the disease.

WRITINGS: "Susceptibility of Monkeys to the Virus of Measles," *J. of Experimental Med.* 33 (1921): 385-412 (with Francis G. Blake); "Observations on the Treatment of Scarlet Fever with Scarlatinal Antistreptococci Serum," *JAMA* 82 (1924): 712-14; "Observations on the Epidemiology of Poliomyelitis with Particular Reference to So-Called Abortive Poliomyelitis," *Trans., Assoc. of Am. Physicians* 47 (1932): 116-22 (with John R. Paul); "Poliomyelitis Virus in Human Stools," *JAMA* 111 (1938): 6-11 (with John

R. Paul and A. J. Vignee). REFERENCES: *BHM* (1975-79), 127; *DAB*, Supplement 3: 774-75; Miller, *BHM*, p. 113; *NCAB*, 31: 468-69; *N.Y. Times*, May 25, 1942.

S. Galishoff

TRUDEAU, EDWARD LIVINGSTON (October 5, 1848, New York, N.Y.-November 15, 1915, Saranac Lake, N.Y.). *Physician; Tuberculosis.* Son of James, physician, and Céphise (Berger) Trudeau. Married Charlotte G. Beare, 1871; four children. EDUCATION: 1871, M.D., College of Physicians and Surgeons (Columbia). CAREER: 1871-72, practiced medicine, Long Island and New York City; 1873-80, became seriously ill with consumption and went to the Adirondack Mountain area of N.Y. State to recover; *post* 1880, began practicing medicine again, Saranac Lake (N.Y.), specializing in tuberculosis; president: 1904, National Association for the Study and Prevention of Tuberculosis (later National Tuberculosis Association); 1905, Association of American Physicians; and 1910, Congress of American Physicians and Surgeons. CONTRIBUTIONS: Pioneered in the development of clinical and laboratory methods for combatting tuberculosis. Established the Adirondack Cottage Sanitarium for treatment of incipient tuberculosis in working men and women (1884), the first American sanitarium; therapy consisted mainly of rest, fresh air, and a nutritious diet; directed and financed the center almost single-handedly for 30 years; became a model and the stimulus for the establishment of numerous other sanitariums. Established Saranac Laboratory for the Study of Tuberculosis (1894), the first laboratory of its kind in the United States. Did important research there on immunity, tuberculin, and the effectiveness of fresh air therapy.

WRITINGS: "Artificial Immunity in Experimental Tuberculosis," *Trans., Assoc. of Am. Physicians* 8 (1903): 97; *An Autobiography* (1916, posthumously). REFERENCES: *BHM* (1964-69), 262; (1970-74), 170; *DAB*, 19: 2-4; K. E. Harrod, *Man of Courage* (1959); Kelly and Burrage (1928), 1227-29; Miller, *BHM*, p. 114; *NCAB*, 13: 564; *Who Was Who in Am.*, 1: 1255.

S. Galishoff

TUFTS, COTTON (May 31, 1731, Medford, Mass.-December 8, 1815, Weymouth, Mass.). *Physician.* Son of Simon, physician, and Abagail (Smith) Tufts. Married Lucy Quincy (d. 1785), 1755, one child; Susanna Warner, 1789. EDUCATION: Harvard College: 1749, A.B.; and 1752, A.M.; 1785, M.D. (hon.), Harvard Medical School; studied under older brother, Dr. Simon Tufts (1727-86). CAREER: 1752-c. 1805, medical practitioner, Weymouth, Mass.; member: 1784, Mass. General Court (state senate); and 1788, U.S. Constitutional Convention (supported the Constitution); president, Society for the Reformation of Morals; 1765, planned the first Mass. medical society (unsuccessfully); 1780, incorporator, American Academy of Arts and Sciences; 1781, founder, Massachusetts Medical Society; 1785-87, vice-president, Massachusetts Medical Society; 1787-95, president, Massachusetts Medical Society. CONTRIBUTIONS: Scientific publication, a clinical discussion of the symptoms and treatment of a cattle disease, clearly indicates that veterinary medicine was frequently a part of his practice. Although early reputation was based on skill in curing putrid sore throat (diphtheria), eminence appears to have stemmed more from his political, moral, and missionary activities than from his medical achievements. Religious fervor pervaded many spheres of interest which shaped career. In therapeutic encounters, sought to heal the "inner man" as well as the outward body by including "instruction in righteousness" in prescription for health.

WRITINGS: "An Account of the Horn-Distemper in Cattle, with Observations on That Disease," *Mem. Am. Acad. of Arts and Sci.* 1 (1783): 529-36; *An Oration, in Honor of the Memory of General George Washington, Who Died December 14, 1799, in the 68th Year of His Age* (1800); "Letter to James Humphrey" (against the Stamp Act), *Weymouth Hist. Soc. Publ.* 2 (1885): 296-99. REFERENCES: *DAB*, 10, Supplement 2: 49-50; "Diaries of Rev. William Smith and Cotton Tufts," *Proc., Mass. Hist. Soc.* 42 (1908-9): 444-78; Kelly and Burrage (1920), 1164-65; Clifford K. Shipton, "Cotton Tufts," *Sibley's Harvard Graduates, 1749-1750*, 12 (1962): 493-500; James Thacher, *Am. Med. Biog.* 2 (1828): 149-52.

M. H. Warner

TUNNICLIFF, RUTH MAY (May 1, 1876, Macomb, Ill.-September 22, 1946, Chicago, Ill.). *Physician; Bacteriology.* Daughter of Damon George, lawyer and jurist, and Sarah Alice (Bacon) Tunnicliff. Never married. EDUCATION: 1896, A.B., Vassar College; 1903, M.D., Rush Medical College, Chicago; 1903-4, intern, hospital of the John McCormick Institute for Infectious Diseases, Chicago. CAREER: 1903-40, research staff, McCormick Institute; 1918, contract surgeon (clinical laboratory work), U.S. Army; 1934-40, research staff, Foundation for Dental Research, Chicago College of Dental Surgery of Loyola University. CONTRIBUTIONS: Contributed extensively to the bacteriology of scarlet fever, erysipelas, dental caries, and other conditions. Studied the pathogenicity of streptococci and of host immunological responses; made investigations (with George H. Weaver) of the practical value of antistreptococcal serums. Became convinced (1920s) of the streptococcal etiology in measles and influenza. The so-called Tunnicliff toxin of measles was actually produced by *Corynebacterium diphtheriae*. Made important studies of bacterial dissociation, morphology, and life cycle and of the presence of antibodies in colostrum and milk.

WRITINGS: "The Streptococco-opsonic Index in Scarlatina," *J. Infect. Dis.* 4 (1907): 304; "Further Studies of Antistreptococcus Serum," *ibid.*, 9 (1911): 130 (with G. H. Weaver); "Specific Nature of the Hemolytic Streptococcus of Scarlet Fever," *JAMA* 74 (1920): 1386. REFERENCES: Ludwig Hektoen, *Proc., Inst. Med., Chicago* 16 (1947): 298-99; *JAMA* 132 (1946): 466.

L. P. Rubin

TUPPER, HENRY MARTIN (April 11, 1831, Monson, Mass.-November 12, 1893, Raleigh, N.C.). *Educator.* Son of Earl and Permelia (Norris) Tupper. Married Sarah Baker, 1864. EDUCATION: Monson Academy; 1859, A.B., Amherst College; 1862, A.M., Newton Theological Institution (Mass.); 1886, D.D.,

Wake Forest College. CAREER: 1862, ordained a Baptist minister; 1862-65, fought and did chaplain's work in Union Army in South, primarily Va. and Miss.; 1865, commissioned by the American Baptist Home Mission Society as missionary to choose site of his work in the South; 1865-93, founder and president, Shaw University, Raleigh. CONTRIBUTIONS: Established and fostered development of Leonard Medical College, the medical department of Shaw University (1882-93). Conceived the idea of training black physicians at Shaw (1860s) and pursued that goal with the Board of Trustees, the American Baptist Home Mission Society, and northern philanthropists until it reached fruition. When Leonard closed (1918), it had graduated over 400 black physicians. Organized all aspects of the medical school, convinced local white physicians to teach there, and continually raised funds to keep the school, which was always in financial danger of becoming insolvent. REFERENCES: H. L. Morehouse, *H.M. Tupper, D.D.—A Narrative of Twenty-Five Years' Work in the South* (1890); *NCAB*, 1: 270; *Twentieth Century Biographical Dictionary of Notable Americans*, vol. 10.

T. L. Savitt

TURNER, DELOS ASHLEY (December 9, 1877, Pioche, Nev.-January 1945, Ill.). *Physician; Surgeon.* Son of Ephraim and Mary Katherine Turner. EDUCATION: M.D., 1901, University of Illinois College of Physicians and Surgeons; intern, Cook County Hospital, Chicago, Ill. CAREER: 1904-16, chief surgeon, Goldfield Mine Operators Association; chief officer, U.S. Veterans Bureau, Reno, Nev.; 1937, staff, Veterans Administration Facility, Reno; 1938-44, staff member, Veterans Administration hospital, Hines, Ill. CONTRIBUTIONS: Served the miners in Nev. (1904-16), and the U.S. Veterans' Administration (1937-44). Served in the military medical branch in World War I.

J. Edwards

TURNER, JOHN PATRICK (November 1, 1885, Raleigh, N.C.-September 14, 1958, Detroit, Mich.). *Physician; Surgeon.* Son of Jesse Edward and Jennie Virginia (Edwards) Turner. Married Marian Carmencita Harris, 1908; one child. EDUCATION: 1900-1903, City College of New York; 1906, M.D., Leonard Medical College; 1920-21, postgraduate surgical studies, University of Pennsylvania Medical School; 1930, study of hospital techniques and management at hospitals in major European cities; 1920s, postgraduate studies in internal medicine, Jefferson Medical College and Philadelphia General Hospital; and in contagious diseases, Municipal Hospital (Philadelphia, Pa.). CAREER: 1906-48, staff, Mercy-Douglass Hospital, Philadelphia: last 25 years, president of staff; and 1935-48, chief of surgery; 1912-31, medical inspector, Philadelphia Public Schools; 1931-58, surgeon, Philadelphia Police Department. CONTRIBUTIONS: Deeply involved black pioneer in medicine and civic affairs of Philadelphia. Founded Pennsylvania State Medical, Dental, and Pharmaceutical Association (black) (1921) and served as its president. President, NMA (1921), and served on editorial board,

JNMA (until 1958). First black appointed a police surgeon in Philadelphia. Devoted much time to treatment of narcotic addiction.

WRITINGS: *Ringworm and Its Successful Treatment* (1921); several other pamphlets. Writings listed in *JNMA* 51 (1959): 161. REFERENCES: W. Montague Cobb, "John Patrick Turner, M.D., 1885-1958," *JNMA* 51 (1959): 160-61; "Our President-Elect," *JNMA* 11 (1919): 159-60; *WWICA* 7 (1950): 518.

T. L. Savitt

TUTHILL, ALEXANDER MACKENZIE (September 22, 1871, South Lebanon, N.Y.-May 25, 1958, Phoenix, Ariz.). *Physician; Surgeon.* Son of William H., businessman, and Christina (Mackenzie) Tuthill. Married May E. Heimann, 1896; two children. EDUCATION: 1895, M.D., University of Southern California; 1895-96, intern, Los Angeles County Hospital and assistant physician, San Bernardino County Hospital; 1905, 1911, 1919, post graduate work, New York Post-Graduate Medical School and Hospital. CAREER: 1895-98, practice, Los Angeles, Calif.; 1898, became a physician, Detroit Copper Company, Morenci, Ariz.; 1903-16, chief surgeon, Detroit Copper Co; *post* 1919, practice in Phoenix. CONTRIBUTIONS: Organized a troop and became captain in the Arizona National Guard (1903). Promoted through ranks to major general before retiring (1952). State director, selective service, in World War II. With American Expeditionary Forces in World War I. Member, Ariz. Constitutional Convention (1910). State superintendent of health (1921-22). Specialized in general and industrial surgery. Pioneered in the use of metal bone plates in traumatic surgery. REFERENCES: *Arizona Republic* (Phoenix), May 26, 1958; James H. McClintock, *Arizona* (1916); *NCAB*, 44: 373; *Who's Who in Arizona, 1938-1940.*

J. S. Goff

TWITCHELL, AMOS (April 11, 1781, Dublin, N.H.-May 26, 1850, Keene, N.H.). *Surgeon.* Son of Samuel T., farmer, and Alice (Willson) Twitchell. Married Elizabeth Goodhue, 1815; no children. EDUCATION: 1802, New Ipswich Academy; Dartmouth: 1805, A.M. and B.M.; and 1811, M.D. CAREER: Practiced, Norwich, Vt., and Marlborough, N.H., before settling in Keene (1810), where he practiced until death; although offered professorships in surgery at three medical schools, including Dartmouth, declined them all; founder, American Medical Association; and president, 1829-30, New Hampshire Medical Society. CONTRIBUTIONS: Seems to have been the second surgeon to ligate the common carotid artery successfully, for the victim of a pistol accident, on October 8, 1807; this was eight months before Astley Cooper's case, the first to be published, and four years after the true first case, which was not published until 1817. Did not report his case until 1842. Published very little on his own, but expertise was widely recognized, as attested by his election to honorary membership, Massachusetts Medical Society (1838).

WRITINGS: "Gun-Shot Wound of the Face and Neck—Ligature of the Carotid Artery," *New Eng. Q. J. of Med. & Surg.* 1 (1842-43): 188-93. Other medical articles are reprinted in Henry I. Bowditch's *Memoir of Amos Twitchell* (1851) but without their bibliographic citations. REFERENCES: *BHM* (1964-69), 263; (1980), 39; Bowditch, *Memoir of Amos Twitchell*; *DAB* 10, pt. 1: 84-85; Kelly and Burrage (1928), 1235-36; Francis R. Packard, *History of Medicine in the United States* 2 (1931): 1105-7.

J. W. Estes

TYSON, JAMES (October 26, 1841, Philadelphia, Pa.-February 21, 1919, Philadelphia, Pa.). *Physician; Educator*. Son of Henry, physician, and Gertrude (Haviland) Tyson. Married Fanny Bosdevex, 1865; two children. EDUCATION: Haverford College: 1861, B.A.; and 1864, M.A.; read medicine under his father, Henry; Dr. John Brooke, Reading, Pa.; and Dr. John Neill, Philadelphia; 1863, M.D., University of Pennsylvania; 1863-64, resident, Pennsylvania Hospital. CAREER: 1865, acting assistant surgeon, U.S. Army; 1868-70, lecturer on microscopy and urinary chemistry, University of Pennsylvania Medical School; 1870-78, professor of physiology and microscopy, Pennsylvania College of Dental Surgery; at University of Pennsylvania Medical School: 1874-76, lecturer, pathological anatomy and morbid anatomy; 1876-89, professor of general pathology and morbid anatomy; 1888-92, dean, medical faculty; 1889-1910, professor, practice of medicine; and 1910-19, professor emeritus; president: 1907-8, Association of American Physicians; and 1907-10, College of Physicians of Philadelphia. CONTRIBUTIONS: Authored several influential medical textbooks during the latter decades of the nineteenth century. A founder, Association of American Physicians (1886).

WRITINGS: *The Cell Doctrine: It History and Present State* (1870); *A Guide to the Practical Examination of Urine* (1875); *A Treatise on Bright's Disease and Diabetes* (1881); *Manual of Physical Diagnosis* (1891); *The Practice of Medicine* (1896). REFERENCES: George W. Corner, *Two Centuries of Medicine* (1965), 107; *NCAB*, 9: 356; *DAB*, 19: 103.

N. Gevitz

U

UNDERWOOD, FELIX JOEL (November 21, 1882, Nettleton, Miss.-January 9, 1959, Jackson, Miss.). *Physician; State health official.* Son of Marion Milton and Amanda Capitola (Battle) Underwood. Married Sarah Beatrice Tapscott, 1904; two children. EDUCATION: Public schools, Nettleton; 1908, M.D., University of Tennessee. CAREER: Began practice of medicine, Nettleton, and was part-time health officer, Monroe County (Miss.), until 1915; 1912-25, secretary, Northeast Mississippi Thirteen Counties Medical Society; 1912-19, member of council (chairman, 1915-19), Mississippi State Medical Association; 1917-20, director, Monroe County Health Department; 1919-20, president, Mississippi State Medical Association; 1920-23, member, Miss. Governor Russell's staff; 1920-24, director, Bureau of Child Hygiene, Mississippi State Board of Health; 1921-27, councilor, Miss., Southern Medical Association; 1924-58, secretary and executive officer, Mississippi State Board of Health; 1924-retirement, secretary, Board of Trustees, Mississippi State Tuberculosis Sanatorium; 1928-retirement, member, Board of Trustees (president since 1941), Mississippi Children's Home Society; 1930, president, Southern Medical Association and State and Provincial Health Authorities; 1931-retirement, member of the staff, Mississippi Baptist Hospital, and president, State Board of Examiners for Nurses; 1937, president, Mississippi Public Health Association; member: 1938-40, Board of Science Directors, Rockefeller Foundation; and 1939, planning committee and report committees, White House Conference on Children in a Democracy; 1944, president, American Public Health Association. CONTRIBUTIONS: A leading public health official in the nation for over three decades. At one time mentioned for appointment as Surgeon General of the United States. Mississippi State Board of Health building in Jackson is named in his honor.

WRITINGS: *Public Health and Medical Licensure in Mississippi, 1798-1948*, 2 vols. (1941, 1948, with R. N. Whitfield); numerous articles in medical journals. REFERENCES:

J. Kobler, "He Saved a Million Lives," *Am. Mag.* 158 (Sept. 1954): 45-46; A. Rankin, "Mississippi's Medical Giant," *Coronet* 36 (Oct. 1954): 149-52; *Who Was Who in Am.*, 3: 868.

M. S. Legan

V

VAN HOOSEN, BERTHA (March 26, 1863, Stony Creek, Mich.-June 7, 1952, Romeo, Mich.). *Obstetrician; Surgeon.* Daughter of Joshua, farmer, and Sarah Ann (Taylor) Van Hoosen, teacher. Never married. EDUCATION: University of Michigan: 1884, A.B.; and 1888, M.D.; 1888-92, clinical training, Woman's Hospital, Detroit, Mich.; Kalamazoo State Hospital for the Insane in Mich.; and the New England Hospital for Women and Children, Boston, Mass. CAREER: 1892, opened a private obstetrical practice, Chicago, Ill.; 1893-1902, anatomy and embryology faculty, Northwestern University Woman's Medical School, Chicago; 1902-12, clinical gynecology faculty, Illinois University Medical School; held a number of hospital appointments; 1913, became chief of the gynecological staff, Cook County Hospital, the first time a woman had received this appointment, which was granted on the basis of a competitive civil service exam; 1920, became chief of obstetrics, Cook County; 1918-37, professor and head of obstetrics, Loyola University Medical School. CONTRIBUTIONS: First woman to head a medical division at a co-educational university (Loyola). An outstanding surgeon (known as the dean of women surgeons in America) who devoted her skill to the benefit of women and children and a demanding but revered teacher who trained scores of women surgeons (whom she referred to as her "surgical daughters") and a number of male surgeons as well. Traveled extensively, performing surgery in a number of countries, where her innovative techniques and surgical skill captured the respect of those in attendance. Organized (1915) the first national medical women's association in the country (today known as the American Medical Women's Association). Pioneered in the use of scopolamine-morphine anesthesia (twilight sleep) in childbirth (*post* 1904). Gave public lectures on sex hygiene to women and their daughters (*post* 1907). Developed better methods of prenatal care and created the first human breast milk bank in Chicago (1930).

WRITINGS: Over 50 articles on various topics in obstetrics and gynecology, about women physicians, and about her travels around the world; an autobiography, *Petticoat*

Surgeon (1947). Manuscript and published copies of articles and presentations are available in the Archives and Special Collections on Women in Medicine, The Medical College of Pennsylvania, Philadelphia, Pa. REFERENCES: *BHM* (1964-69), 265; *Notable Am. Women*, 4: 706-7; *Petticoat Surgeon* (1947); Van Hoosen Collection, Archives and Special Collections on Women in Medicine, The Medical College of Pennsylvania, Philadelphia.

S. L. Chaff

VAN INGEN, PHILIP (July 31, 1875, Washington, Conn.-March 28, 1953, New York, N.Y.). *Physician; Pediatrics*. Son of E. H., businessman, and Mary L. (McLane) Van Ingen. Never married. EDUCATION: 1897, A.B., Yale University; 1901, M.D., College of Physicians and Surgeons (Columbia); 1901-4, house physician, Presbyterian and Foundling hospitals (N.Y.); 1904-5, studied pediatrics in Vienna. CAREER: *Post* 1905, practiced medicine, N.Y.; 1921-30, clinical pediatrics faculty, College of Physicians and Surgeons; *post* 1921, consulting physician, Willard Parker Hospital; *post* 1938, consultant on pediatrics, Roosevelt Hospital; 1929, chairman, committee on the medical care of children, White House Conference on Child Health and Protection; 1930-33, member, committee to investigate maternal mortality, New York Academy of Medicine; president: American Pediatrics Society, American Academy of Pediatrics, and American Child Hygiene Association. CONTRIBUTIONS: Played a major role in the movement to improve infant and child welfare in the United States during the early decades of the twentieth century. Led the fight to get New York City to establish well-baby clinics throughout the city. A prominent figure in the Society for the Study and Prevention of Infant Mortality (later American Child Hygiene Association); served as its secretary (1912) and president (1917) and prepared its annual reports and charts, which called attention to the nation's high infant mortality rate and how it could be reduced. Induced the Commonwealth Fund to sponsor demonstration projects in four cities that showed what local health agencies could accomplish in child health conservation if staffed with competent personnel and given adequate finances. Wrote some of the first histories of the American child health movement.

WRITINGS:"The History of Child Welfare in the United States," in Mazyck Porcher Ravenel, ed., *A Half Century of Public Health; Jubilee Historical Volume of the American Public Health Association* (1921), 290-322; *The Story of the American Child Health Association* (1936); *History of the New York Academy of Medicine—Its First 100 Years* (1949). REFERENCES: *N.Y. Times*, March 29, 1953; Borden Smith Veeder, "Philip Van Ingen (1875-1952)," in B. S. Veeder, ed., *Pediatric Profiles* (1957), 182-188; *Who Was Who in Am.*, 3: 874.

S. Galishoff

VAN SLYKE, DONALD DEXTER (March 29, 1883, Pike, N.Y.-May 4, 1971, Garden City, N.Y.). *Biological chemist*. Son of Lucius Lincoln, agricultural chemist, and Lucy (Dexter) Van Slyke. Married Rena Mosher, 1907; Else von Bardenfleth Brock, 1948; two children by first marriage. EDUCATION: University of Michigan: 1905, B.S.; and 1907, Ph.D. CAREER: 1907-14, research chemist, biochemical laboratory, Rockefeller Institute for Medical Research; 1914-49, chief chemist, Hospital of the Rockefeller Institute for Medical Research; 1922-23, visiting professor of biochemistry, Peking Union Medical College; 1941-47, president, American Bureau for Medical Aid to China; 1949-51, deputy director of biology and medicine, Brookhaven National Laboratory (Upton, N.Y.); 1951-56, served part time as counselor for research grants, Eli Lilly and Company; 1956-71, research biochemist, department of medicine, Brookhaven National Laboratory. CONTRIBUTIONS: Internationally famous for major discoveries in chemistry, physiology, and medicine. Conducted extensive research in the applications of chemistry to clinical and investigative medicine. Perhaps best known for studies on acidosis; defined *acidosis* as a decrease in the bicarbonate concentration of the blood and developed a diagnostic test; revolutionized the treatment of diabetes, in which heretofore acidotic coma had been a grave risk. Made long-term studies of renal physiology that clarified the mechanism of renal excretion and the diagnosis of kidney disease. Made scientific contributions in the areas of amino acid and protein chemistry, the transport of oxygen and carbon dioxide in the blood stream, and acid-base, gas, fluid, and electrolyte equilibriums in body fluids and the relation of these equilibriums to disease states; research resulted in many new analytical methods and apparatus. Discovered and identified the amino acid hydroxylysine. With John Peters, wrote *Quantitative Clinical Chemistry* (1931-32), an authoritative work that was widely used by medical students and biochemical investigators throughout the world. Edited *Journal of Biological Chemistry* (1914-25). Trained a large number of physicians in the chemical approach to clinical investigation who distinguished themselves in academic medicine and biochemistry.

WRITINGS: "Studies of Acidosis. XIII. A Method for Titrating the Biocarbonate Content of the Plasma," *J. Biol. Chem.* 38 (May 1919): 167-78 (with E. Stillman and G. E. Cullen); *Cyanosis* (1923, with Christen Lundsgaard); *Factors Affecting the Distribution of Electrolytes, Water, and Gases in the Animal Body* (1926); *Observations on the Courses of Different Types of Bright's Disease and on the Resultant Changes in Renal Anatomy* (1930, with others); *Micromanometric Analyses* (1961, with John Plazin). REFERENCES: *BMNAS*, 48 (1976): 309-35; *DSB*, 13: 574-75; *NCAB*, 56: 68-69; *N.Y. Times*, May 6, 1971.

S. Galishoff

VAUGHAN, GEORGE TULLY (June 27, 1859, Arrington, Va.-April 26, 1948, Washington, D.C.). *Surgeon.* Son of James Walter Washington Lafayette, physician, and Frances Ellen (Shields) Vaughan. Married May Townsend Venable, June 27, 1883; two children. EDUCATION: Private schools and Kenmore University High School, Amherst, Va.; 1879, M.D., University of Virginia; 1880, M.D., Bellevue Hospital Medical College; postgraduate courses: 1883, New York Polyclinic Medical School and Hospital; 1894-95, University of Berlin; and 1905-6, Jefferson Medical College. CAREER: 1880-88, began private practice, Lowesville and Farmville, Va.; 1888, until he resigned, 1906, in the

U.S. Marine Hospital Service: 1888, assistant surgeon; 1900, surgeon; and 1902, assistant surgeon-general; 1897-1933, professor and head, Department of Surgery, Georgetown University Medical School; 1897-1933, chief surgeon, Georgetown University Hospital; consulting surgeon at various area hospitals; until retirement in 1943, maintained private surgical practice. CONTRIBUTIONS: Pioneering work on surgery of the heart and blood vessels and on typhoid perforation. Founder-member, American College of Surgeons. Fellow, International Surgical Association. Member, numerous medical, surgical, and scientific societies. Recipient of many medals and other honors. Navy surgeon aboard the USS *Leviathan* (1917-19).

WRITINGS: More than 100 articles in medical journals and two books: *The Principles and Practice of Surgery* (1903) and *Papers on Surgery and other Subjects* (1932). REFERENCES: D. S. Lamb et al., *History of the Medical Society of the District of Columbia, 1817-1909* (1909), 386-87; *NCAB*, 38: 43-44; *Who Was Who in Am.* 2, 546.

R. Kondratas

VAUGHAN, VICTOR CLARENCE (October 27, 1851, Mount Airy, Mo.-November 21, 1929, Richmond, Va.). *Biochemist; Medical administrator; Microbiology; Public health.* Son of John and Adeline (Dameron) Vaughan. Married Dora Catherine Taylor, 1877; five children. EDUCATION: 1872, B.S., Mount Pleasant College (Mo.); University of Michigan: 1875, M.S.; 1876, Ph.D.; and 1878, M.D.; 1888, studied bacteriology in Berlin under Robert Koch. CAREER: At University of Michigan Medical School: 1875-87, physiological chemistry faculty; 1883-87, therapeutics and materia medica faculty; 1887-1909, director, hygienic laboratory; 1887-1921, hygiene and physiological chemistry faculty; and 1891-1921, dean; member: 1883-95, 1901-18, Michigan State Board of Health; and 1898, Typhoid Fever Board, U.S. Army; 1917-18, in charge of communicable diseases, U.S. Surgeon General's Office; 1919-27, member, Board of Directors, International Health Board, Rockefeller Foundation; 1921-22, 1925-26, chairman, Division of Medical Sciences, National Research Council; president: 1909-10, Association of American Physicians; 1914-15, American Medical Association; and 1919-20, National Tuberculosis Association. CONTRIBUTIONS: With Frederick G. Novy (q.v.), established the first laboratory course in bacteriology in an American university (1888). With Novy, made important biochemical investigations of food poisons. With Walter Reed (q.v.) and Edward O. Shakespeare (q.v.), showed that much of the incidence of typhoid in army camps during the war with Spain was attributable to contact infection and transmission of the disease by flies. Active in public health and co-authored a widely used textbook on the subject. Made the University of Michigan Medical School one of the best in the nation; lengthened the course of instruction and raised entrance requirements; assembled a distinguished faculty, increased the size of the library, and improved clinical facilities. Nationally renowned as a medico-legal expert in toxicology. Founded and managing editor for some time, *Phy-*

sician and Surgeon (1879) and *Journal of Laboratory and Clinical Medicine* (1915). First editor, *Hygeia* (1922).

WRITINGS: *Textbook of Physiological Chemistry* (1878); *Ptomaines and Leucomaines* (1888, with F. G. Novy); *Origin and Spread of Typhoid Fever in U.S. Military Camps* (1904); *Epidemiology and Public Health* (1922-23, with Henry F. Vaughan and George T. Palmer). Bibliography is in *J. of Lab. and Clin. Med.* (Jun. 1930). REFERENCES: *BHM* (1970-74), 172; *DAB*, 19: 236-37; Miller, *BHM*, p. 115; *NCAB*, 29: 434-35; *Who Was Who in Am.*, 1: 1275.

S. Galishoff

VEDDER, EDWARD BRIGHT (June 28, 1878, New York City-January 30, 1952, Washington, D.C.). *Physician; Military medicine; Deficiency diseases.* Son of Henry Clay, clergyman, and Minnie (Lingham) Vedder. Married Lily Sheldrake Norton, 1903; two children. EDUCATION: 1898, Ph.B., University of Rochester; 1902, M.D., University of Pennsylvania; postgraduate studies at the Army Medical School, Washington, D.C., as assistant surgeon in the U.S. Army Medical Corps; 1904, M.D., Army Medical School. CAREER: 1904-13, military service, primarily in the Philippines; 1913-19, professor of pathology, Army Medical School; 1919-22, director of the Southern Department Laboratory at Fort Sam Houston, Texas; 1922-25, chief of medical research, Edgewood (Md.) Arsenal; 1925-29, senior member of the Army Board for Medical Research, Manila; 1930, commandant, Army Medical School; 1933, retired from military service and became professor of experimental medicine, George Washington University; 1942-47, director of medical education, Alameda County (Calif.) Hospital and laboratory director at Highland County Hospital (Oakland). Retired in 1947. CONTRIBUTIONS: Discovered that beriberi is a deficiency disease. Work on scurvy helped lead the way to the discovery (by others) that ascorbic acid was a vitamin. Researched and wrote on medical aspects of chemical warfare (1925).

WRITINGS: *Beriberi* (1913); *The Prevalence of Syphilis in the Army* (1915); *Sanitation for Medical Officers* (1917); *Syphilis and Public Health* (1918); *The Medical Aspects of Chemical Warfare* (1925); *Medicine: Its Contribution to Civilization* (1929). REFERENCES: *DAB*, Supplement 5: 710-11; *NCAB*, 41: 229; *N.Y. Times*, February 2, 1952.

M. Kaufman

VEEDER, BORDEN SMITH (August 21, 1883, Fonda, N.Y.-June 24, 1970, St. Louis, Mo.). *Pediatrician.* Son of James and Jennie (Smith) Veeder. Married Vera Giannini Angert, 1930; Lillie deLeuw, 1960. EDUCATION: 1901, B.A., Colgate; 1907, M.D., University of Pennsylvania. CAREER: 1909-11, instructor in pathology, University of Pennsylvania; 1911-12, instructor in pediatrics, Washington University School of Medicine; 1912-17, assistant professor, pediatrics, and acting chief of staff, St. Louis Children's Hospital; 1917-19, lieutenant colonel and commanding officer, Base Hospital 21, U.S. Army; 1919-52, professor of clinical pediatrics, Washington University School of Medicine; 1952-70, professor emeritus; at *Journal of Pediatrics*: 1932-47, co-editor; and

1948-58, editor; founding member: 1932, American Academy of Pediatrics; and 1933, American Board of Pediatrics; president: 1934, American Pediatric Society; 1943, American Academy of Pediatrics; and 1946-50, National Board of Medical Examiners. CONTRIBUTIONS: Primary contributions were in the organization of pediatrics as a medical specialty. Active in the early development of the Department of Pediatrics, Washington University School of Medicine, and served as chief of staff, St. Louis Children's Hospital, after John Howland's (q.v.) abrupt departure as chairman of pediatrics, Washington University School of Medicine (1911). Interested in the improvement of medical education in pediatrics and in the general upgrading of the field. Instrumental in the formation of a National Board of Pediatrics (1934). President of many important medical organizations and edited *Journal of Pediatrics* for decades. Skills as an organizer and conciliator, as well as a clinician, were recognized by colleagues, who accorded him the title "pediatric statesman" in his 1960 Festschrift. Always interested in the social aspects of medicine, last published article (1961) dealt with the delicate issue of medical ethics in pediatrics—an issue that received increasing attention in medical literature in succeeding decades.

WRITINGS: "Child Hygiene and the Private Physician," *JAMA* 79 (1922): 2228-29; "Pediatrics and the Child," *ibid.*, 81 (1923): 517-18; "The Trend of Pediatrics," *Arch. of Ped.* 41 (1924): 5-12; "The Relation of Hospital Residency to Graduate Education in Pediatrics," *Hospitals*, 11 (1937): 91-95; Presidential Address, American Academy of Pediatrics, *J. Pediat.* 23 (1943): 632-39; "The Influence of David Edsall on Pediatrics in the United States," *ibid.*, 47 (1955): 808-16; "A Pediatric Ethical Question," *ibid.*, 58 (1961): 604-5. An unpublished paper on the formation of the American Board of Pediatrics is in the Washington University Medical School Archives, St. Louis, Mo. REFERENCES: See *Festschrift* in Honor of Borden S. Veeder, *J. Pediat.* 56 (1960): 2, esp. Park J. White, "Borden S. Veeder," pp. 139-46; *Who Was Who in Am.*, 7: 587.

M. Hunt

VEST, WALTER (January 20, 1882, Floyd County, Va.-January 28, 1962, Huntington, W.Va.). *Physician.* Son of William Madison and Mary Susan (Boone) Vest. Married Saddie Pearl Blankinship, 1910; one child. EDUCATION: 1902, A.B., William and Mary College; 1909, M.D., Medical College of Virginia; 1909-1910, intern, Memorial Hospital, Richmond, Va. CAREER: Practice: 1910-15, Meherrin, Va.; *post* 1915, Huntington; during World War I, chief of medical service, base hospital, Camp Wadsworth, S.C. CONTRIBUTIONS: Editor, *West Virginia Medical Journal.* Improved it to the point where it became recognized as a quality publication. President, West Virginia State Medical Association (1930), Southern Medical Association (1938-39) and Federation of Medical Licensing Boards of the United States (1952-53). Member, editorial board, *Today's Health.* REFERENCES: *Who Was Who in Am.*, 4: 970.

K. Nodyne and R. Murphy

VIKO, LOUIS EINDRED (August 25, 1896, Park City, Utah-January 17, 1968, Salt Lake City, Utah). *Physician; Cardiology; Public health.* Son of

Eindred, physician, and Margaret (Carney) Viko. Married La Vaun Clark, 1927; two children. EDUCATION: 1913-15, student at University of Utah; 1920, M.D., Harvard Medical School; 1921-22, research resident in cardiology under Paul Dudley White (q.v.), Massachusetts General Hospital; 1929-30, research resident in cardiology under Thomas Lewis, University College Hospital, London; 1931, studied in Vienna. CAREER: 1922-67, practiced internal medicine, Inter-Mountain Clinic, Salt Lake City; 1931-67, staff, Latter Day Saints and University hospitals; 1932-35, Salt Lake City health commissioner; 1961-65, member, Utah State Board of Health (chairman, 1963-65); president: 1937, Utah Public Health Association; 1943, Utah State Medical Association; and 1951, Utah Heart Association; 1937, governor, American College of Physicians; 1949-67, clinical professor of medicine, University of Utah Medical School. CONTRIBUTIONS: A leader in changing the two-year University of Utah Medical School to a four-year school (1941-42). Studied cardiac disorders, adding to the literature. Significantly developed the Salt Lake City Board of Health and achieved enforcement of regulations.

WRITINGS: "Disorders of the Heart Beat," *Med. Clinics North America* 5 (Mar. 1922): 1479-1508 (with Paul D. White); "Cardiac Neurosis Associated with Rheumatic Valvular Heart Disease," *Am. Heart J.* 1 (Jun. 1926): 539-45; "Heart Disease in Rocky Mountain Region," *ibid.*, 6 (Dec. 1930): 264-73; "Prognosis in Arteriosclerotic Heart Disease," *JAMA* 103 (Aug. 25, 1934): 553-58; "Modern Treatment of Heart Disease," *Med. Record* 148 (Oct. 5, 1938): 260-63; "The Utah Plan for Evaluating Industrial Cardiac Cases," in Paul B. Boeber, ed., *Work and the Heart* (1959). REFERENCES: Joseph R. Morrell, M.D., *Utah's Health and You* (1956), 108-10; *NCAB*, 54 (1973): 343-44.

H. Bauman

VINCENT, UBERT CONRAD (January 5, 1892, Raleigh, N.C.-December 18, 1938, New York, N.Y.). *Surgeon; Urologist*. Son of Andrew Conrad, minister and professor of theology, and Cora F. Vincent, teacher. Married Naomi Tulane, 1920; four children. EDUCATION: 1914, A.B., Shaw University (Raleigh); 1914-15, Leonard Medical College; 1915-18, M.D., University of Pennsylvania; 1918-19, intern, Bellevue Hospital, N.Y. (admitted only after pressure was applied, owing to racial prejudice); 1919-20, resident in urology, Bellevue Hospital. CAREER: 1920-38, private practice, Harlem district of New York City; 1925-30, 1933-36, urology attending staff, Harlem Hospital, N.Y.; 1929-30, director, Vincent's Sanitorium, Harlem. CONTRIBUTIONS: Developed improved procedure for surgical repair of varicocele (1918 or 1919). Established a community hospital, Vincent's Sanitorium, to serve the needs of Harlem residents for a good private hospital facility (1929-30); failed because of Vincent's sudden illness and the stock market crash. Succeeded in breaking racial barrier at Bellevue Hospital, N.Y., to become an intern at that institution (1918).

WRITINGS: "The Open Operation," *Surg. Gyn. & Obst.* 5 (1929): 558-65. REFER-

ENCES: W. Montague Cobb, "Ubert Conrad Vincent, B.S., M.D., 1892-1938," *JNMA* 67 (1975): 73-80.

T. L. Savitt

VINSONHALER, FRANK (April 14, 1864, Graham, Mo.-September 1, 1942, Little Rock, Ark.). *Physician; Ophthalmology.* Son of George, farmer, and Sarah (Rea) Vinsonhaler. Married Wrennetta Beidelman, 1898; three children. EDUCATION: Northwestern Normal School, Oregon, Mo.; 1885, M.D., College of Physicians and Surgeons, Columbia University; 1892, student extraordinary, University of Vienna; 1892-93, postgraduate study, Royal Ophthalmic Hospital, London. CAREER: Private practice: 1885-91, northwestern Nebraska; 1893, St. Louis, Mo.; and 1893-1927, Little Rock; medical faculty: 1893, Missouri Medical College; and 1893-1918, 1920-42, University of Arkansas medical department; 1918-19, U.S. Army Medical Corps; 1927-39, dean, University of Arkansas School of Medicine. CONTRIBUTIONS: Promoted state medical organization as secretary (1898-1900) and president (1901-2), Arkansas Medical Society. Guided University of Arkansas School of Medicine, while its dean, through the financial difficulties of depression years and helped it survive by obtaining a grant for a new building (1935) and a lease of the City Hospital for teaching purposes (1939). Chaired a committee appointed by the Arkansas Legislative Council (1929) to prepare legislation requiring examination in basic sciences for all applicants for medical licensure; toured the state at own expense to gain support for the bill and assure its enactment. Wrote the major part of a history of the state medical society, published by the society after his death.

WRITINGS: *History of the Arkansas Medical Society* (1943). REFERENCES: W. David Baird, *Medical Education in Arkansas* (1979), 144-72; *Who Was Who in Am.*, 2 (1950): 548.

D. Konold

VOEGTLIN, CARL (July 28, 1879, Zofingen, Switzerland-April 9, 1960, Washington, D.C.). *Chemist; Biochemistry; Pharmacology; Oncology.* Son of Carl Voegtlin, physician. Married Lillian Kreuter, 1912; one child. EDUCATION: Studied at universities of Basel, Munich, Geneva, and Freiburg; 1904, Ph.D., University of Freiburg; 1905, went to the United States. CAREER: 1905, chemistry faculty, University of Wisconsin; 1906-13, pharmacology faculty, Johns Hopkins Medical School; 1913-39, chief, Division of Pharmacology, U.S. Hygienic Laboratory (later National Institutes of Health); 1938-42, chief, National Cancer Institute; 1943-45, consultant to the medical section of the Manhattan District; 1943-50, lecturer in pharmacology, University of Rochester Medical School; chairman or president: 1927-30, American Society for Pharmacology and Experimental Therapeutics; 1928, American Federation for Experimental Biology; and 1941, American Association for Cancer Research. CONTRIBUTIONS: Directed the first biochemical research laboratory to be established in an American medical school (Johns Hopkins, 1906). With William G. MacCallum (q.v.), discovered the relation of tetany to the parathyroid glands and to calcium metabolism. Made important studies of the relation of diet to pellagra and the diagnosis and prevention of T.N.T. poisoning (1913-20). Developed toxicity standards for the arsphenamines that were used in the administration of the Biologics Act and demonstrated the existence of Ehrlich's hypothetical "arsenic receptor" (1917-24). Contributed to knowledge of the biochemistry of tumors. First director of cancer research, Public Health Service, and first chief, National Cancer Institute. Participated in and directed investigation of the toxicology of uranium compounds (1943-49).

WRITINGS: "On the Relation of Tetany to the Parathyroid Glands and to Calcium Metabolism," *J. of Experimental Med.* 11 (1909): 118 (with William G. MacCallum); "Trinitrotoluene Poisoning—Its Nature, Diagnosis and Prevention," *Hygienic Laboratory Bull.* 126 (1920): 7 (with C. W. Hooper and J. M. Johnson); "Viscosity and Toxicity of Arsphenamine Solutions," *Public Health Reports* 39 (1924): 179 (with J. M. Johnson and H. Dyer); "The Chemistry of Carcinogenesis and Tumor Growth," Fifth Frank Billings Lecture, *Proc., Inst. Med., Chicago* 14 (1943): 454; *Pharmacology and Toxicology of Uranium Compounds* (1949, with Harold C. Hodge). A bibliography is in *J. National Cancer Instit.* REFERENCES: *BHM* (1977), 34; *J. National Cancer Instit.* 25, no. 4 (1960): iii-xv; *Who Was Who in Am.*, 6: 418.

S. Galishoff

VON BÉKÉSY, GEORG (June 3, 1899, Budapest, Hungary-June 13, 1972, Honolulu, Hawaii). *Physicist; Acoustics.* Son of Alexander, diplomat, and Paula (Mazaly) Von Békésy. Never married. EDUCATION: 1916-20, studied at University of Bern, Switzerland; 1923, Ph.D., University of Budapest. CAREER: 1924-46, engineer, Royal Hungarian Institute for Research in Telegraphy; 1926-27, at central laboratory of Siemens and Halske A.G., Berlin; 1932-46, experimental physics faculty, University of Budapest; 1946-47, at Karolinska Institute, Stockholm; 1949-66, at Psycho-Acoustic Laboratory, Harvard University; 1966-72, sensory sciences faculty, University of Hawaii. CONTRIBUTIONS: Discovered how the ear distinguishes the pitch of sounds. Showed that the cochlea converts the mechanical vibration of sounds into electrical nerve impulses of varying strength that are received by the brain, enabling it to distinguish pitch. Led to the development of new diagnostic procedures and treatments for impaired hearing. Invented an audiometer for determining whether deafness in individual cases is caused by damage to the ear or to the brain, but was primarily interested in research rather than practical applications. For discoveries concerning the physical mechanics of acoustic stimulation of the inner ear, was awarded the 1961 Nobel Prize for physiology or medicine, the first physicist to be so honored.

WRITINGS: "Zur Theorie des Hörens; die Schwingungsform der Basilarmembran," *Physikalische Zeitschrift* 29 (1928): 793-810; "Über den Knall und die Theorie des Hörens," *ibid.*, 34 (1933): 577-82; *Experiments in Hearing*, trans. and ed. Ernest G. Wever (1960); *Sensory Inhibition* (1967). A bibliography is in *BMNAS*. REFERENCES:

BMNAS, 48 (1976): 25-49; *Current Biog.* (1962), 36-38; *McGraw-Hill Modern Men of Sci.* 1 (1966): 30-31.

S. Galishoff

VON MANSFELDE, ALEXANDER SIEDSCHLAG (December 21, 1845, Neumark, Prussia-June 17, 1928, Ashland, Nebr.). *Physician; Surgeon.* Son of Herman, landowner, and Augusta (Tapp) von Mansfelde. Married Julia Labhart, October 22, 1868 (d. January 1916), eight children; Sylvia A. Butts, May 29, 1917. EDUCATION: 1863-66, studied and worked as a pharmacist; studied medicine under A. B. Hunt, M.D., and B. S. Woodworth, M.D., Ft. Wayne, Ind.; 1872, M.D., Rush Medical College. CAREER: 1872-75, practice of medicine and lecturer, Rush Medical College, Chicago, Ill.; 1875-78, practice of medicine, Lincoln, Nebr.; 1878-1928, medical practice, Ashland; 1881-85, professor of pathology and histology, Omaha Medical College; in Nebraska State Medical Society: 1881, an organizer; 1887-1889, secretary; and 1893, president and chairman, Medico-Legal Defense Committee; at *Omaha Clinic*: 1885-92, associate editor; and 1892-99, editor; organizer and president, Nebraska Railroad Surgeons' Society; in Missouri Valley Medical Society: 1888, secretary; and 1891-92, president; 1896, president, Nebraska Academy of Sciences. CONTRIBUTIONS: A dominant figure in organized medicine in Nebr. Either drafted or sponsored every Nebr. statute affecting health and medical practice. Influential in national health-related legislation, particularly in regard to compensation of participants in yellow-fever conquest. An early advocate of county medical societies as qualification for State Medical Society membership and (1894) suggested this plan as basis for national association membership. Performed surgery in his home, part of which was set up as a hospital. Wife served as the anesthetist with chloroform as the anesthetic.

WRITINGS: "Tuberculosis Pulmonum, Acute and Chronic: Its Nature and Treatment," *JAMA* 6, no. 12 (1886): 309-13, 342-45; "The Nebraska State Medical Society: Its History for the First One-Third of a Century," *Western Med. Rev.* 7, no. 5 (May 15, 1902): 127-40 (with H. W. Orr); "History of Medicine in Nebraska," *Bull. Univ. of Nebraska Coll. of Med.* 1, no. 4 (Oct. 1906): 161-71. REFERENCES: H. W. Orr, "Nebraska Medical Pioneers: Dr. Alexander S. von Mansfelde," *Western Med. Rev.* 6, no. 12 (Dec. 16, 1901): 363-65; A. E. Sheldon, *Nebraska, the Land and the People* 3 (1931): 130-31; A. T. Tyler and E. F. Auerbach, *History of Medicine in Nebraska*, enlarged by B. M. Hetzner (1977), 74-76.

B. M. Hetzner

W

WAHL, HARRY ROSWELL (May 5, 1886, Minnesota City, Minn.-June 18, 1956, Kansas City, Kans.). *Physician; Pathologist.* Son of Henry S., physician, and Clara E. (Waterman) Wahl, schoolteacher. Married Elizabeth Emery, 1916, three children; after her death, Katherine Bell, 1940, one child. EDUCATION: University of Wisconsin: 1908, A.B.; and 1910, M.A.; 1912, M.D., Johns Hopkins; and house physician, Mt. Wilson Sanitarium, Baltimore; 1912-13, research fellow, Western Reserve School of Medicine. CAREER: At Western Reserve: 1913-15, instructor in pathology; and 1915-19, associate professor; 1916-19, directed laboratories, Mt. Sinai Hospital (Cleveland, Ohio); 1916-19, rose to rank of major in Medical Corps; 1919-51, at University of Kansas School of Medicine: 1924-27, acting dean; and 1927-48, dean; and headed department of pathology and was superintendent of the teaching hospital. CONTRIBUTIONS: Principal contributions were in administration and teaching. Presided over the University of Kansas School of Medicine during the lean years while the people of Kans. were slowly deciding to support the expensive business of moving medical education from the realm of theory to the costly classrooms of hospital and laboratory. Held together a small cadre of dedicated and excellent full-time physician-educators who placed the school in a good position to take advantage of the period of rapid growth beginning with the 1950s.

WRITINGS: "Neuroblastomata . . ." *J. of Med. Research* 25 (1914): 205-6; "Gaucher's Disease . . .," *Johns Hopkins Hosp. Bull.* 27 (1916): 1-25. REFERENCES: *NCAB*, 45: 261.

R. Hudson

WAKSMAN, SELMAN ABRAHAM (July 22, 1888, Priluka, Russia-August 16, 1973, Hyannis, Mass.). *Biochemist; Soil bacteriologist; Microbiology; Chemotherapy.* Son of Jacob, merchant, and Fradia (London) Waksman. Went to United States, 1910; naturalized, 1916. Married Bertha Deborah Mitnik, 1916; one child. EDUCATION: Rutgers University: 1915, B.S.; and 1916, M.S.; 1918,

Ph.D., University of California. CAREER: 1917-18, research biochemist, Cutter Biological Laboratories (Berkeley, Calif.); 1942-58, soil microbiology faculty, Rutgers University; 1918-54, microbiologist, New Jersey Agricultural Experiment Station; 1919-20, bacteriologist, Takamine Laboratories (Clifton, N.J.); 1930-42, marine bacteriologist, Woods Hole Oceanographic Institute; 1949-58, director, Rutgers Institute of Microbiology; 1942, president, Society of American Bacteriologists. CONTRIBUTIONS: Did earliest research on soil conservation, being especially known for work on peat and humus. Became interested in the possible therapeutic uses of actinomycetes, a genus of soil fungi, which were known to inhibit the growth of pathogenic bacteria; coined the term *antibiotic* for the chemical products of microorganisms that could destroy harmful bacteria; searched for antibiotics in the soil that would not be too toxic for man and found one (1943) which he called "streptomycin"; was widely used to fight diseases that could not be treated by penicillin, including tularemia, bacterial meningitis, endocarditis, pulmonary and urinary tract infections, and, most important, tuberculosis; awarded the 1952 Nobel Prize in medicine or physiology for this accomplishment. Used royalties from the sale of streptomycin to establish the Rutgers Institute of Microbiology. With his colleagues at the institute, developed other antibiotics from actinomycetes including neomycin and candicidin.

WRITINGS: *Principles of Soil Microbiology* (1927); *Streptomycin, Its Nature and Applications* (1949); *Neomycin, Nature and Application* (1958); *The Actinomycetes* (1959-62). REFERENCES: *BHM* (1964-69), 273; (1975-79), 131; *Current Biog.* (1946), 615-17; H. A. Lechevalier and M. Solotorovsky, *Three Centuries of Microbiology* (1965), 475-87; *McGraw-Hill Modern Men of Sci.* (1966) 1: 505-6; Miller, *BHM*, p. 116; NCAB, 1: 312-13; S. A. Waksman, *My Life with the Microbes* (1954); *Who Was Who in Am.*, 6: 420.

S. Galishoff

WALD, LILLIAN D. (March 10, 1867, Cincinnati, Ohio-September 1, 1940, Westport, Conn.). *Public health nurse; Settlement leader; Social reformer.* Daughter of Max D., merchant, and Minnie (Schwarz) Wald. Never married. EDUCATION: 1891, graduated from New York Hospital school for nurses; 1893, Woman's Medical College (N.Y.). CAREER: 1892, nurse, New York Juvenile Asylum; 1893-1933, co-founder and head, Nurses' Settlement (later Henry Street Settlement House). CONTRIBUTIONS: Founded public health nursing in the United States. With Mary Brewster, opened the Henry Street Settlement on Manhattan's Lower East Side; provided visiting nurse service as well as settlement services to the poor residents of that community; inspired the organization of similar services elsewhere. With Lina Rogers, initiated the first public school nursing service in the world (New York City, 1902). Persuaded life insurance companies, beginning with Metropolitan Life Insurance Company (1909), to organize nursing programs for their policyholders. Conceived the idea of the Federal Children's Bureau, which, at her urging, was established in 1912. Originated the plan for town and country nursing adopted by the American Red Cross (1912). Helped found and was first president, National Organization for Public Health Nursing (1912). Fought a lifetime battle to end slums, regulate sweatshops, and abolish child labor.

WRITINGS: *The House on Henry Street* (1915); *Windows on Henry Street* (1934). REFERENCES: *BHM* (1964-69), 273; (1970-74), 176; *Biog. Index*, 1: 982; 3: 991; 5: 744; 8: 705; *DAB*, Supplement 2: 687-88; Miller, *BHM*, p. 116; *Notable Am. Women*, 3: 526-29; *N.Y. Times*, September 2, 1940.

S. Galishoff

WALKER, DELOS (October 19, 1836, Crawford, County, Pa.-July 30, 1910, Oklahoma City, Okla.). *Physician*. Married Emerette Greenfield, 1860; two children. EDUCATION: 1858, after graduating from an academy, studied medicine under Dr. James Dunn; 1861, entered the medical department, University of Michigan; schooling was interrupted to serve with volunteer regiments in Civil War; 1864, M.D., Michigan. CAREER: 1865, organized a volunteer company and served as lieutenant-colonel during spring and summer; after war, established practice in Pa.; and served as surgeon, Pennsylvania and Erie railroads, and pension examiner for the government; 1867-89, practice, Greeley County, Kans.; 1889, he and son made the run into Okla. Territory when it was opened for settlement and began practice, Oklahoma City. CONTRIBUTIONS: First president, Oklahoma Territory Medical Association. Worked to improve ethical standards of the profession in the new state. Served as Oklahoma City superintendent of health. President, Oklahoma City Board of Health and Oklahoma Medical Society. First president, Oklahoma City School Board. REFERENCES: William F. Browne and R. Palmer Howard, "The Role of the Oklahoma County Medical Society in Territorial Medicine, 1904-1905," *Journal of the Oklahoma State Medical Association* 7, no. 3 (Mar. 1977): 92-98; "Delos Walker" file, History of Medicine Collection, University of Oklahoma Health Sciences Center Library, Oklahoma City, Okla.; Mark R. Everett, *Medical Education in Oklahoma: The University of Oklahoma School of Medicine and Medical Center 1900-1931* (1972); R. Palmer Howard and Rose C. Gideon, "The Beginning of Medical Organization in Oklahoma, 1889-1893," *Journal of the Oklahoma State Medical Association* 67, no. 2 (Nov. 1974): 45-54.

V. Allen

WALKER, MARY EDWARDS (November 26, 1832, Oswego Town, N.Y.-February 21, 1919, Oswego Town). *Physician; Woman's rights advocate*. Daughter of Vesta (Whitcomb), schoolteacher and educator, and Alvah Walker, farmer, educator, physician. Briefly married to Albert E. Miller, physician, 1855. EDUCATION: Preparatory education at a family-founded free school conducted by her parents and sisters on their farm near Oswego and at Falley Seminary, Fulton, N.Y.; 1855, M.D., Syracuse Medical College; 1862, M.D., New York Hygeio-Therapeutic College. CAREER: 1855, reputed to have practiced medicine, Columbus, Ohio; 1855-59, practiced medicine, Rome, N.Y., with husband and former medical school classmate, Albert E. Miller; 1861-64, organized and trained nurses for the Union army and provided medical care to the wounded soldiers, Patent Office Hospital, Washington, D.C.; 1864-65, assistant surgeon, Union army (first woman so commissioned in U.S. Army); 1865, awarded Congressional Medal of Honor for work in the Civil War (rescinded 1917, restored by Congress 1977), first and only woman to receive this award; 1865, limited practice, Washington, D.C.; 1866-67, European lecture tour: lectured on dress reform, women's suffrage, capital punishment, evils of strong drink and tobacco, and life as a medical officer during the Civil War; *post* 1867, became actively involved in women's suffrage campaign in the United States and dress reform. CONTRIBUTIONS: Sought to improve the health and hygiene of women through reformation of female apparel. Designed practical outfits for women's outer wear (which usually involved some form of trousers and over-garment), because she felt that conventional female dress was unhygienic and caused suffering and invalidism. Designed a dress reform undersuit to improve women's health and discourage rape. Other contributions during the Civil War period included organizing and training nurses for the northern army; founding Woman's Relief Organization, Washington, D.C., for women going to the city to look for relatives and friends among the wounded soldiers; and exerting influence to establish a foundling hospital in New York City for single pregnant women.

WRITINGS: *Hit* (1871); *Unmasked, Or the Science of Immorality* (1878); *Crowning Constitutional Argument of Mary E. Walker, M.D. (1907): Woman's Franchise . . . Final Argument*; numerous articles on dress reform for the *Sibyl*, a fortnightly woman's magazine and voice of the Dress Reform Movement. REFERENCES: James A. Brussel, "Pants, Politics, Postage, and Physic," *Psychiatric Q. Suppl.* 35, pt. 1 (1969): 332-45 (quasi-analysis of Mary Walker's personality); *DAB*, 10, pt. 1: 352; Linden F. Edwards, "Dr. Mary Edwards Walker (1832-1919): Charlatan or Martyr?" pts. 1 and 2, *Ohio State Med. J.* 54 (1958): 1160-62, 1296, 1298; *NCAB*, 13: 99; Lida Poynter Manuscript and Notes in the Archives and Special Collections on Women in Medicine, The Medical College of Pennsylvania, Philadelphia, Pa.; Charles McCool Snyder, *Dr. Mary Walker: The Little Lady in Pants* (1962); Robert Werlich, "Mary Walker: From Union Army Surgeon to Sideshow Freak," *Civil War Times Illustrated* 6 (Jun. 3, 1967): 46-49.

S. L. Chaff

WALL, JOHN PERRY (Sept. 17, 1836, Jasper, Hamilton County, Fla.-April 19, 1895, Gainesville, Fla.). *Physician; Sanitation and public health.* Son of Judge Perry Green and Mrs. Nancy (Hunter) Wall. Married Pressie Eubanks, 1862 (d. 1871), five children; Matilda McKay, 1872 (d. 1893), three children; Louisa Williams, 1894. EDUCATION: Local schools, Brooksville, Hernando County, Fla.; 1858, M.D., Medical College of South Carolina. CAREER: Practice: 1859-60, Brooksville, Fla., partner of Dr. Thomas P. Gary (q.v.); 1860-61, Fernandina, Fla., partner of Dr. Edward Seabrook; 1861-64, medical service, Confederate States of America, Florida Hospital, Richmond, Va.; 1864-65, field service as surgeon, Eighth Florida Battalion, Hq., Brooksville; practice: 1865-71, Brooksville; and 1871-95, Tampa, Fla.; 1878, mayor, Tampa; 1885, delegate, Fla. Constitutional Convention; 1878-82, editor, Tampa *Sunland Tribune*; 1884-85, president, Florida Medical Association. CONTRIBUTIONS: Possibly Fla.'s most highly esteemed and widely known nineteenth century physician. Considered an authority on sanitation and yellow fever. Constant supporter of rigid licensing requirements and high ethical standards. Showed disdain for homeopathy.

WRITINGS: "Modern Medicine," *Proc., Fla. Med. Assoc.* (1877), 41-54; "Congenital Absence of Eyeballs," *Med. Record* 19 (1881): 358; "Observations on Yellow Fever," *JAMA* 11 (1888): 691-95; "Yellow Fever in Tampa, Plant City, Manatee and Palmetto," *Rept. Surg. Gen., Marine Hosp.* (1889), 60-76; "Puerperal Eclampsia," *Proc., Fla. Med. Assoc.* (1890), 81-86. REFERENCES: Karl Grismer, *Tampa* (1950), 130; James M. Ingram, "John Perry Wall—A Man for All Seasons," *J. Fla. Med. Assoc.* 53 (1966): 709-17; *NCAB*, 4: 94; *Proc., Fla. Med. Assoc.* (1896), 41-45; *Tribune* (Tampa), April 20, 1895.

E. A. Hammond

WALSH, JAMES JOSEPH (April 12, 1865, Archbald, Pa.-March 1, 1942, New York, N.Y.). *Physician; Medical historian*. Son of Martin J. and Bridget (Golden) Walsh. Married Julia Huelot Freed, 1915; two children. EDUCATION: Sisters of Mercy, Wilkes Barre, Pa.; Fordham University: 1884, A.B.; 1885, A.M.; and 1889, Ph.D.; 1895, M.D., University of Pennsylvania; 1895-97, Pasteur Institute, Paris, and Virchow's Laboratory, Berlin. CAREER: 1898-1907, medical faculty, New York Polyclinic School of Medicine; 1907-13, medical faculty and dean, Fordham Medical School; faculty, Cathedral College; medical editor, *New York Herald*; contributing editor, *JAMA* and *New York State Journal of Medicine*. CONTRIBUTIONS: A pioneer in the teaching of medical history to medical students. Wrote extensively on the history of medicine in N.Y. and on the history of science.

WRITINGS: *History of the Medical Society of the State of New York* (1907); *The Popes and Science* (1908); *History of Medicine in New York*, 5 vols. (1919). REFERENCES: H. W. Kirwin, "J. J. Walsh," *Catholic Hist. Rev.* 45 (1960): 409-35; *NCAB*, 46: 349; *N.Y. Times*, March 2, 1942; *WWAPS*, p. 1246.

D. O. Powell

WARE, JOHN (December 19, 1795, Hingham, Mass.-April 29, 1864, Boston, Mass.). *Physician; Educator*. Son of Henry, pastor, and Mary (Clark) Ware. Married Helen Lincoln, 1822, widowed; Mary Green Chandler, 1862; eight children. EDUCATION: Harvard: 1813, B.A.; and 1816, M.D. CAREER: 1817, began practice, Boston, as physician and dentist; 1823-25, physician, Boston Almshouse; 1824-27, co-editor, *New England Journal of Medicine and Surgery*; 1828, editor, *Boston Medical and Surgical Journal*; 1832-36, instructor; 1836-

64, Hersey Professor of the Theory and Practice of Physic, Harvard Medical School; 1848-52, president, Massachusetts Medical Society; active in the field of natural history. CONTRIBUTIONS: Wrote first important work on delirium tremens in America (1831) and provided one of the earliest specific descriptions of what became known as diphtheria (1842). Mid-nineteenth-century advocate of higher educational standards.

WRITINGS: *Remarks on the History and Treatment of Delirium Tremens* (1831); *Discourse on Medical Education and the Medical Profession* (1847): *Contributions to the History and Diagnosis of the Croup* (1850); *On Hemoptysis as a Symptom* (1860). REFERENCES: Henry K. Beecher and Mark D. Altschule, *Medicine at Harvard* (1977), 73-77; *DAB*, 19: 449-50; G. E. Gifford, "John Ware and the Book of Nature," *Harvard Med. Alum. Bull.* 43 (Winter 1969): 9-16; Kelly and Burrage (1928), 1257-58.

N. Gevitz

WARFIELD, WILLIAM ALONZA (November 17, 1866, Hyattstown, Md.-December 18, 1951, Washington, D.C.). *Physician; Surgeon*. Son of William R. and Rachel (Lyles) Warfield. Married Violet B. Thompson, 1901; two children. EDUCATION: 1891, A.B., Centenary Biblical Institute (now Morgan State College); 1894, M.D., Howard University; 1894-95, intern, Freedmen's Hospital, Washington, D.C. CAREER: At Freedmen's Hospital: 1895-1901, assistant surgeon; and 1901-36, surgeon-in-chief (chief administrator); 1895-1936, faculty, Howard University Medical School; 1936-51, emeritus status, Freedmen's Hospital and Howard University. CONTRIBUTIONS: As surgeon-in-chief, developed Freedmen's Hospital and its residency program from a weak, struggling position to one of size and stature. Set tone for training of black nurses and physicians at Freedmen's Hospital by own example during 42 years of service. Regularly obtained U.S. government funds to build Freedmen's Hospital from one building shared with Howard Medical School to a 322-bed, six-wing institution. Oversaw growth and development of Freedmen's during its crucial transitional years as it continued to be the leading black institution for training black physicians.

WRITINGS: "Some Educational Advantages of the Freedmen's Hospital and Asylum, Now a Prime Factor in Training Physicians and Nurses," *JNMA* 22 (1930): 141-42; three others listed in *JNMA* 44 (1952): 219. REFERENCES: W. Montague Cobb, "William Alonza Warfield, M.D., 1866-1951," *JNMA* 44 (1952): 207-19; *WWCR* 1 (1915): 276.

T. L. Savitt

WARING, GEORGE EDWIN (July 4, 1833, Pound Ridge, N.Y.-October 29, 1898, New York, N.Y.). *Agriculturist; Sanitary engineer*. Son of George Edwin, farmer, and Sarah (Burger) Waring. Married Euphemia Johnston Blunt, 1855; Virginia Clark, 1865; Mrs. Louise E. Yates, 1898; at least two children. EDUCATION: 1847-49, Bartlett's School (College Hill), Poughkeepsie, N.Y.; 1853, studied agricultural chemistry under James J. Mapes. CAREER: 1854-55, lectured on scientific agriculture to farmers in Maine and Vt.; 1855-57, manager, Horace Greeley's farm, Chappaqua, N.Y.; 1857-61, drainage engineer, Central

Park, New York City; 1861, officer, Garibaldi Guards, U.S. Army; 1862-65, commander, Fourth Missouri Cavalry, U.S. Volunteers; 1867-77, manager, Ogden Farm, near Newport, R.I.; *post* 1877, sanitary engineer; established engineering firm of Waring, Chapman, and Farquhar in New York City; 1879-83, member, National Board of Health; special agent in charge of social statistics of cities, Tenth Census (1880) of the United States; 1895-98, commissioner of street cleaning, New York City. CONTRIBUTIONS: Implemented numerous sanitary improvements, chiefly in connection with the drainage of houses and towns. Upon recommendation of the National Board of Health, designed and supervised the construction of a sewer system in Memphis, Tenn. (1880), which was widely credited with having brought about a major improvement in its public health; provided impetus in the following decades to the development of municipal sewer systems throughout the nation, several of which he designed. First used different size sewers to carry off rainwater and sewage but later adopted the more practical combined sewerage system. Revamped the New York City Department of Street Cleaning; improved the morale and efficiency of the force by placing it under civil service and by outfitting it in white uniforms; rooted out slothfulness and corruption. Required householders to separate their wastes into three categories—garbage, rubbish, and ashes—to facilitate final disposition; resulted in a marked improvement in the cleanliness of city streets. Continued to support the theory that filth was the primary and direct cause of disease despite mounting evidence (1880s, 1890s) that microorganisms were responsible for most epidemic diseases.

WRITINGS: *The Sanitary Drainage of Houses and Towns* (1876); *The Sewerage of Memphis* (1881); *Street Cleaning and the Disposal of a City's Wastes* (1897). REFERENCES: *BHM* (1977), 34; James H. Cassedy, "The Flamboyant Colonel Waring: An Anti-Contagionist Holds the American Stage in the Age of Pasteur and Koch," *Bull. Hist. Med.* 36 (Mar.-Apr. 1962): 163-76; *DAB*, 19: 456-57; Martin V. Melosi, *Pragmatic Environmentalist: Sanitary Engineer George E. Waring, Jr.* (1977); *NCAB*, 6: 157; *N.Y. Times*, October 30, 1898; *Who Was Who in Am.*, Hist. Vol.: 634.

S. Galishoff

WARNER, HULBERT HARRINGTON (January 19, 1842, Van Buren, N.Y.-January 27, 1923, Minneapolis, Minn.). *Proprietary medicine manufac turor.* Son of Willlam and Electa Harrington. Married Martha Keeney, 1864; Olive Emily Stoddard, 1872; some children. EDUCATION: Private academy, Elbridge, N.Y. CAREER: 1865-70, stove and hardware business, Mich.; 1870-84, sale of safes nationwide from Rochester, N.Y.; 1879-94, developed worldwide proprietary medicine business from Rochester; 1895-1923, various unsuccessful business ventures in many places. CONTRIBUTIONS: Claiming to have been cured of kidney disease by a proprietary medicine, bought formula and marketed it as Warner's Safe Kidney and Liver Cure using picture of a safe as trademark. Numerous other proprietaries followed under the Safe and the Log Cabin labels. Developed marketing outlets throughout the United States, Europe, and the

Orient. Sold business (1890) to an English corporation, although retaining many shares, but went bankrupt in Panic of 1893. Promoted medicines by boasting of own conspicuous gestures. Spent $750,000 annually in newspaper advertising, pamphlets, and almanacs promoting diabetes cure, asthma cure, nervine tonic, bitters, and other nostrums. Credited with originating the newshead advertisement, which simulated ordinary newspaper reading matter. Warner's brand names, with "cure" demoted to "remedy" and with therapeutic claims in labeling deflated as a result of the 1906 Food and Drugs Act, survived in marketplace long after their originator's loss of ownership. REFERENCES: E. C. Atwater, "Hulbert Harrington Warner," *N.Y. Hist.* 56 (1975): 154-90; Henry W. Holcombe, *Patent Med. Tax Stamps* (1979), 538-48; Blake McKelvey, *Rochester the Flower City* (1949), 241-43, 321, 336-37; obituary, *Printers' Ink* 122 (Feb. 1, 1923): 140; Charles W. Oleson, *Secret Nostrums*, 5th ed. (1891), 187; W. F. Peck, *Semi-Centennial Hist.. . .of Rochester* (1884), 681-85; Frank S. Presbrey, *Hist. and Development of Advertising* (1929), 294; various Rochester newspapers.

J. H. Young

WARNSHUIS, FREDERICK COOK (June 16, 1880, Alton, Ia.-January 6, 1946, Windsor, Ontario, Canada). *Surgeon; General surgery.* Son of Rev. John W. Warnshuis, Dutch Reformed minister. His mother died soon after his birth. Married Calla Ewing Botsford, 1906; two children. EDUCATION: Hope College (Holland, Mich.); 1902, M.D., Grand Rapids Medical College (Mich.); 1903, New York Post-Graduate Medical School; 1905, attended clinics, Johns Hopkins University Hospital. CAREER: 1902-34, general surgical practice, Grand Rapids, Mich.; 1913-34, secretary, Michigan State Medical Society; and editor, Michigan State Medical Society *Journal*; 1914-20, secretary, Michigan State Board of Registration in Medicine; 1918, commanding officer, Base Hospital Ninety-Nine, American Expeditionary Forces; 1922-35, speaker, American Medical Association House of Delegates; 1932-33, president, Aero-Medical Association of the United States; 1934-38, secretary-treasurer, California Medical Association; 1938-41, founding president, American Medico-Legal Association; and founding editor, *American Journal of Law and Medicine*; 1941-46, surgeon, U.S. Public Health Service, Windsor, Ontario, where he ended his own life. CONTRIBUTIONS: In 13 years as spokesman, AMA House of Delegates, and 21 years as editor, Mich. profession's organ, led the attempt of general practitioners to limit and regulate the growing specialization of American medicine and became spokesman for the early hard-line opponents of government health insurance. Later, helped create the professional organizations of two new medical specialties: aviation medicine and medical jurisprudence.

WRITINGS: *Principles of Surgical Nursing* (1918); "Who Shall Be Permitted to Continue Practice of Medicine," *Proc., Annual Congress of Med. Educators* (1931), 95-96. REFERENCES: C. B. Burr, *Medical History of Michigan* 2 (1930): 429; James Burrow, *AMA: Voice of American Medicine* (1963), 157, 163; *Detroit Free Press*, January 9, 1946, p. 18; E. B. Fisher, *Grand Rapids and Kent County* 2 (1918): 390-91; *Grand Rapids Spectator*, February 8, 1930; *JAMA* 130 (1946): 166; Michigan State Med. Soc.,

J. 34 (1935): 508; 45 (1946): 232; Rosemary Stevens, *American Medicine and the Public Interest* (1971), 206.

M. S. Pernick

WARREN, EDWARD (January 22, 1828, Tyrrell County, N.C.-September 16, 1893, Paris, France). *Surgeon.* Son of William Christian, physician, and Harriet (Alexander) Warren. Married Elizabeth Cotton Johnstone, 1857; four children. EDUCATION: c. 1843-45, Fairfax Institute, Alexandria, Va.; apprentice to father; 1850, M.D., University of Virginia; 1851, M.D., Jefferson Medical College; 1854-55, studied medicine in Paris hospitals. CAREER: 1851-54, 1855-60, general medical practice with father, Edenton, N.C.; 1860-61, professor of materia medica and therapeutics, University of Maryland; 1861-65, served successively as member, Confederate States Medical Examining Board; medical director, Department of Cape Fear (N.C.); and surgeon-general, N.C.; 1865-73, surgical practice, Baltimore, Md.; 1867-71, professor of surgery and director, Washington University Medical School, Baltimore; 1872-73, professor of surgery, College of Physicians and Surgeons of Baltimore; 1873-75, chief surgeon of general staff of the Khedive of Egypt; 1875-93, medical and surgical practice, Paris, France. CONTRIBUTIONS: Conceived idea of injecting a solution of morphia under the skin with a lancet puncture and an Anel's syringe while earning a second M.D. in Philadelphia (1851) and therefore claimed priority in inventing technique. Established a national reputation as correspondent from Paris to leading American medical journals, including the prestigious *American Journal of the Medical Sciences* (1854-55), and as a fine practitioner. Won the Fiske Prize of the Rhode Island Medical Society for essay "The Influence of Pregnancy on the Development of Tubercles" (1856), later published as a book. This award caused him to be elected member, Boston Gynecological Society, and to be named delegate, American Medical Society of Paris, to the AMA. Served as first editor, *Medical Journal of North Carolina* (1857-60). Founded and edited *Baltimore Journal of Medicine* (1861). A strong advocate for improving and organizing the N.C. medical profession (1855-60), including establishment of a board of medical examiners (1856). Came under fire during Civil War for advocacy of maintaining high standards in examining candidates for medical practice. Book *An Epitome of Practical Surgery for Field and Hospital* (1863) was used by every Confederate medical officer. Reorganized and revived the defunct Washington University School of Medicine, Baltimore (1867), and greatly improved its reputation, serving as teacher and director. Elected to first Maryland Board of Medical Examiners and to vice-presidency of state medical society (1871-72). Founded and edited *Medical Bulletin*, official organ of state medical society (1868-70). Co-founded College of Physicians and Surgeons of Baltimore (1872). Won recognition and honors in Europe and America for surgical work, outspoken criticism of conservative physicians, and autobiography. Invented a splint for treatment of fracture of the clavicle (1872).

WRITINGS: *An Epitome of Practical Surgery for Field and Hospital* (1863); *A Doctor's Experience in Three Continents* (1885); many articles in *American Journal of the Medical Sciences, The Lancet* (London), *Medical Journal of North Carolina*, and *Medical Bulletin* (Maryland). REFERENCES: *Biographical Dict. of the Confederacy* (1977), 428-29; Eugene F. Cordell, *The Medical Annals of Maryland, 1799-1899* (1903), 610; Dorothy Long, ed., *Medicine in North Carolina* (1972), 57-58, 92, 110, 186, 217, 218, 219, 277; *NCAB*, 33: 169-70; Edward Warren, *A Doctor's Experience in Three Continents* [autobiography] (1885).

T. L. Savitt

WARREN, JOHN (July 27, 1753, Roxbury, Mass.-April 4, 1815, Boston, Mass.). *Physician; Anatomist; Surgeon; Medical educator*. Son of Joseph, prosperous farmer, and Mary (Stevens) Warren. Married Abigail Collins, 1777; 17 children. EDUCATION: 1771, A.B., Harvard College; studied medicine with his brother Joseph, the Revolutionary War hero; 1786, M.D. (hon.), Harvard University. CAREER: 1774-75, began a brief and not entirely successful practice at Salem, Mass.; 1775-77, hospital surgeon, siege of Boston and the N.Y.-N.J. campaign; 1777-82, in charge of the Continental Army hospital, Boston; 1780-82, gave three series of anatomical lectures, the last two sponsored by the Boston Medical Society; 1782-1815, member, original faculty, Harvard Medical School; and first Hersey Professor of Anatomy and Surgery; 1804-15, president, Massachusetts Medical Society; active in community affairs as grand master, Massachusetts Lodge of Free and Accepted Masons; a founder and president, Massachusetts Humane Society; a founder, Anthology Club; manager and trustee, Massachusetts Charitable Society; trustee, Massachusetts Agricultural Society; member, editorial board, *Boston Magazine*; and fellow, American Academy of Arts and Sciences. CONTRIBUTIONS: Single most important figure in the early institutionalization of Boston medicine, being a founder, Boston Medical Society (1780); an incorporator, Massachusetts Medical Society (1781), and later its president; and author of the plan that led to the establishment of Harvard Medical School (1782). Possessing a lifelong passion for anatomy, was an early member and possibly the founder of a semisecret anatomical society (the Spunks or Spunkers) while an undergraduate at Harvard. Gave public lectures on anatomy toward the end of the Revolution and became the first professor of anatomy, Harvard Medical School. A gifted surgeon, amputating at the shoulder joint (1781), doing an abdominal resection (1785), and excising the parotid gland (1804). Although stridently ambitious and disagreeably self-righteous, a gifted anatomist, an innovative surgeon, and an exciting teacher who dominated Boston medicine (1777-death in 1815).

WRITINGS: *A View of the Mercurial Practice in Febrile Diseases* (1813). REFERENCES: *BHM* (1975-79), 132; *DAB*, 10, pt. 1: 479-80; James Jackson, *A Eulogy on the Character of John Warren, M.D.* (1815); Kelly and Burrage (1920), 1193-96; Miller, *BHM*, pp. 116-17; *NCAB*, 10: 288; C. K. Shipton, "John Warren," *Sibley's Harvard Graduates*

7: 655-69; Rhoda Truax, *The Doctors Warren of Boston: First Family of Surgery* (1968); Edward Warren, *The Life of John Warren, M.D.* (1874).

P. Cash

WARREN, JOHN COLLINS (August 1, 1778, Boston, Mass.-May 4, 1856, Boston). *Physician; Educator.* Son of John (q.v.), Revolutionary War physician, and Abigail (Collins) Warren. Married Susan Powell, 1803, six children; Anne Winthrop, 1843. EDUCATION: Boston Latin School; 1793-97, Harvard College, B.A., 1797; apprentice to his father; 1799-1802, study in London, Paris, and Edinburgh, where he received degree. CAREER: 1802, began medical practice, Boston, with increasingly surgical orientation; at Harvard Medical School: 1809, adjunct in anatomy and surgery; 1815-47, full professor; and 1816-19, dean. CONTRIBUTIONS: With James Jackson (q.v.), founded the Massachusetts General Hospital (1821) and was its senior surgeon (until late 1840s). Collected scientific materials that formed the basis for the Warren Museum of Harvard Medical School. Devoted much time and effort to the reconstruction of a mastodon. With Jackson, founded the Medical Improvement Society and *New England Journal of Medicine and Surgery* (1812). Best remembered for technical contributions to surgery: first in United States to operate for strangulated hernia; the surgeon who performed (1846) the first recorded operation under anesthesia administered by William T. G. Morton (q.v.).

WRITINGS: *Cases of Organic Diseases of the Heart* (1809); *A Comparative View of the Sensorial and Nervous Systems in Men and Animals* (1822); *Inhalation of Etheral Vapor for the Prevention of Pain in Surgical Operations* (1846); *Surgical Observations on Tumors. . .*(1837); *Etherization; with Surgical Remarks* (1848). REFERENCES: *DAB* 10, pt. 1: 480-81; *Life of John C. Warren* (1860); *NCAB*, 6: 426; R. Truax, *The Doctors Warren of Boston* (1968).

G. C. Sanchez

WARREN, J[OHN] COLLINS (May 4, 1842, Boston, Mass.-November 3, 1927, Boston). *Surgeon; Educator.* Son of Jonathan Mason and Annie (Crowninshield) Warren. Married Amy Shaw, 1873; two sons. EDUCATION: Boston Latin School and Mr. Dixwell's School; 1859-62, Harvard College; 1863-64, studied at Jefferson Medical College and the University of Pennsylvania; 1866, M.D., Harvard Medical School; postgraduate studies, Europe. CAREER: 1869, returned from Europe to Boston to begin surgical practice and serve on faculty, Harvard (professor, 1893-1907); 1876, appointed visiting surgeon, Massachusetts General Hospital; taught surgical pathology with Reginald Fitz (q.v.). CONTRIBUTIONS: Brought antiseptic techniques from Europe. Performed one of the earliest operations in the United States "strictly according to the directions of Lister," a mastectomy (1869). Active in the campaign to move Harvard Medical School to Boylston Street (*post* 1874) and more active still when (*post* 1899) it was decided to move it to its present location on Longwood Avenue. Editor, *Boston Medical and Surgical Journal* (1873-80). President, American Surgical

Association (1896). Largely due to his efforts that the Collis P. Huntington Hospital for Cancer Research was built (1913).

WRITINGS: *The Healing of Arteries after Ligature in Man and Animals* (1886); *Surgical Pathology and Therapeutics* (1895); *To Work in the Vineyard of Surgery*, ed. Edward Churchill (1958). REFERENCES: *BHM* (1964-69), 274; (1975-79), 132; Churchill, *To Work in the Vineyard of Surgery*; *DAB* 10, pt. 1: 481-82; Miller, *BHM*, p. 117; R. Truax, *The Doctors Warren of Boston* (1968).

G. C. Sanchez

WARREN, JOSEPH, III (June 11, 1741, Roxbury, Mass.-June 17, 1775, Bunker Hill, Mass.). *Physician; Soldier*. Son of Joseph II, farmer, and Mary (Stevens) Warren. Married Elizabeth Hooten, 1764; four children. EDUCATION: Harvard College: 1759, B.A.; and 1762, M.A.; 1760-64, studied medicine under Dr. James Lloyd (q.v.), Boston, Mass. CAREER: 1764-75, practiced medicine, Boston, and taught private classes in anatomy, surgery, and general medicine. Became involved in the struggle against British rule during the imposition of the Stamp Act (1765); 1775, was chosen president, Provincial Congress, and major-general, Mass. armed forces; shot and killed at Battle of Bunker Hill. CONTRIBUTION: Helped train a number of physicians, including brother John (q.v.), who became important figures in American medicine after the Revolution. REFERENCES: *BHM* (1964-69), 275; John H. Cary, *Joseph Warren: Physician, Politician, Patriot* (1961); *DAB*, 10, pt. 1: 482-83; R. Frothingham, *Life and Times of Joseph Warren* (1865); Miller, *BHM*, p. 117; R. Truax, *The Doctors Warren of Boston* (1968).

N. Gevitz

WASHBURN, VICTOR DUKE (July 16, 1882, New York, N.Y.-Sept. 24, 1966, Wilmington, Del.). *Physician; Urology; Public health*. Son of Victor D. and Carlotta (Sorino) Washburn. Married Margaret Elliot, 1915, two children; Helen Crittendon, 1961. EDUCATION: 1905, M.D., Southern Homeopathic College. CAREER: 1905-51, private practice, Wilmington; 1907, joined staff, Wilmington Homeopathic Hospital (later became Memorial Hospital); 1917-19, U.S. Army Medical Corps; 1951-59, medical director, Memorial Hospital. CONTRIBUTIONS: Fought successfully for a number of public health measures including the fluoridation of water and medical examination of food handlers in Wilmington. City health commissioner, Wilmington (1948-52). Successfully developed methods to combat the spread of athlete's foot in Del.'s public schools; methods were later copied in a number of public schools across the nation. President, Medical Society of Delaware (1953). REFERENCES: *Who Was Who in Am.*, 4: 986; *Wilmington Morning News*, September 26, 1966; September 30, 1966.

W. H. Williams

WATERHOUSE, BENJAMIN (March 4, 1754, Newport, R.I.-October 2, 1846, Boston, Mass.). *Physician; Vaccinator; Medical educator; Botanist*. Son of Timothy, a chair maker who is said to have been a judge of the Court of Common Pleas and on the Governor's Council, and Hannah (Proud) Waterhouse.

Married Elizabeth Oliver, 1788, six children; Louisa Lee, 1819, no children. EDUCATION: Academy founded by Bishop Berkeley; studied medicine with Dr. John Halliburton and Judge Robert Lightfoot, Newport; 1775-78, studied medicine and science at Edinburgh (nine months) and in London with kinsman Dr. John Fothergill; 1780, M.D., Leyden (spent another year there studying history and the law of nations); 1786, M.D. (hon.), Harvard University. CAREER: 1782, began practicing, Newport, and elected to Board of Fellows, College of Rhode Island (Brown); 1783-1812, member, original faculty, Harvard Medical School; and first Hersey Professor of the Theory and Practice of Physic; forced to resign because of incompatibility with the rest of the medical faculty and role in trying to establish a new medical society that probably would have led to the founding of another medical school; 1807-9, chief physician, U.S. Marine Hospital, Charlestown, Mass.; generated substantial improvements but was dismissed amidst charges of petty graft; 1813-20, served first as a hospital surgeon and then as medical superintendent of all military posts in New England; 1820s, strong supporter of Samuel Thomson (q.v.) and his medical system; later life largely confined to literary pursuits. CONTRIBUTIONS: Played a leading role in the introduction of vaccination in the United States (1799-1802). During this time, tried to maintain a monopoly over the cowpox vaccine, partly for selfish financial reasons and partly to keep the practice of vaccination from falling into incompetent or fraudulent hands, as sometimes had been the case with inoculation. Induced the Boston Board of Health to sponsor an especially well thought-out, controlled clinical experiment in which 19 vaccinated and 2 unvaccinated boys were exposed to smallpox under the same conditions, with the unvaccinated succumbing to the disease while the vaccinated remained immune. More interested in science than medicine, gave lectures on natural history (biology and mineralogy), first at Rhode Island College (1786-87) and then at Harvard (1788-1806). This was the first systematic treatment of these subjects at Harvard. Established a mineralogical and zoological cabinet and a botanical garden at Harvard. A strong moralist, published Harvard lecture (November 20, 1804) warning against the increased use of alcohol and tobacco, and it became his most popular work. Basically a misplaced *philosophe*, constantly stirred up trouble wherever he was but did much more good than harm.

WRITINGS: *A Synopsis of a Course of Lectures on the Theory and Practice of Medicine. In Four Parts* (1786); *The Rise, Progress, and Present State of Medicine* (1792); *A Prospect of Exterminating the Small Pox, Part I* (1800), *Part II* (1802); *Cautions to Young Persons Concerning Health. . .Showing the Evil Tendency of the Use of Tobacco. . .with Observations on the Use of Ardent and Vinous Spirits* (1805); *Information Respecting the Origin, Progress, and Efficacy of the Kine Pock Inoculation* (1810); *The Botanist, Being the Botanical Part of a Course of Lectures on Natural History. . .Together with a Discourse on the Principles of Vitality* (1811). REFERENCES: J. B. Blake, "Benjamin Waterhouse, Harvard's First Professor of Physic," *J. of Med. Ed.* 33 (1958): 771-82; idem, *Benjamin Waterhouse and the Introduction of Vaccination: A Reappraisal* (1957); *NCAB*, 9: 254; J. C. Trent, "The London Years of Benjamin Waterhouse," and

"Benjamin Waterhouse (1754-1846)," *J. Hist. Med.* 1 (1946): 25-40, 357-64; *DAB*, 19:529-32.

P. Cash

WATKINS, WILLIAM WOODBURY (August 3, 1846, Warner, N.H.-August 4, 1901, Moscow, Idaho). *Physician.* Son of Jason, farmer and merchant, and Phoebe (Abbott) Watkins. Married Caroline A. Woodhouse, 1873; three children. EDUCATION: 1872, M.D., Washington University, St. Louis, Mo. CAREER: 1880-87, practice, St. Louis; 1887, settled in Moscow, Idaho; chief of surgery, Latah County Hospital. CONTRIBUTIONS: Instrumental in organizing the Idaho State Medical Association (later Society) in meetings he called beginning in 1890. Elected its first president (1893) and reelected (1894). Served the state and city as regent, University of Idaho; president, Moscow Chamber of Commerce; and chairman, State Republican Convention. REFERENCES: R. Z. Johnson, *History of Idaho* (1899), 534; *Who Was Who in Am.*, 1: 1307.

A. A. Hart

WATSON, BERIAH ANDRÉ (March 26, 1836, Lake George, N.Y.-December 22, 1892, Jersey City, N.J.). *Physician.* Son of Percy, farmer, and Marios (Place) Watson. Married Phebe A. Traphagen, 1868; two children. EDUCATION: Warren County (N.Y.) district schools; tutored privately; State Normal School, Albany, N.Y.; apprentice to Dr. James Reilly (Succasunna, N.J.); 1861, M.D., New York University Medical School. CAREER: 1861-62, private practice, White House, N.J.; 1862-65, surgeon, U.S. Army; 1865-92, private practice, Jersey City; surgical staff: 1869-92, Jersey City Hospital; 1873-92, St. Francis Hospital, Jersey City; and 1885-92, Christ's Hospital, Jersey City. CONTRIBUTIONS: Helped found the Jersey City Hospital. Provided the stimulus for the N.J. legislature legalizing the dissection of human cadavers (1895).

WRITINGS: *Amputations and Their Complications* (1885). Writings listed in *Trans., Med. Soc. N.J.* (1893), 188-89. REFERENCES: *Appleton's CAB*, 6: 390; *Biographical Encyclopaedia of N.J.* (1877), 96-97; Kelly and Burrage (1928), 1271; Roy Inglis, "Beriah Andre Watson, M.D.," *Trans., Med. Soc. N.J.* (1893), 186-90.

W. Barlow

WEATHERLY, JOB SOBIESKI (July 8, 1828, Bennettsville, S.C.-June 29, 1891, Montgomery, Ala.). *Physician.* Married Eliza Taliaferro, 1852; six children. EDUCATION: 1849, M.D., University of New York. CAREER: 1851-56, practiced, Palmetta, Ala.; 1857-92, first vice-president, American Medical Association; president: 1869, 1870, 1879, Montgomery Medical Society; and 1874-75, Medical Association of the State of Alabama; 1869-79, chairman, AMA Committee on Education. CONTRIBUTIONS: Instrumental in helping to reunite northern and southern physicians in the AMA following the Civil War. As chairman, AMA Committee on Education, urged reform. In Ala., worked for the control of malaria through the drainage of swamps and helped push through the legislature a bill establishing a board of health.

WRITINGS: "Diseases of the City and County of Montgomery," *Trans., Med. Assoc. State of Ala.* (1870), 415-17; "Report of the Chairman of the Committee on Education," *TAMA* 23 (1871): 17-21; "Pres. Address," *Trans., Med. Assoc. State of Ala.* (1875), 58-80. REFERENCES: Emmett Carmichael, "Job Sobieski Weatherly," *J. Med. Assoc. Ala.* 33 (1964): 340-43; "Dr. J. S. Weatherly," in *Representative Men of the South* (1880), 173-86; T. M. Owen, *History of Alabama* 4 (1921): 1735-36.

N. Gevitz

WEBSTER, NOAH (October 16, 1758, West Hartford, Conn.-May 28, 1843, New Haven, Conn.). *Epidemiologist; Educator; Lexicographer; Philologist.* Son of Noah, farmer, and Mercy (Steele) Webster. Married Rebecca Greenleaf, 1789; eight children. EDUCATION: Yale: 1778, B.A.; and 1781, M.A.; 1781, admitted to Conn. bar. CAREER: A strong nationalist and intellectual activist of enormous energy and multiple talents, Webster worked at various times as a farmer, lawyer, teacher, journalist, editor, political pamphleteer, essayist, and lexicographer; a founder, Amherst College. CONTRIBUTIONS: Although chiefly noted for *Grammatical Institute of the English Language* and an *American Dictionary of the English Language*, has been hailed as the father of American epidemiology. This claim is based on three works: *A Collection of Papers on the Subject of Bilious Fever, Prevalent in the United States for A Few Years Past* (1795), an assemblage of responses to a circular letter sent out by Webster to prominent physicians in an attempt to determine the origin and nature of the yellow-fever epidemics that had been ravaging American coastal cities; *Letters on Yellow Fever Addressed to Dr. William Currie* (1797), a collection of 25 public letters addressed to Dr. Currie, Philadelphia, Pa., a strong contagionist and bitter opponent of Benjamin Rush (q.v.), that contain the first full statement of Webster's theory that epidemics are generated by the interaction of a given state of the atmosphere with local factors and urging personal hygiene and public sanitation as a defense; *A Brief History of Epidemic and Pestilential Diseases*, 2 vols. (1799), called by William Osler (q.v.) "the most important medical work written in this country by a layman," this was a pioneering effort to synthesize epidemiological fact and theory through the use of history and statistical inference, which determined that the ultimate source of epidemic disease was the electrical quality of the atmosphere as influenced by celestial phenomena such as meteors and comets, natural disasters such as volcanic eruptions and floods, excessive heat and cold, and plant and animal diseases.

WRITINGS: *A Collection of Papers on the Subject of Bilious Fever, Prevalent in the United States for a Few Years Past* (1796); *Letters on Yellow Fever Addressed to Dr. William Currie* (1797) *with an Introductory Essay by Benjamin Spector*, Supplement No. 9 of the *Bulletin of the History of Medicine* (1947); *A Brief History of Epidemic and Pestilential Diseases; with the Principal Phenomenon of the Physical World Which Precede and Accompany Them, and Observations Deduced from the Facts Stated*, 2 vols. (1799); Emily E. F. Skeel, *A Bibliography of the Writings of Noah Webster*, ed. E. H. Carpenter, Jr. (1958). REFERENCES: *DAB*, 10, pt. 1: 594-97; Emily E. F. Ford, *Notes on the Life of Noah Webster*, 2 vols., ed. Emily E. F. Skeel (1912); *NCAB*, 2: 394;

George Rosen, "Noah Webster, Historical Epidemiologist," *J. Hist. Med.* 20 (1965): 97-114; H. R. Warfel, *Noah Webster: Schoolmaster to America* (1936); A. S. Warthin, "Noah Webster As Epidemiologist," *JAMA* 80 (1923): 755-64; C.-E. A. Winslow, "The Epidemiology of Noah Webster," *Trans., Conn. Acad. of Arts and Sci.* 32 (1934): 21-109.

P. Cash

WEED, GIDEON ALLEN (b. March 1833, New Providence, N.J.). *Physician.* Married Adaline M. Willis, 1857; two children. EDUCATION: 1855-56, studied medicine, N.Y. medical school; M.D., Rush Medical School. CAREER: Private practice: 1858-60, Salem, Oreg.; 1861-67, Washoe City, Nev.; 1867-69, Crystal Peak and Truckee, Nev.; 1869-70, Vallejo, Calif.; and *post* 1870, Seattle, Wash. CONTRIBUTIONS: A leading practitioner in Washington during late nineteenth century. Organized, with ten other physicians, the Medical Society of Washington Territory (1873) of which he was an active and prominent member. The State Medical Society was formed from this organization (1889). Organized and served as first president, King County Medical Society (Seattle, 1888). Promoted and secured a provision in the state constitution requiring the legislature to make laws for the regulation of medical practice, a provision not found in other state constitutions. Secured passage of law establishing State Medical Board. Engaged in civic life of Seattle, both as active private citizen and as mayor (1876-77). Served for ten years as a regent, Territorial University. REFERENCES: Biographical sketch in Julian Hawthorne, ed., *History of Washington* 2 (1893): 655-57.

T. L. Savitt

WEED, LEWIS HILL (November 15, 1886, Cleveland, Ohio-December 21, 1952, Reading, Pa.). *Physician; Anatomy; Medical education.* Son of Charles Henry, ironmaster and banker, and Mary Frances (Lewis) Weed. Never married. EDUCATION: Yale University: A.B., 1908; and A.M., 1909; 1912, M.D., Johns Hopkins University; 1912-14, surgical fellow, Peter Bent Brigham Hospital (Boston, Mass.). CAREER: At Johns Hopkins Medical School: 1914-47, anatomy faculty; 1923-29, dean; and 1929-46, director; 1917-19, Medical Corps, U.S. Army; and director, U.S. Army Neurosurgical Laboratory, Johns Hopkins Medical School; at National Research Council: 1935-39, member, Medical Fellowship Board; 1939-49, chairman, Division of Medical Sciences; and 1941-47, member and vice-chairman, Committee on Medical Research, Office of Scientific Research and Development; 1943-47, chairman, Medical and Health Advisory Committee, American Red Cross; trustee: *post* 1930, Institute for Advanced Study; and *post* 1935, Carnegie Institution of Washington. CONTRIBUTIONS: Investigated cerebral structure. Traced the embryonic development of the cerebrospinal spaces (1917). Discovered the origin of the cerebrospinal fluid and mapped out its circulation. Work led to two important clinical developments: the experimental production of hydrocephalus, which provided insight into the development of this condition in human infants; and the injection of a hypertonic saline solution to lower intracranial tension caused by swelling of brain tissues after injury or surgical intervention. Trained several of the leading anatomists of his time. Merged the existing medical collections at Johns Hopkins into one great medical library (Welch Library) and established the Institute of the History of Medicine, the first modern medical history department in the United States. During World War II, held major government administrative positions, in which capacity he played a leading role in planning the great advances in medical science that were made during that conflict.

WRITINGS: "Studies on Cerebrospinal Fluid. III. The Pathways of Escape from the Subarachnoid Spaces with Particular Reference to the Arachnoid Villi," *J. of Med. Research* 31 (Sept. 1914): 51-117; *The Development of the Cerebrospinal Spaces in Pig and Man* (1917); *The Experimental Production of an Internal Hydrocephalus* (1919); "Pressure Changes in the Cerebrospinal Fluid Following Intravenous Injection of Solutions of Various Concentrations," *Am. J. of Physiol.* 48 (Apr. 1, 1919): 512. REFERENCES: *DAB*, Supplement 5: 733-34; A. McGehee Harvey, *Research and Discovery in Medicine* (1981), 181-87; *N.Y. Times*, December 22, 1952; *Who Was Who in Am.*, 3: 898.

S. Galishoff

WEEDON, LESLIE WASHINGTON (April 27, 1860, Sandersville, Ga.-November 12, 1937, Tampa, Fla.). *Physician; Eye, ear, nose, and throat specialist.* Son of William Henry Harrison and Augusta (Renfroe) Weedon. Married Blanche Henderson, 1889; four children. EDUCATION: Georgia public schools; M.D., 1885, New York University College of Medicine. CAREER: 1885-1917, practice, Tampa, except for brief intervals of public health service elsewhere; 1891, 1893, postdoctoral study, New York Polyclinic; owner, Weedon Drug Store, a successful business venture, Tampa. CONTRIBUTIONS: A serious, reflective physician, came early to national attention for knowledge of yellow fever. Firmly believed rigid quarantine the only effective preventive measure. As Tampa's city physician (1888), imposed strict quarantine, thought to have spared Tampa an epidemic so deadly in other Fla. towns. Dispatched to New Orleans, La., by U.S. Bureau of Public Health (1894) to assist in dealing with epidemic, to Honduras as health commissioner following year for further observation of disease. An organizer of Hillsborough County Medical Society and assistant state health officer (1889-90). Organized city health department, Tampa. Instrumental in establishing Tampa Emergency Hospital, of which he was chief physician.

WRITINGS: "Hypertrophic Rhinitis," *Proc., Fla. Med. Assoc.* (1893), 138-47. REFERENCES: *NCAB*, 28: 181; *Proc., Fla. Med. Assoc.* (1887, and subsequent years); R. P. Rerick, *Memoirs of Florida* 2 (1902): 745-46; *Tampa Tribune*, November 13, 1937; Weedon Family Papers, in possession of Mrs. Mary Weedon Keen, Tallahassee, Fla.

E. A. Hammond

WEEKS, JOHN ELMER (August 9, 1853, Painesville, Ohio-February 2, 1949, LaJolla, Calif.). *Physician; Ophthalmology.* Son of Seth R., house painter, and Deborah Ann (Blydenburgh) Weeks. Married Jennie Post Parker, 1890; one child. EDUCATION: 1881, M.D., University of Michigan; 1881-82, intern, New York Almshouse and Workhouse Hospital; 1882, postgraduate study, Ophthalmic and Aural Institute, N.Y.; 1883-85, resident physician, New York State Emigrant Hospital; 1884-85, studied ophthalmic surgery, pathology, and bacteriology, Berlin; 1885-87, intern, Ophthalmic and Aural Institute. CAREER: 1870s, painter and repairman in a railroad shop; 1887-1927, practiced medicine, N.Y.; 1886-88, ophthalmology faculty, New York University Medical College; 1888-90, ophthalmological staff, Vanderbilt Clinic, N.Y.; 1890-1920, surgical and pathological staffs, New York Eye and Ear Infirmary; ophthalmology faculty: 1890-92, 1900-1920, Bellevue Hospital Medical College (later part of New York University-Bellevue Medical Center); and 1891-1900, Women's Medical College of New York Infirmary for Women and Children; 1917-18, U.S. Army Medical Reserve Corps; 1921, president, American Ophthalmological Society. CONTRIBUTIONS: Shortly after Robert Koch discovered the bacillus of two forms of infectious conjunctivitis (Egyptian ophthalmia), discovered (1886) the same organism to be the cause of "pink-eye"; organism has become known as the Koch-Weeks bacillus. With George S. Dixon, developed a method for using X-rays to locate foreign bodies in the eye that was used for some 50 years. Developed an operation for inserting an artificial eye into the eye socket. Devised a new instrument for cataract extraction and advanced surgical treatment of trachoma and glaucoma. A founder, American Board of Ophthalmology. A benefactor, University of Oregon Medical School, and played a leading role in the establishment of its medical library which was named after him.

WRITINGS: "The Bacillus of Acute Conjunctival Catarrh or 'Pink-Eye,' " Arch. Ophthal. 15 (1886): 441-51; Diseases of the Eye, Ear, Throat, and Nose (1892, with Frank E. Miller and James P. McEvoy); A Treatise on Diseases of the Eye (1910). A bibliography is in his Autobiography (1954). REFERENCES: DAB, Supplement 4: 864-66; NCAB, 38: 364-65; N.Y. Times, February 4, 1949; Who Was Who in Am., 2: 564.

S. Galishoff

WEIBLE, RALPH EMERSON (December 21, 1878, Tidioute, Pa.-November 8, 1942, Prescott, Wis.). *Physician; Surgeon.* Son of James Samuel, farmer, and Mary Augusta (Sniffen) Weible. Married Mary Hope Darrow, 1905; four children. EDUCATION: 1901, M.D., Rush Medical College; postgraduate study, Edinburgh, N.Y., and Vienna. CAREER: Physician and surgeon: 1901-02, Grandin, N.Dak.; and 1902-40, Fargo, N.Dak.; 1919, co-founder, Dakota Clinic, Fargo. CONTRIBUTIONS: Expert surgeon specializing in thyroid and gallbladder disorders; established Dakota Clinic, one of N.Dak.'s most important medical facilities (1919). A founder and fellow of the American College of Surgeons.

WRITINGS: "Volvulus," J.-Lancet 36 (1916); "Visible Changes in the Liver in Chronic Cholecystitis," Surg., Gyn. and Obst. 40 (1925); "Acute Diverticulitis of Colon," Minnesota Med. 20 (1937); "Pseudocysts of the Pancreas," J.-Lancet 59 (1939). Writings listed in *Quarterly Cumulated Index Medicus, 1916-42*. REFERENCES: *Fargo Forum*, November 10, 1942, p. 2; *NCAB*, 38: 474.

L. Remele

WEISKOTTEN, HERMAN GATES (September 22, 1884, Syracuse, N.Y.-February 13, 1972, Syracuse). *Physician; Educator*. Son of Eugene and Clara (Mercer) Weiskotten. Married Kathryn Harrer, 1912; two children. EDUCATION: 1906, Ph.B., Syracuse University; 1909, M.D., Syracuse University College of Medicine; 1909-10, resident in pathology, Hospital of Good Shepherd, Syracuse. CAREER: At Syracuse University College of Medicine: 1910-12, instructor in pathology and bacteriology; 1912-13, assistant professor of pathology; 1913-17, associate professor of pathology; 1917-50, professor of pathology; and 1925-50, dean and director, University Hospital; 1926-28, commissioner of health, Syracuse; on AMA Council on Medical Education and Hospitals: 1942-43, secretary; and 1946-57, chairman. CONTRIBUTIONS: Responsible for a comparative study of medical schools that sought to develop objective and subjective indicators measuring quality of programs (1940). Led post-World War II AMA efforts to strengthen medical education nationally.

WRITINGS: *Medical Education in the United States, 1934-1939* (1940, with others); *Medical Care of the Discharged Hospital Patient* (1944, with Frode Jenson and Margaret Thomas); "The Present and Future Status of the Hospital Phase of Medical Education," *J. of Med. Ed.* 38 (1963): 737-41. REFERENCES: "Obituary—Herman G. Weiskotten," *JAMA* 221 (1972): 422; "Herman G. Weiskotten," *Bull. Onondaga Med. Soc.* 36 (Mar. 1972): 4.

N. Gevitz

WEISS, SOMA (Janaury 27, 1899, Bestercze, Hungary-January 31, 1942, Cambridge, Mass.). *Physician; Pharmacology; Physiology*. Son of Ignac, architect and engineer, and Leah (Kahan) Weiss. Married Elizabeth Sachs, 1928; three children. EDUCATION: Royal Hungarian University, Budapest; 1921, A.B., Columbia University; 1923, M.D., Cornell University Medical School; 1923-25, intern, Bellevue Hospital, N.Y.; 1925-27, research fellow in medicine, Harvard Medical School. CAREER: 1921-23, assistant, Department of Pharmacology, Cornell University Medical School; 1925-29, worked in Thorndike Memorial Laboratory, Boston City Hospital; at Harvard University: 1927-39, medicine faculty; and 1939-42, Hersey Professor of the Theory and Practice of Physic; medical staff: 1932-39, Boston City Hospital; and 1939-42, Peter Bent Brigham Hospital, Boston, Mass.; served on the committee for the revision of the U.S. Pharmacopoeia and on the Council on Pharmacy and Chemistry of the American Medical Association. CONTRIBUTIONS: With Herrman L. Blumgart, pioneered in the biological use of radioactive tracers and made classic studies of velocity of human blood flow. With Frederick Parker, described changes in the pulmonary vessels caused by mitral stenosis and the changes in renal vessels caused by pyelonephritis. Made major contributions to knowledge of pathophysiology of left ventricular failure and acute pulmonary edema. With Robert W. Wilkins, described (1936) the relation between cardiovascular disturbances and vitamin deficiencies, especially in the disease beriberi. Investigated many other subjects, including the autonomic nervous system, the toxemia of pregnancy, scleroderma heart disease, and the causes and pathophysiology of syncope, shock, and sudden death.

WRITINGS: "Studies in the Velocity of Blood Flow," *J. Clin. Invest.* 4 (1927): 1-13, 15-31, 149-71, 173-97, 199-209, 389-425, 555-74 (with Herrman Ludwig Blumgart); "The Significance of the Afferent Impulses from the Skin in the Mechanism of Visceral Pain: Skin Infiltration as a Useful Therapeutic Measure," *Am. J. of Med. Sci.* 176 (Oct. 1928): 517-36 (with D. Davis); "The Velocity of Blood Flow in Health and Disease as Measured by the Effect of Histamine on the Minute Vessels," *Am. Heart J.* 4 (1929): 664-91 (with G. P. Robb and H. L. Blumgart); "The Carotid Sinus in Health and Disease: Its Role in the Causation of Fainting and Convulsions," *Medicine* 12 (Sept. 1933): 297-354 (with J. P. Baker). REFERENCES: *DAB*, Supplement 3: 805-6; *N.Y. Times*, February 1, 1942.

S. Galishoff

WELCH, WILLIAM HENRY (April 8, 1850, Norfolk, Conn.-April 30, 1934, Baltimore, Md.). *Pathologist; Bacteriologist; Health educator.* Son of William Wickham, physician, and Emeline (Collin) Welch. Bachelor. EDUCATION: 1870, A.B., Yale University; 1870-72, apprentice to father; 1872-75, M.D., College of Physicians and Surgeons of New York; 1875-76, intern, Bellevue Hospital; 1876-78, medical studies, Germany and Austria; 1884-85, study in Germany with Koch and disciples. CAREER: 1878-84, professor of pathological anatomy and general pathology, Bellevue Hospital Medical College; 1884-1916, professor of pathology, Johns Hopkins Medical School; 1889-1916, pathologist, Johns Hopkins Hospital; 1893-98, dean, Johns Hopkins Medical School; 1918-26, director, Johns Hopkins School of Hygiene and Public Health; 1926-31, professor of the history of medicine, Johns Hopkins Institute for the History of Medicine. CONTRIBUTIONS: Among first Americans to recognize significance of Koch's work and to introduce his bacteriological technique into American medical schools; organized first laboratory course in pathology in America. Worked with John Shaw Billings (q.v.) in creating an outstanding faculty and staff for the Johns Hopkins Medical School and Hospital; insisted on high admission standards for medical students, emphasized need for study in the basic sciences, and made laboratory research and clinical work a major aspect of medical training. Under his direction, Johns Hopkins set pattern for American medical schools in the twentieth century. Through outstanding work at Johns Hopkins and influence with men of wealth, became the dominant medical figure of his age. Convinced Rockefeller Foundation to support the first school of public health, Johns Hopkins Institute for Hygiene and Public Health. Served for more than 30 years as president, Maryland State Board of Health.

WRITINGS: *General Pathology of Fever* (1888); *Biology of Bacteria, Infection and Immunity* (1894); *Bacteriology of Surgical Infections* (1895); *Thrombosis and Embolism*

(1899); *Collected Papers and Addresses*, 3 vols. (1920). For complete list, see Walter Cleveland Burket, *Bibliography of William Henry Welch, M.D., LL.D.* (1917). REFERENCES: *BMNAS* 22 (1943): 215-31; *DAB*, 19: 621-24; *DSB*, 14: 248-50; Donald Fleming, *William H. Welch and the Rise of Modern Medicine* (1954); Simon Flexner, "William Henry Welch—A Biographical Sketch," *Sci.* 52 (1920): 417; Simon Flexner and James Thomas Flexner, *William Henry Welch and the Heroic Age of American Medicine* (1941); *JAMA* (1934), 1513-14; *NCAB*, 26: 6; *Sun* (Baltimore), May 1, 1934.

J. Duffy

WELLS, H[ARRY] GIDEON (July 21, 1875, Fair Haven, Conn.-April 26, 1943, Chicago, Ill.). *Physician; Pathology; Biochemistry; Immunology.* Son of Romanta, pharmacist, and Emma Townsend (Tuttle) Wells. Married Bertha Robbins, 1902; one child. EDUCATION: 1895, Ph.B., Sheffield Scientific School (later part of Yale University); 1898, M.D., Rush Medical College; 1903, Ph.D. (pathology), University of Chicago; 1898-99, intern, Cook County Hospital; 1904-5, postgraduate study, University of Berlin. CAREER: c.1900, practiced medicine, Chicago; 1901-40, pathology faculty, University of Chicago; 1911-40, first director, Otho S. A. Sprague Memorial Institute, Chicago; 1917-19, member, American Red Cross mission to Roumania; president: 1915-16, 1919-20, American Association for Cancer Research; 1919, American Association of Pathologists and Bacteriologists; and 1923, American Association of Immunologists. CONTRIBUTIONS: Leading American authority on the chemical aspects of pathology and immunology. Advanced knowledge of fat necrosis, tissue staining, enzyme action, pathologic calcification, and degenerative processes and tissue necrosis. Book *Chemical Pathology* (1907) was for many years the standard reference in its field. As director, Sprague Memorial Institute, promoted research in many fields, including the chemotherapy of tuberculosis and the role of heredity in cancer. An outstanding morbid anatomist and tissue pathologist; investigations included studies of adrenal gland atrophy, muscle degeneration, postoperative pulmonary embolism, and the pathology of the liver. With Thomas B. Osborne (q.v.), studied the chemistry of immunity and anaphylaxis; investigations of protein sensitivity established the dependence of reaction specificity on the chemistry of proteins rather than their biologic origin.

WRITINGS: "Primary Carcinoma of the Liver," *Trans., Chicago Path. Soc,* 5 (1901): 11; "Fatal Pulmonary Embolism During Convalescence from a Simple Appendectomy," ibid., 5 (1902): 134; "Experimental Fat Necrosis," *J. of Med. Research* 9 (1903): 70; *The Chemistry of Tuberculosis* (1923, with Lydia DeWitt and Esmond R. Long); *The Chemical Aspects of Immunity* (1924). A bibliography is in *BMNAS*. REFERENCES: *BMNAS* 26 (1951): 233-63; *DAB*, Supplement 3: 806-8; *NCAB*, 37: 110-11; *N.Y. Times*, April 27, 1943; *Who Was Who in Am.*, 2: 566.

S. Galishoff

WELLS, HORACE (January 21, 1815, Hartford, Vt.-January 24, 1848, New York, N.Y.). *Dentist; Anesthetist.* Son of Horace, farmer, and Betsy (Heath) Wells. Married Elizabeth Wales, 1838; one son. EDUCATION: Private schools,

Hopkinton and Walpole, N.H., and academy, Amherst, Mass.; 1834-36, studied dentistry under preceptors in Boston, Mass. CAREER: 1836-48, practiced dentistry, Hartford, Conn. CONTRIBUTIONS: Noted for discovery of anesthesia (December 1844). After observing exhibition of "laughing gas" (nitrous oxide), noted that the subject injured himself but experienced no pain. The next day, after inhaling nitrous oxide, Wells had a tooth extracted and experienced not even a "prick of pain." In January 1845, went to Boston to demonstrate the phenomenon to the Harvard medical faculty. The gas bag was prematurely removed and the patient cried out, eliciting jeers from his audience. Returned to Hartford deeply discouraged. Was shocked when former student and partner Dr. W.T.G. Morton (q.v.) and Professor Charles T. Jackson (q.v.) announced the discovery of their "compound Letheon" (sulphuric ether aromatized) as an anesthetic after a successful demonstration in the Massachusetts General Hospital. Controversy developed over who was the real discoverer of anesthesia, with the French Academy of Medicine finally voting Wells the honor and bestowing upon him the honorary title of M.D. (1848).

WRITINGS: *An Essay on Teeth, Comprising a Brief Description of Their Formation, Diseases, and Proper Treatment* (1838); *A History of the Discovery of the Application of Nitrous Oxide Gas, Ether and Other Vapors to Surgical Operations* (1847). REFERENCES: *DAB*, 10, pt. 1: 640-41; Henry Wood Erving, "The Discoverer of Anesthesia: Dr. Horace Wells of Hartford," *Yale J. Biol. & Med.* 5 (May 1933): 421-30; Walter H. Jacobs, D.D.S., "Horace Wells," *Conn. State Med. J.* 8 (Nov. 1944): 729-35; *NCAB*, 6:438; Max E. Soifer, D.D.S., "Dr. Horace Wells, the Discoverer of Anesthesia: A Centenary Tribute," *Bull. Conn. State Dental Assoc.* (May 26-27, 1944), 4-10.

J. W. Ifkovic

WENDE, ERNEST (July 23, 1853, Millgrove, N.Y.-February 11, 1910, Buffalo, N.Y.). *Physician; Dermatologist; Health officer.* Son of Bernard P., farmer, and Susan (Kirk) Wende. Married Frances Harriett Cutler, 1881; three children. EDUCATION: Buffalo High School; 1875-76, U.S. Military Academy; apprentice to Dr. Hubbard A. Foster (Buffalo) and Dr. Henry Lapp (Clarence, N.Y.); 1878, M.D., University of Buffalo; 1881-82, College of Physicians and Surgeons; University of Pennsylvania: 1884, M.D.; and 1885, B.S.; 1885-86, Berlin and Vienna. CAREER: Private practice: 1878-84, Alden, N.Y.; and 1884-1910, Buffalo; at University of Buffalo: 1887-1910, medical faculty; and 1890-1910, pharmacy faculty; medical staff, Buffalo General Hospital and University of Buffalo Dispensary; 1895-1910, associate editor, *Buffalo Medical Journal*; 1892-1902, 1907-10, health commissioner, Buffalo. CONTRIBUTIONS: Introduced the germ theory of disease to Buffalo medicine and public health. Pioneered in the control of contagious diseases by requiring vaccination and quarantine and by founding a hospital for such diseases. Established sanitary inspection of milk, water, plumbing, markets, hotels, and restaurants.

WRITINGS: *The Microscope in the Diagnosis of Diseases of the Skin* (1887); *Municipal Restriction of Disease* (1899); *Report on the Cause and Prevention of Infant Mortality* (1900). REFERENCES: *DAB*, 10, pt. 1: 648-49; *JAMA* 54 (1910): 723; Adelbert Moot,

"Ernest Wende: A Memoir," *Pub. of the Buffalo Hist. Soc.* 22 (1918): 127-44; *Morning Express* (Buffalo), February 12, 1910; *NCAB*, 4: 381.

D. O. Powell

WERNER, WALTER IGNACIO (February 6, 1898, Cleveland, Ohio-August 22, 1954, in an air crash near Rochester, Minn.). *Internist; Tuberculosis; Asthma.* Son of Conrad F. and Catherine (Steidle) Werner. Married to Dr. Freida Wally-Sternburg, Berlin, an M.D. specializing in pediatrics; one child. EDUCATION: 1922-23, student extern, Bay View City Hospital, Baltimore, Md.; 1923, M.D., University of Maryland Medical School; 1923-24, intern, Mt. Sinai Hospital, Cleveland, Ohio; 1925, resident house officer, Union Printers Home, Colorado Springs, Colo.; 1925-30, senior resident, William H. Maybury Sanatorium, Northville, Mich. CAREER: 1924-25, went west to Denver, Colo., seeking a cure for TB, which he had contracted; 1930-34, medical director, Oakland County Tuberculosis Sanatorium, Pontiac, Mich.; 1934, out because of illness; 1935, director, Maytag Laboratories-Institute Tuberculosis Research, Southwestern Presbyterian Sanatorium, Albuquerque, N.Mex.; 1938, associate, American College of Physicians; 1939, certified, American Board of Internal Medicine; 1941, fellow, American College of Physicians. CONTRIBUTIONS: Started a testing program for TB among N.Mex. schoolchildren. Ran a pneumo clinic at Southwestern Presbyterian Sanatorium and gave pneumothorax treatment free to the poor. With decrease in the incidence of TB due to antibiotics, went into allergy research and cardiology.

WRITINGS: Published many articles on pulmonary tuberculosis, including "Rest and Exercise in the Treatment of Pulmonary Tuberculosis," *Michigan State Med. J.* (Jan. 1928); "The Significance of Positive and Negative Sputum Findings in Pulmonary Tuberculosis," *Am. Rev. of Tuberculosis* (Oct. 1928); "Childhood Type Tuberculosis," *Southwestern Med.* (Feb. 1935); "The Problem of Tuberculosis in New Mexico," *ibid.* (1940). Also wrote "Hay-Fever Plants of Albuquerque, New Mexico. A Preliminary Report," *Annals of Allergy* (Jan.-Feb. 1947). REFERENCES: Interview with Evalena Stormfels, Werner's former associate and laboratory assistant at Southwestern Presbyterian Sanatorium, Albuquerque, N.Mex.; newspaper clipping file kept by E. Stormfels.

C. L. Cutter

WESSELHOEFT, CONRAD (March 23, 1834, Weimar, Germany-December 17, 1904, Newton, Mass.). *Homeopathic physician; Educator.* Son of Robert, physician, and Ferdinanda Emilia (Hecker) Wesselhoeft, who migrated to America while Conrad was young. Married Elizabeth Foster Pope, 1863; one child. EDUCATION: Sent by his parents to Germany for his preliminary education; 1853, graduated from the Nicolai Gymnasium, Leipzig; 1856, M.D., Harvard Medical School. CAREER: 1856-63, medical practice, Dorchester, Mass.; 1863, practice in Boston; 1873-1904, professor of materia medica and then of pathology and therapeutics, Boston University School of Medicine; 1855-1904, member of the medical staff, Homeopathic Hospital, Boston. CONTRIBUTIONS: An early convert to homeopathy and a founder of the Boston University (homeopathic) School of

Medicine. President, American Institute of Homeopathy, 1879. Tried to keep homeopathy in line with the development of modern scientific medicine.

WRITINGS: Translated into English, Samuel Hahnemann's *Organon*; various articles in homeopathic medical journals; co-editor of the *Homeopathic Pharmacopoeia of the United States*. REFERENCES: *DAB*, 10, pt. 2: 4; Kelly and Burrage (1928), 1285; W. H. King, *Hist. of Homeopathy . . .* (1905), vol. 4; *Trans. of the Am. Instit. of Homeopathy*, (1905).

M. Kaufman

WEST, ARCHA K. (1865, Miss.-1925, Oklahoma City, Okla.). *Physician*. EDUCATION: 1894, M.D., Memphis Hospital Medical College. CAREER: Practice, Tex., before arriving in Oklahoma City, 1899; professor and dean, Epworth College of Medicine; 1912, when Epworth merged with the University of Oklahoma, became head, Department of Medicine, serving until death, 1925. CONTRIBUTIONS: Active member, Oklahoma Territory Medical Association. A strong proponent of medical ethics. Leader in medical education and in efforts to establish a medical school in Oklahoma City (1903, Epworth College of Medicine). Worked to strengthen licensing requirements in Okla. Territory. Through influence on state and other governmental authorities, gave greater strength to the organized medical profession. An important leader in the medical profession during the transitional phase from territory to state and a prominent physician in Oklahoma City.

WRITINGS: "Vesica Vaginal Fistula," *Okla. Med. News J.* 11 (Aug. 1903): 286; "Medical Education," ibid., 14 (Jul. 1906): 145-50; "Modern Research—A Criticism and a Suggestion with Special Reference to Typhoid Fever," *J. Okla. State Med. Assoc.* 3: 77-82. REFERENCES: William F. Browne and R. Palmer Howard, "The Role of the Oklahoma County Medical Society in Territorial Medicine, 1904-1905," *Journal of the Oklahoma State Medical Association* 7, no. 3 (March 1977): 92-98; Mark R. Everett, *Medical Education in Oklahoma: The University of Oklahoma School of Medicine and Medical Center, 1900-1931* (1972); R. Palmer Howard and Rose C. Gideon, "The Beginning of Medical Organization in Oklahoma, 1889-1893," *Journal of the Oklahoma State Medical Association* 67, no. 2 (November 1974): 45-54; R. Palmer Howard and Richard E. Martin, "The Contributions of B. F. Fortner, LeRoy Long, and Other Early Surgeons in Oklahoma," *Journal of the Oklahoma State Medical Association* (November 1968): 541-49; "Archa West" file, History of Medicine Collection, University of Oklahoma Health Sciences Center Library, Oklahoma City, Okla.

V. Allen

WEST, HAROLD DADFORD (July 16, 1904, Flemington, N.J.-March 5, 1974, Nashville, Tenn.). *Medical educator; Biochemist*. Son of George H. and Mary Ann (Joney) West. Married Jessie Juanita Penn, 1927; two children. EDUCATION: University of Illinois: 1925, B.S.; 1930, M.S.; and 1937, Ph.D. CAREER: 1925-27, professor of chemistry and head, Department of Science, Morris Brown College, Atlanta, Ga.; 1927-52, 1965-69, faculty, Meharry Medical College: 1927-38, associate professor; 1938-52, professor and chairman; 1965-69, professor, Department of Biochemistry; and 1952-65, president. CON-TRIBUTIONS: First black president of Meharry Medical College (1952-65) and first Ph.D. to join the Meharry faculty (1927). Considered an excellent, concerned teacher and effective administrator. Involved in many biochemical research proj-ects of medical significance, including the discovery of the antibiotic biocerin, the synthesis and large scale preparation of the essential amino acid threonine, and the relationship in blacks between serum calcium levels and tuberculosis. REFERENCES: W. Montague Cobb and Calvin C. Sampson, "Harold Dadford West, Ph.D., LL.D., F.A.I.C.," *JNMA* 66 (1974): 448-49; *Who's Who in Am.* 38 (1974-75): 3265; *Am. Men and Women of Sci.*, 12 (1973): 6829-30; *JNMA* 55 (1963): 245-46.

T. L. Savitt

WESTMORELAND, JOHN GRAY (June 4, 1816, Monticello, Ga.-March 3, 1887, Atlanta, Ga.). *Physician; Educator.* Son of Robert Westmoreland. Married Annie Buchanan; two children. EDUCATION: Fayetteville Academy; read medicine with a country physician; 1843, M.D., Medical College of Georgia. CAREER: Early 1850s, moved to Atlanta from Pike County, Ga.; 1854-55, was the driving force behind the establishment of the Atlanta Medical College; at Atlanta Medical College: *post* 1855, professor of materia medica and therapeu-tics, while brother Willis Furman Westmoreland was professor of surgery (having secured his M.D. from Jefferson Medical College, 1850); and dean of the faculty; 1855-76, with brother, established and edited or co-edited the *Atlanta Medical and Surgical Journal*, Ga.'s best medical journal following the demise of Au-gusta's *Southern Medical and Surgical Journal*, 1867; founder, Brotherhood of Physicians, a group from which the Fulton County Medical Society emerged, and is credited with establishing the first bona fide hospital in Atlanta; 1855, elected for one term to the Georgia House of Representatives. CONTRIBUTIONS: The most important founder, Atlanta Medical College, from whence came the Atlanta College of Physicians and Surgeons. The latter school was one of the essential components that went together to make up the Emory University School of Medicine. Role in founding and editing *Atlanta Medical and Surgical Journal* was noteworthy.

WRITINGS: Writings about ecology, therapeutics, and aspects of medical and chemical pharmacy are in *Atlanta Med. and Surg. J*. REFERENCES: F. Phinizy Calhoun, "The Founding and the Early History of the Atlanta Medical College, 1854-1875," *Georgia Hist. Q.* 9 (1925): 34-54; *Index Catalogue* 16 (1895): 403; Kelly and Burrage (1920), 1219-20; and for information on Willis F. Westmoreland see *ibid.*, pp. 1220-21, and *Memoirs of Georgia* 2 (1893): 40-42.

P. Spalding

WHEELER, JOHN BROOKS (1853, Stowe, Vt.-May 1, 1942, Burlington, Vt.). *Physician; Surgeon.* Son of John Brooks, attorney, and Eliza Jane (Hunter) Wheeler. Orphaned at early age, lived with grandfather, Rev. John Wheeler, president, University of Vermont. Married Anna Sanford, 1884; two children. EDUCATION: 1875, A.B., Vermont; 1878, M.D., Harvard (degree actually awarded 1879 after serving as house officer, Mass. General Hospital, 1878-79); 1879-81, study in Vienna, Austria; Strassburg, France; and Berlin, Germany. CAREER: 1881-1942, surgical practice, Burlington; at University of Vermont: 1881-92, instructor of surgery; 1892-1900, professor of clinical and minor surgery; 1900-1924, professor of surgery; and 1924-42, emeritus. CONTRIBUTIONS: The most prominent surgeon of Burlington for most of his 60 years of practice. Tenure spanned the early acceptance of antiseptic methods, the performance of most operations in patients' homes, to the era of the modern hospital operating room. Kept up to date, practicing and teaching new methods as they were developed, and was responsible for most of the surgical instruction of generations of medical students. Introduced (1886) intubation for diphtheria (while visiting physician, St. Joseph's Orphanage) and, in the same year, the use of cocaine for local anesthesia to the Burlington medical community. Member, founder's group, American College of Surgeons (1913), and New England Surgical Society (1916), and president (1917-18).

WRITINGS: "Antiseptic Surgery in the Country," *Phila. Times and Register*, November 23, 1889 (to show antisepsis is possible "in a back woods shanty"); "Appendicitis," *N.Y. Med. J.* (Nov. 3, 1894); *Memoirs of a Small Town Surgeon* (1935). REFERENCES: *NCAB*, 34: 547.

L. J. Wallman

WHIPPLE, ALLEN OLDFATHER (September 2, 1881, Urmia, Persia (later Risaiyeh, Iran)-April 6, 1963, Princeton, N.J.). *Physician; Surgery; Medical education*. Son of William, Presbyterian clergyman, and Mary (Allen) Whipple. Married Mary Neales, 1912; three children. EDUCATION: 1904, B.S., Princeton University; 1908, M.D., College of Physicians and Surgeons (Columbia); 1908-10, intern, Roosevelt Hospital (New York City). CAREER: 1911-17, practiced medicine, New York City; 1911-12, surgical staff, Sloane Hospital (New York City); 1911-46, surgical faculty, College of Physicians and Surgeons (Columbia); 1911-46, surgical staff, Presbyterian Hospital (New York City); during World War II, member, National Research Council's Committee on Surgery; 1946-51, clinical director, Memorial Hospital (New York City); president: 1933-35, New York Surgical Society; 1935-37, Society for Clinical Surgery; and 1939-40, American Surgical Association; trustee: 1941-57, American University of Beirut; and 1951-63, Princeton University. CONTRIBUTIONS: A leader in abdominal, spleen, and gallbladder surgery. Eponymously known for triad of criteria for hyperinsulinism with islet tumors and for operation for carcinoma of the pancreas. Most important contribution was the creation of the spleen clinic in the surgery department, Columbia University, from which came many important advances, including prosthetic materials for aortic grafting and the measurement and treatment of portal hypertension. After retirement from Columbia, revised the medical training program at Memorial Hospital, New York City (1946-51) and at American University, Beirut, Lebanon (1952). Editor-in-chief, *Nelson's Loose-Leaf Surgery*, for 20 years, and member, editorial board, *Annals of Surgery* (1932-46).

WRITINGS: "Adenoma of the Islet-Cells with Hyperinsulinism: A Review," *Annals of Surg*. 101 (Jun. 1935): 1299-1335 (with V. K. Frantz); "Treatment of Carcinoma of the Ampulla of Vater," ibid., 102 (Oct. 1935): 763-79 (with W. B. Parsons and C. R. Mullins); "Surgical Treatment of Carcinoma of the Ampullary Region and Head of the Pancreas," *Am. J. of Surg*. 40 (Apr. 1938): 260-63; *Evolution of Surgery in the United States* (1963); *The Story of Wound Healing and Wound Repair* (1963). REFERENCES: *NCAB*, 51: 503; *N.Y. Times*, April 17, 1963; Mark M. Ravitch, *A Century of Surgery*, 2 vols. (1981); Fordyce B. St. John, "Allen Oldfather Whipple, 1881-1963," *Trans., Am. Surg. Assoc*. 82 (1964): 471-72; *Who Was Who in Am.*, 4: 1002.

S. Galishoff

WHIPPLE, GEORGE HOYT (August 28, 1878, Ashland, N.H.-February 1, 1976, Rochester, N.Y.). *Pathologist; Medical educator*. Son of Ashley Cooper, physician, and Frances Anna (Hoyt) Whipple. Married Katherine Ball Waring, 1914; two children. EDUCATION: 1900, A.B., Yale University; 1905, M.D., Johns Hopkins University; 1909, 1911, studied in Europe. CAREER: 1905-14, pathology faculty, Johns Hopkins Medical School; 1906-7, pathology staff, Ancon Hospital, Panama; University of California Medical School: 1914-21, research medicine faculty and director, Hooper Foundation for Medical Research; and 1920-21, dean; at University of Rochester School of Medicine and Dentistry: 1921-55, pathology faculty; and 1921-53, dean. CONTRIBUTIONS: Studied the effects of various foods on blood regeneration in dogs with experimentally induced anemia; found that liver was one of the best foods for the production of new, hemoglobin-filled, red blood cells (1918-25); gave George R. Minot (q.v.) and William P. Murphy the idea of using a liver diet to treat pernicious anemia in man; for this work, the three men were awarded the 1934 Nobel Prize in medicine or physiology. For over 30 years, was the first dean, Rochester School of Medicine and Dentistry, which he developed into a medical center of the first rank. Began the modern study of protein metabolism with investigations of the body's methods for storing and releasing proteins (1940s, 1950s) Did significant research on tuberculosis, pancreatitis, regeneration of plasma protein, chloroform poisoning in animals, intestinal lipodystrophy ("Whipple's disease"), and blackwater fever (a severe form or complication of malaria).

WRITINGS: "Blood Regeneration in Severe Anemia. II. Favorable Influence of Liver, Heart and Skeletal Muscle in Diet," *Am. J. of Physiol*. 72 (1925): 408-18 (with Frieda S. Robscheit-Robbins); *The Dynamic Equilibrium of Body Proteins. Hemoglobin, Plasma Proteins, Organ and Tissue Proteins* (1956). A bibliography is in G. W. Corner, *George Hoyt Whipple and His Friends* (1963). REFERENCES: *Am. Philos. Soc. Yearbook* (1976), 135-40; *BHM* (1970-74), 178; (1978), 31; Corner, *George Hoyt Whipple and His Friends* (1963); A. McGehee Harvey, *Adventures in Medical Research* (1976), 46-48; *McGraw-*

Hill Modern Men of Sci. 2 (1966): 595-96; Miller, *BHM*, p. 122; *Trans., Assoc. of Am. Physicians* 89 (1976); *Who Was Who in Am.*, 6: 433-34.

S. Galishoff

WHITE, ELLEN GOULD (HARMON)   (November 26, 1827, Gorham, Maine-July 16, 1915, St. Helena, Calif.). *Spiritual leader; Health reformer.* Daughter of Robert, hatter, and Eunice (Gould) Harmon. Married James White, 1846; four children. EDUCATION: Brackett Street School and Westbrook Seminary (Portland, Maine). CAREER: Co-founder, Seventh-day Adventist Church; 1855-81, Battle Creek, Mich.; 1881-85, Calif.; and 1885-87, Europe; 1887-91, returned to United States; 1891-1900, mission to Australia and New Zealand; 1900-15, St. Helena. CONTRIBUTIONS: Following the disappointment of William Miller's millennial prophecies (1844), founded what was to become the Seventh-day Adventist Church. After receiving a "vision" on health in 1863, made health reform an integral part of the Adventist message, establishing the Western Health Reform Institute at Battle Creek (1866) which evolved into the Battle Creek Sanitarium and College of Medical Evangelists, Loma Linda, Calif. (1906). Her health doctrines, which she believed were revealed to her by God, shared much with similar health and moral reform movements of her time; they included avoiding stimulants and meats, while promoting exercise, fresh air, water, and dress reform. Many of her ideas were shared with Dr. John Harvey Kellogg (q.v.), medical director, Battle Creek Sanitarium; although the two split (1907) over Kellogg's growing skepticism about the nature of White's revelations.

WRITINGS: Produced more than 50 books and pamphlets and several thousand articles; later medical views were well presented in *The Ministry of Healing* (1905). Writings listed in *Comprehensive Index to the Writings of Ellen G. White*, 3 vols. (1962-63). REFERENCES: *DAB*, 20: 98-99; *Notable Am. Women*, 3: 585-88; Ronald L. Numbers, *Prophetess of Health* (1976); Arthur L. White, Ellen G. White, 6 vols. planned (1981-); Ellen G. White, *Life Sketches of Ellen G. White* (1915).

M. S. Pernick

WHITE, JAMES CLARKE   (July 7, 1833, Belfast, Maine-January 5, 1916, Boston, Mass.). *Physician; Dermatology.* Son of James Patterson, shipowner, and Mary Ann (Clarke) White. Married Martha Anna Ellis, 1862; three children. EDUCATION: Harvard University: 1853, B.A.; and 1856, M.D.; 1856-57, postgraduate work, Vienna; studied under Ferdinand von Hebra. CAREER: At Harvard Medical School: 1858-63, instructor in chemistry; 1866-71, adjunct professor of chemistry; 1871-1902, professor of dermatology; and 1902-16, professor emeritus; president: 1877-87, American Dermatological Association; and 1892, Massachusetts Medical Society; 1867-71, editor, *Boston Medical and Surgical Journal.* CONTRIBUTIONS: Founded, with Benjamin Jeffries, the first dermatological clinic in the United States (1860). Held the first professorship established in his specialty in this country (1871). Helped found the American Dermatological Association (1877).

WRITINGS: *Dermatitis Venenata* (1887); *Sketches from My Life* (1914). REFERENCES: Henry K. Beecher and Mark D. Altschule, *Medicine at Harvard* (1977), 90-93; *DAB*, 20: 100; Kelly and Burrage (1928), 1224-26; *NCAB*, 19: 358.

N. Gevitz

WHITE, JAMES PLATT (March 14, 1811, Austerlitz, N.Y.-September 28, 1881, Buffalo, N.Y.). *Physician; Obstetrician; Gynecologist.* Son of David Pierson, farmer, and Anna (Platt) White. Married Mary Elizabeth Penfield, 1835; one adopted child. EDUCATION: Middlebury Academy; apprentice to Dr. Josiah Trowbridge (Buffalo); 1830-33, College of Physicians for the Western District; 1834, M.D., Jefferson Medical College; 1834-35, Edinburgh, Paris, Vienna. CAREER: 1835-81, private practice, Buffalo; 1846-81, medical faculty and president, University of Buffalo Medical College; medical staff, Sisters of Charity, Buffalo General, Providence Retreat, and Maternity and Foundling hospitals. CONTRIBUTIONS: Founded the University of Buffalo Medical College. Conducted the first clinical demonstrations in obstetrics in the United States (1850). Modified obstetrical forceps, reduced an inversion of the uterus (1856), and advocated anesthesia in childbirth. A founder, American Gynecological Society and several Buffalo hospitals.

WRITINGS: *Remarks on the Construction of Obstetrical Forceps* (1849); *Report on a Case of Inversion of the Uterus* (1858); *Chronic Inversion of the Uterus* (1877). REFERENCES: Carl T. Javert, "James Platt White, A Pioneer in American Obstetrics and Gynecology," *J. Hist. Med. & Allied Sci.* 3 (1948): 489-506; Oliver P. Jones, "A Bench Mark for Obstetric History in the United States," *Obst. and Gyn.* 43 (1974): 784-91; idem, "Our First Professor of Obstetrics: James Platt White," *The Buffalo Physician* (Spring 1974): 42-47; Kelly and Burrage (1928), 1292-93; *NCAB*, 7: 277.

D. O. Powell

WHITE, PAUL DUDLEY (June 6, 1886, Roxbury, Mass.-October 31, 1973, Boston, Mass.). *Physician; Cardiology.* Son of Herbert, physician, and Elizabeth A. (Dudley) White. Married Ina Reid, 1924; two children. EDUCATION: 1908, A.B., Harvard College; 1911, M.D., Harvard Medical School; 1911-13, intern, Massachusetts General Hospital; 1913-14, graduate student, University College Hospital Medical School, London; 1914-17, 1919-20, resident in medicine, Massachusetts General Hospital; 1928-29, Moseley Traveling Fellow, Vienna. CAREER: 1914-56, faculty, Harvard Medical School; 1916-19, medical officer, British and American Expeditionary Forces, France; 1911-48, staff, Massachusetts General Hospital; 1955, physician to President Eisenhower; in American Heart Association: founder; and 1942-44, president; 1970, nominated for Nobel Peace Prize. CONTRIBUTIONS: Pioneer in the diagnosis, treatment, and prevention of diseases of the heart and circulatory system. A founder of cardiology in America, a field in which he stressed clinical observation and research. Introduced electrocardiology in the United States (1914). Well-known advocate of diet, exercise, and weight control for both the prevention and treatment of cardiac disease.

WRITINGS: *Heart Disease* (1931, and subsequent editions) and numerous other works. For White's bibliography, see *Am. J. of Cardiology* 15 (1965): 581-602. REFERENCES: E. Grey Dimond and J. Willis Hurst, eds., "Paul Dudley White, A Portrait," *Am. J. Cardiology* 15 (1965): 433-603; "Dr. Paul Dudley White Is Dead at 87," *N.Y. Times*, November 1, 1973, p. 40; *NCAB*, 58: 169; Paul Dudley White (with the assistance of Margaret Parton), *My Life and Medicine: An Autobiographical Memoir* (1971).

M. H. Warner

WHITE, WILLIAM ALANSON (January 24, 1870, Brooklyn, N.Y.-March 7, 1937, Washington, D.C.). *Psychiatrist; Hospital superintendent*. Son of Alanson and Harriet (Hawley) White. Married Lola Thurston, 1918; stepdaughter. EDUCATION: 1889, A.B., Cornell University; 1891, M.D., Long Island Medical College. CAREER: 1891, medical staff, Eastern District Hospital, Brooklyn and Alms and Workhouse Hospital on Blackwell's Island, N.Y.; 1892-1903, medical staff, Binghamton State Hospital, N.Y.; 1903-37, superintendent, St. Elizabeth's Hospital, Washington, D.C., appointed by President Theodore Roosevelt; 1903, appointed professor of nervous and mental disease, Medical School, Georgetown University; 1904, appointed professor of psychiatry, George Washington University; president: American Psychiatric Association, American Psychoanalytic Association, American Psychopathological Association, and First International Congress of Mental Hygiene (1930); active in forensic psychiatry; appeared as a psychiatrist for the defense in the Loeb-Leopold murder trial; developed a close friendship with Dr. Smith Ely Jelliffe (q.v.), and their collaboration produced significant results, notably the Nervous and Mental Disease Monograph Series, and *Diseases of the Nervous System* (1915) which went through five editions; 1913, founded *The Psychoanalytic Review*, the first English language journal devoted to psychoanalysis. CONTRIBUTIONS: As an efficient organizer and administrator, transformed St. Elizabeth's Hospital (officially known until 1917 as the Government Hospital for the Insane) into a modern treatment center for the mentally ill. A constant source of innovation, offering inspiration and encouragement to the staff. Established a psychological lab, neuropathological lab, and division of internal medicine. Applied psychotherapeutic and psychoanalytic principles to the treatment of the institutionalized mentally ill. A major synthesizer and promoter of psychoanalysis and actively involved in the mental hygiene movement, devoting much of his writing to educating the public.

WRITINGS: A prolific writer: more than 275 articles, 19 books, 379 book reviews. Most important books include *Outlines of Psychiatry* (1907), *The Principles of Mental Hygiene* (1917), *Foundations of Psychiatry* (1921), *Essays in Psychopathology* (1925), *Twentieth Century Psychiatry: Its Contribution to Man's Knowledge of Himself* (1936). Major writings listed in Arcangelo R. T. D'Amore, *William Alanson White, the Washington Years, 1903-1937* (1976). REFERENCES: *DAB*, Supplement 2: 711-12; D'Amore, *William Alanson White*; *NCAB* , 38: 565; *Who Was Who in Am.*, 1: 1336.

L. V. Bell

WHITEHEAD, PETER FLANAGAN (June 9, 1838, Winchester, Ky.-September 5, 1878, Vicksburg, Miss.). *Physician*. Married Irene Cowan, 1865; no children. EDUCATION: Winchester (Ky.) Academy; 1857, apprenticed to Dr. H. Taylor, Winchester; 1859, M.D., Jefferson Medical College, Philadelphia, Pa. CAREER: 1859, physician, Blockley Hospital (Philadelphia, Pa.); 1861, moved to Independence, Mo., and began practice; when Civil War began, enlisted as a private in Capt. Eugene Erwin's Company, Independence; shortly thereafter, was commissioned as a surgeon, Missouri State Guard, and assigned to duty at Gen. Sterling Price's headquarters as a surgeon in the general's escort; served in Missouri State Guard until mustered out; 1862, reenlisted at Corinth, Miss., as private in a regiment of Mo. troops, but soon appointed as a surgeon in the Confederate service; assigned to duty, Third Louisiana Regiment, and served through the siege of Vicksburg; later served as chief surgeon of Gen. William Wing Loring's Division in which position he surrendered at Greensboro, N.C., in Apr. 1865; after war, returned to Vicksburg, married, and practiced medicine until death in the yellow-fever epidemic of 1878. CONTRIBUTIONS: 1874-75, president, Mississippi State Medical Association; 1875, represented association at the American Medical Association convention; 1875, suggested that a Miss. State board of health be organized; 1877, named member, first Mississippi State Board of Health.

M. S. Legan

WHITEHEAD, WILLIAM MASSIE (October 21, 1905, Lovington, Va.-November 11, 1966, Chichagoff Island, Alaska). *Physician; General practitioner; Surgeon.* Son of Stuart B. and Susan (Massie) Whitehead. Married Dorothy Johnson, September 23, 1934; five children. EDUCATION: 1931, M.D., University of Virginia School of Medicine; 1931-32, intern, Virginia Mason Hospital, Seattle, Wash. CAREER: 1932-34, surgeon, American Mail Line vessels; 1934, entered Alaska at Wrangell; 1935-66, private practice, Juneau, Alaska; 1936-1965, member of staff, St. Ann's Hospital, Juneau. CONTRIBUTIONS: With W. W. Council (q.v.), helped to establish the Juneau Medical and Surgical Clinic (1936-65). Delivered 4,000 babies. Secretary, Alaska Board of Medical Examiners (1943-66). President, Alaska Territorial Medical Association (1945) and Alaska Medical Association (1958-59). Member, senior editorial staff, *Western Journal of Surgery, Obstetrics and Gynecology.* Chairman, first Alaska Judicial Council (1959). Member, Alaska House of Representatives (1963). Appointed to the Board of Regents, University of Alaska (1965).

WRITINGS: "A Handy Device for the Identification of Medications" in *Alaska Med.* (Sept. 1959); various other articles of interest to the practitioner in Alaska. REFERENCES: *Alaska Med.* 8, no. 4 (Dec. 1966): 83; personal correspondence.

A. R. C. Helms

WHITEHEAD, WILLIAM RIDDICK (December 15, 1831, Suffolk, Va.-October 13, 1902, Denver, Colo.). *Surgeon.* Son of William Boykin and Emeline (Riddick) Whitehead. Married Eliza Benton, 1863; four children. EDUCATION: 1851, graduated from Virginia Military Institute; 1853, M.D., University of

Pennsylvania; 1854-60, studied in Paris and Vienna; 1860, M.D., École de Médecine, Paris. CAREER: 1855, as a Russian Army surgeon under Pirogov, served at Sevastopol; awarded Imperial Russian Order of St. Stanislaus; 1860-61, professor of clinical medicine, New York Medical College; 1861-63, surgeon, 44th Virginia Infantry; cared for Stonewall Jackson at Chancellorsville; left behind at Gettysburg to attend Confederate wounded; captured by Union troops and held prisoner in an enclosure adjoining Fort McHenry, Baltimore, Md.; escaped, and by way of N.Y., Canada, and Bermuda, finally reached Richmond, Va., where Surgeon-General Moore, Confederate States of America, appointed him president of a board for the examination of conscripts and disabled soldiers; after the war, practiced surgery, New York City; 1872, moved to Colo.; 1874, elected to the Denver, Colo., City Council; president: 1877, Denver Medical Society; and 1884, Colorado Medical Society; 1881-83, professor of anatomy and of diseases of the genito-urinary system, University of Denver; 1883-86, first professor of anatomy, University of Colorado. CONTRIBUTIONS: Known for cleft-palate operations for which he designed instruments and techniques that were widely used. Reported many cases during the period 1868-86.

WRITINGS: Partial listing in *Medical Coloradoana* (1922). REFERENCES: [Editorial], "The Death of Dr. William R. Whitehead," *Colorado Med. J.* 8 (1902): 488-90; *NCAB*, 10: 267; Wm. R. Whitehead, *The Autobiography of a Western Surgeon* (1890; includes bibliographical addendum).

F. B. Rogers

WHITMAN, MARCUS (September 4, 1802, Rushville, N.Y.-November 29, 1847, Waiilatpu, Wash.). *Physician; Medical missionary.* Son of Beza, tanner and currier, and Alice (Green) Whitman. Married Narcissa Prentiss, 1836; one child. EDUCATION: Hallock School, Plainfield, Mass.; 1823-25, apprentice to Dr. Ira Bryant, Rushville, N.Y.; 1825-26, 1831-32, College of Physicians and Surgeons of the Western District of N.Y., Fairfield, M.D., 1832. CAREER: 1823-25, schoolteacher, Rushville; practiced medicine: for two months in 1827, Sugargrove, Pa.; 1827-30, Gainsboro, Upper Canada; and 1832-35, Wheeler, N.Y.; 1835, made missionary reconnaissance of Oregon Territory for American Board of Commissioners for Foreign Missions (Presbyterian, Congregational, Dutch Reform churches); 1836-47, missionary and physician to Cayuse Indians (and to white settlers), Waiilatpu, near Fort Walla Walla, Wash.; 1847, killed by Cayuse Indians angry that he could not prevent deaths of their people from measles as he could whites during an epidemic and suspicious that he had been poisoning them. CONTRIBUTIONS: One of the first physicians in Wash. Served the white and Indian populations medically and spiritually for 12 years. Helped open up Wash. to white settlement. A key figure in the early medical and political history of Washington. REFERENCES: *DAB*, 10, pt. 2: 141-43; Clifford M. Drury, *Marcus and Narcissa Whitman and the Opening of Old Oregon*, 2 vols. (1973); *NCAB*, 11: 112; W. H. Rice, comp., *The Work of Marcus Whitman, Missionary Physician to*

Oregon from 1835 until His Cruel Death at the Hands of the Cayuse Indians, November 29, 1847, as Shown by Government Documents (1895).

T. L. Savitt

WHITMAN, ROYAL (October 24, 1857, Portland, Maine-August 19, 1946, New York, N.Y.). *Physician; Orthopedic surgery.* Son of Royal Emerson, soldier and inventor, and Lucretia Octavia (Whitman) Whitman. Married Julia Lombard Armitage, 1886; one child. EDUCATION: 1882, M.D., Harvard Medical School; c. 1883, intern, Boston City Hospital; late 1880s, studied at Cook's School of Anatomy, London, England; 1889, received diploma, Royal College of Surgeons. CAREER: Mid-late 1880s, practiced medicine, Boston, Mass.; 1889-1929, surgical staff, Hospital for the Ruptured and Crippled, New York City; served as adjunct professor of orthopedic surgery, College of Physicians and Surgeons (Columbia); and professor, New York Polyclinic Medical School; 1895, president, American Orthopedic Association. CONTRIBUTIONS: An early specialist in surgery of deformities and diseases of the joints. Developed several techniques for treatment of disorders of the foot and hip that quickly became standard; devised a special metal plate, still known as the Whitman plate, for the treatment of flat foot (1889); developed an astragalectomy operation for stabilizing the paralytic foot, especially the foot with calcaneus deformity (1901); originated the "abduction treatment" for fracture of the neck of the femur (1904); pioneered in the reconstruction operation for ununited fracture of the hip (1916). Exerted great influence through his clinical teaching and through his textbook *A Treatise on Orthopaedic Surgery* (1901), which in 1930 was in its ninth edition.

WRITINGS: "Observations on Forty-five Cases of Flat-foot with Particular Reference to Etiology and Treatment," *Boston Med. and Surg. J.* 118 (Jun. 14, 1888): 598-601; (Jun. 21, 1888): 616-20; "The Operative Treatment of Paralytic Talipes of the Calcaneus Type," *Am. J. of Med. Sci.* 122 (Nov. 1901): 593-601; "A New Method of Treatment of Fracture of the Neck of the Femur, Together with Remarks on Coxa Vara," *Annals of Surg.* 36 (Nov. 1902): 746-61; "The Reconstruction Operation for Ununited Fracture of the Neck of the Femur," ibid., 73 (Feb. 1921): 245-47; and *Surg. Gyn. & Obst.* 32 (Jun. 1921): 479-86. REFERENCES: *DAB*, Supplement 4: 886-88; *N.Y. Times*, August 20, 1946; *Who Was Who in Am.*, 2: 574.

S. Galishoff

WHITTICO, JAMES MALACHI (September 23, 1893, Ridgeway, W.Va.-August 10, 1975, Huntington, W.Va.). *Physician.* Son of Hezekiah Jink, farmer, and Letitia (Pace) Whittico. Married Nannie L. Cobbs, 1914 (divorced 1936), one child; Lafadia Belle Dickerson, 1939, one child. EDUCATION: Walden University (Nashville, Tenn.); 1912, M.D., Meharry Medical College. CAREER: During childhood and again while at Meharry, worked in W.Va. and Ky. coal mines to help support family and later to pay for medical education; 1912-75, private practice, Williamson, W.Va.; during World War I, served in France with American Expeditionary Forces. CONTRIBUTIONS: Served blacks and large numbers of whites in the mining community of Williamson for more than 60 years.

Encountered and successfully fought against open white racism (e.g., Ku Klux Klan activities) in Williamson area. Helped financially troubled blacks purchase land, businesses, homes, farm equipment. Aided aspiring black pharmacists, dentists, and physicians with their careers. Served NMA as sergeant-at-arms, House of Delegates, for many years. REFERENCES: A. B. Caldwell, *History of the American Negro* 7 (1923): 268-71; W. Montague Cobb, "James Malachi Whittico, Sr., M.D., 1893-1975," *JNMA* 68 (1976): 441-43.

T. L. Savitt

WICKES, STEPHEN (March 17, 1813, Jamaica, N.Y.-July 8, 1889, Orange, N.J.). *Physician; Medical historian.* Son of Van Wyck, businessman, and Eliza (Herriman) Wickes. Married Mary Whitney Heyer, 1835, one child; Lydia Matilda (Howard) Van Sinderen, 1841; two children. EDUCATION: Union Hall Academy, Jamaica; Union College: 1831, A.B.; and 1834, M.A.; 1832, studied natural sciences, Rensselaer Polytechnic Institute; apprentice to Dr. Thomas W. Blatchford (Troy, N.Y.); 1834, M.D., University of Pennsylvania Medical School. CAREER: Private practice: 1835, New York City; 1835-52, Troy; and 1852-86, Orange; 1873-86, medical staff, Orange Memorial Hospital; 1883, president, Medical Society of New Jersey. CONTRIBUTIONS: First medical historian of N.J. Edited (1861-82) the *Transactions of the Medical Society of New Jersey*, which included articles on the medical history of the state, and the "old *Transactions*," covering 1766-1800.

WRITINGS: *Water-Cure in Orange* (1861); *The Rise, Minutes, and Proceedings of the New Jersey Medical Society, Established July 23d, 1766* (1875); *History of Medicine in New Jersey, and of Its Medical Men, from the Settlement of the Province to A.D. 1800* (1879); Writings listed in *Appleton's Cyclopaedia*, 6: 498. REFERENCES: *Appleton's CAB*, 6: 498; *Biographical Encyclopaedia of N.J.* (1877), 480; *DAB*, 10, pt. 2: 181; *Evening News* (Newark), July 8, 1889; Kelly and Burrage (1928), 1299; *Med. News* (Jul. 13, 1889); *N.Y. Times*, July 9, 1889; S. H. Pennington, "Stephen Wickes, M.D.," *Trans., Med. Soc. N.J.* (1890): 335-39; Stephen Wickes, *Thomas Weekes Emigrant to America and the Lineage of His Descendant Thomas Wickes of Huntington, Long Island* (1904), 58-59.

W. Barlow

WIESENTHAL, CHARLES FREDERICK (1726, Prussia-June 1, 1789, Baltimore, Md.). *Physician.* Naturalized in 1771 and soon thereafter married a woman from York, Pa.; one son and two daughters. CAREER: Family tradition suggests he was physician to Frederick the Great (he was at least associated with the Prussian army); 1762, a prominent Lutheran, helped insure the erection of their first church in Baltimore; January 1775, selected member, Committee of Observation of Baltimore County; 1775, superintendent of the manufacture of saltpeter, Baltimore; 1776, medical purveyor, Maryland Troops; 1776, state examining surgeon; March 2, 1776, commissioned surgeon-major, Smallwood's First Maryland Battalion; 1777, Md. troops' surgeon-general; after the Revolution, taught medical students at the hospital and dissecting room he built on his own Baltimore property during the war; September 17, 1784, elected president and physician, German Immigrant Society, Baltimore; December 26, 1788, elected president, Medical Society of Baltimore. CONTRIBUTIONS: Known as "The Sydenham of Baltimore" because of his "rare and singular virtues and his nobility of character." In "Remarks Concerning the Future Treatment of the Sick in Our Troops" (April 10, 1776), called for both a "moving or flying hospital" and a "Fix't Hospital" for troops on and off the front, respectively. As surgeon-general to the Md. troops, established a hospital in Baltimore (the "first medical school in Maryland, a private undertaking, which existed up to the year 1817") that included a dissecting room, which was mobbed (1788) as he and students dissected a murderer's body. A strong proponent of medical reform and regulation to guard against quackery, was a central organizer of the short-lived Medical Society of Baltimore (November 27, 1788). Eleven years later, his then defunct society proved the nucleus for the Medical and Chirurgical Faculty of Maryland. REFERENCES: E. F. Cordell, "Charles Frederick Wiesenthal, Medicinae Practicus, the Father of the Medical Profession of Baltimore," *Johns Hopkins Hosp. Bull.* 11 (Jul.-Aug. 1900): 170-74; idem, "Dr. Charles Frederick Wiesenthal's Medical Reports," ibid., 16, no. 177 (Dec. 1905): 407-9; Dieter Cunz, "Wiesenthal's Pioneer Medical Work," *American-German Review* 9, no. 1 (Oct. 1942): 13-14; Kelly and Burrage (1928), 1300-1301; J. R. Quinan, *Medical Annals of Baltimore. . .* , (1884), 178.

C. Donegan

WIGGERS, CARL JOHN (May 28, 1883, Davenport, Ia.-April 27, 1963, Cleveland, Ohio). *Physician; Physiology; Cardiovascular research.* Son of Jürgen, a farmer, and Anna Margaretha (Kuendel) Wiggers. Married Minerva E. Berry, 1907; two children. EDUCATION: 1906, M.D., University of Michigan; 1912, research under Otto Frank, Ludwig Maximilian University Physiological Institute, Munich, Germany. CAREER: 1905-11, instructor of physiology, University of Michigan; 1911-18, instructor and assistant professor, Cornell University Medical College; 1918, contract surgeon, U.S. Army, General Hospital, Lakewood, N.J.; 1918-53, professor of physiology, Western Reserve University; 1953, professor emeritus. CONTRIBUTIONS: Internationally known cardiologist. Pioneered research in electroshock resuscitation, heart sounds, shock, cardiodynamics of valvular lesions. Devised a training course to teach methods of cardiovascular studies on animals and patients. Editor, *Circulation Research.*

WRITINGS: *Brief Text of Physiology* (1910); *Circulation in Health and Disease* (1915); *Pressure Pulses in the Cardiovascular System* (1928); *Principles and Practice of Electrocardiography* (1929); *Physiology in Health and Disease* (1934); *Physiology of Shock* (1950); *Circulatory Dynamics: Physiologic Studies* (1952). Contributed many articles to medical journals. REFERENCES: *BMNAS* 48 (1976): 363-97; Harold Feil, "Carl Wiggers, M.D. (1883-1963)," *Case Western Reserve Med. Alumni Bull.* 35 (3rd quarter, 1971):

7-9; *NCAB*, 50: 615; Carl J. Wiggers, *Reminiscences and Adventures in Circulation Research* (1958).

G. P. Jenkins

WILBUR, HERVEY BACKUS (August 18, 1820, Wendell, Mass.-May 1, 1883, Syracuse, N.Y.). *Physician; Educator.* Son of Hervey, clergyman, and Ann (Toppan) Wilbur. Married Harriet Holden, 1847; Emily Petheram, 1874; six children. EDUCATION: Newburyport (Mass.) High School; 1834-36, Dartmouth College; Amherst College: 1838, A.B.; and 1841, A.M.; 1843, M.D., Berkshire Medical College. CAREER: 1843-51, private practice, Lowell, Dana, and Barre, Mass.; 1848-51, head, Barre School for Idiots; 1851-54, superintendent, New York State School for Idiots, Albany, N.Y.; 1854-83, superintendent, New York State Asylum for Idiots, Syracuse; 1876-83, faculty, Syracuse University; 1872-76, medical faculty, Syracuse College of Medicine; president, National Association for Protection of the Insane and Prevention of Insanity. CONTRIBUTIONS: Established the first school for the retarded in the United States (1848). Pioneered in the treatment, care, and education of the feebleminded and urged the organization and improvement of state institutions for the insane. Founded Custodial Asylum for Adult Idiots and Feeble-Minded Females, Newark, N.Y.

WRITINGS: *Aphasia* (1867); *Report on the Management of the Insane in Great Britain* (1876); *Buildings for the Insane* (1877). REFERENCES: *Alumni Record and General Catalogue of Syracuse University* (1899), 162-63; *Amherst College Biographical Record* (1973), 47; *DAB*, 10, pt. 2: 199-200; *J. of Nervous and Mental Diseases* 10 (1883): 658-62; *Evening Herald* (Syracuse), May 1, 1883; *NCAB*, 10: 450.

D. O. Powell

WILBUR, RAY LYMAN (April 13, 1875, Boonesboro, Ia.-June 26, 1949, Palo Alto, Calif.). *Physician; Educator.* Son of Dwight Locke, lawyer and land developer, and Edna Maria (Lyman) Wilbur. Married Marguerite Blake, 1898; five children. EDUCATION: Leland Stanford Jr. University: 1896, A.B.; and 1897, A.M.; 1899, M.D., Cooper Medical College; 1903, studied at Frankfurt and London; 1909, study in Munich, Germany. CAREER: At Cooper Medical College: 1899-1900, lecturer in physiology; and 1900-1903, assistant professor of physiology; until 1909, practiced medicine, San Francisco, Calif.; at Stanford University: 1909, professor of medicine; 1911, dean of the medical faculty; 1915, named president; and 1943, chancellor; 1929, secretary, U.S. Department of the Interior, named by President Herbert Hoover. CONTRIBUTIONS: Chief, U.S. Food Administration Conservation Division during World War I. Appointed to the AMA Council on Medical Education and Hospitals (1920), serving as chairman (1929-46). President, AMA (1923-24). Chairman, Committee on the Cost of Medical Care (1927-35). President: American Social Hygiene Association, American Academy of Medicine, and California Academy of Medicine. Recognized as a progressive thinker in the fields of education, medicine, and statesmanship until 1929, but regarded as conspicuously conservative thereafter.

WRITINGS: *The Hoover Policies* (1937, with Arthur M. Hyde); *Human Hopes* (1937); *The March of Medicine* (1938); *Papers on Education, Citizenship, and Social Problems* (1940). Writings listed in *The Memoirs of Ray Lyman Wilbur* (1960). REFERENCES: *DAB*, Supplement 4: 891-95; *NCAB*, 15: 353; E. E. Robinson and P. C. Edwards, eds., *The Memoirs of Ray Lyman Wilbur, 1875-1949* (1960).

Y. V. O'Neill

WILEY, HARVEY WASHINGTON (October 18, 1844, Jefferson County, Ind.-June 30, 1930, Washington, D.C.). *Physician; Educator; Chemist; Reformer*. Son of Preston, farmer and teacher, and Lucinda (Maxwell) Wiley. Married Anna Kelton, 1911; two children. EDUCATION: 1867, A.B., Hanover College; 1871, M.D., Indiana Medical College; 1873, B.S., Harvard; 1878, study of chemistry, physiology, pathology, and food adulteration, Germany. CAREER: At Northwestern Christian University (now Butler University): 1868-71, instructor of Latin and Greek; and 1873-74, professor of chemistry; professor of chemistry: 1873-75, Indiana Medical College; and 1874-83, Purdue University; 1874-1883, Indiana state chemist; 1883-1912, chief chemist, U.S. Department of Agriculture; 1899-1914, professor of agricultural chemistry, George Washington University; 1912-29, director, Bureau of Foods, Sanitation, and Health, *Good Housekeeping* magazine. CONTRIBUTIONS: The "muckraker" responsible for publicizing the scandalous situation in America's drug and food processing industries, resulting in the passage of the Pure Food and Drug Act of 1906.

WRITINGS: Scores of governmental bulletins and scientific papers and the following books: *Foods and Their Adulteration* (1907); *1001 Tests of Foods, Beverages, and Toilet Accessories; Good and Otherwise; Why They Are So* (1914); *Not by Bread Alone: The Principles of Human Nutrition* (1915); *Beverages and Their Adulteration* (1919); *Harvey W. Wiley: An Autobiography* (1930). REFERENCES: O. E. Anderson, *Health of a Nation* (1958); R. E. Bants, *Indiana Authors and Their Books* (1949); *DAB*, 10, pt. 2: 215-16; *DSB*, 14: 357-58; *NCAB*, 21: 72; *Harvey W. Wiley: An Autobiography*.

C.A. Bonsett

WILKERSON, VERNON ALEXANDER (August 21, 1901, Fort Scott, Kans.-May 24, 1968, Washington, D.C.). *Physician; Biochemist*. Married; three children by first wife, none by second wife. EDUCATION: 1921, A.B., University of Kansas; 1925, M.D., University of Iowa; 1925-26, intern, Kansas City Hospital Number 2; 1926-27, house surgeon, Wheatley-Provident Hospital, Kansas City, Mo.; 1929-32, studied biochemistry, University of Minnesota, under General Education Board Fellowship; 1932, Ph.D., University of Minnesota (biochemistry). CAREER: 1927-29, assistant surgeon, Kansas City Hospital No. 2; 1927-29, private practice, Kansas City; 1932-66, biochemistry faculty (chair 1934-48), Howard University Medical School; early 1940s-mid 1960s, private practice, Washington, D.C. CONTRIBUTIONS: Built biochemistry department at

Howard (1932-48). Recognized as excellent teacher of biochemistry (1932-66). Performed research on chemistry of embryonic growth, chemistry of human skin, and proteins in body fluids (1932-46). Provided medical care to black ghetto residents of Washington, D.C. (1940s-60s).

WRITINGS: Several, including "Chemistry of Human Epidermis: Amino Acid Content of Stratum Corneum and Its Comparison with Other Human Keratins," *J. Biol. Chem.* 107 (1934): 377-81; "The Chemistry of the Human Skin, III. The Occurrence of Methionine in Human Skin," ibid., 23 (1939): 165-70. Writings listed in *JNMA* 60 (1968): 345. REFERENCES: Obituary, *JNMA* 60 (1968): 344-45.

T. L. Savitt

WILLIAMS, DANIEL HALE (January 18, 1858, Hollidaysburg, Pa.-August 4, 1931, Idlewild, Mich.). *Surgeon; Hospital administrator.* Son of Daniel, Jr., in real estate, and Sarah (Price) Williams. Married Alice D. Johnson, 1898; no children. EDUCATION: 1877, classical academy, Janesville, Wis.; 1878-80, apprentice to Dr. Henry Palmer, Janesville; 1883, M.D., Chicago Medical College; 1883-84, intern, Mercy Hospital, Chicago, Ill. CAREER: 1884-94, 1898-1912, practice of medicine and surgery, Chicago; 1885-89, demonstrator of anatomy, Northwestern University School of Medicine; surgeon: 1884-91, South Side (Chicago) Dispensary; and 1891-93, 1898-1912, Provident Hospital, Chicago; 1893-98, surgeon-in-chief, Freedmen's Hospital, Washington, D.C.; 1900-1906, attending surgeon, Cook County Hospital, Chicago; 1907-31, associate attending surgeon, St. Luke's Hospital, Chicago. CONTRIBUTIONS: Outstanding Negro physician and medical scientist. Founder, Provident Hospital (1891), first hospital in the United States operated by blacks. Founded training school association (for nurses). Established internship program, Freedmen's Hospital, that became important source of postgraduate training for black physicians. Promoted medical education for blacks by many trips and educational programs. Pioneer in suturing spleen (1904) and pericardium (1897). Inaugurated annual surgical teaching clinics at Meharry (1899). Opened surgery rooms of Freedmen's Hospital to the public to demonstrate skill of Negro surgeons (1890s). First black physician to serve on faculty of medical school other than Meharry or Howard. Charter member, American College of Surgeons, and the only black member for years (1913). A founder, National Medical Association, and first vice-president. Had a profound influence on black medicine and black physicians of his time.

WRITINGS: "Penetrating Wounds of the Chest, Perforating the Diaphragm and Involving the Abdominal Viscera; Case of Successful Spleen Suture for Traumatic Haemorrhage," *Annals of Surg.* 40 (1904): 675-85; "Stab Wound of the Heart and Pericardium—Suture of the Pericardium—Recovery—Patient Alive Three Years Afterward," *Med. Record* (N.Y.) 51 (1897): 437-39; "Ovarian Cysts in Colored Women. . .," *Chicago Med. Record* 20 (1901): 47-57. Writings listed in Helen Buckler, *Daniel Hale*

Williams: Negro Surgeon (1968), 366-68. REFERENCES: Buckler, *Daniel Hale Williams*; *Chest* 60 (1971): 175-82; W. Montague Cobb, in *JNMA* 45 (1953): 379-85; *DAB* 10, pt. 2: 252-53.

W. K. Beatty

WILLIAMS, ELKANAH (December 19, 1822, Lawrence County, Ind.-October 5, 1888, Hazlewood, Pa.). *Physician; Ophthalmology.* Son of Isaac, farmer and pioneer settler in Ind., and Amelia (Gibson) Williams. Married Sarah L. Farmer (d. 1851), December 1847, two children; Sally B. McGrew, April 7, 1857, no children. EDUCATION: Bedford Academy, Bedford, Ind.; 1847, A.B., Indiana Asbury University (now DePauw); studied medicine with Dr. Isaac Denson, Bedford, Ind.; 1850, M.D., University of Louisville, also private student of Dr. T. G. Richardson; 1851, attended third course of lectures, University of Louisville, with Professor S. D. Gross (q.v.); 1852-53, 18 months' study, Paris, London, Prague, Vienna, and Berlin. CAREER: 1850-52, practiced medicine, Bedford; 1852, moved to Cincinnati before going to Europe for further training; 1855, returned to Cincinnati and opened a practice devoted solely to diseases of the eye; founded a charitable clinic for eye care attached to Miami Medical College, where he was also clinical lecturer on diseases of ear and eye; during Civil War, was assistant surgeon, U.S. Marine Hospital, Cincinnati, Ohio; 1865, appointed professor of ophthalmology, Miami Medical College, the first chair of this specialty in the United States; 1862-73, served on the staff of Cincinnati Hospital; 1867-73, editor, *Lancet and Observer*, Cincinnati; elected president: 1875, Ohio Medical Society; 1876, International Ophthalmological Congress, N.Y.; and American Ophthalmological Society. CONTRIBUTIONS: One of the first Americans to specialize in diseases of the eye. Helped to introduce the ophthalmoscope to American physicians and, through his teaching, furthered the trend to specialize in ophthalmology. A founder, Cincinnati Academy of Medicine.

WRITINGS: Published nearly 50 articles on ophthalmology, mostly in the *Lancet and Observer* (Cincinnati). "The Ophthalmoscope," *London Med. Times and Gazette*, July 1, 1854, and July 8, 1854; "Injuries and Diseases of the Eyes and Their Appendages," in *Internat. Encyclopedia of Surg.* 5 (1884). REFERENCES: *DAB*, 10, pt.2: 258-59; Kelly and Burrage (1920); *NCAB*, 3: 524; Richard F. Stone, *Biog. of Eminent Am. Physicians and Surgeons* (1894).

M. H. Dawson

WILLIAMS, FRANCIS HENRY (April 15, 1852, Uxbridge, Mass.-June 22, 1936, Boston, Mass.). *Physician; Roentgenology.* Son of Henry Willard, physician (q.v.), and Elizabeth (Dewé) Williams. Married Anna Dunn Phillips, 1891; no children. EDUCATION: 1873, B.S., Massachusetts Institute of Technology; 1877, M.D., Harvard University; 1877-79, studied in Europe. CAREER: 1874, assistant member, U.S. Transit of Venus Expedition to Japan; *post* 1879, practiced medicine, Boston; 1884-91, materia medica and therapeutics faculty,

Harvard Medical School; *post* 1896, medical staff, Boston City Hospital. CON-
TRIBUTIONS: Showed the importance of X-rays for medicine; used them to detect
enlargement of the heart, diagnose early cases of pulmonary tuberculosis, locate
foreign bodies in the eye, and treat skin cancer; summarized findings in *The
Roentgen Rays in Medicine and Surgery, as an Aid in Diagnosis and as a
Therapeutic Agent* (1901) which became a classic in its field. With the physicist
William Rollins, devised instruments that contributed greatly to diagnostic radiology and radium therapy. Was an early experimenter with the therapeutic
uses of beta rays from radium, especially in cases of diseased tonsils and diseases
of the eye (*post* 1904). First Boston physician to make bacteriological investigations in suspected cases of diphtheria (1892) and first to use diphtheria antitoxin
(1894).

WRITINGS: *Radium Treatment of Skin Diseases, New Growths, Diseases of the Eyes,
and Tonsils* (1935). REFERENCES: *DAB*, Supplement 2: 717-18; *NCAB*, 32: 411; Charles
Snyder, "The Williams Brothers and the Roentgen Ray," *Arch. Ophthal.* 73 (1965):
749-52; *Who Was Who in Am.*, 1: 1351; Murray Watnick, "The Seventy-Fifth Anniversary
of Francis Henry Williams' Clinical Application of the X-Ray," *Rhode Island Med. J.*
54 (1971): 422-23, 432.

S. Galishoff

WILLIAMS, HENRY WILLARD (December 11, 1821, Boston, Mass.-June
13, 1895, Boston). *Ophthalmologist*. Son of Willard and Elizabeth (Osgood)
Williams. Married Elizabeth Dewé, 1848; Elizabeth Adeline Low, 1860; at least
six children. EDUCATION: Attended Boston Latin School and Salem Latin School;
1845-46, attended Harvard Medical School; 1847-49, study in Europe, became
interested in new specialty of ophthalmology; 1849, M.D., Harvard Medical
School; 1850, private practice in Boston; 1866-71, lecturer in ophthalmology,
Harvard Medical School; 1871, first professor of ophthalmology, Harvard Medical School; 1864-91, ophthalmologic surgeon, Boston City Hospital. CONTRI-
BUTIONS: A pioneering ophthalmologist. A founder of the American
Ophthalmological Society (1864) and its president (1868-75). Contributed to the
knowledge of the specialty by writing on operations for cataract, the use of
anesthetic in eye surgery, and the use of atropine as a treatment for iritis. Among
the first in the U.S. to recognize the value of the ophthalmoscope (invented in
1851 by Hermann von Helmholtz). President of the Mass. Medical Society,
1880-82.

WRITINGS: *A Practical Guide to the Study of the Diseases of the Eye* (1862); *Our
Eyes, and How to Take Care of Them* (1871); *The Diagnosis and Treatment of the Diseases
of the Eye* (1881). REFERENCES: *Boston Med. and Surg. J.*, June 27, 1895; *DAB*, 10,
pt. 2: 265-66; Kelly and Burrage (1920).

M. Kaufman

WILLIAMS, JOHN WHITRIDGE (January 26, 1866, Baltimore, Md.-Oc-
tober 21, 1931, Baltimore). *Physician; Obstetrics; Medical education*. Son of
Philip C., physician, and Mary Cushing (Whitridge) Williams. Married Mar-

garetta Stewart Brown, 1891; three children; Caroline (Theobold) Pennington, 1930. EDUCATION: Baltimore City College; 1886, A.B., Johns Hopkins University; 1888, M.D., University of Maryland; 1887-89, studied, Vienna and Berlin; 1889-96, resident in gynecology, Johns Hopkins Hospital. CAREER: At Johns Hopkins University School of Medicine: 1896-99, associate professor of obstetrics; 1899-1931, professor of obstetrics; and 1911-23, dean. CONTRIBUTIONS: Helped establish obstetrics as an academic discipline in America with scientific writings, textbook (1903), and many leaders in the specialty whom he trained. Played an important role in the development of prenatal care and the founding of the American Association for Study and Prevention of Infant Mortality. As dean, Johns Hopkins, led the development of the full-time system for medical faculty.

WRITINGS: *Obstetrics: A Textbook for the Use of Students and Practitioners*, 6 eds. (1903). Writings listed in J. Morris Slemons, *John Whitridge Williams, Academic Aspects and Bibliography* (1935). REFERENCES: *DAB*, 10: 280; Alan F. Guttmacher, "Recollections of John Whitridge Williams," *Bull. Hist. Med.* 3 (1935): 19-30; Howard A. Kelly, "John Whitridge Williams (1866-1931)," *Am. J. Surg.* 15 (1932): 169-74; Lawrence D. Longo, "John Whitridge Williams and Academic Obstetrics in America," *Trans. and Studies of the Coll. of Physicians of Phila.*, 5th series, 3 (1981): 221-54; Slemons, *John Whitridge Williams*.

L. D. Longo

WILLIAMS, STEPHEN WEST (March 27, 1790, Deerfield, Mass.-July 6, 1855, Laona, Ill.). *Physician.* Son of William Stoddard, physician, and Mary (Hoyt) Williams. Married Harriet T. Goodhue, 1818; four children. EDUCATION: Apprentice to his father and one term of lectures at the medical school of Columbia College (1812-13). CAREER: 1813-53, general practice, Deerfield. CONTRIBUTIONS: Published the second major biographical study of American physicians (1844), thereby continuing the pioneering work of James Thacher (q.v.). Lectured on medical jurisprudence at several medical schools (1823-31). Wrote a history of the medical practices in Franklin County (Mass.) and served as the first president, Franklin County Medical Society (1851).

WRITINGS: *A Catechism of Medical Jurisprudence* (1835); *American Medical Biography* (1844). REFERENCES: Whitfield J. Bell, Jr., "Lives in Medicine: The Biographical Dictionaries of Thacher, Williams, and Gross," *Bull. Hist. Med.* 42 (1968): 101-20; *DAB*, 10, pt. 2: 291; *NCAB*, 1: 182.

C. Burns

WILLIAMS, WILLIAM CARLOS (September 17, 1883, Rutherford, N.J.-March 4, 1963, Rutherford). *Physician; Poet; Author.* Son of William George, water company employee, and Raquel Helene (Hoheb) Williams, Puerto Rican artist. Married Florence Herman; two sons. EDUCATION: Attended public schools in Rutherford; 1897-99, Chateau de Lancy (near Geneva, Switzerland) and Lycee Condorcet (in Paris); 1899-1902, Horace Mann High School, New York City; 1902-6, University of Pennsylvania Medical School, M.D., 1906; 1906-9, intern at French Hospital and at the Nursery and Child's Hospital, New York City; 1909-10, postgraduate study at the University of Leipzig. CAREER: 1910, medical practice, Rutherford; 1920, appointed as medical inspector of schools; 1924, appointed to the medical staff of Passaic General Hospital. CONTRIBUTIONS: Well-known American poet and author of the early 20th century. Some writings had a medical theme as in the novel *A Voyage to Pagany* (1928) which described an American physician's response to the cultural life of Europe, and his epic poem *Paterson* (1946-58) which focused on the search of a physician-poet for meaning in the history of his environment. During McCarthy period, was accused of being a Communist sympathizer but was cleared of all charges in 1953. Received the first National Book Award for poetry (1950) and the Pulitzer Prize in poetry (1963, posthumously).

WRITINGS: Listed in Emily M. Wallace, *A Bibliography of William Carlos Williams* (1968). REFERENCES: James E. Breslin, *William Carlos Williams: An American Artist* (1970); *DAB*, supp. 7: 788-91; Reed Whittemore, *William Carlos Williams: Poet from Jersey* (1975).

M. Kaufman

WILSON, FRANK NORMAN (November 19, 1890, Livonia, Mich.-September 11, 1952, Stockbridge, Mich.). *Physician; Cardiology.* Son of Norman Orlando, farmer, and Mary (Holtz) Wilson. Married Juel A. Mahoney, 1913; one child. EDUCATION: University of Michigan: 1911, B.S.; 1913, M.D.; and 1913-14, intern. CAREER: 1914-16, 1921-52, internal medicine faculty, University of Michigan Medical School; 1917-19, Medical Corps, U.S. Army; 1916-20, medicine faculty, University of Washington Medical School. CONTRIBUTIONS: Inaugurated modern studies of the electrical phenomena of the heart. Made fundamental contributions to the theory of electrocardiography and the interpretation of electrocardiograms. Demonstrated that the common type of bundle branch block was left branch block and the rare type right branch block and not the reverse as was commonly believed. Advanced the diagnosis of myocardial infarction by elucidating the phenomena of normal and abnormal ventricular excitation. Trained students from all over the world in electrocardiography.

WRITINGS: "The Order of Ventricular Excitation in Bundle Branch Block," *Am. Heart J.* 7 (1932): 305-30 (with A. G. MacLeod and P. S. Barker); "The Distribution of the Action Currents Produced by Heart Muscle and Other Excitable Tissues Immersed in Extensive Conducting Media," *J. of General Physiology* 16 (1933): 423-56 (with A. G. MacLeod and P. S. Barker); "The Electrocardiogram in Myocardial Infarction with Particular Reference to the Initial Deflections of the Ventricular Complex," *Heart* 16 (Jun. 1933): 155-99 (with others); "The Precordial Electrocardiogram," *Am. Heart J.* 27 (1944): 19-85 (with others). A bibliography is in Franklin D. Johnston and Eugene Lepeschkin, eds., *Selected Papers of Dr. Frank N. Wilson* (1954). REFERENCES: Thomas M. Durant, "Dr. Frank N. Wilson: A Biographical Sketch," *Trans. and Studies of the Coll. of Physicians of Phila.* 25 (1958): 160-66; George R. Herrmann, "An Appreciation of Frank N. Wilson, M.D.,'' *Am. Heart J.* 40 (1950): 647-49; *Trans., Assoc. of Am. Physicians* 66 (1953): 18-19; *Who Was Who in Am.*, 3: 926.

S. Galishoff

WILSON, LOUIS BLANCHARD (December 22, 1866, Pittsburgh, Pa.-October 5, 1943, Rochester, Minn.). *Physician; Pathology; Medical education.* Son of Henry Harrison and Susan E. Harbach (or Harbaugh) Wilson. Married Mary Elizabeth Stapleton, 1891; Mrs. Anne Maud (Headline) Mellish, 1924; Grace Greenwood McCormick, 1935; two children by first marriage. EDUCATION: 1886, graduated from State Normal School, California, Pa.; 1896, M.D., University of Minnesota. CAREER: Late 1880s, early 1890s, taught science, California, Pa.; Des Moines, Ia.; and St. Paul, Minn.; 1896-1905, practiced medicine, St. Paul; assistant to Frank Westbrook, director, bacteriological laboratory, Minnesota State Board of Health; and pathology and bacteriology faculty, University of Minnesota; 1905-37, director, laboratories for pathologic and bacteriologic studies, Mayo Clinic; 1915-37, first director, Mayo Foundation for Medical Education and Research (later Mayo Graduate School of Medicine), and pathology faculty, Graduate School of the University of Minnesota; during World War I, assistant director, Laboratory Division, American Expeditionary Force, Dijon, France; president: 1931-33, Association of American Medical Colleges; 1934-37, Advisory Board of Medical Specialties. CONTRIBUTIONS: Developed (1905) a frozen-tissue method for rapid and accurate histologic diagnosis to facilitate the immediate laboratory analysis of specimens removed in surgical operations; has been used widely by surgeons ever since then. With Henry S. Plummer and Edward C. Kendall (q.v.), provided a valuable classification of thyroid disease. Made greatest mark in medical education, especially in his capacity as first director (1915-37) of the Mayo Graduate School of Medicine, which he made one of the largest and best institutions of its kind.

WRITINGS: ''A Method for the Rapid Preparation of Fresh Tissues for the Microscope,'' *JAMA* 45 (1905): 1737; ''Graduate Instruction in Medicine,'' *St. Paul Med. J.* 14 (1912): 287-95; ''Staining Sections of Living Tissue, Unfixed,'' *J. Lab. and Clin. Med.* 1 (1915): 40-45; ''The Pathologic Classification of Lesions of the Thyroid Gland,'' *Annals of Clinical Med.* 1 (1922): 44-50. A bibliography is in *Physicians of the Mayo Clinic and the Mayo Foundation* (1937), 1485-91. REFERENCES: *DAB*, Supplement 3: 831-33; *NCAB*, 40: 268; *N.Y. Times*, October 6, 1943; *Who Was Who in Am.*, 2: 584.

S. Galishoff

WINSLOW, CHARLES-EDWARD AMORY (February 4, 1877, Boston, Mass.-January 8, 1957, New Haven, Conn.). *Leader in public health movement.* Son of Erving, merchant and author, and Catherine Mary (Reignolds) Winslow. Married Anne Fuller Rogers, 1907; one daughter. EDUCATION: 1898, B.S., 1899, M.S., Massachusetts Institute of Technology. CAREER: 1902-10, Massachusetts Institute of Technology: 1902-9, sanitary bacteriology faculty; 1903-10, biologist in charge of sanitary research laboratory; 1910, bacteriology faculty, University of Chicago; 1910-14, associate professor of biology, New York City College;

1910-22, curator of public health, American Museum of Natural History; 1914-15, director, Bureau of Public Health Education, New York State Health Department; 1915-45, Anna M. R. Lauder Professor of Public Health and chairman of department, Yale Medical School; 1932-57, director, John B. Pierce Laboratory of Hygiene. CONTRIBUTIONS: Published the first American textbook on the elements of water bacteriology (with Professor Samuel C. Prescott [q.v.]). Took an active part in the founding of the *Journal of Bacteriology* and was its first editor (1916-44). Founded the Yale Department of Public Health (1915), serving as department chairman until retirement (1945). Expert health assessor, Health Committee, League of Nations (1927-30). Later played a leading part in the league's Committee on the Hygiene of Housing. President, American Public Health Association (1926). Editor, *American Journal of Public Health* (1944-54), contributing more than 430 editorials and eight manuscripts. Played a leading role in the founding of the Yale School of Nursing (1923), placing great emphasis on public health nursing. Chairman, first national committee to study and make recommendations for the improvement of the education of nurses (1918); work resulting in the famous Winslow-Goldmark report. Chairman of the board, New Haven Demonstration Health Center (1919-23), which clearly established the effectiveness of generalized public health nursing. Helped organize the Committee on the Costs of Medical Care (1926) and guided its survey work.

WRITINGS: *The Evolution and Significance of the Modern Public Health Campaign* (1923); *The Conquest of Epidemic Disease* (1943); *The Cost of Sickness and the Price of Health* (1951). A yearly listing of writings for 1896-1945 is in the *Yale J. of Biol. & Med.* 19 (1947): 779-800. REFERENCES: Reginald M. Atwater, M.D., Dr.P.H., F.A.P.H.A., "C.-E. A. Winslow: An Appreciation of a Great Statesman," *Am. J. of Public Health* 47 (Sept. 1957): 1065-70; bibliography, *Yale J. of Biol. & Med.* 19 (1947): 779-800; *British Med. J.* 1 (Feb. 9, 1957): 345; *DAB*, Supplement 6: 701-3; Haven Emerson et al., "Charles-Edward Amory Winslow, February 4, 1877-January 8, 1957, A Memorial," *Am. J. of Public Health* 47 (Feb. 1957): 153-67; John F. Fulton, "C. E. A. Winslow, Leader in Public Health," *Sci.* 125 (Jan.-Jun. 1957): 1236; Ira V. Hiscock, "Charles-Edward Amory Winslow, February 4, 1877-January 8, 1957," *J. of Bacteriology* 73 (Jan.-Jun. 1957): 295-96; *NCAB*, D: 443.

                                                                                                      J. W. Ifkovic

WINTERNITZ, MILTON CHARLES (February 19, 1885, Baltimore, Md.-October 3, 1959, Havover, N.H.). *Physician; Pathology*. Son of L. Carl, physician, and Jennie (Kittner) Winternitz. Married Helen Watson, 1913; five children; Pauline Webster Whitney, 1932. EDUCATION: 1903, A.B., Johns Hopkins University; 1907, M.D., Johns Hopkins Medical School. CAREER: 1907-17, fellow, assistant instructor, and associate professor of pathology, Johns Hopkins Medical School; 1910-13, assistant resident pathologist, Johns Hopkins Hospital; at Yale Medical School: 1913-17, associate pathologist; 1917-20, professor of pathology and bacteriology; 1920-35, dean; 1935-50, professor of pathology; and 1950-59, professor emeritus. CONTRIBUTIONS: Helped to develop the Yale Medical School to its present eminence. Appointed outstanding faculty, partly by raising the funds necessary for the chairs in internal medicine, surgery, and pediatrics. Introduced the "full-time" system in clinical departments. The Yale Plan of medical education was established, which included opportunity for elective study and the experience of a close association in the laboratory with members of the faculty in the preparation of a thesis. Introduced the system of cutting horizontally across individual departmental lines. A successful example was the Neurological Study Unit, which involved the Departments of Anatomy, Physiology, Pathology, Internal Medicine, and Surgery. Introduced a building program appropriate to the rebirth of the medical school. Most challenging idea was that of the Institute of Human Relations, founded on the ideal that medicine should deal with the whole person in his social and economic environment. On its board were lawyers, physicians, clergymen, sociologists, psychiatrists, and psychologists. An Oral Pathology Unit was also organized at the Medical School to relate the problems of the dentist and physician. Encouraged the founding of the School of Nursing (1923). In World War I, served as chief of pathology, Chemical Warfare Research Laboratory, Army Medical Reserve Corps, and compiled an important work on the pathology of war gas poisoning. During World War II, directed a series of important studies on the pathology of shock. Chairman, National Research Council's Committee on Treatment of Gas Casualties, and was largely instrumental in securing appropriations for the Medical Research Laboratory, Edgewood Arsenal, Md., and in organizing a coordinating center for information dealing with chemical agents in insect and rodent control. After the war, remained active in the National Research Council.

WRITINGS: *The Pathology of Influenza* (1920); *The Pathology of War Gas Poisoning* (1920); *The Biology of Arteriosclerosis*, (1938, with Robert M. Thomas and Philip Le Compte). A full bibliography is in the *Yale J. of Biol. & Med.* 32 (Dec. 1959): 165-71. REFERENCES: Averill A. Liebrow and Levin L. Waters, "Milton Charles Winternitz, February 19, 1885-October 3, 1959," *Yale J. of Biol. & Med.* 32 (Dec. 1959): 143-64; Robert E. Mellors, M.D., "M. C. Winternitz, M.D. (1885-1959)," *Cancer* 13 (1961): 4; *N.Y. Times*, October 4, 1959; John R. Paul, "Dean Winternitz and the Rebirth of the Yale Medical School in the 1920's," *Yale J. of Biol. & Med.* 43 (Oct. 1970): 110-19; *Who Was Who in Am.*, 3: 931.

J. W. Ifkovic

WISHARD, WILLIAM NILES (October 10, 1851, Greenwood, Ind.-January 22, 1941, Indianapolis, Ind.). *Surgeon; Administrator; Educator.* Son of William, physician, and Harriet (Moreland) Wishard. Married Alice Woolen, 1880; Frances Scoville, 1896, five children. EDUCATION: Southport, Ind., public schools; 1870-72, Wabash College, Ind.; 1874, M.D., Indiana Medical College; 1876, M.D., Miami Medical College; 1887-90, postgraduate study, Chicago, Ill.; New York, N.Y.; London, England; and Berlin, Germany. CAREER: 1874-75, practice of medicine with his father, Southport, Ind.; 1876-79, general practice, Indianapolis, and deputy coroner; 1879-87, superintendent, Indianapolis City Hospital; 1887-90, general practice; at Medical College of Indiana: 1883, appointed to the chair of general medicine; and 1887-1936, professor and head, Department of Genito-Urinary Surgery. CONTRIBUTIONS: As superintendent, Indianapolis City Hospital, established the first training school for nurses in Ind. and pursued an active construction campaign. Developed a rubber catheter bearing his name, as well as other specialized catheters and numerous instruments for genito-urinary (G-U) surgery. Author of the Medical Practice Act in Ind., passed 1897. One of the first surgeons to perform perineal prostatectomy, first to apply cautery under visual observation for reduction of enlarged prostate (1890). Author of numerous articles on G-U surgery. President: Indianapolis Surgical Society (1890), Mississippi Valley Medical Association (1895), Indiana State Medical Association (1898), and American Urological Association (1905). Surgeon-general, Indiana National Guard (1890-92). Member, Indiana State Board of Health (1900-1911; chairman at time of resignation).

WRITINGS: See *J. of the Indiana State Med. Assoc.* 34 (1941). REFERENCES: *J. of the Indiana State Med. Assoc.* 34 (1941); *NCAB*, F: 540; 30: 5.

C. A. Bonsett

WISTAR, CASPAR (September 13, 1761, Philadelphia, Pa.-January 22, 1818, Philadelphia). *Physician; Anatomy.* Son of Richard and Sarah (Wyatt) Wistar. Married Isabella Marshall, 1788, no children; Elizabeth Mifflin, three children. EDUCATION: Penn Charter School; apprentice to Dr. John Redman (q.v.); 1782, B.M., University of Pennsylvania; 1783-87, study in Europe; 1786, M.D., University of Edinburgh. CAREER: 1789-92, professor of chemistry, College of Philadelphia; 1793-1808, adjunct professor, University of Pennsylvania; 1808-10, professor of anatomy and midwifery; 1810-18, professor of anatomy; 1793-1810, staff of Pennsylvania Hospital. CONTRIBUTIONS: As an anatomist, published the first American text in the field. Described the correct anatomical relation between the ethmoid and sphenoid bones. Founded a society for the promotion of vaccination (1809). President, American Philosophical Society (1815-18), succeeding Thomas Jefferson in that position. Upon his death, family donated his anatomical collection to the University of Pennsylvania, which became the basis for what later became the Wistar-Horner Museum. Held open houses for members of the American Philosophical Society and visiting dignitaries, and after his death, the "Wistar Parties" continued to be a Philadelphia tradition.

WRITINGS: *System of Anatomy* (1811). REFERENCES: *DAB*, 10, pt. 2: 433-34; *DSB*, 14: 451-57; W. S. Middleton, article in *Annals of Med. Hist.* (1922); *NCAB*, 1: 273.

M. Kaufman

WITHERSPOON, JOHN ALEXANDER (September 13, 1864, Columbia, Maury County, Tenn.-April 28, 1929, Nashville, Tenn.). *Physician; Medical educator.* Son of John McDowell, lawyer and judge, and Mary Talitha (Hanks) Witherspoon. Married Cornelia Dixon, 1888; four children. EDUCATION: W. R.

Moore's School for Boys, Glass, Tenn.; Austin College, Sherman, Tex. (did not graduate due to ill health); read medicine under Dr. Robert Pillow, Columbia, Tenn.; 1887, M.D., University of Pennsylvania; 1895, 1899, 1905, 1909, 1913, postgraduate study, Europe. CAREER: 1887-95, practice of medicine, Columbia, Tenn.; 1895-1929, practice, Nashville; 1888-94, professor of physiology and later professor of medicine, University of Tennessee, Nashville; 1895-1929, professor of medicine and clinical medicine, Vanderbilt University; 1895, called upon by the chancellor of Vanderbilt to assist in the establishment of the Vanderbilt School of Medicine; toured Europe, inspecting medical schools and purchasing equipment; 1904, original member, AMA Council on Medical Education, serving 1904-11; 1910-11, president, Association of American Medical Colleges; 1908-10, founder and first editor, *Journal of the Southern Medical Association*; president: 1909, Mississippi Valley Medical Society and Southern Medical Association; 1910, Tennessee State Medical Association; 1913-14, 65th president, American Medical Association. CONTRIBUTIONS: Skilled in teaching and in obtaining funds from philanthropic organizations; contributed to the excellence of Vanderbilt University School of Medicine.

WRITINGS: Published 19 papers in medical journals, mainly on clinical subjects of medical education. REFERENCES: *DAB*, 10, pt. 2: 438-39; Morris Fishbein, *A History of the American Medical Association* (1947), 724-25; *JAMA* 58 (1912): 1861-62; *ibid.*, 92 (1929): 1538.

S. R. Bruesch

WITTHAUS, RUDOLPH AUGUSTUS (August 30, 1846, New York, N.Y.-December 19, 1915, New York, N.Y.). *Chemist; Toxicologist; Forensic medicine*. Son of Rudolph A. and Marie Antoinette (Dunbar) Witthaus. Married Bly-Ella Faustina (Coles) Ranney, 1882. EDUCATION: Columbia University: A.B., 1867, A.M., 1870; 1867-69, 1873, studied in France; 1871, attended Columbia Law School; 1872-73, attended Bellevue Medical College; 1875, M.D., College of Medicine of the University of the City of New York. CAREER: University of the City of New York: chemistry and physiology faculty, 1876-78; physiological chemistry faculty, 1882-86; chemistry and physics faculty, 1886-98; 1878-1900, chemistry and toxicology faculty, University of Vermont; 1882-88, chemistry and toxicology faculty, University of Buffalo; 1898-1911, chemistry and physics faculty, Cornell University. CONTRIBUTIONS: One of the leading American authorities on toxicology, often called as an expert witness in poisoning cases. Wrote a number of important books on medical chemistry, including *General Medical Chemistry for the Use of Practitioners of Medicine* (1881), *Medical Student's Manual of Chemistry* (1883), and *A Laboratory Guide in Urinalysis and Toxicology* (1886). Was best known for his *Medical Jurisprudence, Forensic Medicine and Toxicology* (4 vols., 1894-96), which he edited with T.C. Becker, and to which he contributed the introduction and the entire fourth volume.

REFERENCES: *DAB*, 20: 439; Kelly and Burrage (1928), 1320-21; *NCAB*, 11: 60-61; *Who Was Who in Am.*, 1: 1371.

S. Galishoff

WOLBACH, SIMEON BURT (July 3, 1880, Grand Island, Nebr.-March 19, 1954, Sudbury, Mass.). *Physician; Pathology.* Son of Samuel N., banker and merchant, and Rosa (Stein) Wolbach. Married Anna F. Wellington, 1914; three children. EDUCATION: 1897-99, studied at the Lawrence Scientific School, Harvard University; 1903, M.D., Harvard Medical School; 1903-5, assistant pathologist to Frank B. Mallory (q.v.) and William T. Councilman (q.v.), Boston City Hospital. CAREER: 1905-8, assistant instructor in pathology, Harvard Medical School; 1908-9, faculty, Albany Medical College; and director, Bender Hygienic Laboratory, Albany, N.Y.; 1909-10, lecturer and director of histology laboratory, McGill University; 1910-22, assistant and associate professor of pathology and bacteriology, Harvard Medical School; 1922-47, Shattuck Professor of Pathological Anatomy, Harvard Medical School, (emeritus 1947-54); pathologist-in-chief: 1917-47, Peter Bent Brigham Hospital; and 1915-47, The Children's and Infant's Hospital; 1947-54, director, Division of Nutrition Research, The Children's Hospital, Boston, Mass., and consultant in pathology, Boston Lying-In Hospital, Free Hospital for Women, and Long Island Hospital, Boston Harbor, Mass.; 1951-53, consultant, Atomic Energy Commission.CONTRIBUTIONS: Conducted pioneer research on pathological histology of chronic X-ray dermatitis and early X-ray carcinoma. Identified the causative agent, described the pathological anatomy, and elucidated the role of the tick as biological transmitter of Rocky Mountain spotted fever. Important studies in Gambia of trypanosomiasis (1911). On commission sent by the League of Red Cross Societies to study typhus in Poland; isolated the etiological agent and elucidated the sequence by which lesions appear in typhus (1920). Shifted from studies of rickettsial diseases (*post* 1925) to important studies of specific structural alterations induced by vitamin A and C deficiencies; stressed the value of experimentally induced avitaminosis as a biological research method.

WRITINGS: List of 112 publications in Wolbach's faculty file, Harvard Medical School Archives, Countway Library, Boston, Mass. REFERENCES: Walter B. Cannon, "Foreword," *Arch. Path.* 30 (1940): 1-6; Sidney Farber and Charlotte L. Maddock, "S. Burt Wolbach," ibid., 59 (1955): 624-39; Charles A. Janeway, "S. Burt Wolbach," *Trans., Assoc. of Am. Physicians* 67 (1954): 30-35; Charlotte L. Maddock and Arthur T. Hertig, "S. Burt Wolbach, MD," *Harvard Med. Alumni Bull.* 28 (1954): 41-45; *NCAB*, 46: 274.

J. H. Warner

WOLCOTT, ERASTUS BRADLEY (October 18, 1804, in Benton, Yates County, N.Y.-January 5, 1880, Milwaukee, Wis.). *Physician; Surgery.* Son of Elisha and Anna (Hull) Wolcott. Married Elizabeth Jane Dousman, 1836 (d. 1860), five children; Laura J. Ross, no children. EDUCATION: Public schools,

Yates County, N.Y.; Fairfield Medical College, Fairfield, N.Y.; 1822-25, studied medicine and surgery with Dr. Joshua Lee, surgeon, Ontario, Canada; 1825, diploma, Yates County Medical Society; 1833, M.D., College of Physicians and Surgeons of Western New York. CAREER: After receiving diploma from Yates County Medical Society, worked as surgeon for mining company in N.C. and in private practice, Charleston, S.C., to finance further medical education; after receiving medical degree, enlisted in U.S. Army; 1836, appointed surgeon, Fort Mackinac, Wis.; 1838 or 1839, resigned commission and moved to Milwaukee, where he practiced medicine for 40 years; 1842, appointed surgeon, Wisconsin State Militia; 1846, commissioned as colonel, Regiment of the State Militia; and promoted to major-general, First Division, Wisconsin State Militia; 1850, appointed by governor to the Board of Regents, University of Wisconsin; 1860, appointed surgeon-general, Wis., and held post through the Civil War; he and staff served in the war, wherever Wis. units saw action; 1866, appointed by U.S. Congress to head National Home for Disabled Volunteer Soldiers which he had lobbied to have located in Milwaukee; later in life, was involved in some of the earliest industrial enterprises in Wis.; served on the Board of Trustees, Wisconsin Hospital for the Insane. CONTRIBUTIONS: Not only a busy private practitioner but devoted considerable time during career to public service. For extending consultations and surgical assistance to homeopathic physicians, was barred from most professional societies. As surgeon-general, Wis., helped organize the state's medical service. One of first surgeons to remove the kidney. Never published about the procedure but work was cited in many German works and in the *Philadelphia Medical Reporter*. REFERENCES: Kelly and Burrage (1920), 1253-54; *NCAB*, 16: 24-25; C. L. Stoddard, *Phila. Med. Reporter* 12 (1861-62): 126.

M. H. Dawson

WOLCOTT, LAURA J. (ROSS) (July 16, 1826, Shapleigh, Maine-December 8, 1915, Ravenswood, Ill.). *Physician*. Daughter of James and Lovey (Huntress) Ross. Married Erastus B. Wolcott (q.v.), physician, 1869; no children. EDUCATION: Horace Mann Normal School, Lexington, Mass.; private student of Harvard science professors; 1856, M.D., Woman's Medical College of Pennsylvania; periodically studied in Europe. CAREER: 1857-90, private practice of medicine, Milwaukee, Wis.; consulting physician, Milwaukee institutions, including Industrial School of Girls, Convent of Notre Dame, St. Mary's Hospital, Passavant Hospital, Milwaukee Orphan Asylum, St. John's Home for Aged Women, County Poorhouse and Jail (women's physician). CONTRIBUTIONS: Waged a long battle for admission to the City Medical Society, which she won (1869) and which led to her commitment to the women's suffrage movement. Specialized in the treatment of women and children. Upon marriage to a physician who had defended her right to membership in the City Medical Society, merged practice with his. After his death, gradually gave up practice and became involved in the suffrage movement. One of the first women to practice medicine in Milwaukee and Wis. REFERENCES: *Dict. of Wisconsin Biog. (1960)*, 379-80; L. F. Frank, *Medical*

Hist. of Milwaukee (1915), 35-36; Dennis H. Phillips, "Women in 19th Century Wisconsin Medicine," *Wisconsin Med. J.* 71 (1972): 13-18; Works Progress Administration biography, Archives Division, State Historical Society of Wisconsin, Madison, Wis.

E. B. Keeney

WOLLSTEIN, MARTHA (November 21, 1868, New York, N.Y.-September 30, 1939, New York). *Pathologist; Medical researcher.* Little is known of her family except that parents were born in Germany. Never married. EDUCATION: 1889, M.D., Woman's Medical College of the New York Infirmary; 1890, intern, Babies Hospital, New York City. CAREER: 1892, appointed pathologist, Babies Hospital; 1906, assistant, Rockefeller Institute (under Simon Flexner [q.v.]); 1921-retirement in 1935, devoted to pediatric pathology, Babies Hospital; 1923, appointed head of Pediatric Section, New York Academy of Medicine. CONTRIBUTIONS: Major contributions (1903) on the subject of infant diarrhea. With Simon Flexner, completed the first experimental analysis of polio in the United States (1907). Worked closely with Samuel Meltzer (q.v.) in an experimental study of pneumonia (1910). In collaboration with Harold Amoss, developed a new method (1918) for the rapid preparation of antimeningitis serum and also devised criteria for the standardization of such sera. Attempted to extend Charles Nicolle's research on mumps (1918). First scientist, Rockefeller Institute, to recognize the importance of the bacteriophage discovered by Felix d'Herell. Began classifying different varieties of phage (1920). First woman member, American Pediatric Society (1930). Greatest contributions were in the field of pediatric pathology. Careful pathological studies improved the diagnostic skills of generations of physicians who worked with her at Babies Hospital.

WRITINGS: Wrote one of the first accounts of women's medical education in the United States, "The History of Women in Medicine," *Woman's Med. J.* (Apr. 1908). "The Development of Experimental Pneumonia under Direct Observation of the Lungs in the Living Animal," *Proc., Soc. for Experimental Biol. & Med.* 10 (1913, with S. J. Meltzer); "A Biological Study of the Cerebro-spinal Fluid in Anterior Poliomyelitis," *J. of Experimental Med.* (Jul. 8, 1948). REFERENCES: *Am. Men of Sci.*, 6th ed. (1938); Kate Campbell Hurd-Mead, *Medical Women of America* (1933); *Notable Am. Women, 1607-1950* (1971).

V. Drachman

WOOD, CASEY ALBERT (November 21, 1856, Wellington, Ontario, Canada-January 26, 1942, La Jolla, Calif.). *Physician; Ophthalmology; Ornithology; Bibliophile.* Son of Orrin Cottier, physician, and Rosa Sophia (Leggo) Wood. Married Emma Shearer, October 28, 1886; no children. EDUCATION: 1874, graduated with honors, Ottawa Collegiate Institute; 1877, master of surgery and M.D., University of Bishop's College, Montreal, Quebec, Canada (later merged with McGill University); 1886, training at New York Eye and Ear Infirmary and Post-Graduate School; 1888-89, studied in Berlin, Paris, and Vienna; and two years as clinical assistant, Royal London Ophthalmic Hospital (Moorfields). CAREER: 1877, after graduation, practiced medicine, Montreal, while serving as professor of pathology and chemistry, University of Bishop's College, and attending physician, Western Hospital; 1890, returned from Europe to Chicago, Ill., where he set up practice and worked on staffs of several Chicago hospitals (Cook County, Alexian Brothers, Passavant Memorial, and Post-Graduate Medical School); 1890-99, professor of clinical ophthalmology, Chicago Post-Graduate Medical School; editor: 1896-98, *Annals of Ophthalmology*; and 1897-1918, *Ophthalmic Record*; 1898, elected chairman, Ophthalmology Section, AMA; 1899-1906, 1913-17, professor of clinical ophthalmology, University of Illinois; 1906-8, professor of clinical ophthalmology, Northwestern University; elected president, American Academy of Ophthalmology and Otolaryngology; 1917-20, served in the U.S. Army Medical Corps in hospitals in Ohio and Wash., where he trained workers for dealing with blind soldiers; 1918, appointed to editorial board, *Annals of Medical History*; devoted last 20 years of life to two hobbies: ornithology (becoming an expert on the sight mechanism of birds and participant in collecting expeditions to British Guiana, India, Ceylon, and the South Pacific) and book-collecting (compiling an extensive library of historical works on ophthalmology and translating several texts into English). CONTRIBUTIONS: An influential and popular teacher and a prominent practitioner. Published numerous works in ophthalmological journals, and translated a number of important works on ophthalmology of historical interest.

WRITINGS: *Lessons in the Diagnosis and Treatment of Eye Diseases* (1891); *The Commoner Diseases of the Eye* (1904); *A System of Ophthalmic Therapeutics* (1909); *A System of Ophthalmic Operations,* 2 vols. (1911); *The American Encyclopedia and Dictionary of Ophthalmology*, 18 vols. (1913-21, editor); *Fundis Oculi of Birds* (1917); numerous articles in professional and popular journals. REFERENCES: *Am. J. of Ophthalmology* (May 1942); *DAB*, Supplement 3: 834-36; *JAMA* (Mar. 21, 1942); *NCAB*, 10: 284; *New England J. of Med.* (Jun. 25,1942); obituaries, *Arch. Ophthal.* (Apr. 1942); *Who Was Who in Am.*, vol. 2.

M. H. Dawson

WOOD, GEORGE BACON (March 13, 1797, Greenwich, N.J.-March 30, 1879, Philadelphia, Pa.). *Physician; Educator; Author; Theory and practice of medicine; Materia medica.* Son of Richard, farmer, and Elizabeth (Bacon) Wood. Married Caroline Hahn, 1823; no children. EDUCATION: Private school, N.Y.; University of Pennsylvania: 1815, A.B., and 1818, M.A., M.D.; office student of Dr. Joseph Parrish (q.v.). CAREER: c. 1818, instructor, Dr. Joseph Parrish's private medical school; at Philadelphia College of Pharmacy: 1821-31, professor of chemistry; and 1831-35, professor of materia medica; 1822-44, attending physician (and sometimes president), Institution for the Deaf and Dumb; 1835-59, attending physician, Pennsylvania Hospital; at University of Pennsylvania: 1835-50, professor of materia medica and therapeutics; and 1850-60, professor of the theory and practice of medicine; 1833-41, member, Board of Trustees, Girard College; 1836-43, vice-president, Philadelphia College of Pharmacy; president: 1848-79, College of Physicians of Philadelphia; 1850, 1860, National

Convention on the Revision of the Pharmacopoeia; 1855-56, American Medical Association; and 1859-79, American Philosophical Society; at University of Pennsylvania: 1863-75, trustee; and 1864-75, chairman, Trustees' Committee on Medical Education; 1876-79, Board of Managers, University of Pennsylvania Hospital. CONTRIBUTIONS: With Franklin Bache (q.v.), played the dominant role in the revision and editing of the *Pharmacopoeia of the United States* from the first (Philadelphia) revision (1831) through the fourth revision (1863). With Bache, compiled the monumental and authoritative *Dispensatory of the United States*. This *Dispensatory*, a continuation of which is still being published, went through 14 editions in Wood's lifetime, became indispensable to both the medical and pharmaceutical professions, and is estimated to have sold between 120,000 and 150,000 copies while Wood was alive. An exceptional lecturer and noted for the introduction of "occular demonstrations" of specimens, models, casts, and drawing in materia medica and pathology lectures. Left substantial endowments to the University of Pennsylvania Medical School, the University Hospital, and the College of Physicians of Philadelphia.

WRITINGS: *The Dispensatory of the United States*, 14 eds. (1833-79, with Franklin Bache); *History of the University of Pennsylvania* (1834); *A Treatise on the Practice of Medicine*, 6 eds. (1847-66); *A Treatise on Therapeutics and Pharmacology, or Materia Medica* (1856, 1860, 1868); *Historical and Biographical Memoirs* (1872). REFERENCES: *DAB*, 10, pt. 2: 458-59; J. W. England, ed., *The First Century of the Philadelphia College of Pharmacy* (1922), 81-83, 397-98; H. Hartshorne, "Memoir of George Wood," *Proc., Am. Philos. Soc.* 19 (1880): 118-52; S. Littell, "Memoir of George Wood," *Trans., Coll. of Physicians of Phila.*, 3rd series, 5 (1881): xxv-lxxvi; *NCAB*, 5: 346; W. S.W. Ruschenberger, *Account of the Institution and Progress of the College of Physicians of Philadelphia* (1887), 275-76; G. Sonnedecker, *Kremers and Urdang's History of Pharmacy*, 4th ed. (1976).

D. L. Cowen

WOOD, HORATIO CHARLES (January 13, 1841, Philadelphia, Pa.-January 3, 1920, Philadelphia). *Physician; Naturalist; Pharmacology; Therapeutics*. Son of Horatio Curtis, successful Philadelphia businessman, and Elizabeth Head (Bacon) Wood. Married Eliza H. Longacre, May 10, 1866; four children. EDUCATION: Westtown Boarding School; Friends Select School in Philadelphia; 1862, M.D., University of Pennsylvania; served residency at Blockley and Pennsylvania hospitals. CAREER: Worked as student, National Academy of Science, which published in its proceedings his first article at age 20; after residency, served in the medical service of the Union army; 1865, started private practice, Philadelphia; 1866-76, chair of botany, auxiliary medical faculty, University of Pennsylvania; 1870-88, consulting physician, Philadelphia, Episcopal, University, and Burn Brae hospitals, Philadelphia; 1871-73, editor, *New Remedies*; at University of Pennsylvania: 1876-1901, clinical professor of nervous diseases; and 1875-1906, professor of materia medica and therapeutics; 1873-83, editor, *Philadelphia Medical Times*; *post* 1883, president, Neurological Society; 1884-90, editor, *Therapeutic Gazette*; 1893, lectured on therapeutics, Harvard University; 1902-4, 1906, poor health required that he resign his academic position; president: 1902-4, College of Physicians and Surgeons of Philadelphia; and 1890-1910, U.S. Pharmacopeial Convention. CONTRIBUTIONS: One of the first Americans to advocate the use of laboratory and animal experiments in testing and classifying drugs. Helped transform pharmacology from the empirical clinical science it had been in the nineteenth century into an experimental science.

WRITINGS: A prolific writer not only of medical works but also in botany and entomology, publishing almost 300 pieces. Most important works include *Thermic Fever and Sunstroke* (1872, won Boylston Prize); *A Treatise on Therapeutics* (1874), which went through 13 editions; "Hyoscine: Its Physiological and Therapeutic Action," *Therapeutic Gazette* 9 (1885): 1-10; *Nervous Diseases and Their Diagnoses* (1887); *The Practice of Medicine* (1897). REFERENCES: Concerning Wood's numerous works, the following article was published, "Bibliographic Record 1860-1911," *Trans. and Studies of the Coll. of Physicians of Phila.*, 3rd series, 42 (1920): 242-57; *DAB*, 10, pt. 2: 459-60; *DSB*, 14: 495-97; Hobart Amory Hare, "Horatio C. Wood, the Pioneer in American Pharmacology," *Therapeutic Gazette* 44 (1920): 322-24; *NCAB*, 13: 569; George B. Roth, "An Early American Pharmacologist: Horatio C. Wood," *Isis* 30 (1939): 37-45.

M. H. Dawson

WOOD, JAMES RUSHMORE (September 14, 1813, Mamaroneck, N.Y.-May 4, 1882, New York, N.Y.). *Physician; Surgery.* Son of Elkanah, miller and leather shop owner, and Mary Rushmore Wood. Married Emma Rowe, 1853; three children. EDUCATION: Friends' Seminary, New York City. Studied medicine with Dr. David L. Rogers, New York City, and Dr. William Tully, New Haven, Conn.; College of Physicians and Surgeons, New York City; 1834, M.D., Castleton Medical College, Vt. CAREER: After graduation, appointed demonstrator of anatomy, Castleton Medical College; 1837, set up private practice, New York City; 1847, appointed to Medical Board, Bellevue Hospital; 1856, donated anatomical collection to New York City commissioner of charities, who used it to found the Wood Museum, Bellevue Hospital; 1861, helped found Bellevue Hospital Medical College, where he was appointed professor of operative surgery and surgical pathology; 1868, became professor emeritus; surgeon, St. Vincent's Hospital and New York Ophthalmic Dispensary; consulting surgeon, New York Academy of Medicine; twice president, New York Pathological Institute. CONTRIBUTIONS: One of America's noted surgeons. Among the first to perform many surgical procedures in treating many nervous, muscle, and bone-related problems. Featured prominently in ameliorating conditions in Bellevue Hospital and the creation of the medical and nursing schools. First American to study the periosteal reproduction of human bones. Influential in the passage of the New York law (1857) permitting the unclaimed bodies of vagrants to be used for anatomical dissection.

WRITINGS: Published several articles in the *New York Journal of Medicine*, and the ones listed below were later reissued as separate monographs. *Spontaneous Dislocation of the Head of the Femur,. . .* (1854); "Ligature of the External Iliac Artery, Followed by Secondary Haemorrhaging," *N.J. J. of Med.* (1856); "Removal of the Entire Lower

Jaw for Necrosis Caused by Phosphoric Acid Gas," ibid. (May 1856); "Early History of the Operation of Ligature of the Primitive Carotoid Artery," ibid. (Jul. 1857). REFERENCES: *DAB*, 10, pt. 2: 463; Fredric S. Dennis, *A Memoir of James R. Wood* (1884); Kelly and Burrage (1920), 1257-58; *NCAB*, 9: 357; Richard Stone, *Biog. Eminent Am. Physicians and Surgeons* (1894), 567.

M. H. Dawson

WOOD, THOMAS FANNING (February 23, 1841, Wilmington, N.C.-August 22, 1892, Wilmington). *Physician; Medical editor; Public health*. Son of Robert B. and Mary A. (?) Wood. EDUCATION: Apprentice to Dr. James H. Dickson, Dr. Thomas, and Dr. McBee or McRee, all of Wilmington; learned about drugs while clerk in an antebellum Wilmington drug store; during early part of Civil War, attended one course of lectures, Medical College of Virginia; 1868, M.D. (hon.), University of Maryland. CAREER: 1861-65, hospital steward and then assistant surgeon, N.C. troops; 1865-92, medical practice, Wilmington; 1878-92, editor, *North Carolina Medical Journal*. CONTRIBUTIONS: Founded (1878) and edited (1878-92) the state's only medical journal, *North Carolina Medical Journal*, a major publishing outlet and source of medical information for N.C. physicians. Known as the father of public health in N.C. for role as promoter, organizer, first secretary, and active member, North Carolina Board of Health (1877-92). Considered by state medical historians to be the most important figure in late nineteenth-century N.C. medicine. Active as member and officer, North Carolina Medical Society. A great publicist of proper health practices. Co-founded and served as vice-president (1891), American Public Health Association.

WRITINGS: Numerous articles and editorials in *N.C. Med. J.* REFERENCES: Dorothy Long, ed., *Medicine in North Carolina* (1972); *NCAB*, 9: 276.

T. L. Savitt

WOOD, WILLIAM BARRY, JR. (May 4, 1910, Milton, Mass.-March 9, 1971, Boston, Mass.). *Physician; Microbiology; Immunology*. Son of William Barry, businessman, and Emily Niles (Lockwood) Wood. Married Mary Lee Hutchins, 1932; five children. EDUCATION: 1932, A.B., Harvard University; 1936, M.D., Johns Hopkins University; 1936-39, medical house officer, Johns Hopkins Hospital; 1939-40, National Research Council fellow in bacteriology, Harvard Medical School. CAREER: 1937-42, medicine faculty, Johns Hopkins Medical School; 1942-55, medicine faculty, Washington University School of Medicine; and medical staff, Barnes Hospital; 1955-59, vice-president, Johns Hopkins University and Hospital; 1955-71, microbiology faculty, Johns Hopkins Medical School; member: 1944-55, Board of Overseers, Harvard College; 1950-62, Armed Forces Epidemiological Board; and 1954-71, Board of Trustees, Rockefeller Foundation; president: 1952, American Society for Clinical Investigation; and 1962-63, Association of American Physicians. CONTRIBUTIONS: Made long-term studies of leucocytes (white blood cells) and the pathogenesis of fever. Described surface phagocytosis, a mechanism by which white blood cells destroy encapsulated bacteria in the absence of antibodies; demonstrated that leucocytes played a primary role in recovery from pneumococcal pneumonia and were not merely scavenger cells that cleaned up after antibodies or other defense mechanisms had overcome the invading microorganisms; illuminated the early (preantibody) phase of acute infection. With others, investigated pyrogen, the hormone that acts on the hypothalamus to produce fever; isolated endogenous (white blood cell) pyrogen, as distinguished from various exogenous substances that produce fever; studied its chemistry and identified the mechanisms which trigger its release.

WRITINGS: "Studies on the Mechanism of Recovery in Pneumococcal Pneumonia. IV. The Mechanism of Phagocytosis in the Absence of Antibody," *J. of Experimental Med.* 84 (1946): 387-402 (with M. R. Smith and B. Watson); chapters on pneumococcal pneumonia and other forms of acute bacterial pneumonia, in *Cecil's Textbook of Medicine* (1951), 100-129; "Studies on the Pathogenesis of Fever. IV. The Leucocytic Origin of Endogenous Pyrogen in Acute Inflammatory Exudates," *J. of Experimental Med.* 107, no. 2 (1958): 279-90 (with M. K. King); *From Miasmas to Molecules* (1961); *Microbiology* (1967, with B. D. Davis, R. Dulbecco, H. Eisen, and H. Ginsberg). A bibliography is in *BMNAS*. REFERENCES: *BMNAS*, 51 (1980): 387-407; *McGraw-Hill Modern Men of Sci.* 2 (1966): 618; *N.Y. Times*, March 10, 1971; R. C. Tilghman, "William Barry Wood, Jr., May 4, 1910-March 9, 1971," *Johns Hopkins Med. J.* 129 (Aug. 1971): 111-20; *Who Was Who in Am.*, 5: 796.

S. Galishoff

WOODWARD, JOSEPH JANVIER (October 30, 1833, Philadelphia, Pa.-August 17, 1884, Wawa, Pa.). *Army medical officer; Pathology.* Son of Joseph Janvier and Elizabeth Graham (Cox) Woodward. Married twice; second marriage to Blanche Wendell; at least one child from first marriage. EDUCATION: 1853, M.D., University of Pennsylvania. CAREER: 1853-61, practiced medicine, Philadelphia; surgical faculty, University of Pennsylvania; in U.S. Army Medical Corps: 1861, assistant surgeon; 1862-65, transferred to Surgeon General's headquarters in Washington, D.C., with duties of planning hospital construction, performing surgery, and keeping medical records; and *post* 1865, assistant to curator, Army Medical Museum; 1870-88, in charge of medical section of *Medical and Surgical History of the War of the Rebellion*; 1881, one of the surgeons who cared for President James A. Garfield following his shooting by the assassin Guiteau; and president, American Medical Association. CONTRIBUTIONS: Perfected the technique of photomicrography which he adapted for investigations of normal and pathological histology. With George Alexander Otis, who was responsible for the surgical section, prepared a six-volume medical and surgical history of the Civil War. Helped establish and organize the Army Medical Museum. Made pioneering microscopial studies of cancer (1858-73).

WRITINGS: *Outlines of the Chief Camp Diseases of the United States Armies. . .*(1863); "On Photomicrography with the Highest Powers, as Practiced in the Army Medical Museum," *Am. J. of Med. Sci.*, n.s., 42 (Sept. 1866): 189; *On the Structure of Cancerous*

Tumors and the Mode in Which Adjacent Parts are Invaded, First Toner Lecture, *Smithsonian Miscellaneous Collections No. 266* (1873); "Typho-Malarial Fever: Is It a Special Type of Fever?" *Trans., International Med. Cong., 1876*, p. 305. A bibliography is in *BMNAS*. REFERENCES: *BHM* (1964-69), 282; (1970-74), 181; *BMNAS*, 2 (1886): 297-307; *DAB*, 20: 509-10; L. D. Heaton and J. M. Blumberg, "Lt. Col. Joseph J. Woodward (1833-1884): U.S. Army Pathologist-Researcher-Photomicroscopist," *Military Med.* 131 (1966): 530-38; Kelly and Burrage (1928), 1332; Miller, *BHM*, p. 148; *NCAB*, 11: 518-19; *Who Was Who in Am.*, Hist. Vol.: 668.

S. Galishoff

WOODWARD, SAMUEL BAYARD (June 10, 1787, Torringford, Conn.-January 3, 1850, Northampton, Mass.). *Physician; Asylum superintendent*. Son of Samuel, physician, and Polly (Griswold) Woodward. Married Maria Porter, 1815; 11 children. EDUCATION: Medical apprentice to his father; 1809, diploma, Connecticut State Medical Society; 1822, M.D. (hon.), Yale College. CAREER: 1810-32, general practice, Wethersfield, Conn.; secretary, state medical society; 1827-32, physician, penitentiary at Wethersfield; examiner, Yale Medical School; 1830, elected to Conn. Senate; planner and founder, Hartford Retreat; 1833-46, superintendent, State Lunatic Hospital, Worcester, Mass. CONTRIBUTIONS: One of the "original 13" founding fathers, Association of Medical Superintendents of American Institutions for the Insane, and its first president (1844). A strong advocate of moral treatment, established a high standard of care in public mental institutions. Under his leadership, the State Lunatic Hospital, Worcester, achieved national recognition and became a model for other state asylums. The hospital regimen included psychological as well as medical methods of treatment, notably, individualized care, recreation, occupational therapy, and the avoidance of harsh restraints. His therapeutics produced a significant recovery rate that was widely publicized.

WRITINGS: The Annual Reports of Worcester State Lunatic Hospital, 1833-45, provide the best source for Woodward's ideas and therapeutics. These reports were circulated nationwide and provided guidelines for other physicians interested in improving the lot of the mentally ill. Writings listed in *BHM* and Gerald N. Grob, "Samuel Woodward and the Practice of Psychiatry in Early Nineteenth-Century America," *Bull. Hist. Med.* 36 (1962). REFERENCES: Leland V. Bell, *Treating the Mentally Ill from Colonial Times to the Present* (1980), 16-18; George Chandler, "Life of Dr. Woodward," *Am. J. of Insanity* 8 (1851): 119-35; *DAB*, 10, pt. 2: 511; Grob, "Samuel Woodward," pp. 420-43; idem, *The State and the Mentally Ill: A History of Worcester State Hospital in Massachusetts, 1830-1920* (1966).

L. V. Bell

WOODWARD, THEODORE (July 17, 1788, Hanover, N.H.-October 10, 1840, Brattleboro, Vt.). Son of Jonathan and Rebecca (Smith) Woodward. *Physician; Surgeon*. Married Mary Armington; six children. EDUCATION: 1810, studied medicine with distant cousin, Dr. Nathan Smith (q.v.), then one of two professors at Dartmouth Medical School; 1810-12, in Poultney, Vt., studying with Dr. Adin Kendrick; 1821, M.D. (hon.), Middlebury; 1821, M.D. (hon.), Harvard. CAREER: 1812-38, medical and surgical practice, Castleton, Vt.; 1818-38, professor, Castleton Medical Academy (later called Vermont Academy of Medicine, Castleton Medical College). CONTRIBUTIONS: After having established himself as a preceptor, founded (1818), with Selah Gridley (q.v.), the Castleton Medical Academy and served that institution as vice-president and professor. A popular and influential teacher for 20 years and the mainstay of the college, which graduated more physicians than any other medical college in New England (1820-61). Had first convulsive seizure (1823). In later years, attacks became more frequent, his mind became affected, and he developed paralysis of legs and was forced to resign (by 1838) professorship and successful practice because of disability.

WRITINGS: Only known writings are a series of newspaper articles replying to Benjamin Lincoln (q.v.), University of Vermont, who attacked him for unfair competition in recruiting of medical students. REFERENCES: *Boston Med. and Surg. J.* 23 (1841): 349-52; Kelly and Burrage (1928): 1333-34; F. C. Waite, *The First Medical College in Vermont* (1949), 61-66.

L. J. Wallman

WOODWORTH, JOHN MAYNARD (August 15, 1837, Big Flats, N.Y.-March 14, 1879, Washington, D.C.). *Physician; Public health administrator.* Married Maggie C. Hannahs, 1873. EDUCATION: 1862, M.D., Chicago Medical College; 1865, studied in Berlin and Vienna. CAREER: In U.S. Army: 1862-63, assistant surgeon; 1863, surgeon; and 1863-65, medical inspector and medical director, Army of the Tennessee; *post* 1866, practiced medicine, Chicago, Ill.; 1866, anatomy faculty, Chicago Medical College; 1868, surgeon, Chicago Soldiers' Home; and sanitary inspector, Chicago Board of Health; 1871-79, supervising surgeon-general, Marine Hospital Service. CONTRIBUTIONS: Reformed the Marine Hospital Service; eliminated politics in the appointment and promotion of its medical officers by requiring that all positions be secured through examination; won acceptance for the pavilion plan of hospital construction; replaced the large stone and iron structures then in use which were expensive to build and hard to keep clean. Instilled order and economy in all of the Service's affairs. Charter member, American Public Health Association (1872). Largely responsible for the National Quarantine Act of 1878.

WRITINGS: *Hospitals and Hospital Construction* (1874); *Cholera Epidemic of 1873 in the United States. . .* (1875); *The Safety of Ships and of Those Who Travel in Them* (1877). REFERENCES: Bess Furman, *A Profile of the United States Public Health Service, 1798-1948* (1973), 121-49; Kelly and Burrage (1928), 1334; Richard Stone, *Biog. Eminent Am. Physicians and Surgeons* (1894), 569-70; *TAMA* 30 (1879): 845-47.

S. Galishoff

WOOTEN, THOMAS DUDLEY (March 6, 1829, Barren County, Ky.-August 1, 1906, Eureka Springs, Ark.). *Physician; Surgeon.* Son of Joseph W. Wooten. Married Henrietta C. Goodall, April 21, 1852; 10 children. EDUCATION:

1853, M.D., University of Louisville. CAREER: 1853-61, medical practice, Tompkinsville, Ky., and Springfield, Mo.; 1861-65, surgeon, Confederate Army; practice: 1865-76, Paris, Tex.; and 1876-1906, Austin, Tex.; 1881-99, member, University of Texas Board of Regents: 1886-95, president; and 1895-99, chairman. CONTRIBUTIONS: Excelled as a leader in the overlapping new areas of local and statewide medicine, education, government, and politics. As president and chairman, Board of Regents, University of Texas, made and explained university policies to officials and the public, procured legislative appropriations, and protected and extended endowed land revenues. Honesty, integrity, and unselfishness permitted the plans for the university, first set out by Ashbel Smith (q.v.), to be carried out.

WRITINGS: *A Plea for the Practical Professions* (1880). REFERENCES: *The Alcade* 2 (Nov. 1913): 1-12; L. E. Daniell, *Types of Successful Men in Texas* (1890): 555-59; *Handbook of Texas* 2 (1952): 934; *JAMA* 47 (Aug. 18, 1906): 528; letters and speeches in the Wooten collection, Barker History Center, University of Texas, Austin; *Texas State J. of Med.* 2 (Sept. 1906): 144; 47 (1951): 266, 309, 311.

J. Morris

WRIGHT, ELIPHALET NOTT (April 3, 1858, near Armstrong Academy, Choctaw Nation, Indian Territory-January 10, 1932, Okla.). *Physician*. Son of Rev. Allen, missionary and Choctaw leader, and Mrs. Harriet (Mitchell) Wright, mission teacher. Married Ida Belle Richards, mission teacher, April 26, 1888; three children. EDUCATION: Spencer Academy, Choctaw Nation; Westminster College, Fulton, Mo.; and Union College, N.Y.; 1884, M.D., Albany Medical College, N.Y.; 1894-95, postgraduate work, College of Physicians and Surgeons, New York City. CAREER: 1896, began medical practice, Boggy Creek, Choctaw Nation, Indian Territory; moved to Atoka, Indian Territory, and following example of father, soon became a leader in Choctaw tribal government. CONTRIBUTIONS: Prepared and furthered a law regulating the practice of medicine in the Choctaw Nation. Was appointed to the first Board of Medical Examiners in the nation and was instrumental in removing many unqualified practitioners from the area. An organizer, Indian Territory Medical Association (1889), and worked to pave the way for the formation of a new organization at the time of Okla. statehood. Active in securing proper compensation for timber and coal taken from Choctaw lands and later for proper compensation from outside commercial interests dealing with the tribe. Named resident delegate in Washington (1908), representing the affairs of the Choctaw Nation, and in that capacity, was the first to retain a reputable law firm to represent the nation in dealings with the U.S. government. Throughout life, continued to practiced medicine. REFERENCES: Virginia Allen, ''Medical Practices and Health in the Choctaw Nation, 1831-1885,'' *Chronicles of Oklahoma* 48, no. 1 (Spring 1970:) 60-73; Angie Debo, *The Rise and Fall of the Choctaw Republic* (1934); ''E. N. Wright'' file, History of Medicine Collection, University of Oklahoma Health Sciences Center Library, Oklahoma City,

Okla.; Muriel H. Wright, "A Brief Review of the Life of Eliphalet Nott Wright," *Chronicles of Oklahoma* 10, no. 11 (June 1932): 265-86.

V. Allen

WRIGHT, LOUIS TOMPKINS (July 22, 1891, LaGrange, Ga.-October 8, 1952, New York, N.Y.). *Surgeon.* Son of Ceah Ketcham, minister and physician, and Lula (Tompkins) Wright. Married Corinne M. Cooke, 1918; two children. EDUCATION: 1911, A.B., Clark University (Atlanta); 1915, M.D., Harvard University; 1915-16, intern, Freedmen's Hospital, Washington, D.C. CAREER: 1916-17, general practice, Atlanta, Ga.; 1917-19, U.S. Army Medical Corps, France; 1919-52, private surgical practice, New York City; on staff of Harlem Hospital, N.Y.: 1943-52, surgical director; 1948-52, president, Board of Medical Staff; 1948-52, director, Harlem Hospital Cancer Research Foundation; 1929-52, surgeon, New York City Police Department; 1948-52, member, Advisory Council and Executive Committee, New York City Department of Hospitals. CONTRIBUTIONS: Introduced new method of intradermal vaccination against smallpox (1918). Pioneered use of aureomycin in humans (1948). Invented brace for cervical vertebrae fractures (1936) and blade-plate for operative treatment of fractures about the knee joint. Founded *Harlem Hospital Bulletin* (1948). Chairman, Board of Directors, NAACP (1932-52), and promoted black equality in professional and personal careers. Demonstrated validity of Schick test in Negroes (1917). First black to hold position of police surgeon in a major U.S. city (1929) and first black to be appointed to the staff of a N.Y. hospital (1919). Second black to become fellow, American College of Surgeons (1934). A cofounder and influential member of the strongly antisegregationist Manhattan Central Medical Society (1930s).

WRITINGS: Almost 100 articles. "The Schick Test with Especial Reference to the Negro," *J. Infect. Dis.* 21 (1917): 265-68; "Intradermal Vaccination Against Smallpox," *JAMA* 71 (1918): 654-57; "Aureomycin, a New Antibiotic with Virucidal Properties. A Preliminary Report on Successful Treatment in Twenty-five Cases of Lymphogranuloma Venereum," *JAMA* 138 (1948): 408-12 (with Murray Sanders, Myra A. Logan, Aaron Prigot, and Lyndon M. Hill); "The Treatment of Lymphogranuloma Venereum and Granuloma Inguinale in Humans with Aureomycin," *Annals, N.Y. Acad. of Sci.* 51 (1948): 318-30 (with others). Writings listed in *JNMA* 45 (1953): 146-48. REFERENCES: W. Montague Cobb, "Louis Tompkins Wright, 1891-1952," *JNMA* 45 (1952): 130-48; *J. Negro Hist.* 52 (1967): 169-84; Frank Kingdon, "Patriot and Physician," *The Crisis* 47 (1940): 14-15, 27; *NCAB*, 43: 390-91; *WWAPS* 1 (1938): 1320.

T. L. Savitt

WYLDER, MELDRUM KEPLINGER (May 15, 1877, Macaupin County (on farm), Ill.-January 27, 1962, Albuquerque, N.Mex.). *Physician; Obstetrics; Pediatrics.* Son of Rev. J. L., pioneer Methodist minister, and Sarah Ellen Wylder. Married Elizabeth Coleman, 1904 (d. 1920), one child; Ethel Rost, 1922 (d. 1922); Evadine Alexander, 1927, two children. EDUCATION: B.S., Marion College, Ind.; 1901, M.D., Washington University Medical School, St.

Louis, Mo.; internship, St. Louis City Hospital, St. Louis; while practicing in Albuquerque, took time off to take short courses under pediatric specialists, St. Louis Children's Hospital and Boston Children's Hospital. CAREER: Developed TB; went west seeking cure; 1903, arrived in Albuquerque, expecting to stay two weeks but never left; licensed to practice medicine in N.Mex., and opened office in Albuquerque; for 50 years, tended medical ailments of Albuquerque and a wide area of N.Mex.; delivered more than 15,000 babies; 1925, became member, American College of Physicians; 1930, accepted to newly formed Academy of Pediatrics; an active member, New Mexico State Board of Health, for more than 25 years; president, New Mexico Medical Society. CONTRIBU-TIONS: Lectured to student nurses at St. Joseph's Hospital, Albuquerque (beginning 1904) and taught pediatrics there (since 1923). An active Republican, was elected Bernalillo County commissioner (1918) and used influence to aid in the establishment of New Mexico Department of Public Health (1920). Instrumental in getting bill through the state legislature requiring diphtheria immunizations before children entered school; finally got bill through as war measure—fewer diphtheria cases meant more time for doctors to care for other cases.

WRITINGS: "Differential Diagnosis and Treatment of Duodenal Ulcer," *Southwestern Med. J.* 1 (Apr. 1917); *Rio Grande Medicine Man* (1958), an autobiography of Wylder's long medical career in N.Mex. REFERENCES: Interview with Muriel James, Visiting Nurse Association, Albuquerque, N.Mex.; Meldrum K. Wylder, *Rio Grande Medicine Man* (1958).

C. L. Cutter

WYMAN, JEFFRIES (August 11, 1814, Chelmsford, Mass.-September 4, 1874, Cambridge, Mass.). *Physician; Naturalist; Anatomy; Physiology*. Son of Dr. Rufus Jeffries, physician, and Ann (Morrill) Wyman; brother of Morrill Wyman (q.v.). Married Adeline Wheelwright, 1850 (d.1855), two daughters; Anna Williams Whitney, 1861, (d. 1864 shortly after giving birth to a son). EDUCATION: 1828, Philips Exeter Academy; 1833, A.B., Harvard University; 1834, studied medicine with father, and Dr. John C. Dalton (q.v.); 1836, assistant, Massachusetts General Hospital; 1837, M.D., Harvard Medical School; 1841, went abroad to study medicine and anatomy, Paris and London. CAREER: To support education, worked for Boston Fire Department; 1837, anatomy demonstrator for Dr. John C. Warren (q.v.); 1840, curator and lecturer, Lowell Institute; 1843, professor of anatomy and physiology, Hampton-Sidney College, Richmond, Va.; 1847, Hersey Professor of Anatomy, Harvard University; 1848-49, lecturer, Lowell Institute; 1856, participated in collecting expedition to Surinam; 1857-66, taught in private Cambridge medical school with brother Morrill Wyman and others; 1858, accompanied Capt. J. M. Forbes and George A. Peabody across South America collecting material for Harvard's museums; 1862, conducted experiments like those of Pasteur and Pouchet on spontaneous generation but did not publish results; 1866, curator and head, new Department and Museum of Archeology and Ethnology, Harvard University; 1875, elected president, American Association for the Advancement of Science, but did not assume duties. CONTRIBUTIONS: One of America's most noted anatomists and naturalists. Corresponded with Darwin on evolution and Pasteur on the spontaneous generation debate. An excellent and influential teacher.

WRITINGS: Published 175 papers, mostly on comparative anatomy. REFERENCES: *DAB* 10, pt. 2: 583-84; R. N. Doesch, "Early American Experiments on 'Spontaneous Generation' by Jeffries Wyman (1814-74)," *J. Hist. Med. & Allied Sci.* 17 (1962): 326-32; Asa Gray, in *Proc., Boston Soc. of Natural Hist.* 17 (1875): 96-124; O. W. Holmes, *Atlantic Monthly* (Nov. 1874); *NCAB*, 2: 254; A. S. Packard, "Memoir of Jeffries Wyman," *Biographical Memoirs. National Academy of Sciences* 2 (1886): 75-126; Morrill Wyman, "List of Scientific Papers and Works by Jeffries Wyman," *Animal Mechanics* (1902).

M. H. Dawson

WYMAN, MORRILL (January 25, 1812, Chelmsford, Mass.-January 30, 1903, Cambridge, Mass.). *Physician; Surgery.* Son of Rufus, physician, and Ann (Morrill) Wyman, brother of Jeffries Wyman (q.v.). Married Elizabeth Aspinwall Pulsifer, August 14, 1839; three children. EDUCATION: Graduated from Phillips Exeter Academy; 1833, A.B., Harvard University; 1837, M.D., Harvard Medical School; 1837, house pupil, Massachusetts General Hospital. CAREER: To support education, worked as assistant engineer, Boston & Worcester Railroad; 1838, after graduation, set up private practice which he pursued until a few years before death; 1853-56, adjunct Hersey Professor of the Theory and Practice of Medicine, Harvard Medical School; 1857, with brother Jeffries Wyman and two others, set up private medical school, Cambridge, Mass.; during Civil War, inspector, military hospitals; 1875-87, overseer, Harvard University; 1881, founded Cambridge Hospital and was chairman, Board of Trustees, until 1898; consulting physician, Massachusetts General Hospital, for most of career. CONTRIBUTIONS: A noted practitioner and surgeon, wrote two influential works on the importance of ventilating buildings. In surgery, was the first American to perform a thoracentisis, improving on previous English efforts. Work on hay fever was the first clear description of the allergy.

WRITINGS: *A Practical Treatise on Ventilation* (1846); report on chimneys and ventilators in *Proc., Am. Acad. of Arts and Sci.* 1 (1848): 307ff.; *Autumnal Catarrh (Hay Fever)* (1876). REFERENCES: *Boston Med. and Surg. J.* (Feb. 5, 1903); *Boston Transcript*, January 31, 1903; *DAB*, 10, pt. 2: 584-85; T. F. Harrington, *The Harvard Medical School* 2 (1905); *NCAB*, 28: 308; Morrill Wyman, Jr., *A Brief Record of the Lives and Writings of Dr. Rufus Wyman. . . and His Son Dr. Morrill Wyman* (1913), includes a bibliography of Wyman's works.

M. H. Dawson

WYNN, FRANK BARBOUR (May 28, 1860, near Brookville, Ind.-July 27, 1922, Glacier National Park, Mont.). *Physician; Educator.* Son of James, farmer, and Margaret (Barbour) Wynn. Married Carrie Louise Arnold, 1895; one son. EDUCATION: DePauw: 1885, A.B.; and 1886, A.M.; M.D., 1885, Medical College of Ohio; intern, Good Samaritan Hospital, Cincinnati, Ohio; 1892-93, post-graduate work in gross and microscopical anatomy, Vienna and Berlin. CAREER: Practiced medicine, State Hospital, Dayton, Ohio, and later at the Logansport State Hospital, Ind.; 1893, settled in Indianapolis, Ind.; practice of internal medicine; appointed city sanitarian of Indianapolis; professor of pathology and director of the pathology museum, Indiana Medical College; 1908 to death, professor of medicine, Indiana University School of Medicine. CONTRIBUTIONS: With Dr. William Wishard (q.v.), set up educational exhibit at the AMA annual meeting (1898), thereby originating what became known as the Annual Scientific Exhibit program of the AMA. Served on the committee that worked on the merger of the Indiana Medical College, Central College of Physicians and Surgeons, and Fort Wayne Medical College into the Indiana University School of Medicine. An avid mountain climber and explorer, Mount Wynn in Glacier National Park is named in his honor.

WRITINGS: Most of his articles in *Trans., Indiana State Med. Soc.* and *J. Indiana State Med. Assoc.* REFERENCES: C. A. Bonsett, "Frank B. Wynn, 1860-1922. . . ," *J. Indiana State Med. Assoc.* 65 (1972): 1067-71; *NCAB*, 17: 175.

C. A. Bonsett

Y

YANDELL, LUNSFORD PITTS (July 4, 1805, Hartsville, Sumner County, Tenn.-February 4, 1878, Louisville, Ky.). *Physician; Geologist; Editor; Educator.* Son of Wilson, physician, and Elizabeth (Pitts) Yandell. Married Susan Juliet Wendell, 1825; six children. Married Eliza P. Bland, 1861; no children. EDUCATION: 1821, began the study of medicine under his father; 1823-24, 1825-26, Transylvania University Medical Department, Lexington, Ky.; 1824-25, University of Maryland, Baltimore, Md.; M.D., 1825; 1823-24, private pupil of Drs. Charles Caldwell (q.v.) and Benjamin Dudley (q.v.), Lexington; 1824-25, private house pupil of J. B. Davidge (q.v.), Baltimore; spring 1825, visited medical centers, Philadelphia, Pa.; New York, N.Y.; and New Haven, Conn.; 1830, received instruction in chemistry from Dr. Gerard Troost, Nashville, Tenn. CAREER: 1825-29, practiced with father, Murfreesboro, Tenn.; 1830, practiced, Nashville; 1831-37, professor of chemistry and pharmacology, Transylvania University medical department, Lexington; at Louisville Medical Institute, Louisville: 1837-38, professor of chemistry and materia medica; and 1838-46, professor of chemistry and pharmacy; at University of Louisville medical department, Louisville: 1846-49, professor of chemistry and pharmacy; and 1849-59, professor of physiology and pathological anatomy; 1859-61, professor of theory and practice of medicine, Medical College of Memphis; 1862-67, Presbyterian minister, Dancyville, Tenn.; 1867, returned to Louisville to practice medicine and occasionally preach. CONTRIBUTIONS: First dean, Louisville Medical Institute, Louisville (1837-38). Incorporator, with several students, the student medical society at Louisville Medical Institute known as Louisville Medical Society (1837). Editor, *Transylvania Medical Journal*, Lexington (1832-37). Co-founder and co-editor, *Louisville Journal Medicine and Surgery* (1838). Editor or co-editor, *Western Journal Medicine and Surgery* (1840-55). Devoted to the teaching and practice of medicine. Although he held the chair of chemistry at Transylvania, Louisville Medical Institute, and University of Louisville medical department, did not find the subject his major interest. Received a prize from the Medical Society of Tennessee (May 1841) for the best essay on bilious fever (malaria) in which he urged the use of quinine for treatment. Knowledgeable in the new science of geology and paleontology and contributed to its early development. At least seven Devonian fossil species bear his name.

WRITINGS: "On the Progress of Etherization," *Western J. of Med. & Surg.*, 3rd series, 3 (1849): 1-36; *History of the Medical Department of the University of Louisville, An Introductory Lecture* (1852); *How Louisville Succeeded Lexington as a Center of Medical Education* (1852); "Medical Literature of Kentucky," *Trans., Ky. State Med. Soc.* (1874); *Address on Am. Med. Lit. Delivered Before the International Medical Congress at Philadelphia, September 8, 1876* (1876). REFERENCES: *BHM* (1980), 42; *DAB*, 10, pt. 2: 546-47; E. F. Horine, *Daniel Drake (1785-1852): Pioneer Physician of the Midwest* (1961), 332-33; MSS. Autobiography, 1875, in Yandell Collections, The Filson Club, Louisville, Ky.; *NCAB*, 4: 301; R. Peter, "Doctor Lunsford P. Yandell, Sr.," *Ky. Med. J.* 15 (1917): 74-76.

E. H. Conner

YARROS, RACHELLE (SLOBODINSKY) (May 18, 1869, Berdechev, Russia-March 17, 1946, San Diego, Calif.). *Physician; Reformer.* Daughter of Joachim and Bernice Slobodinsky. Married Victor S. Yarros, 1894; one adopted child. EDUCATION: 1890, College of Physicians and Surgeons, Boston, Mass.; 1893, M.D., Woman's Medical College of Pennsylvania; 1894, intern, New England Hospital for Women and Children, Boston; postdoctoral work in pediatrics, New York Infirmary for Women and Children and Michael Reese Hospital, Chicago, Ill. CAREER: 1895, opened obstetric and gynecological practice, Chicago; 1897, appointed instructor in clinical obstetrics, "College of Physicians and Surgeons" (a clinical staff associated with the University of Illinois Medical School); 1902, advanced to associate professorship and continued there until 1926; 1908, appointed director of an obstetrical dispensary, Chicago; 1926-39, appointed to special professorship in social hygiene, University of Illinois Medical School; associate director, Chicago Lying-in Hospital; president, Westside Branch, Chicago's Social Settlement. CONTRIBUTIONS: Reform career gradually supplanted medical practice, and she became most closely identified with the causes of social hygiene and birth control. Founder, American Social Hygiene Association (1914). President, Illinois Social Hygiene League (1915).

WRITINGS: "Birth Control and Democracy," *World Democracy* (Sept. 1925); "Birth Control and Its Relation to Health and Welfare," *Med. Woman's J.* (Oct. 1925); "Training and Guidance in Recreation," *J. of Social Hygiene* (Feb. 1929); *Modern Women and Sex* (1933), reissued as *Sex Problems in Modern Society* (1938). REFERENCES: *NCAB*, 35: 168; *Notable Am. Women, 1607-1950*, 3: 693-94; Margaret Sanger, *An Autobiography* (1938), 361.

V. Drachman

YOUNG, HUGH HAMPTON (September 18, 1870, San Antonio, Tex.-August 23, 1945, Baltimore, Md.). *Physician; Urology.* Son of William Hugh,

lawyer and real estate developer, and Frances Michie (Kemper) Young. Married
Bessy Mason Colston, 1901; four children. EDUCATION: University of Virginia:
1893, A.B., M.A.; and 1894, M.D.; Johns Hopkins: 1894-95, postgraduate
study; and 1895-98, intern and resident. CAREER: 1898-1942, urology faculty,
Johns Hopkins Medical School; at Johns Hopkins Hospital: 1898-1942, urological surgery staff; and 1915-42, director, Brady Urological Institute; *post* 1908,
chairman, Maryland State Lunacy Commission (later Board of Mental Hygiene
for Maryland); 1917, director of urology, Army Expeditionary Force; president:
1909, American Association of Genito-Urinary Surgeons; and American Urological Association; and 1927, International Association of Urology. CONTRI-
BUTIONS: The founder of modern urology in the United States. Invented numerous
operating instruments and other surgical apparatus; developed an improved cystoscope and the Young Punch, an instrument used to excise the prostate gland.
Devised several new surgical procedures for treating genito-urinary diseases; did
the first perineal prostatectomy (1902), which soon replaced the more dangerous
suprapubic approach, and performed the first radical operation on a cancerous
prostate gland (1904). Made pioneer investigations of hermaphroditism. Trained
many of the leading urologists of his time. Founded (1917) and edited the *Journal
of Urology* until death. Organized urological clinics for the army during World
War I which brought about a marked lowering of venereal disease among servicemen. Developed the drug "mercurochrome" which he used as an intravenous
antiseptic. An early advocate of the use of sulfanilamide and other chemotherapeutic drugs in the treatment of venereal disease.

WRITINGS: *Hypertrophy and Cancer of the Prostate Gland* (1906); *Studies in Urological Surgery* (1906); *Young's Practice of Urology* (1926). REFERENCES: *BHM* (1970-
74), 182; (1975), 28; *DAB*, Supplement 3: 853-54; Miller, *BHM*, p. 126; *NCAB*, 38:
253-54; *N.Y. Times*, August 24, 1945; *Who Was Who in Am.*, 2: 598; H. H. Young, *A
Surgeon's Autobiography* (1940).

                                                                    S. Galishoff

YOUNG, JOHN WILLIAM (October 27, 1846, Carroll County, Miss.-Feb-
ruary 15, 1933, Grenada, Miss.). *Physician.* Son of Samuel Hart and Catherine
W. (Small) Young. Married Mollie I. McCain, 1873; no children. EDUCATION:
Carroll County schools; 1869, M.D., Tulane University. CAREER: At age 16,
joined the Confederate forces; became a member of a cavalry company, Vaiden,
Miss., serving under Nathan Bedford Forrest; served until General Forrest's last
battle, Selma, Ala.; after the war, worked as a tenant farmer while studying
medicine until he could earn money to attend Tulane University; during Reconstruction period, member, Ku Klux Klan; until 1890, practiced medicine, Carroll
County, when he moved to Grenada; 1890 until retirement, practiced medicine,
Grenada. CONTRIBUTIONS: Active member, Mississippi State Medical Association. President, Mississippi State Medical Association (1910-11). Long-time

district surgeon, Illinois Central Railway System. REFERENCES: E. M. Sherwood, "Doctor Young Is 83 Years Old," *Illinois Central Mag.* 18 (May 1930): 6.

M. S. Legan

YOUNT, CLARENCE EDGAR (February 14, 1874, Fort Dodge, Ia.-March 10, 1954, Prescott, Ariz.). *Physician; Surgeon.* Son of Ephraim Myers, employee of U.S. government, and Laura Rebecca (Musselman) Yount. Married Clara M. Criley, 1904; four children. EDUCATION: Public schools, Washington, D.C.; 1896, M.D., Georgetown University. CAREER: Private practice: 1896-1902, Washington, D.C.; and 1902-54, Prescott, Ariz.; 1907, 1st lieutenant, Arizona National Guard; in World War I, served overseas with the Guard; health officer, Prescott, for 18 years. CONTRIBUTIONS: Worked as health officer in frontier Ariz. Said to have owned the first microscope in Ariz.

WRITINGS: *The Sixth International Congress of Tuberculosis*; *Human Myiasis from the Screw Worm Fly*; *Malta Fever in Arizona*. REFERENCES: *Phoenix Gazette*, March 10, 1954; Richard E. Sloan and Ward Adams, *History of Arizona* (1930).

J. S. Goff

Z

ZAKRZEWSKA, MARIE ELIZABETH (September 6, 1829, Berlin, Germany-May 12, 1902, Boston, Mass.). *Physician; Hospital administrator*. Daughter of Martin Ludwig, Prussian army pensioner, and Frederika C. W. (Urban) Zakrzewski, midwife. EDUCATION: 1851, midwifery degree, Charité Hospital, Berlin; 1856, M.D., Western Reserve. CAREER: 1852, chief midwife and professor, Charité; 1857-59, resident physician and general manager, New York Infirmary for Women and Children; 1859-62, professor of obstetrics and diseases of women and children, New England Female Medical College, Boston, Mass.; at New England Hospital for Women and Children: founder; 1862, resident physician; 1863-87, attending physician; and 1887-1902, advisory physician. CONTRIBUTIONS: Provided first-rate institution at which pioneer women physicians could gain needed clinical experience in surgery and obstetrics. Indefatigable feminist and supporter of the cause of women in medicine. Gained grudging respect from Boston's male medical community for high medical standards. Assiduous advocate of quality medical education for women. Important link between Boston reformist community and women physicians at a time when training facilities were few and public support was badly needed.

WRITINGS: *Introductory Lecture Delivered Before the New England Female Medical College* (1859); "Report of One Hundred and Eighty-seven Cases of Midwifery in Private Practice," *Boston Med. and Surg. J.* 121 (1889): 557-60. REFERENCES: John B. Blake, "Marie Elizabeth Zakrzewska," *Notable Am. Women* 3 (1971): 702-4; Caroline H. Dall, *A Practical Illustration of "Woman's Right to Labor"* (1860); Agnes C. Vietor, *A Woman's Quest: The Life of Marie E. Zakrzewska, M.D.* (1924).

R. M. Morantz

ZINSSER, HANS (November 17, 1878, New York, N.Y.-September 4, 1940, New York). *Physician; Microbiology; Immunology*. Son of August, businessman, and Marie Theresia (Schmidt) Zinsser. Married Ruby Handforth Kunz, 1905; two children. EDUCATION: Columbia University: 1899, A.B.; 1903, M.A.

and M.D.; 1903-5, intern, Roosevelt Hospital. CAREER:1905-10, 1913-23, bacteriology faculty, College of Physicians and Surgeons (Columbia); 1907-10, pathology staff, St. Luke's Hospital (N.Y.); 1910-13, bacteriology faculty, Stanford University; 1913-23, bacteriology staff, Presbyterian Hospital (N.Y.); 1915, member, American Red Cross Sanitary Commission to Serbia; 1917-18, sanitary inspector and assistant director, laboratories and infectious diseases, Army Expeditionary Force; 1923-40, bacteriology and immunology faculty, Harvard Medical School; 1925, sanitary commissioner, Russia, health section, League of Nations; 1924-40, bacteriology staff, Children's and Peter Bent Brigham hospitals (Boston, Mass.); president: 1919, American Association for Immunologists; and 1926, Society of American Bacteriologists. CONTRIBUTIONS: One of the world's foremost authorities on rickettsial diseases; showed that Brill's disease, which appeared among immigrants in New York City, was not a type of American murine (endemic) typhus, as was commonly believed, but rather a recrudescence of epidemic exanthematic typhus contracted in Europe (early 1930s). Contributed to the development of an effective vaccine against typhus and added to what was known about the biology of the rickettsiae. Did important work in immunology. Hypothesized that manifestations of infection are caused by sensitization to "residue antigens" (nonprotein substances) of the invading bacteria. Differentiated anaphylaxis and the tuberculin type of allergic reaction. Also studied the measurement of virus size and host resistance to syphilis. First with Philip H. Hiss, Jr. (1910-13), and then with Stanhope Bayne-Jones (q.v., *post* 1913), published *A Textbook of Bacteriology*, which in Zinsser's lifetime went through eight editions and was translated into several languages. Trained numerous physicians and graduate students from all over the world.

WRITINGS: *Infection and Resistance* (1914); "Studies on the Tuberculin Reaction and on Specific Hypersensitiveness in Bacterial Infection," *J. of Experimental Med.* 34 (1921): 495-524; "Varieties of Typhus Fever and the Epidemiology of the American Form of European Typhus Fever (Brill's Disease)," *Am. J. of Hygiene* 20 (1934): 513-32; *Rats, Lice and History* (1935). Bibliography is in *BMNAS* 24 (1947): 323-60. REFERENCES: *BHM* (1970-74), 183; *DAB*, Supplement 2: 744-45; *DSB*, 14: 622-25; Miller, *BHM*, p. 126; *NCAB*, 36: 35-36; *N.Y. Times*, September 5, 1940; *Who Was Who in Am.*, 1: 1396.

S. Galishoff

APPENDIXES

Listing by Date of Birth

1613
Pell, Thomas

1620
Thacher, Thomas

1662
Mather, Cotton*

1675
Belisle, Henri

1679
Boylston, Zabdiel

1684
Kearsley, John

1688
Colden, Cadwallader
Dickinson, Jonathan

1691
Douglass, William*

1700
Tennent, John*

1707
Cadwalader, Thomas*

1708
Lining, John

1709
Hersey, Ezekiel

1710
Bull, William

1713
Bond, Thomas

1714
Thornton, Matthew

1716
Bard, John

1720
Olyphant, David

1722
Redman, John

1726
Wiesenthal, Charles F.

1728
Holyoke, Edward A.
Lloyd, James

1729
Bartlett, Josiah
Hunter, William*
Jones, John
Moultrie, John, Jr.

* Year of birth uncertain

1730

Cochran, John
Craik, James
Garden, Alexander

1731

Tufts, Cotton

1732

McKean, Robert

1733

Brackett, Joshua

1734

Church, Benjamin
Munson, Eneas

1735

Cutter, Ammi R.
Morgan, John

1736

Shippen, William

1739

Jackson, Hall

1741

Archer, John
Kuhn, Adam
Perkins, Elisha
Warren, Joseph, III

1742

Bard, Samuel

1744

Coffin, Nathaniel, Jr.

1745

Bayley, Richard
Elmer, Jonathan
Fayssoux, Peter
Tilton, James

1746

Crawford, John
McClurg, James
Rush, Benjamin

1748

Brown, William

1749

Baynham, William
Ramsay, David

1750

Dexter, Aaron
Hopkins, Lemuel

1752

Barker, Jeremiah

1753

Smith, Peter
Warren, John

1754

Ramsay, Alexander
Thacher, James
Waterhouse, Benjamin

1756

Romayne, Nicholas

1757

Ridgely, Frederick
Sibley, John

1758

Webster, Noah

1760

Greenwood, John

1761

Cogswell, Mason F.
Wistar, Caspar

1762

Durham, James
Smith, Nathan

1763

Physick, Philip S.
Saugrain de Vigne, Antoine F.

1764

Mitchill, Samuel L.
Pomeroy, John
Prevost, Francois M.*

1766

Barton, Benjamin
Post, Wright

1768

Davidge, John B.
Dewees, William P.

1769

Brown, Samuel
Ferguson, Richard B.
Gallup, Joseph A.
Hayden, Horace H.
Hosack, David
Thomson, Samuel
Todd, Eli

1770

Gridley, Selah
Potter, Nathaniel
Seaman, Valentine

1771

McDowell, Ephraim
North, Elisha

1772

Caldwell, Charles

1773

Appleton, Moses
Coxe, John R.
Ewell, James
May, Frederick

1774

Otto, John C.

1775

Drake, Daniel
Spalding, Lyman

1777

Dyott, Thomas W.*
Galt, William C.
Jackson, James

1778

Warren, John C.

1779

Heermann, Lewis
Silliman, Benjamin

1780

Chapman, Nathaniel
Mussey, Reuben D.

1781

Robertson, Felix
Twitchell, Amos

1782

Darlington, William
Guthrie, Samuel

1783

Cooke, John E.
Dorsey, John S.
Shattuck, George C.

1784

Farrar, Bernard G.

1785

Beaumont, William
Dudley, Benjamin W.
Mott, Valentine

1786

Barton, William P. C.
Bigelow, Jacob
Channing, Walter

1787

Delameter, John
Eberle, John
Gallaudet, Thomas
Jackson, Samuel
Oliver, Daniel
Woodward, Samuel B.

1788

Parsons, Usher
Woodward, Theodore

1789

Antony, Milton
Bates, James
Fearn, Thomas
Francis, John W.
Knight, Jonathan

1790

Benites, Jose M.
Brown, Solyman
Galland, Isaac*
Williams, Stephen W.

1791

Beck, T. Romeyn
Pattison, Granville S.*

1792

Bache, Franklin
Clapp, Asahel
Meigs, Charles D.

1793

Cartwright, Samuel A.
Horner, William E.
Mitchell, John K.
Shattuck, Lemuel

1794

Beach, Wooster
Delafield, Edward
Fussell, Bartholomew
Godman, John D.
Graham, Sylvester
Paine, Martyn

1795

March, Alden
Smith, Alban G.
Smith, Lyndon A.
Ware, John

1796

Harrison, John P.
Hays, Isaac
Hodge, Hugh L.
McClellan, George

1797

Curtis, Alva
Fisher, John Dix
Hulse, Isaac
Parmly, Eleazar
Pitcher, Zina
Smith, Nathan R.
Steuart, Richard S.
Sutton, William L.
Wood, George B.

1798

Alcott, William A.
Brigham, Amariah
Dickson, Samuel H.
Dunglison, Robley

1799

Atlee, John L.
Awl, William M.
Dunlap, Livingston
Geddings, Eli
Morton, Samuel G.
Pennock, Caspar W.
Reid, William W.

1800

Burrough, James W.
Crosby, Dixi
Gunn, John C.
Hering, Constantine
Knowlton, Charles
Miller, Henry, Jr.
Parker, Willard

1801

Ford, Lewis D.
Howe, Samuel G.

1802

Dix, Dorothea
Green, Horace
Lincoln, Benjamin
Whitman, Marcus

1803

Gorrie, John
Jarvis, Edward
Judd, Gerrit P.
Monette, John W.
Phelps, Edward E.

1804

Bartlett, Elisha
Nott, Josiah C.
Parker, Peter
Storer, David H.
Wolcott, Erastus B.

1805

Gross, Samuel D.
Hunt, Harriot K.
Jackson, Charles T.

McDowell, Joseph N.
Pancoast, Joseph
Peter, Robert
Smith, Ashbel
Yandell, Lunsford P.

1806

Bedford, Gunning
Bell, Luther V.
Dugas, Louis A.
Eve, Paul F.
Harris, Chapin A.
Hooker, Worthington
Jackson, John B. S.
Miller, Thomas
Toland, Hugh H.

1807

Brandreth, Benjamin
Davis, Henry G.
Fenner, Erasmus D.
Kirkwood, James P.
Ray, Isaac

1808

Arnold, Richard D.
Atlee, Washington
Bowditch, Henry I.
Bowling, William K.
Carpenter, Walter
Gibbons, Henry
Maynard, David S.
Stone, Warren

1809

Armsby, James H.
Bobbs, John S.
Earle, Pliny
Gerhard, William W.
Griscom, John H.
Holmes, Oliver W.
Kirkbride, Thomas S.

1810

Frissell, John
Hall, William W.
Hullihen, Simon P.
Jackson, James, Jr.
Nichols, Mary S.N.G.
Ruggles, David

1811

Baldwin, Abel S.
Jackson, James C.
Parrish, Isaac
White, James P.

1812

Brainard, Daniel
Bush, Lewis P.
Delany, Martin R.
Flint, Austin
Seguin, Edouard
Still, James
Trall, Russell T.
Wyman, Morrill

1813

Cabell, James
Garcelon, Alonzo
Gregory, Samuel
King, John
Lozier, Clemence S.
Main, John H. T.
McCready, Benjamin W.
Moore, Samuel P.
Preston, Ann
Shattuck, George C., Jr.
Sims, J. Marion
Smith, James McC.
Stillé, Alfred
Wickes, Stephen
Wood, James R.

1814

Evans, John
McKee, William H.
Moore, Edward M.
Wyman, Jeffries

1815

Blake, James
Long, Crawford W.
Morse, John F.
Palmer, Alonzo B.
Sutherland, Earl W.
Wells, Horace

1816

Brown, William W.*
Buckingham, Richard G.
Griffin, John S.
Shew, Joel

Thomas, Mary F. M.
Westmoreland, John G.

1817

Bayless, George W.
Byford, William H.
Davis, Nathan S.
Dibrell, James A.
Phares, David L.
Procter, William, Jr.
Thayer, Samuel W.

1818

Agnew, David H.
Ayer, James C.
Baldwin, William O.
Barker, B. Fordyce
Bigelow, Henry J.
Faget, Jean C.
Hargis, Robert B.
Meigs, John F.
Newton, Robert S.
Parrish, Joseph
Pittman, Newsome J.
Pope, Charles A.

1819

Favill, John
Longshore, Hannah E. M.
Mayo, William W.
Morton, William T. G.
Pinkham, Lydia E.
Squibb, Edward R.

1820

Anderson, William H.
Bell, Simeon B.
Blaney, James V.
Clarke, Edward H.
Cooper, Elias S.
Elwell, John J.
Sayre, Lewis A.
Snow, Edwin M.
Wilbur, Hervey B.

1821

Barton, Clara
Blackwell, Elizabeth
Den, Richard S.
Eddy, Mary Baker
Hillebrand, Wilhelm
Howard, William T.
Hughes, John C.

Krackowizer, Ernst
Livermore, Mary A. R.
Palmer, Thomas M.
Passavant, William A.
Williams, Henry W.

1822

Gunn, Moses
Lindsley, John B.
Purple, Samuel S.
Williams, Elkanah

1823

Brodie, William
Leidy, Joseph
Lewis, Dio
McCaw, James B.
Smith, Stephen

1824

Andrews, Edmund
Bentley, Edwin
Campbell, Henry F.
Harris, Elisha
Kerr, John G.
Letterman, Jonathan
Sanford, John F.

1825

Augusta, Alexander
Bozeman, Nathan
Dalton, John Call
Gray, John P.
Haywood, Edmund B.
Ketchum, George A.
Merrick, Myra
Porcher, Francis P.
Rock, John S.
Steele, Henry K.
Toner, Joseph M.

1826

Blackwell, Emily
Hodgen, John T.
Remond, Sarah P.
Rogers, William E.
Wolcott, Laura J. R.

1827

Dana, Israel T.
Hitchcock, Homer O.
Livingston, Robert R.
Smith, Job L.

Taylor, Charles F.
White, Ellen G.

1828

Battey, Robert
Briggs, William T.
Busey, Samuel C.
Daniel, Richard P.
Garretson, James E.
Hammond, William A.
Hitchcock, Edward
Rauch, John H.
Still, Andrew T.
Warren, Edward
Weatherly, Job S.

1829

Cleveland, Emeline H.
Cole, Richard B.
Dolley, Sarah R. A.
Mitchell, S. Weir
Parvin, Theophilus
Scudder, John M.
Thompson, Mary H.
Wooten, Thomas D.
Zakrzewska, Marie E.

1830

Chaillé, Stanford
Chisolm, Julian J.
Hartman, Samuel B.
Hunt, Ezra M.
Jacobi, Abraham
Lane, Levi C.
Storer, Horatio R.

1831

Bartholow, Roberts
Bodine, James M.
Cheever, David W.
Cochran, Jerome
Gilman, Daniel C.
Greene, Cordelia
Hoyt, John W.
Loomis, Alfred L.
Lothrop, Charles H.
Mitchell, Robert W.
Robertson, William S.
Thomas, T. Gaillard
Tupper, Henry M.
Whitehead, William R.

1832

Brinton, John H.
Crosby, Alpheus B.
Knapp, (J.) Hermann
Walker, Mary E.

1833

Brackett, Cyrus F.
Da Costa, Jacob M.
Gihon, Albert L.
Helmuth, William T.
Hooper, Philo O.
Jenks, Edward W.
Jones, Joseph
Kane, John K.
Reyburn, Robert
Steele, William L.
Waring, George E.
Weed, Gideon A.
White, James C.
Woodward, Joseph J.

1834

Bancroft, Frederick
Bryce, Peter
Eliot, Charles W.
Klebs, Theodore A.
Maury, Richard B.
Reeve, James T.
Swain, Clara
Wesselhoeft, Conrad

1835

Gary, Thomas P.
Henry, Morris H.
Hewitt, Charles N.
McGuire, Hunter H.
Phillips, Josiah L.
Smith, Albert H

1836

Black, Greene V.
Carmalt, William H.
Chandler, Charles F.
Finfrock, John H.
Flint, Austin, Jr.
Mills, Hiram F.
Walker, Delos
Wall, John P.
Watson, Beriah A.

1837

Abbott, Anderson
Baker, Henry B.
Black, John J.
Gross, Samuel W.
Keen, William W., Jr.
Lyster, Henry F. L.
Schuyler, Louise L.
Shrady, George F.
Skene, Alexander
Smith, Andrew H.
Woodworth, John M.

1838

Billings, John S.
Holton, Henry D.
Leavitt, Erasmus
Noon, Adolphus H.
Post, George E.
Potter, William W.
Solis-Cohen, Jacob D.
Sternberg, George M.
Whitehead, Peter F.

1839

Beard, George M.
Coffman, Victor H.
McGraw, Theodore A.

1840

Baruch, Simon
Bowditch, Henry P.
Fenger, Christian
Owens-Adair, Bethenia A.

1841

Delafield, Francis
Hubbard, George W.
Janeway, Edward G.
Kempster, Walter
O'Dwyer, Joseph
Peck, Washington F.
Richards, Linda
Smith, Thomas J.
Souchon, Edmund
Stevenson, Sarah A. H.
Tyson, James
Wood, Horatio C.
Wood, Thomas F.

1842

Eastman, Joseph
Fabrique, Andrew H.

Fitzbutler, (W.) Henry
Gruening, Emil
Jacobi, Mary P.
Maghee, Thomas G.
Purvis, Charles B.
Rutherford, Frances A.
Warner, Hulbert H.
Warren, J. Collins

1843

Bosworth, Franke H.
Connor, Leartus
Cordell, Eugene F.
Fitz, Reginald H.
Hurd, Henry M.
Keyes, Edward L.
Lamb, Daniel S.
McKay, Read J.
Pepper, William
Ripley, Martha G.
Seguin, Edward C.

1844

Ah Fong, C. K.
Atwater, Wilbur O.
Gilliam, David T.
Hall, G. Stanley
Handy, John C.
Putnam, Charles P.
Senn, Nicholas
Wiley, Harvey W.

1845

Calhoun, Abner W.
Denison, Charles
Duhring, Louis A.
Gerrish, Frederic
Gorgas, William C.
McBurney, Charles
Mills, Charles K.
Palmer, Daniel D.
Pilcher, Lewis S.
Solly, S. Edwin
Von Mansfelde, Alexander S.

1846

Brown, Charlotte
Dibrell, James A., Jr.
Lefferts, George M.
Mosher, Eliza M.
Putnam, James J.
Shakespeare, Edward O.
Spalding, James A.

Towne, Solon R.
Watkins, William W.
Witthaus, Rudolph
Young, John W.

1847

Broomall, Anna E.
Dimock, Susan
Fairchild, David S.
Fortner, Benjamin
Hamilton, John B.
Marshall, Clara
Mathews, Joseph M.
McCormack, Joseph N.
McKinney–Steward, Susan M. S.
Porter, Joseph Y.
Shipp, Ellis R.

1848

Bradford, Edward H.
Fowler, George R.
Hocker, William A.
Howe, Lucien
Hughes, Henry A.
Magruder, George L.
Martin, Henry N.
Porter, Henry R.
Straus, Nathan
Trudeau, Edward L.

1849

Benjamin, Dowling
Holt, Erastus E.
Lloyd, John U.
McGillycuddy, Valentine
Ohage, Justus
Osler, William
Prudden, T. M.
Riis, Jacob A.
Rotch, Thomas M.

1850

Dennis, Frederic S.
Foster, Eugene
Grassick, James
Kober, George M.
Lenow, James H.
Meigs, Arthur V.
Meserve, Charles F.
Parsons, Mary A.
Salmon, Daniel D. E.
Welch, William H.

1851

Donaldson, Mary E.
Dorsette, Cornelius
Huntington, George
Johnson, Peter A.
Meltzer, Samuel J.
Mergler, Marie J.
Millspaugh, Joseph G.
Reed, Walter
Richardson, Maurice H.
Vaughan, Victor C.
Wishard, William N.

1852

Carter, Henry R.
Dana, Charles L.
Gant, Harris A.
Halsted, William S.
Hurty, John N.
Kellogg, John H.
Minot, Charles S.
Park, Roswell
Shadd, Furman J.
Simmons, George H.
Spitzka, Edward C.
Williams, Francis H.

1853

Freeman, John W.
Gates, Frederick
Jayne, Walter A.
Price, Joseph
Weeks, John E.
Wende, Ernest
Wheeler, John B.

1854

Billings, Frank
Carroll, James
Coit, Henry L.
Councilman, William T.
Fulton, Mary H.
Haralson, Hugh H.
Prince, Morton
Takamine, Jokichi

1855

Bradford, Claudius
Darrow, Edward M.
Deaver, John B.
Goodfellow, George E.
Harison, Beverly D.

Holt, L. Emmett
Jarvis, William C.
McClennan, Alonzo C.
Milroy, William F.
Sedgwick, William T.
Sewall, Henry
Spafford, Frederick
Stickney, Victor H.

1856

Andrews, Edward W.
Babcock, James W.
Caverly, Charles S.
Chapin, Charles V.
Chittenden, Russell H.
Collister, George
Flick, Lawrence F.
Jackson, Edward
Mossell, Nathan F.
Mouritz, Arthur A.
Smith, Andrew C.
Thompson, William G.
Tinkham, Henry C.
Wood, Casey A.

1857

Abel, John J.
Donaldson, Henry H.
Gardiner, Charles F.
Gibson, Samuel C.
Holmes, Christian
Huson, Florence
Koller, Carl
Martin, Franklin H.
Murphy, John B.
Solis-Cohen, Solomon
Whitman, Royal

1858

Boyd, Robert F.
De Schweinitz, George E.
Dock, Lavinia L.
Engstad, John E.
Flower, Benjamin O.
Fordyce, John A.
Gifford, Harold
Kelly, Howard A.
Koplik, Henry
Lathrop, Julia C.
Meyer, Willy
Miller, William S.
Nutting, Mary A.
Osborne, John E.

Pettigrew, George A.
Rodman, William L.
Sachs, Bernard
Summers, John E., Jr.
Williams, Daniel H.
Wright, Eliphalet

1859

Biggs, Hermann M.
Buxton, Lauren H.
De Witt, Lydia M.
Hall, Josiah N.
Kelley, Florence
Ladd, Edwin F.
Loeb, Jacques
Long, Francis A.
Mackenzie, Kenneth A. J.
Osborne, Thomas B.
Smith, Theobold
Vaughan, George T.

1860

Dock, George
Favill, Henry B.
Howell, William H.
Hunter, John F.
Kinyoun, Joseph J.
Matas, Rudolph
Patrick, Hugh T.
Randall, Edward
Richardson, Rodney H.
Robb, Isabel A. H.
Weedon, Leslie W.
Wynn, Frank B.

1861

Anderson, John W.
Barber, Amos
Bevan, Arthur D.
Dickinson, Robert L.
Fite, Francis B.
Heg, Elmer E.
Herrick, James B.
Leonard, Charles L.
Lilienthal, Howard
Mayo, William J.
McLean, Mary H.
Smith, Clarence A.
Spivak, Charles D.

1862

Biddle, Andrew P.
Butler, Henry R.

Campbell, Elizabeth
Coakley, Cornelius
Coley, William B.
Crumbine, Samuel J.
Delano, Jane A.
Eagleson, James B.
Einhorn, Max
Gamble, Henry F.
Hill, Luther L.
Hood, William H.
Hutchinson, Woods
Mall, Franklin P.
Mallory, Frank B.
Menninger, Charles F.
Nuttall, George H. F.
Porter, William T.
Rose, Wickliffe
Tait, F. Dudley

1863

Abrams, Albert
Beatty, Theodore
Finney, John M.
Flexner, Simon
Gillette, Arthur J.
Hektoen, Ludvig
Johnston, George P.
McCaw, Walter D.
Moore, Aaron M.
Mumford, James G.
Munsterberg, Hugo
Park, William H.
Thoms, Adah B.
Van Hoosen, Bertha

1864

Crile, George W.
Hall, George C.
Harper, Cornelius
Hemmeter, John C.
Howe, Percy R.
McGee, Anita N.
Majors, Monroe A.
Novy, Frederick G.
Roman, Charles V.
Schwyzer, Arnold
Thayer, William S.
Tibbals, Frank B.
Vinsonhaler, Frank
Witherspoon, John A.

1865

Dyer, Isadore
Evans, William A., Jr.
Gundersen, Adolf
Heath, Lillian
Herter, Christian
Hoffman, Frederick
Jackson, Chevalier
Kremers, Edward
Lambright, Middleton
Lommen, Christian
Mayo, Charles H.
Montezuma, Carlos
Picotte, Susan La F.
Pusey, William A.
Scott, Arthur C.
Walsh, James J.
West, Archa K.

1866

Blesh, Abraham L.
Cushny, Arthur R.
Ewing, James
Flexner, Abraham
Jackson, James M., Jr.
Jelliffe, Smith Ely
Jordan, Edwin O.
Lazear, Jesse W.
Lusk, Graham
Manning, Isaac H.
Meyer, Adolf
Morgan, Thomas H.
Warfield, William A.
Williams, John W.
Wilson, Louis B.

1867

Abt, Isaac A.
Barker, Lewellys
Bloodgood, Joseph C.
Folin, Otto
Folks, Homer
Harris, William H.
Jermain, Louis F.
Kiefer, Guy L.
Lyon, Elias P.
McKenzie, Robert T.
Mead, Kate C. H.
Meriwether, Clinton P.
Stiles, Charles W.
Wald, Lillian D.

1868

Barlow, Walter J.
Bierring, Walter L.
Cabot, Richard C.
Cogswell, William F.
Copeland, Royal S.
Cullen, Thomas S.
Curtis, Austin M.
Findley, Palmer
Hatcher, Robert A.
Howard, William F.
Landsteiner, Karl
Macfadden, Bernarr
Smith, Morgan
Wollstein, Martha

1869

Abbott, Maude
Bilderback, Joseph B.
Cannon, George E.
Carter, William S.
Codman, Ernest A.
Coffey, Robert C.
Covington, Benjamin J.
Cushing, Harvey W.
De Lee, Joseph B.
Dodd, Walter J.
Edsall, David Linn
Ellett, Edward C.
Hamilton, Alice
Hazen, Allen
Healy, Henry H.
Healy, William
Loeb, Leo
Long, Leroy
Moeur, Benjamin B.
North, Charles E.
Rosenau, Milton J.
Simpson, John
Yarros, Rachelle

1870

Benedict, Francis G.
Brödel, Max
Caldwell, Eugene W.
Colwell, Nathan P.
Eddy, Harrison P.
Garrison, Fielding
Harris, Seale
Harrison, Ross G.
Hertzler, Arthur E.
Holt, Winifred

Hunt, Reid
Lovejoy, Esther P.
Minton, Henry M.
Packard, Francis R.
Perry, John E.
Quain, Eric P.
Russell, Frederick
Schamberg, Jay F.
Thompson, Solomon H.
White, William A.
Young, Hugh H.

1871

Bardeen, Charles R.
Behle, Augustus
Blair, Vilray P.
Brown, Lawrason
Cannon, Walter B.
Cooley, Thomas B.
Dickerson, Spencer C.
Lynk, Miles V.
Potter, Ellen C.
Ricketts, Howard T.
Sabin, Florence R.
Tuthill, Alexander

1872

Allen, Lyman
Bingham, Arthur W.
Blumer, George
Cabot, Hugh
Cary, Edward H.
Cole, Rufus
Cowie, David M.
Cramp, Arthur J.
Davis, John S.
Evans, Matilda A.
Fuller, Solomon C.
Gies, William J.
Haggard, William D., Jr.
Knox, James H. M., Jr.
Kolle, Frederick S.
Libman, Emanuel
McCormack, Arthur T.
Mendel, Lafayette B.
Moore, Phoebia G.
Prescott, Samuel C.
Ramsey, Walter R.
Robinson, John L.
Romig, Joseph H.
Taussig, Frederick

1873

Ashford, Bailey K.
Baker, S. Josephine
Carrel, Alexis
Dean, Lee W.
Frederick, Rivers
French, Harley E.
Frisbie, Evelyn F.
Goldwater, Sigismund
Henderson, Yandell
Hinson, Eugene T.
Howland, John
Opie, Eugene L.
Shore, Clarence
Streeter, George L.

1874

Brill, Abraham A.
Carter, C. Dana
Chase, Will H.
Clinton, Fred S.
Emerson, Haven
Erlanger, Joseph
Gay, Frederick
Goldberger, Joseph
Hargrave, Frank S.
Jervey, James W.
Kenney, John A.
Leathers, Waller
MacCallum, William G.
Mendenhall, Dorothy R.
Perkins, Roger G.
Plummer, Henry S.
Quain, Fannie A.
Snow, William F.
Sollmann, Torald H.
Timme, Walter
Yount, Clarence E.

1875

Auer, John
Brown, Percy
Coca, Arthur F.
Hess, Alfred F.
Lumsden, Leslie L.
Moorman, Lewis J.
Pittenger, Fred A.
Poynter, Charles W. M.
Ramstad, Niles O.
Rubinow, Isaac M.
Van Ingen, Philip

Wells, Harry G.
Wilbur, Ray L.

1876

Abell, Irvin
Barringer, Emily D.
Beard, Mary
Beers, Clifford
Burch, Frank E.
Cole, Fern M.
Jones, Noble W.
Minoka-Hill, Lillie R.
Noguchi, Hideya
Northcross, David C.
Palmer, Erroll P.
Richards, Alfred N.
Southard, Elmer E.
Timberlake, Gideon
Tracy, Martha
Tunnicliff, Ruth M.

1877

Avery, Oswald T.
Beecher, Clarence H.
Blake, Francis G.
Cannon, Ida M.
Davis, Abraham I.
Downey, Hal
Goldmark, Josephine
Krebs, Ernest
Longcope, Warfield T.
Macfarlane, Catharine
Orr, Hiram W.
Schick, Bela
Sullivan, John J.
Turner, Delos A.
Winslow, Charles-E. A.
Wylder, Meldrum K.

1878

Hale, John H.*
Henderson, Lawrence
Jackson, Algernon
Jean, Sally L.
Lattimore, John A.*
McNeill, William C.
Moten, Pierce S.
Robinson, G. Canby
Stastny, Olga F.
Steindler, Arthur
Vedder, Edward B.
Weible, Ralph E.

Whipple, George H.
Zinsser, Hans

1879

Cohn, Alfred E.
Cox, George W., Jr.
Davis, George G.
Davis, Michael M.
Dearholt, Hoyt E.
Espinosa, Tobias
Garrison, Charles W.
Hirschfelder, Arthur D.
McCollum, Elmer V.
Morrell, Joseph R.
Orton, Samuel T.
Pearl, Raymond
Rous, Peyton
Sanger, Margaret
Sleyster, Rock
South, Lillian H.
Voegtlin, Carl

1880

Alexander, Walter G.
Blanton, Wyndham B.
Campbell, Willis C.
Cheatham, Anderson
Cooke, Robert A.
Frost, Wade H.
Gesell, Arnold L.
Ladd, William E.
Lahey, Frank H.
Marine, David
Matson, Ralph C.
Matson, Ray W.
Neal, Josephine B.
Ranson, Stephen W.
Richards, Ralph T.
Sprague, Edward W.
Warnshuis, Frederick C.
Wolbach, Simeon B.

1881

Alcock, Nathaniel
Beebe, James
Dick, George F.
Dick, Gladys
Levy, Julius
Macnider, William
Palmer, Bartlett J.
Shaffer, Philip A.
Swift, Homer F.

Sydenstricker, Edgar
Whipple, Allen O.

1882

Carson, Simeon L.
Council, Walter W.
Dochez, Alphonse
Du Bois, Eugene F.
Forbes, Alexander
Mason, James T.
Schloss, Oscar M.
Taylor, Eugene T.
Underwood, Felix J.
Vest, Walter
Washburn, Victor D.

1883

Blackfan, Kenneth D.
Crowe, Samuel J.
Gamble, James L.
Graham, Evarts A.
Hinton, William A.
Just, Ernest E.
Lovelace, William R.
Martland, Harrison S.
Nixon, Pat I.
Papanicolaou, George N.
Richards, George T.
Rowntree, Leonard G.
Rubin, Isidore C.
Scammon, Richard E.
Smith, Warren G.
Van Slyke, Donald D.
Veeder, Bordon S.
Wiggers, Carl J.
Williams, William C.

1884

Benedict, Stanley R.
Boswell, Henry
Brunk, Andrew S.
Clendening, Logan
Lennox, William G.
Major, Ralph H.
Marshall, Hyrum L.
Meyer, Karl F.
Moursund, Walter H.
Murphy, James B.
Orr, Thomas G.
Robins, Charles A.
Ross, Julian W.
Sellards, Andrew W.

Smith, Philip E.
Weiskotten, Herman G.

1885

Adams, Numa P. G.
Bousfield, Midian O.
Burgess, Alexander
Dailey, Ulysses G.
Francis, Grossi H.
Hare, Lyle
Horine, Emmet F.
Horney, Karen
Koch, William
Marriott, W. McKim
Minot, George R.
Pearce, Louise
Quinland, William S.
Todd, Thomas W.
Turner, John P.
Winternitz, Milton C.

1886

Anderson, William H.
Brinkley, John R.*
Dandy, Walter E.
Dillehunt, Richard B.
Donahoe, William E.
Goodpasture, Ernest W.
Kendall, Edward C.
Kenny, Elizabeth
Kline, Benjamin S.
Roberts, Carl G.
Scott, James R.
Shoulders, Harrison
Smillie, Wilson G.
Wahl, Harry R.
Weed, Lewis H.
White, Paul D.

1887

Barnes, William H.
Brown, William E.
Coller, Frederick
Leighton, Adam P.
Lynch, Kenneth M.
Mann, Frank C.

1888

Aldrich, Charles A.
Bayne-Jones, Stanhope
Chesney, Alan M.
Cutler, Elliott C.
Gardner, Leroy U.

Gasser, Herbert S.
Maloney, Arnold H.
Murray, Peter M.
Rivers, Thomas M.
Smith, Fred M.
Waksman, Selman A.

1889

Bertner, Ernst W.
Bishop, George H.
Fishbein, Morris
Hill, Frederick
Hume, Edgar E.
Mahoney, John F.
Marshall, E. K., Jr.
Maxcy, Kenneth F.
Reid, Mont R.
Smith, Relliford S.
Toomey, John A.

1890

Becker, Harry F.
De Kruif, Paul H.
Donnell, Clyde H.
Garvin, Charles H.
Giles, Roscoe C.
Graham, Helen T.
Greenberg, Morris
Hartmann, Alexis F.
Kelly, George L.
Larsen, Nils P.
Middleton, William S.
Muller, Hermann J.
Smith, Alonzo D.
Spray, Robb S.
Trask, James D.
Wilson, Frank N.

1891

Alexander, Franz G.
Foley, Frederick
McMaster, Philip D.
McQuarrie, Irvine
Sigerist, Henry E.
Wright, Louis T.

1892

Allen, Edgar
Burton, De Witt
Cohn, Edwin J.
Craig, Winchell
Davison, Wilburt C.
Gifford, Sanford R.

Hall, James L.
Lawless, Theodore K.
Parran, Thomas
Rappleye, Willard C.
Richards, Paul S.
Sullivan, Harry S.
Tillett, William S.
Vincent, Ubert C.

1893

Barron, Moses
Dibble, Eugene H.
Dragstedt, Lester
Freedlander, Samuel O.
Garland, Joseph
Padgett, Earl C.
Paul, John R.
Shryock, Richard H.
Tildon, Toussaint
Whittico, James

1894

Beck, Claude S.
Callister, Alfred C.
Johnson, A. Holmes
Lam, Frederick K.

1895

Churchill, Edward D.
Glasser, Otto
Loeb, Robert F.
Raab, Wilhelm
Richards, Dickinson W.
Rovenstine, Emery A.
Smith, Harry P.
Smith, Homer W.

1896

Branche, George C.
Cori, Gerty
Hench, Philip S.
Smith, Margaret
Stokes, Joseph, Jr.
Viko, Louis E.

1897

Blakemore, Arthur H.
Bronk, Detlev W.
Keefer, Chester S.
Reich, Wilhelm

1898

Baird, David W. E.
Clark, Sam L.
Gathings, Joseph G.
Larson, Leonard W.
Robinson, Paul T.
Werner, Walter I.

1899

Blalock, Alfred
Fulton, John F.
Long, Perrin H.
Menninger, William C.
Osgood, Edwin E.
Theiler, Max
Von Békésy, Georg
Weiss, Soma

1900

Albright, Fuller
Dameshek, William
Evans, George
Francis, Thomas, Jr.

1901

Elvehjem, Conrad A.
Gage, E. Lyle
Greene, Clarence S.
Haight, Cameron
Long, Cyril N. H.
Morman, William D.
Shope, Richard E.
Wilkerson, Vernon A.

1902

Hoerr, Normand L.
Rousselot, Louis M.

1903

Blanton, William P.
Farber, Sidney
Gibbon, John H., Jr.
Pincus, Gregory G.
Thomas, William M.

1904

Beecher, Henry K.
Drew, Charles R.
McGee, Lemuel
O'Leary, James L.
Stanley, Wendell M.
West, Harold D.

1905

Davidson, Henry A.
Harkins, Henry N.
Marshall, Hubert
Whitehead, William M.

1906

Flocks, Rubin H.
Horsfall, Frank L., Jr.
Merritt, John W.
Stubbs, Frederick D.

1907

Laurey, James R.
Lovelace, William R. II
Payne, Howard M.

1908

Johnson, John B.
Moore, Carl V.

1909

MacLeod, Colin M.
Tatum, Edward L.

1910

Wood, William B., Jr.

1914

Pride, Maynard P.

1915

Sutherland, Earl W., Jr.

1917

Hume, David M.

1920

Clement, Kenneth W.

1923

Maddock, William O.

1927

Dooley, Thomas A.

Listing by Place of Birth

ARGENTINA

Parvin, Theophilus   1829

AUSTRALIA

Kenny, Elizabeth   1886

AUSTRIA

Brill, Abraham A.	1874
Krackowizer, Ernst	1821
Landsteiner, Karl	1868
Raab, Wilhelm	1895
Reich, Wilhelm	1897
Rubin, Isidore C.	1883

BERMUDA

Meigs, Charles D.   1792

CANADA

Abbott, Anderson	1837
Abbott, Maude	1869
Avery, Oswald T.	1877
Barker, Lewellys	1867
Cogswell, William F.	1868
Cowie, David M.	1872
Cullen, Thomas S.	1868
Evans, George	1900
Fitzbutler, (W.) Henry	1842
Healy, Henry H.	1869
Livingston, Robert R.	1827
MacCallum, William G.	1874
Mackenzie, Kenneth A. J.	1859

MacLeod, Colin M.	1909
McKenzie, Robert T.	1867
Mead, Kate C. H.	1867
Mossell, Nathan F.	1856
Nutting, Mary A.	1858
Osler, William	1849
Palmer, Daniel D.	1845
Ramsey, Walter R.	1872
Robb, Isabel A. H.	1860
Rowntree, Leonard G.	1883
Wood, Casey A.	1856

CHINA

Ah Fong, C. K.	1844
Sydenstricker, Edgar	1881

CZECHOSLOVAKIA

Cori, Gerty	1896
Koller, Carl	1857

DENMARK

Fenger, Christian	1840
Holmes, Christian	1857
Riis, Jacob A.	1849

ENGLAND

Blackwell, Elizabeth	1821
Blackwell, Emily	1826
Blake, James	1815
Blumer, George	1872
Brandreth, Benjamin	1807
Brodie, William	1823

Carroll, James	1854	Mergler, Marie J.	1851
Cramp, Arthur J.	1872	Meyer, Willy	1858
Dodd, Walter J.	1869	Munsterberg, Hugo	1863
Dunglison, Robley	1798	Ohage, Justus	1849
Dyott, Thomas W.	1777*	Sollmann, Torald H.	1874
Healy, William	1869	Steindler, Arthur	1878
Henry, Morris H.	1835	Straus, Nathan	1848
Hutchinson, Woods	1862	Von Mansfelde, Alexander S.	1845
Jacobi, Mary P.	1842	Wesselhoeft, Conrad	1834
Kearsley, John	1684	Wiesenthal, Charles F.	1726
Kempster, Walter	1841	Zakrzewska, Marie E.	1829
Long, Cyril N. H.	1901		
Mayo, William W.	1819		
Merrick, Myra K.	1825	**GREECE**	
Mouritz, Arthur**	1856	Papanicolaou, George N.	1883
Noon, Adolphus H.	1838		
Pell, Thomas	1613		
Peter, Robert	1805	**HUNGARY**	
Pott, John	*	Alexander, Franz G.	1891
Simmons, George H.	1852	Goldberger, Joseph	1874
Solly, S. Edwin	1845	Schick, Bela	1877
Tennent, John	1700*	Von Békésy, Georg	1899
Thacher, Thomas	1620	Weiss, Soma	1899
Todd, Thomas W.	1885		

FRANCE

IRAN

Belisle, Henri	1675	Whipple, Allen O.	1881
Carrel, Alexis	1873		
Prevost, Francois M.	1764*		
Saugrain deVigne, Antoine F.	1763	**IRELAND**	
Seguin, Edouard	1812	Colden, Cadwallader	1688
Seguin, Edward C.	1843	Crawford, John	1746
Sigerist, Henry E.	1891	Den, Richard S.	1821
		Ferguson, Richard B.	1769
GERMANY		Lyster, Henry F. L.	1837
Brodel, Max	1870	Martin, Henry N.	1848
Glasser, Otto	1895	Thornton, Matthew	1714
Heermann, Lewis	1779		
Hering, Constantine	1800	**JAPAN**	
Hillebrand, Wilhelm	1821		
Hoffman, Frederick	1865	Noguchi, Hideya	1876
Horney, Karen	1885	Takamine, Jokichi	1854
Jacobi, Abraham	1830		
Klebs, Theodore A.	1834	**LIBERIA**	
Knapp, (J.) Hermann	1832	Fuller, Solomon C.	1872
Kober, George M.	1850		
Kolle, Frederick S.	1872		
Loeb, Jacques	1859	**NORWAY**	
Loeb, Leo	1869		

* Year of birth uncertain
**Place of birth uncertain

Engstad, John E.	1858
Gundersen, Adolf	1865

POLAND

Baruch, Simon	1840
Gruening, Emil	1842

RUMANIA

Greenberg, Morris	1890

RUSSIA

Barron, Moses	1893
Dameshek, William	1900
Einhorn, Max	1862
Meltzer, Samuel J.	1851
Rubinow, Isaac M.	1875
Spivak, Charles D.	1861
Waksman, Selman A.	1888
Yarros, Rachelle	1869

SCOTLAND

Brown, William	1748
Craik, James	1730
Cushny, Arthur R.	1866
Douglass, William	1691*
Garden, Alexander	1730
Grassick, James	1850
Hunter, William	1729*
Kirkwood, James P.	1807
Lining, John	1708
Middleton, Peter	1700*
Olyphant, David	1720
Pattison, Granville S.	1791
Ramsay, Alexander	1754
Reyburn, Robert	1833
Skene, Alexander J. C.	1837

SOUTH AFRICA

Theiler, Max	1899

SWEDEN

Folin, Otto	1867
Larsen, Nils P.	1890
Quain, Eric P.	1870

SWITZERLAND

Meyer, Adolf	1866
Meyer, Karl F.	1884
Schwyzer, Arnold	1864

Senn, Nicholas	1844
Voegtlin, Carl	1879

WEST INDIES

DaCosta, Jacob M.	1833
Francis, Grossi H.	1885
Gorrie, John	1803
Maloney, Arnold H.	1888
Quinland, William S.	1885

UNITED STATES

Alabama

Baldwin, William O.	1818
Boswell, Henry	1884
Bozeman, Nathan	1825
Cary, Edward H.	1872
Evans, William A., Jr.	1865
Gorgas, William C.	1845
Haralson, Hugh H.	1854
Hill, Luther L.	1862
Johnson, John B.	1908
Pope, Charles A.	1818

Arizona

Montezuma, Carlos	1865

Arkansas

Dibrell, James A., Jr.	1846
Hooper, Philo O.	1833
Meriwether, Clinton P.	1867
Robinson, Paul T.	1898
Smith, Morgan	1868

California

Abrams, Albert	1863
Dochez, Alphonse	1882
Erlanger, Joseph	1874
Goodfellow, George E.	1855
Haight, Cameron	1901
Hirschfelder, Arthur D.	1879
Krebs, Ernest	1877
Nuttall, George H. F.	1862
Tait, F. Dudley	1862

Colorado

Allen, Edgar	1892
Espinosa, Tobias	1879
Lennox, William G.	1884
Sabin, Florence R.	1871
Smillie, Wilson G.	1886

| Smith, Homer W. | 1895 |
| Tatum, Edward L. | 1909 |

Connecticut

Alcott, William A.	1798
Ayer, James C.	1818
Bancroft, Frederick	1834
Bayley, Richard	1745
Beach, Wooster	1794
Beard, George M.	1839
Beaumont, William	1785
Beers, Clifford	1876
Bentley, Edwin	1824
Brown, Solyman	1790
Chittenden, Russell H.	1856
Cleveland, Emeline H.	1829
Cogswell, Mason F.	1761
Coley, William B.	1862
Gallup, Joseph A.	1769
Gardner, Leroy U.	1888
Gilman, Daniel C.	1831
Graham, Sylvester	1794
Gridley, Selah	1770
Hayden, Horace H.	1769
Herter, Christian	1865
Hopkins, Lemuel	1750
Kendall, Edward C.	1886
Knight, Jonathan	1789
Lusk, Graham	1866
McClellan, George	1796
Munson, Eneas	1734
North, Elisha	1771
Osborne, Thomas B.	1859
Park, Roswell	1852
Perkins, Elisha	1741
Potter, Ellen C.	1871
Prudden, T. M.	1849
Ruggles, David	1810
Sedgwick, William T.	1855
Silliman, Benjamin	1779
Smith, Ashbel	1805
Smith, Clarence A.	1861
Todd, Eli	1769
Trall, Russell T.	1812
Van Ingen, Philip	1875
Webster, Noah	1758
Welch, William H.	1850
Wells, Harry G.	1875
Woodward, Samuel B.	1787

Delaware

| Beebe, James | 1881 |
| Black, John J. | 1837 |

Blaney, James V.	1820
Bush, Lewis P.	1812
Garretson, James E.	1828
Gibbons, Henry	1808
Handy, Margaret I.	1889
Smith, Alban G.**	1795
Squibb, Edward R.	1819
Stubbs, Frederick D.	1906
Tilton, James	1745

District of Columbia

Ashford, Bailey K.	1873
Drew, Charles R.	1904
Garrison, Fielding	1870
Greene, Clarence S.	1901
McGee, Anita N.	1864
Magruder, George L.	1848
Maury, Richard B.	1834
Payne, Howard M.	1907
Shadd, Furman J.	1852

Florida

Garvin, Charles H.	1890
Jackson, James M., Jr.	1866
Merritt, John W.	1906
Porter, Joseph Y.	1847
Wall, John P.	1836

Georgia

Arnold, Richard D.	1808
Battey, Robert	1828
Blalock, Alfred	1899
Calhoun, Abner W.	1845
Campbell, Henry F.	1824
Dugas, Louis A.	1806
Eve, Paul F.	1806
Fite, Francis B.	1861
Foster, Eugene	1850
Gunn, John C.	1800
Harris, Seale	1870
Harris, William H.	1867
Jones, Joseph	1833
Kelly, George L.	1890
Ketchum, George A.	1825
Long, Crawford W.	1815
Morman, William D.	1901
Rivers, Thomas M.	1888
Ross, Julian W.	1884
Smith, Relliford S.	1889
Weedon, Leslie W.	1860
Westmoreland, John G.	1816
Wright, Louis T.	1891

Hawaii

Lam, Frederick K.	1894

Illinois

Abt, Isaac A.	1867
Andrews, Edward W.	1856
Beatty, Theodore	1863
Becker, Harry F.	1890
Behle, Augustus	1871
Bevan, Arthur D.	1861
Black, Greene V.	1836
Churchill, Edward D.	1895
Cole, Fern M.	1876
Davis, George G.	1879
Dillehunt, Richard B.	1886
Flower, Benjamin O.	1858
Freeman, John W.	1853
Graham, Evarts A.	1883
Hamilton, John B.	1847
Herrick, James B.	1861
Hinton, William A.	1883
Hoerr, Normand L.	1902
Lathrop, Julia C.	1858
Laurey, James R.	1907
Loeb, Robert F.	1895
Novy, Frederick G.	1864
Poynter, Charles W. M.	1875
Romig, Joseph H.	1872
Smith, Fred M.	1888
Snow, William F.	1874
Stevenson, Sarah A. H.	1841
Tunnicliff, Ruth M.	1876
Wylder, Meldrum K.	1877

Indiana

Billings, John S.	1838
Dick, George F.	1881
Francis, Thomas, Jr.	1900
French, Harley E.	1873
Jackson, Algernon	1878
Maghee, Thomas G.	1842
Mann, Frank C.	1887
Menninger, Charles F.	1862
Roberts, Carl G.	1886
Rovenstine, Emery A.	1895
Stanley, Wendell M.	1904
Wiley, Harvey W.	1844
Williams, Elkanah	1822
Wishard, William N.	1851
Wynn, Frank B.	1860

Iowa

Bierring, Walter L.	1868
Carter, C. Dana	1874
Colwell, Nathan P.	1870
Dean, Lee W.	1873
Findley, Palmer	1868
Frisbie, Evelyn F.	1873
Graham, Helen T.	1890
Hertzler, Arthur E.	1870
Johnson, A. Holmes	1894
Mall, Franklin P.	1862
Palmer, Bartlett J.	1881
Robins, Charles A.	1884
Robinson, John L.	1872
Shipp, Ellis R.	1847
Shope, Richard E.	1901
Smith, Harry P.	1895
Warnshuis, Frederick C.	1880
Wiggers, Carl J.	1883
Wilbur, Ray L.	1875
Yount, Clarence E.	1874

Kansas

Beecher, Henry K.	1904
McCollum, Elmer V.	1879
Menninger, William C.	1899
Padgett, Earl C.	1893
Sellards, Andrew W.	1884
Sutherland, Earl W.	1915
Wilkerson, Vernon A.	1901

Kentucky

Abell, Irvin	1876
Bayless, George W.	1817
Bodine, James M.	1831
Briggs, William T.	1828
Brown, William W.	1816*
Flexner, Abraham	1866
Flexner, Simon	1863
Gamble, James L.	1883
Hall, William W.	1810
Harrison, John P.	1796
Henderson, Yandell	1873
Hocker, William A.	1848
Hodgen, John T.	1826
Horine, Emmet F.	1885
Hume, Edgar E.	1889
McCormack, Arthur T.	1872
McCormack, Joseph N.	1847
McDowell, Joseph N.	1805
Mathews, Joseph M.	1847
Miller, Henry, Jr.	1800

Moorman, Lewis J.	1875
Morgan, Thomas H.	1866
Pusey, William A.	1865
Rodman, William L.	1858
South, Lillian H.	1879
Sutherland, Earl W., Jr.	1915
Sutton, William L.	1797
Whitehead, Peter F.	1838
Wooten, Thomas D.	1829

Louisiana

Bayne-Jones, Stanhope	1888
Dailey, Ulysses G.	1885
Faget, Jean C.	1818
Frederick, Rivers	1873
Lawless, Theodore K.	1892
Matas, Rudolph	1860
Murray, Peter M.	1888
Phares, David L.	1817
Souchon, Edmund	1841

Maine

Barker, B. Fordyce	1818
Bates, James	1789
Brackett, Cyrus F.	1833
Coffin, Nathaniel, Jr.	1744
Cutler, Elliott C.	1888
Cutter, Ammi R.	1735
Davis, Henry G.	1807
Dix, Dorothea L.	1802
Garcelon, Alonzo	1813
Gerrish, Frederic	1845
Hill, Frederick	1889
Holt, Erastus E.	1849
Howe, Lucien	1848
Jordan, Edwin O.	1866
Ladd, Edwin F.	1859
Leighton, Adam P.	1887
Lincoln, Benjamin	1802
Maxcy, Kenneth F.	1889
Mills, Hiram F.	1836
Neal, Josephine B.	1880
Parsons, Usher	1788
Phillips, Josiah L.	1835
Storer, David H.	1804
White, Ellen G.	1827
White, James C.	1833
Whitman, Royal	1857
Wolcott, Laura J. R.	1826

Maryland

Archer, John	1741
Bartholow, Roberts	1831

Bedford, Gunning	1806
Benjamin, Dowling	1849
Bond, Thomas	1713
Brown, Lawrason	1871
Busey, Samuel C.	1828
Chesney, Alan M.	1888
Councilman, William T.	1854
Davidge, John B.	1768
Gies, William J.	1872
Godman, John D.	1794
Hammond, William A.	1828
Hemmeter, John C.	1864
Howell, William H.	1860
Jean, Sally L.	1878
Lazear, Jesse W.	1866
Longcope, Warfield T.	1877
Longshore, Hannah E. M.	1819
Main, John H. T.	1813
Marine, David	1880
Marriott, W. McKim	1885
Parran, Thomas	1892
Potter, Nathaniel	1770
Procter, William, Jr.	1817
Richardson, Rodney H.	1860
Ridgely, Frederick	1757
Robinson, G. Canby	1878
Rous, Peyton	1879
Sachs, Bernard	1858
Steuart, Richard S.	1797
Thomas, Mary F. M.	1816
Warfield, William A.	1866
Williams, John W.	1866
Winternitz, Milton C.	1885

Massachusetts

Aldrich, Charles A.	1888
Armsby, James H.	1809
Barker, Jeremiah	1752
Bartlett, Josiah	1729
Barton, Clara	1821
Bigelow, Henry J.	1818
Bigelow, Jacob	1786
Bowditch, Henry I.	1808
Bowditch, Henry P.	1840
Boylston, Zabdiel	1679
Bradford, Edward H.	1848
Brigham, Amariah	1798
Brown, Percy	1875
Cabot, Hugh	1872
Cabot, Richard C.	1868
Chandler, Charles F.	1836
Clapp, Asahel	1792
Clarke, Edward H.	1820

Codman, Ernest A.	1869	Pomeroy, John	1764
Cooke, John E.	1783	Prince, Morton	1854
Dalton, John Call	1825	Putnam, Charles P.	1844
Dana, Israel T.	1827	Putnam, James J.	1846
Dexter, Aaron	1750	Ray, Isaac	1807
Dickinson, Jonathan	1688	Remond, Sarah P.	1826
Earle, Pliny	1809	Richardson, Maurice H.	1851
Eddy, Harrison P.	1870	Shattuck, George C.	1783
Eliot, Charles W.	1834	Shattuck, George C., Jr.	1813
Fisher, John Dix	1797	Shattuck, Lemuel	1793
Fitz, Reginald H.	1843	Sibley, John	1757
Flint, Austin	1812	Smith, Nathan	1762
Flint, Austin, Jr.	1836	Southard, Elmer E.	1876
Forbes, Alexander	1882	Storer, Horatio R.	1830
Garland, Joseph	1893	Thacher, James	1754
Gay, Frederick	1874	Thayer, William S.	1864
Greenwood, John	1760	Tufts, Cotton	1731
Guthrie, Samuel	1782	Tupper, Henry M.	1831
Hall, G. Stanley	1844	Ware, John	1795
Hall, Josiah N.	1859	Warren, J. Collins	1842
Henderson, Lawrence	1878	Warren, John	1753
Hersey, Ezekiel	1709	Warren, John C.	1778
Hitchcock, Edward	1828	Warren, Joseph, III	1741
Holmes, Oliver W.	1809	White, Paul D.	1886
Holyoke, Edward A.	1728	Wilbur, Hervey B.	1820
Hooker, Worthington	1806	Williams, Francis H.	1852
Howe, Samuel G.	1801	Williams, Henry W.	1821
Hunt, Harriot K.	1805	Williams, Stephen W.	1790
Jackson, Charles T.	1805	Winslow, Charles-E. A.	1877
Jackson, James	1777	Wood, William B., Jr.	1910
Jackson, James, Jr.	1810	Wyman, Jeffries	1814
Jackson, John B. S.	1806	Wyman, Morrill	1812
Jarvis, Edward	1803		
Knowlton, Charles	1800	*Michigan*	
Ladd, William E.	1880	Bardeen, Charles R.	1871
Lahey, Frank H.	1880	Biddle, Andrew P.	1862
Leonard, Charles L.	1861	Cooley, Thomas B.	1871
Livermore, Mary A. R.	1821	Copeland, Royal S.	1868
Lothrop, Charles H.	1831	Davison, Wilburt C.	1892
McBurney, Charles	1845	De Kruif, Paul H.	1890
March, Alden	1795	De Witt, Lydia M.	1859
Mather, Cotton	1662*	Folks, Homer	1867
May, Frederick	1773	Hall, George C.	1864
Meserve, Charles F.	1850	Hood, William H.	1862
Miller, William S.	1858	Hume, David M.	1917
Minot, Charles S.	1852	Hurd, Henry M.	1843
Minot, George R.	1885	Huson, Florence	1857
Morton, William T. G.	1819	Kellogg, John H.	1852
Oliver, Daniel	1787	Kiefer, Guy L.	1867
Osgood, Edwin E.	1899	Koch, William	1885
Parker, Peter	1804	Lyon, Elias P.	1867
Pearce, Louise	1885	McGraw, Theodore A.	1839
Pinkham, Lydia E.	1819	Millspaugh, Joseph G.	1851

Pilcher, Lewis S.	1845	Vaughan, Victor C.	1851
Tibbals, Frank B.	1864	Vinsonhaler, Frank	1864
Van Hoosen, Bertha	1863		
Wilson, Frank N.	1890	*Montana*	

Minnesota		Dragstedt, Lester	1893
		Harkins, Henry N.	1905
Foley, Frederick	1891		
Fulton, John F.	1899	*Nebraska*	
Gillette, Arthur J.	1863		
Larson, Leonard W.	1898	Dick, Gladys	1881
Lommen, Christian	1865	Gifford, Sanford R.	1892
Mayo, Charles H.	1865	Hare, Lyle	1885
Mayo, William J.	1861	Picotte, Susan La F.	1865
Plummer, Henry S.	1874	Spray, Robb S.	1890
Ranson, Stephen W.	1880	Stastny, Olga F.	1878
Wahl, Harry R.	1886	Summers, John E., Jr.	1858
		Wolbach, Simeon B.	1880

Mississippi			
		Nevada	
Anderson, William H.	1886		
Campbell, Willis C.	1880	Sullivan, John J.	1877
Chaillé, Stanford	1830	Turner, Delos A.	1877
Davis, Abraham I.	1877		
Finney, John M.	1863	*New Hampshire*	
Hunter, John F.	1860		
Palmer, Erroll P.	1876	Appleton, Moses	1773
Underwood, Felix J.	1882	Beard, Mary	1876
West, Archa K.	1865	Bell, Luther V.	1806
Young, John W.	1846	Brackett, Joshua	1733
		Carpenter, Walter	1808
Missouri		Cheever, David W.	1831
		Crosby, Alpheus B.	1832
Anderson, John W.	1861	Crosby, Dixi	1800
Blair, Vilray P.	1871	Curtis, Alva	1797
Bousfield, Midian O.	1885	Eddy, Mary Baker	1821
Bradford, Claudius	1855	Hubbard, George W.	1841
Caldwell, Eugene W.	1870	Jackson, Hall	1739
Clendening, Logan	1884	Leavitt, Erasmus	1838
Dandy, Walter E.	1886	Mussey, Reuben D.	1780
Dooley, Thomas A.	1927	Nichols, Mary S. N. G.	1810
Fishbein, Morris	1889	Parker, Willard	1800
Gibson, Samuel C.	1857	Parsons, Mary A.	1850
Hartmann, Alexis F.	1890	Pearl, Raymond	1879
Hatcher, Robert A.	1868	Prescott, Samuel C.	1872
Lovelace, William R.	1883	Smith, Lyndon A.	1795
Lovelace, William R., II	1907	Smith, Nathan R.	1797
McLean, Mary H.	1861	Spalding, James A.	1846
Macfadden, Bernarr	1868	Spalding, Lyman	1775
McKay, Read J.	1843	Thomson, Samuel	1769
Major, Ralph H.	1884	Twitchell, Amos	1781
Moore, Carl V.	1908	Watkins, William W.	1846
Orr, Thomas G.	1884	Whipple, George H.	1878
Owens-Adair, Bethenia A.	1840	Woodward, Theodore	1788
Scammon, Richard E.	1883		

New Jersey

Bard, John	1716
Bell, Simeon B.	1820
Brown, William E.	1887
Carter, William S.	1869
Coit, Henry L.	1854
Cooke, Robert A.	1880
Coxe, John R.	1773
Davidson, Henry A.	1905
Dennis, Frederic S.	1850
Dickinson, Robert L.	1861
Drake, Daniel	1775
Edsall, David Linn	1869
Elmer, Jonathan	1745
Ford, Lewis D.	1801
Handy, John C.	1844
Hunt, Ezra M.	1830
Janeway, Edward G.	1841
Jayne, Walter A.	1853
Johnson, Peter A.	1851
Kelly, Howard A.	1858
Levy, Julius	1881
Lindsley, John B.	1822
Lozier, Clemence S.	1813
Martland, Harrison S.	1883
Moore, Edward M.	1814
Otto, John C.	1774
Pancoast, Joseph	1805
Pincus, Gregory G.	1903
Richards, Dickinson W.	1895
Rock, John S.	1825
Salmon, Daniel E.	1850
Sayre, Lewis A.	1820
Smith, Alonzo D.	1890
Smith, Peter	1753*
Smith, Thomas J.	1841
Still, James	1812
Stokes, Joseph, Jr.	1896
Tracy, Martha	1876
Weed, Gideon A.	1833
West, Harold D.	1904
Williams, William C.	1883
Wood, George B.	1797

New York

Albright, Fuller	1900
Atwater, Wilbur O.	1844
Auer, John	1875
Baker, S. Josephine	1873
Baldwin, Abel S.	1811
Barlow, Walter J.	1868
Barringer, Emily D.	1876
Beck, T. Romeyn	1791
Beecher, Clarence H.	1877
Biggs, Hermann M.	1859
Blackfan, Kenneth D.	1883
Brainard, Daniel	1812
Bronk, Detlev W.	1897
Buckingham, Richard G.	1816
Burrough, James W.	1800
Caverly, Charles S.	1856
Chase, Will H.	1874
Coakley, Cornelius	1862
Cohn, Alfred E.	1879
Cohn, Edwin J.	1892
Connor, Leartus	1843
Davis, Michael M.	1879
Davis, Nathan S.	1817
De Lee, Joseph B.	1869
Delafield, Edward	1794
Delafield, Francis	1841
Delameter, John	1787
Delano, Jane A.	1862
Donaldson, Henry H.	1857
Du Bois, Eugene F.	1882
Dunlap, Livingston	1799
Eastman, Joseph	1842
Emerson, Haven	1874
Farber, Sidney	1903
Favill, John	1819
Flocks, Rubin H.	1906
Fowler, George R.	1848
Francis, John W.	1789
Gardiner, Charles F.	1857
Gates, Frederick	1853
Giles, Roscoe C.	1890
Goldmark, Josephine	1877
Goldwater, Sigismund	1873
Greene, Cordelia	1831
Griscom, John H.	1809
Gunn, Moses	1822
Halsted, William S.	1852
Hamilton, Alice	1869
Harison, Beverly D.	1855
Harris, Chapin A.	1806
Hess, Alfred F.	1875
Holt, L. Emmett	1855
Holt, Winifred	1870
Hosack, David	1769
Howland, John	1873
Hulse, Isaac	1797
Huntington, George	1851
Jackson, James C.	1811
Jelliffe, Smith Ely	1866
Jenks, Edward W.	1833

Jones, John	1729	Spitzka, Edward C.	1852
Judd, Gerrit P.	1803	Sprague, Edward W.	1880
King, John	1813	Sternberg, George M.	1838
Koplik, Henry	1858	Stiles, Charles W.	1867
Lefferts, George M.	1846	Streeter, George L.	1873
Lewis, Dio	1823	Sullivan, Harry S.	1892
Libman, Emanuel	1872	Swain, Clara	1834
Lilienthal, Howard	1861	Swift, Homer F.	1881
Lloyd, James	1728	Taussig, Frederick J.	1872
Lloyd, John U.	1849	Thompson, Mary H.	1829
McCready, Benjamin W.	1813	Thompson, William G.	1856
McKinney-Steward, Susan M. S.	1847	Timme, Walter	1874
Mendel, Lafayette B.	1872	Trask, James D.	1890
Milroy, William F.	1855	Trudeau, Edward L.	1848
Minoka-Hill, Lillie R.	1876	Tuthill, Alexander M.	1871
Mitchill, Samuel L.	1764	Van Slyke, Donald D.	1883
Mosher, Eliza M.	1846	Vedder, Edward B.	1878
Mott, Valentine	1785	Veeder, Bordon S.	1883
Muller, Hermann J.	1890	Walker, Mary E.	1832
Mumford, James G.	1863	Waring, George E.	1833
North, Charles E.	1869	Warner, Hulbert H.	1842
Osborne, John E.	1858	Washburn, Victor D.	1882
Palmer, Alonzo B.	1815	Watson, Beriah A.	1836
Park, William H.	1863	Weiskotten, Herman G.	1884
Peck, Washington F.	1841	Wende, Ernest	1853
Perkins, Roger G.	1874	White, James P.	1811
Pitcher, Zina	1797	White, William A.	1870
Porter, Henry R.	1848	Whitman, Marcus	1802
Post, George E.	1838	Wickes, Stephen	1813
Post, Wright	1766	Witthaus, Rudolph A.	1846
Potter, William W.	1838	Wolcott, Erastus B.	1804
Purple, Samuel S.	1822	Wollstein, Martha	1868
Reeve, James T.	1834	Wood, James R.	1813
Reid, William W.	1799	Woodworth, John M.	1837
Richards, Alfred N.	1876	Zinsser, Hans	1878
Richards, Linda	1841		
Romayne, Nicholas	1756	*North Carolina*	
Rousselot, Louis M.	1902	Branche, George C.	1896
Russell, Frederick F.	1870	Brinkley, John R.	1886*
Rutherford, Frances A.	1842	Butler, Henry R.	1862
Sanger, Margaret H.	1879	Caldwell, Charles	1772
Schuyler, Louise L.	1837	Carson, Simeon L.	1882
Scott, James R.	1886	Coffey, Robert C.	1869
Seaman, Valentine	1770	Council, Walter W.	1882
Shew, Joel	1816	Curtis, Austin M.	1868
Shrady, George F.	1837	Dimock, Susan	1847
Smith, Andrew H.	1837	Donnell, Clyde H.	1890
Smith, James McC.	1813	Dorsette, Cornelius	1851
Smith, Job L.	1827	Fenner, Erasmus D.	1807
Smith, Stephen	1823	Hargis, Robert B.	1818
Smith, Theobold	1859	Hargrave, Frank S.	1874
Smith, Warren G.	1883	Haywood, Edmund B.	1825
Solis-Cohen, Jacob D.	1838	Kinyoun, Joseph J.	1860

Lattimore, John A. C.	1878*	Long, Perrin H.	1899
Long, Leroy	1869	Mallory, Frank B.	1862
McKee, William H.	1814	Mendenhall, Dorothy R.	1874
McNeill, William C.	1878	Newton, Robert S.	1818
MacNider, William de B.	1881	O'Dwyer, Joseph	1841
Manning, Isaac H.	1866	Orton, Samuel T.	1879
Moore, Aaron M.	1863	Patrick, Hugh T.	1860
Murphy, James B.	1884	Pittenger, Fred A.	1875
Pittman, Newsome J.	1818	Porter, William T.	1862
Rogers, William E.	1826	Pride, Maynard P.	1914
Shore, Clarence A.	1873	Ricketts, Howard T.	1871
Tillett, William S.	1892	Sanford, John F.	1824
Turner, John P.	1885	Schloss, Oscar M.	1882
Vincent, Hubert C.	1892	Scudder, John M.	1829
Warren, Edward	1828	Steele, Henry K.	1825
Wood, Thomas F.	1841	Toomey, John A.	1889
		Wald, Lillian D.	1867
North Dakota		Weed, Lewis H.	1886
Quain, Fannie A. D.	1874	Weeks, John E.	1853
		Werner, Walter I.	1898
Ohio			
Abel, John J.	1857	*Oklahoma*	
Benedict, Stanley R.	1884	Clinton, Fred S.	1874
Bosworth, Franke H.	1843	Wright, Eliphalet N.	1858
Brunk, Andrew S.	1884	*Oregon*	
Byford, William H.	1817		
Campbell, Elizabeth	1862	Baird, David W. E.	1898
Coffman, Victor H.	1839	*Pennsylvania*	
Cole, Rufus	1872		
Collister, George	1856	Agnew, David H.	1818
Cooper, Elias S.	1820	Atlee, John L.	1799
Craig, Winchell	1892	Atlee, Washington	1808
Crile, George W.	1864	Awl, William M.	1799
Cushing, Harvey W.	1869	Bache, Franklin	1792
Eagleson, James B.	1862	Barber, Amos	1861
Elwell, John J.	1820	Bard, Samuel	1742
Evans, John	1814	Barnes, William H.	1887
Finfrock, John H.	1836	Barton, Benjamin	1766
Fordyce, John A.	1858	Barton, William P. C.	1786
Freedlander, Samuel O.	1893	Beck, Claude S.	1894
Fulton, Mary H.	1854	Bilderback, Joseph B.	1869
Galland, Isaac	1790*	Blake, Francis G.	1877
Gilliam, David T.	1844	Blesh, Abraham L.	1866
Gross, Samuel W.	1837	Bobbs, John S.	1809
Howard, William F.	1868	Brinton, John H.	1832
Hoyt, John W.	1831	Broomall, Anna E.	1847
Hughes, Henry A.	1848	Brown, Charlotte	1846
Hunt, Reid	1870	Cadwalader, Thomas	1707*
Hurty, John N.	1852	Carmalt, William H.	1836
Johnston, George P.	1863	Coca, Arthur F.	1875
Jones, Noble W.	1876	Cochran, John	1730
Kerr, John G.	1824	Crumbine, Samuel J.	1862
Lane, Levi C.	1830	Darlington, William	1782

de Schweinitz, George E.	1858	Mills, Charles K.	1845
Deaver, John B.	1855	Mitchell, S. Weir	1829
Dewees, William P.	1768	Morgan, John	1735
Dock, George	1860	Morton, Samuel G.	1799
Dock, Lavinia L.	1858	Orr, Hiram W.	1877
Dolley, Sarah R. A.	1829	Packard, Francis R.	1870
Dorsey, John S.	1783	Parrish, Isaac	1811
Downey, Hal	1877	Parrish, Joseph	1818
Duhring, Louis A.	1845	Passavant, William A.	1821
Durham, James	1762	Paul, John R.	1893
Eberle, John	1787	Pennock, Caspar W.	1799
Ewing, James	1866	Pepper, William	1843
Flick, Lawrence F.	1856	Physick, Philip S.	1763
Fussell, Bartholomew	1794	Preston, Ann	1813
Gallaudet, Thomas	1787	Purvis, Charles B.	1842
Gerhard, William W.	1809	Ramsay, David	1749
Gibbon, John H., Jr.	1903	Rauch, John H.	1828
Gihon, Albert L.	1833	Redman, John	1722
Gray, John P.	1825	Robertson, William S.	1831
Gross, Samuel D.	1805	Roman, Charles V.	1864
Harrison, Ross G.	1870	Rosenau, Milton J.	1869
Hartman, Samuel B.	1830	Rotch, Thomas M.	1849
Hays, Isaac	1796	Rush, Benjamin	1746
Helmuth, William T.	1833	Schamberg, Jay F.	1870
Hench, Philip S.	1896	Shakespeare, Edward O.	1846
Hinson, Eugene T.	1873	Shippen, William	1736
Hodge, Hugh L.	1796	Shryock, Richard H.	1893
Hughes, John C.	1821	Smith, Albert H.	1835
Hullihen, Simon P.	1810	Smith, Margaret G.	1896
Jackson, Chevalier	1865	Solis-Cohen, Solomon	1857
Jackson, Edward	1856	Stillé, Alfred	1813
Jackson, Samuel	1787	Toner, Joseph M.	1825
Kane, John K.	1833	Tyson, James	1841
Keefer, Chester S.	1897	Walker, Delos	1836
Keen, William W., Jr.	1837	Walsh, James J.	1865
Kelley, Florence	1859	Weible, Ralph E.	1878
Kirkbride, Thomas S.	1809	Williams, Daniel H.	1858
Kline, Benjamin S.	1886	Wilson, Louis B.	1866
Knox, James H. M., Jr.	1872	Wistar, Caspar	1761
Kuhn, Adam	1741	Wood, Horatio C.	1841
Lamb, Daniel S.	1843	Woodward, Joseph J.	1833
Leidy, Joseph	1823		
Letterman, Jonathan	1824	*Rhode Island*	
Long, Francis A.	1859		
MacFarlane, Catharine	1877	Bartlett, Elisha	1804
McKean, Robert	1732	Channing, Walter	1786
McMaster, Philip D.	1891	Chapin, Charles V.	1856
Marshall, Clara	1847	Church, Benjamin	1734
Matson, Ralph C.	1880	Howe, Percy R.	1864
Matson, Ray W.	1880	Waterhouse, Benjamin	1754
Meigs, Arthur V.	1850		
Meigs, John F.	1818	*South Carolina*	
Middleton, William S.	1890	Babcock, James W.	1856
		Bryce, Peter	1834

Bull, William	1710
Cannon, George E.	1869
Chisolm, Julian J.	1830
Daniel, Richard P.	1828
Dibble, Eugene H.	1893
Dickson, Samuel H.	1798
Evans, Matilda A.	1872
Fayssoux, Peter	1745
Gary, Thomas P.	1835
Geddings, Eli	1799
Jervey, James W.	1874
Just, Ernest E.	1883
Keyes, Edward L.	1843
Lambright, Middleton H.	1865
McClennan, Alonzo C.	1855
Marshall, E. K., Jr.	1889
Minton, Henry M.	1870
Moore, Samuel P.	1813
Moultrie, John, Jr.	1729
Nott, Josiah C.	1804
Palmer, Thomas M.	1821
Porcher, Francis P.	1825
Sims, J. Marion	1813
Steele, William L.	1833
Thomas, T. Gaillard	1831
Toland, Hugh H.	1806
Weatherly, Job S.	1828

South Dakota

Coller, Frederick	1887
Donahoe, William E.	1886
Smith, Philip E.	1884

Tennessee

Boyd, Robert F.	1858
Burton, De Witt	1892
Cheatham, Anderson	1880
Clark, Sam L.	1898
Cochran, Jerome	1831
Dibrell, James A.	1817
Ellett, Edward C.	1869
Gant, Harris A.	1852
Goodpasture, Ernest W.	1886
Haggard, William D., Jr.	1872
Hale, John H.	1878*
Lenow, James H.	1850
Lynk, Miles V.	1871
Mitchell, Robert W.	1831
Moeur, Benjamin B.	1869
Robertson, Felix	1781
Rose, Wickliffe	1862
Shoulders, Harrison	1886

Witherspoon, John A.	1864
Yandell, Lunsford P.	1805

Texas

Bertner, Ernst W.	1889
Blanton, William P.	1903
Covington, Benjamin J.	1869
Cox, George W., Jr.	1879
Dickerson, Spencer C.	1871
Dyer, Isadore	1865
Fortner, Benjamin	1847
Garrison, Charles W.	1879
Gathings, Joseph G.	1898
Hall, James L.	1892
Lynch, Kenneth M.	1887
McGee, Lemuel C.	1904
Majors, Monroe A.	1864
Moten, Pierce S.	1878
Moursund, Walter H.	1884
Nixon, Pat I.	1883
Perry, John E.	1870
Randall, Edward	1860
Scott, Arthur C.	1865
Taylor, Eugene T.	1882
Thomas, William M.	1903
Tildon, Toussaint T.	1893
Young, Hugh H.	1870

Utah

Callister, Alfred C.	1894
McQuarrie, Irvine	1891
Marshall, Hyrum L.	1884
Morrell, Joseph R.	1879
Richards, George G.	1883
Richards, Paul S.	1892
Richards, Ralph T.	1880
Viko, Louis E.	1896

Vermont

Allen, Lyman	1872
Andrews, Edmund	1824
Baker, Henry B.	1837
Burgess, Alexander	1885
Buxton, Lauren H.	1859
Dana, Charles L.	1852
Denison, Charles	1845
Fabrique, Andrew H.	1842
Fairchild, David S.	1847
Green, Horace	1802
Gregory, Samuel	1813
Harris, Elisha	1824
Hazen, Allen	1869
Hewitt, Charles N.	1835

Hitchcock, Homer O.	1827
Holton, Henry D.	1838
Loomis, Alfred L.	1831
Maynard, David S.	1808
Morse, John F.	1815
Paine, Martyn	1794
Parmly, Eleazar	1797
Pettigrew, George A.	1858
Phelps, Edward E.	1803
Ripley, Martha G.	1843
Snow, Edwin M.	1820
Spafford, Frederick A.	1855
Stickney, Victor H.	1855
Stone, Warren	1808
Taylor, Charles F.	1827
Thayer, Samuel W.	1817
Tinkham, Henry C.	1856
Towne, Solon R.	1846
Wells, Horace	1815
Wheeler, John B.	1853

Virginia

Adams, Numa P. G.	1885
Alexander, Walter G.	1880
Anderson, William H.	1820
Antony, Milton	1789
Augusta, Alexander	1825
Baynham, William	1749
Blakemore, Arthur H.	1897
Blanton, Wyndham B.	1880
Bowling, William K.	1808
Brown, Samuel	1769
Cabell, James	1813
Carter, Henry R.	1852
Cartwright, Samuel A.	1793
Chapman, Nathaniel	1780
Clement, Kenneth W.	1920
Cole, Richard B.	1829
Crowe, Samuel J.	1883
Davis, John S.	1872
Dudley, Benjamin W.	1785
Ewell, James	1773
Farrar, Bernard G.	1784
Fearn, Thomas	1789
Frost, Wade H.	1880
Galt, William C.	1777
Gamble, Henry F.	1862
Griffin, John S.	1816
Horner, William E.	1793
Howard, William T.	1821
Jarvis, William C.	1855
Kenney, John A.	1874
Leathers, Waller S.	1874

Lumsden, Leslie L.	1875
McCaw, James B.	1823
McCaw, Walter D.	1863
McClurg, James	1746
McDowell, Ephraim	1771
McGuire, Hunter H.	1835
Mason, James T.	1882
Miller, Thomas	1806
Monette, John W.	1803
Opie, Eugene L.	1873
Price, Joseph	1853
Reed, Walter	1851
Reid, Mont R.	1889
Sewall, Henry	1855
Still, Andrew T.	1828
Thoms, Adah B. S.	1863
Timberlake, Gideon	1876
Vaughan, George T.	1859
Vest, Walter	1882
Whitehead, William M.	1905
Whitehead, William R.	1831

Washington

Horsfall, Frank L., Jr.	1906
Lovejoy, Esther P.	1870
Maddock, William O.	1923

West Virginia

Cordell, Eugene F.	1843
Delany, Martin R.	1812
Marshall, Hubert	1905
Mitchell, John K.	1793
Moore, Phoebia G.	1872
Shaffer, Philip A.	1881
Simpson, John	1869
Thompson, Solomon H.	1870
Whittico, James M.	1893

Wisconsin

Alcock, Nathaniel	1881
Benedict, Francis G.	1870
Billings, Frank	1854
Bingham, Arthur W.	1872
Bishop, George H.	1889
Bloodgood, Joseph C.	1867
Burch, Frank E.	1876
Cannon, Ida M.	1877
Cannon, Walter B.	1871
Darrow, Edward M.	1855
Dearholt, Hoyt E.	1879
Donaldson, Mary E.	1851
Elvehjem, Conrad A.	1901
Favill, Henry B.	1860

Gage, E. Lyle	1901	McGillycuddy, Valentine T.	1849
Gasser, Herbert S.	1888	Mahoney, John F.	1889
Gesell, Arnold L.	1880	Martin, Franklin H.	1857
Gifford, Harold	1858	Murphy, John B.	1857
Harper, Cornelius	1864	O'Leary, James L.	1904
Heath, Lillian	1865	Ramstad, Niles O.	1875
Heg, Elmer E.	1861	Rappleye, Willard C.	1892
Hektoen, Ludvig	1863	Sleyster, Rock	1879
Jermain, Louis F.	1867	Smith, Andrew C.	1856
Kremers, Edward	1865	Steenbock, Harry	1886

Listing by State Where Prominent

Alabama

Anderson, William H. (b. 1820)
Baldwin, William O.
Bozeman, Nathan
Branche, George C.
Bryce, Peter
Cochran, Jerome
Dibble, Eugene H.
Dorsette, Cornelius
Fearn, Thomas
Harris, Seale
Hill, Luther L.
Kenney, John A.
Ketchum, George A.
Moten, Pierce S.
Nott, Josiah C.
Quinland, William S.
Sims, J. Marion
Tildon, Toussaint T.
Weatherly, Job S.

Alaska

Blanton, William P.
Chase, Will H.
Council, Walter W.
Davis, George G.
Johnson, A. Holmes
Maddock, William O.
Romig, Joseph H.
Whitehead, William M.

Arizona

Goodfellow, George E.
Handy, John C.
Hughes, Henry A.

Moeur, Benjamin B.
Noon, Adolphus H.
Palmer, Erroll P.
Tuthill, Alexander M.
Yount, Clarence E.

Arkansas

Bentley, Edwin
Dibrell, James A.
Dibrell, James A., Jr.
Garrison, Charles W.
Hooper, Philo O.
Lenow, James H.
Main, John H. T.
Meriwether, Clinton P.
Smith, Morgan
Vinsonhaler, Frank

California

Abrams, Albert
Barker, Lewellys
Barlow, Walter J.
Benites, Jose M.
Blake, James
Brown, Charlotte
Burrough, James W.
Cole, Richard B.
Cooper, Elias S.
Den, Richard S.
Gay, Frederick
Gibbons, Henry
Griffin, John S.
Kinyoun, Joseph J.
Krebs, Ernest
Lane, Levi C.
Letterman, Jonathan

Loeb, Jacques
Meyer, Karl F.
Morgan, Thomas H.
Morse, John F.
Smith, Philip E.
Snow, William F.
Stanley, Wendell M.
Tait, F. Dudley
Tatum, Edward L.
Thomas, William M.
Toland, Hugh H.
Whipple, George H.
White, Ellen G.
Wilbur, Ray L.

Colorado

Bancroft, Frederick
Buckingham, Richard G.
Denison, Charles
Evans, John
Gardiner, Charles F.
Hall, Josiah N.
Jackson, Edward
Jayne, Walter A.
Sabin, Florence R.
Sewall, Henry
Solly, S. Edwin
Spivak, Charles D.
Steele, Henry K.
Whitehead, William R.

Connecticut

Allen, Edgar
Atwater, Wilbur O.
Bayne-Jones, Stanhope
Beers, Clifford
Benedict, Francis G.
Blake, Francis G.
Blumer, George
Carmalt, William H.
Chittenden, Russell H.
Cogswell, Mason F.
Fulton, John F.
Gallaudet, Thomas
Gesell, Arnold L.
Harrison, Ross G.
Henderson, Yandell
Hooker, Worthington
Hopkins, Lemuel
Knight, Jonathan
Long, Cyril N. H.
Mead, Kate C. H.
Mendel, Lafayette B.

Munson, Eneas
North, Elisha
Osborne, Thomas B.
Paul, John R.
Pell, Thomas
Perkins, Elisha
Silliman, Benjamin
Smith, Nathan
Tatum, Edward L.
Todd, Eli
Trask, James D.
Webster, Noah
Wells, Horace
Winslow, Charles-E. A.
Winternitz, Milton C.
Woodward, Samuel B.

Delaware

Beebe, James
Black, John J.
Bush, Lewis P.
Handy, Margaret I.
Kane, John K.
McGee, Lemuel C.
McKay, Read J.
Tilton, James
Washburn, Victor D.

District of Columbia

Abbott, Anderson
Adams, Numa P. G.
Augusta, Alexander
Barton, Clara
Bayne-Jones, Stanhope
Billings, John S.
Busey, Samuel C.
Carroll, James
Carson, Simeon L.
Curtis, Austin M.
Drew, Charles R.
Garrison, Fielding
Gathings, Joseph G.
Greene, Clarence S.
Hall, James L.
Hamilton, John B.
Hammond, William A.
Jackson, Algernon
Johnson, John B.
Just, Ernest E.
Kinyoun, Joseph J.
Kober, George M.
Lamb, Daniel S.
Laurey, James R.

Lumsden, Leslie L.
Magruder, George L.
Maloney, Arnold H.
Maxcy, Kenneth F.
May, Frederick
McGee, Anita N.
McNeill, William C.
Miller, Thomas
Parker, Peter
Parsons, Mary A.
Payne, Howard M.
Purvis, Charles B.
Reed, Walter
Reyburn, Robert
Ross, Julian W.
Rousselot, Louis M.
Russell, Frederick F.
Shadd, Furman J.
Smith, Alonzo D.
Smith, Theobold
Sternberg, George M.
Stiles, Charles W.
Sullivan, Harry S.
Sydenstricker, Edgar
Toner, Joseph M.
Vaughan, George T.
Vedder, Edward B.
Walker, Mary E.
Warfield, William A.
White, William A.
Wiley, Harvey W.
Wilkerson, Vernon A.
Williams, Daniel H.
Woodward, Joseph J.

Florida

Baldwin, Abel S.
Daniel, Richard P.
Gary, Thomas P.
Gorrie, John
Hargis, Robert B.
Hulse, Isaac
Jackson, James M., Jr.
Merritt, John W.
Moultrie, John, Jr.
Palmer, Thomas M.
Porter, Joseph Y.
Wall, John P.
Weedon, Leslie W.

Georgia

Antony, Milton
Arnold, Richard D.

Battey, Robert
Butler, Henry R.
Calhoun, Abner W.
Campbell, Henry F.
Dugas, Louis A.
Eve, Paul F.
Ewell, James
Ford, Lewis D.
Foster, Eugene
Harris, William H.
Jones, Joseph
Kelly, George L.
Long, Crawford W.
Smith, Relliford S.
Westmoreland, John G.

Hawaii

Hillebrand, Wilhelm
Judd, Gerrit P.
Lam, Frederick K.
Larsen, Nils P.
Mouritz, Arthur A.
Von Békésy, Georg

Idaho

Ah Fong, C. K.
Cole, Fern M.
Collister, George
Donaldson, Mary E.
Howard, William F.
Pittenger, Fred A.
Robins, Charles A.
Watkins, William W.

Illinois

Abbott, Anderson
Abt, Isaac A.
Aldrich, Charles A.
Alexander, Franz G.
Andrews, Edmund
Andrews, Edward W.
Bevan, Arthur D.
Billings, Frank
Black, Greene V.
Blaney, James V.
Bousfield, Midian O.
Brainard, Daniel
Byford, William H.
Colwell, Nathan P.
Cooper, Elias S.
Dailey, Ulysses G.

Davis, Nathan S.
De Lee, Joseph B.
De Witt, Lydia M.
Dick, George F.
Dick, Gladys
Dickerson, Spencer C.
Dock, Lavinia L.
Donaldson, Henry H.
Dragstedt, Lester
Evans, John
Evans, William A., Jr.
Favill, Henry B.
Fenger, Christian
Fishbein, Morris
Gifford, Sanford R.
Giles, Roscoe C.
Hall, George C.
Hall, James L.
Hamilton, Alice
Hamilton, John B.
Healy, William
Hektoen, Ludvig
Herrick, James B.
Hoerr, Normand L.
Jordan, Edwin O.
Kelley, Florence
Klebs, Theodore A.
Lathrop, Julia C.
Lawless, Theodore K.
Livermore, Mary A.
Loeb, Jacques
Majors, Monroe A.
Martin, Franklin H.
Mergler, Marie J.
Montezuma, Carlos
Murphy, John B.
Patrick, Hugh T.
Pusey, William A.
Ranson, Stephen W.
Rauch, John H.
Ricketts, Howard T.
Roberts, Carl G.
Senn, Nicholas
Simmons, George H.
Stevenson, Sarah A. H.
Thompson, Mary H.
Tunnicliff, Ruth M.
Van Hoosen, Bertha
Wells, Harry G.
Williams, Daniel H.
Wood, Casey A.
Woodworth, John M.
Yarros, Rachelle S.

Indiana

Bobbs, John S.
Clapp, Asahel
Dunlap, Livingston
Eastman, Joseph
Evans, John
Hurty, John N.
Parvin, Theophilus
Thomas, Mary F. M.
Wiley, Harvey W.
Wishard, William N.
Wynn, Frank B.

Iowa

Alcock, Nathaniel
Bierring, Walter L.
Dean, Lee W.
Fairchild, David S.
Flocks, Rubin H.
Galland, Isaac
Hughes, John C.
Lothrop, Charles H.
Orton, Samuel T.
Palmer, Bartlett J.
Palmer, Daniel D.
Peck, Washington F.
Robertson, William S.
Sanford, John F.
Smith, Fred M.
Smith, Harry P.
Steindler, Arthur

Kansas

Bell, Simeon B.
Brinkley, John R.
Clendening, Logan
Crumbine, Samuel J.
Fabrique, Andrew H.
Hertzler, Arthur E.
Major, Ralph H.
Menninger, Charles F.
Menninger, William C.
Orr, Thomas G.
Padgett, Earl C.
Thompson, Solomon H.
Wahl, Harry R.

Kentucky

Abell, Irvin
Bayless, George W.
Bodine, James M.

Brown, Samuel
Caldwell, Charles
Cooke, John E.
Drake, Daniel
Dudley, Benjamin W.
Ferguson, Richard B.
Fitzbutler, (W.) Henry
Flexner, Abraham
Galt, William C.
Gross, Samuel D.
Harrison, John P.
Horine, Emmet F.
Lattimore, John A. C.
McCormack, Arthur T.
McCormack, Joseph N.
McDowell, Ephraim
Mathews, Joseph M.
Miller, Henry, Jr.
Peter, Robert
Ridgely, Frederick
Rodman, William L.
Smith, Alban G.
South, Lillian H.
Sutton, William L.
Yandell, Lunsford P.

Louisiana

Cartwright, Samuel A.
Chaillé, Stanford
Durham, James
Dyer, Isadore
Faget, Jean C.
Fenner, Erasmus D.
Frederick, Rivers
Jones, Joseph
Matas, Rudolph
Prevost, Francois M.
Robinson, Paul T.
Sibley, John
Souchon, Edmund
Stone, Warren

Maine

Appleton, Moses
Barker, Jeremiah
Bates, James
Coffin, Nathaniel, Jr.
Dana, Israel T.
Garcelon, Alonzo
Gerrish, Frederic
Hill, Frederick
Holt, Erastus E.
Leighton, Adam P.

Pearl, Raymond
Ramsay, Alexander
Reich, Wilhelm
Smith, Nathan
Spalding, James A.

Maryland

Abel, John J.
Archer, John
Barker, Lewellys
Billings, John S.
Blalock, Alfred
Bloodgood, Joseph C.
Brodel, Max
Chesney, Alan M.
Chisolm, Julian J.
Cordell, Eugene F.
Crawford, John
Crowe, Samuel J.
Cullen, Thomas S.
Dandy, Walter E.
Davidge, John B.
Dock, Lavinia L.
Finney, John M.
Flexner, Simon
Frost, Wade H.
Garrison, Fielding
Gilman, Daniel C.
Halsted, William S.
Harris, Chapin A.
Harrison, Ross G.
Hayden, Horace H.
Hemmeter, John C.
Hirschfelder, Arthur D.
Howard, William T.
Howell, William H.
Howland, John
Hurd, Henry M.
Jean, Sally L.
Kelly, Howard A.
Knox, James H. M., Jr.
Lazear, Jesse W.
Long, Perrin H.
Longcope, Warfield T.
MacCallum, William G.
Mall, Franklin P.
Marshall, E. K., Jr.
Martin, Henry N.
Maxcy, Kenneth F.
Mead, Kate C. H.
Meyer, Adolf
Nuttall, George H.
Nutting, Mary A.

Osler, William
Pattison, Granville S.
Pearl, Raymond
Potter, Nathaniel
Robb, Isabel A. H.
Rowntree, Leonard
Sabin, Florence R.
Shryock, Richard H.
Sigerist, Henry E.
Smith, Nathan R.
Steuart, Richard S.
Stiles, Charles W.
Streeter, George L.
Sullivan, Harry S.
Thayer, William S.
Timberlake, Gideon
Voegtlin, Carl
Warren, Edward
Weed, Lewis H.
Welch, William H.
Wiesenthal, Charles F.
Williams, John W.
Wood, William B., Jr.
Young, Hugh H.

Massachusetts

Albright, Fuller
Alcott, William A.
Ayer, James C.
Bartlett, Elisha
Beard, Mary
Beecher, Henry K.
Bell, Luther V.
Bigelow, Henry J.
Bigelow, Jacob
Blackfan, Kenneth D.
Bowditch, Henry I.
Bowditch, Henry P.
Boylston, Zabdiel
Bradford, Edward H.
Brown, Percy
Cabot, Hugh
Cabot, Richard C.
Cannon, Ida M.
Cannon, Walter B.
Channing, Walter
Cheever, David W.
Church, Benjamin
Churchill, Edward D.
Clarke, Edward H.
Codman, Ernest A.
Cohn, Edwin J.
Councilman, William T.

Cushing, Harvey W.
Cutler, Elliott C.
Dameshek, William
Davis, Michael M.
Delameter, John
Dexter, Aaron
Dimock, Susan
Dix, Dorothea
Dodd, Walter J.
Douglass, William
Earle, Pliny
Eddy, Harrison P.
Eddy, Mary Baker
Edsall, David Linn
Eliot, Charles W.
Farber, Sidney
Fisher, John Dix
Fitz, Reginald H.
Folin, Otto
Forbes, Alexander
Fuller, Solomon C.
Gamble, James L.
Garland, Joseph
Graham, Sylvester
Gregory, Samuel
Hall, G. Stanley
Hamilton, Alice
Hazen, Allen
Henderson, Lawrence
Hersey, Ezekiel
Hinton, William A.
Hitchcock, Edward
Holmes, Oliver W.
Holyoke, Edward A.
Howe, Percy R.
Howe, Samuel G.
Hume, David M.
Hunt, Harriot K.
Hunt, Reid
Jackson, Charles T.
Jackson, James
Jackson, James, Jr.
Jackson, John B. S.
Jarvis, Edward
Keefer, Chester S.
Kirkwood, James P.
Knowlton, Charles
Ladd, William E.
Lahey, Frank H.
Lennox, William G.
Lewis, Dio
Livermore, Mary A.
Lloyd, James

Mallory, Frank B.
Mather, Cotton
Meyer, Adolf
Mills, Hiram F.
Minot, Charles S.
Minot, George R.
Morton, William T. G.
Mumford, James G.
Munsterberg, Hugo
Pincus, Gregory G.
Pinkham, Lydia E.
Porter, William T.
Prescott, Samuel C.
Prince, Morton
Purvis, Charles B.
Putnam, Charles P.
Putnam, James J.
Remond, Sarah P.
Richards, Linda
Richardson, Maurice H.
Rock, John S.
Rosenau, Milton J.
Rotch, Thomas M.
Ruggles, David
Schloss, Oscar M.
Sedgwick, William T.
Sellards, Andrew W.
Shattuck, George C.
Shattuck, George C., Jr.
Shattuck, Lemuel
Smillie, Wilson G.
Smith, Theobold
Southard, Elmer E.
Storer, David H.
Storer, Horatio R.
Thacher, James
Thacher, Thomas
Theiler, Max
Thomson, Samuel
Tufts, Cotton
Von Békésy, Georg
Ware, John
Warren, J. Collins
Warren, John
Warren, John C.
Warren, Joseph, III
Waterhouse, Benjamin
Weiss, Soma
Wesselhoeft, Conrad
White, James C.
White, Paul D.
Wilbur, Hervey B.
Williams, Francis H.

Williams, Henry W.
Williams, Stephen W.
Wolbach, Simeon B.
Woodward, Samuel B.
Wyman, Jeffries
Wyman, Morrill
Zakrzewska, Marie E.
Zinsser, Hans

Michigan

Andrews, Edmund
Baker, Henry B.
Becker, Harry F.
Belisle, Henri
Biddle, Andrew P.
Brodie, William
Brunk, Andrew S.
Burton, De Witt
Cabot, Hugh
Coller, Frederick
Connor, Leartus
Cooley, Thomas B.
Copeland, Royal S.
Cowie, David M.
Cushny, Arthur R.
De Kruif, Paul H.
De Witt, Lydia M.
Dock, George
Francis, Thomas, Jr.
Gunn, Moses
Haight, Cameron
Harison, Beverly D.
Hitchcock, Homer O.
Hurd, Henry M.
Huson, Florence
Jenks, Edward W.
Kellogg, John H.
Kiefer, Guy L.
Koch, William
Lyster, Henry F. L.
McGraw, Theodore A.
Mosher, Eliza M.
Northcross, David C.
Novy, Frederick G.
Palmer, Alonzo B.
Pitcher, Zina
Rutherford, Frances A.
Tibbals, Frank B.
Vaughan, Victor C.
Warnshuis, Frederick C.
White, Ellen G.
Wilson, Frank N.

Minnesota

Aldrich, Charles A.
Barron, Moses
Burch, Frank E.
Cabot, Hugh
Craig, Winchell
Downey, Hal
Foley, Frederick
Gillette, Arthur J.
Hench, Philip S.
Hewitt, Charles N.
Hirschfelder, Arthur D.
Kendall, Edward C.
Kenny, Elizabeth
Lyon, Elias P.
McQuarrie, Irvine
Mann, Frank C.
Mayo, Charles H.
Mayo, William J.
Mayo, William W.
Ohage, Justus
Plummer, Henry S.
Ramsey, Walter R.
Ripley, Martha G.
Rowntree, Leonard G.
Scammon, Richard E.
Schwyzer, Arnold
Wilson, Louis B.

Mississippi

Anderson, William H. (b. 1886)
Boswell, Henry
Cartwright, Samuel A.
Evans, William A., Jr.
Gant, Harris A.
Haralson, Hugh H.
Hunter, John F.
Leathers, Waller S.
Monette, John W.
Phares, David L.
Underwood, Felix J.
Whitehead, Peter F.
Young, John W.

Missouri

Allen, Edgar
Auer, John
Beaumont, William
Bishop, George H.
Blair, Vilray P.
Cheatham, Anderson
Cori, Gerty

Dean, Lee W.
Dock, George
Erlanger, Joseph
Farrar, Bernard G.
Gasser, Herbert S.
Graham, Evarts A.
Graham, Helen T.
Hartmann, Alexis E.
Helmuth, William T.
Hodgen, John T.
Lambright, Middleton H.
Loeb, Leo
McLean, Mary H.
McDowell, Joseph N.
Marriott, W. McKim
Moore, Carl V.
Morman, William D.
O'Leary, James L.
Opie, Eugene L.
Perry, John E.
Pope, Charles A.
Porter, William T.
Robinson, G. Canby
Saugrain de Vigne, Antoine F.
Shaffer, Philip A.
Smith, Margaret G.
Still, Andrew T.
Sutherland, Earl W.
Taussig, Frederick J.
Taylor, Eugene T.
Veeder, Bordon S.
Wood, William B., Jr.

Montana

Cogswell, William F.
Leavitt, Erasmus
Steele, William L.

Nebraska

Coffman, Victor H.
Findley, Palmer
Gifford, Harold
Gifford, Sanford R.
Livingston, Robert R.
Long, Francis A.
Milroy, William F.
Orr, Hiram W.
Picotte, Susan La F.
Poynter, Charles W. M.
Stastny, Olga F.
Summers, John E., Jr.
Towne, Solon R.
Von Mansfelde, Alexander S.

Nevada

Gibson, Samuel C.
Hood, William H.
Richardson, Rodney H.
Robinson, John L.
Sullivan, John J.
Turner, Delos A.

New Hampshire

Bartlett, Josiah
Bell, Luther V.
Brackett, Joshua
Crosby, Alpheus B.
Crosby, Dixi
Cutter, Ammi R.
Jackson, Hall
Mussey, Reuben D.
Oliver, Daniel
Phelps, Edward E.
Smith, Nathan
Spalding, Lyman
Thomson, Samuel
Thornton, Matthew
Twitchell, Amos

New Jersey

Alexander, Walter G.
Benjamin, Dowling
Bingham, Arthur W.
Brackett, Cyrus F.
Cannon, George E.
Cochran, John
Coit, Henry L.
Davidson, Henry A.
Dickinson, Jonathan
Dix, Dorothea
Elmer, Jonathan
Hargrave, Frank S.
Hosack, David
Hunt, Ezra M.
Kenney, John A.
Levy, Julius
McKean, Robert
Martland, Harrison S.
Parrish, Joseph
Potter, Ellen C.
Seguin, Edouard
Shope, Richard E.
Smith, Lyndon A.
Smith, Peter
Smith, Thomas J.
Sprague, Edward W.

Still, James
Trall, Russell T.
Waksman, Selman A.
Watson, Beriah A.
Wickes, Stephen
Williams, William C.

New Mexico

Espinosa, Tobias
Frisbie, Evelyn F.
Lovelace, William R.
Lovelace, William R., II
Scott, James R.
Smith, Warren G.
Werner, Walter I.
Wylder, Meldrum K.

New York

Armsby, James H.
Auer, John
Avery, Oswald T.
Baker, S. Josephine
Bard, John
Bard, Samuel
Barker, B. Fordyce
Barringer, Emily D.
Bartlett, Elisha
Baruch, Simon
Bayley, Richard
Beard, George M.
Beaumont, William
Beck, T. Romeyn
Bedford, Gunning
Benedict, Stanley R.
Biggs, Hermann M.
Billings, John S.
Blackwell, Elizabeth
Blackwell, Emily
Blakemore, Arthur H.
Bosworth, Franke H.
Bozeman, Nathan
Brigham, Amariah
Brill, Abraham A.
Brown, Lawrason
Brown, Solyman
Caldwell, Eugene W.
Chandler, Charles F.
Coakley, Cornelius
Coca, Arthur F.
Cochran, John
Cohn, Alfred E.
Colden, Cadwallader
Cole, Rufus

Murphy, James B.
Murray, Peter M.
Neal, Josephine B.
Newton, Robert S.
Noguchi, Hideya
North, Charles E.
Nutting, Mary A.
O'Dwyer, Joseph
Opie, Eugene L.
Orton, Samuel T.
Paine, Martyn
Papanicolaou, George N.
Park, Roswell
Park, William H.
Parker, Willard
Parmly, Eleazar
Parran, Thomas
Pattison, Granville S.
Pearce, Louise
Pilcher, Lewis S.
Post, Wright
Potter, William W.
Prudden, T. M.
Purple, Samuel S.
Rappleye, Willard C.
Reich, Wilhelm
Reid, William W.
Richards, Alfred N.
Richards, Dickinson W.
Riis, Jacob A.
Rivers, Thomas M.
Robinson, G. Canby
Romayne, Nicholas
Rous, Peyton
Rousselot, Louis M.
Rovenstine, Emery A.
Rubin, Isidore C.
Rubinow, Isaac M.
Sabin, Florence R.
Sachs, Bernard
Sanger, Margaret
Sayre, Lewis A.
Schick, Bela
Schloss, Oscar M.
Schuyler, Louisa L.
Seaman, Valentine
Seguin, Edouard
Seguin, Edward C.
Shew, Joel
Shope, Richard E.
Shrady, George F.
Sims, J. Marion
Skene, Alexander J.

Smillie, Wilson G.
Smith, Alban G.
Smith, Alonzo D.
Smith, Andrew H.
Smith, Homer W.
Smith, James McC.
Smith, Job L.
Smith, Philip E.
Smith, Stephen
Smith, Theobold
Spitzka, Edward C.
Squibb, Edward R.
Stanley, Wendell M.
Straus, Nathan
Swift, Homer F.
Tatum, Edward L.
Taylor, Charles F.
Theiler, Max
Thomas, T. Gaillard
Thompson, William G.
Thoms, Adah B.
Tillett, William S.
Timme, Walter
Tracy, Martha
Trall, Russell T.
Trudeau, Edward L.
Van Ingen, Philip
Van Slyke, Donald D.
Vincent, Ubert C.
Voegtlin, Carl
Wald, Lillian D.
Walker, Mary E.
Walsh, James J.
Waring, George E.
Warner, Hulbert H.
Weeks, John E.
Weiskotten, Herman G.
Wende, Ernest
Whipple, Allen O.
Whipple, George H.
White, James P.
Whitman, Royal
Wilbur, Hervey B.
Witthaus, Rudolph A.
Wollstein, Martha
Wood, James R.
Wright, Louis T.
Zinsser, Hans

North Carolina

Davison, Wilburt C.
Donnell, Clyde H.
Hargrave, Frank S.

Haywood, Edmund B.
Howard, William T.
McKee, William H.
MacNider, William
Manning, Isaac H.
Meserve, Charles F.
Moore, Aaron M.
Pittman, Newsome J.
Rosenau, Milton J.
Shore, Clarence A.
Tupper, Henry M.
Warren, Edward
Wood, Thomas F.

North Dakota

Darrow, Edward M.
Engstad, John E.
French, Harley E.
Grassick, James
Healy, Henry H.
Ladd, Edwin F.
Larson, Leonard W.
Millspaugh, Joseph G.
Porter, Henry R.
Quain, Eric P.
Quain, Fannie A.
Ramstad, Niles O.
Stickney, Victor H.
Weible, Ralph E.

Ohio

Awl, William M.
Bayless, George W.
Beach, Wooster
Beck, Claude S.
Campbell, Elizabeth
Clement, Kenneth W.
Crile, George W.
Curtis, Alva
Delameter, John
Drake, Daniel
Elwell, John J.
Freedlander, Samuel O.
Garvin, Charles H.
Gilliam, David T.
Glasser, Otto
Gross, Samuel D.
Harrison, John P.
Hoerr, Normand L.
Holmes, Christian
Kerr, John G.
King, John
Kline, Benjamin S.

Lambright, Middleton H.
Lloyd, John U.
McKinney-Steward, Susan M. S.
Marine, David
Merrick, Myra K.
Newton, Robert S.
Perkins, Roger G.
Reid, Mont R.
Scudder, John M.
Smith, Peter
Sollmann, Torald H.
Sutherland, Earl W., Jr.
Todd, Thomas W.
Toomey, John A.
Wiggers, Carl J.
Williams, Elkanah

Oklahoma

Blesh, Abraham L.
Bradford, Claudius
Buxton, Lauren H.
Clinton, Fred S.
Davis, Abraham I.
Fite, Francis B.
Fortner, Benjamin
Long, Leroy
Moorman, Lewis J.
Walker, Delos
West, Archa K.
Wright, Eliphalet N.

Oregon

Baird, David W. E.
Bilderback, Joseph B.
Coffey, Robert C.
Dillehunt, Richard B.
Jones, Noble W.
Lovejoy, Esther P.
Mackenzie, Kenneth A. J.
Matson, Ralph C.
Matson, Ray W.
Osgood, Edwin E.
Owens-Adair, Bethenia A.
Smith, Andrew C.
Whitman, Marcus

Pennsylvania

Abbott, Maude
Agnew, David H.
Atlee, John L.
Atlee, Washington
Bache, Franklin
Barnes, William H.

Barton, Benjamin
Barton, William P. C.
Bond, Thomas
Brinton, John H.
Bronk, Detlev W.
Broomall, Anna E.
Cadwalader, Thomas
Chapman, Nathaniel
Cleveland, Emeline H.
Coxe, John R.
Da Costa, Jacob M.
Darlington, William
de Schweinitz, George E.
Deaver, John B.
Delany, Martin R.
Dewees, William P.
Donaldson, Henry H.
Dorsey, John S.
Duhring, Louis A.
Dunglison, Robley
Dyott, Thomas W.
Eberle, John
Flick, Lawrence F.
Fussell, Bartholomew
Garretson, James E.
Gerhard, William W.
Gibbon, John H., Jr.
Godman, John D.
Gross, Samuel D.
Gross, Samuel W.
Hays, Isaac
Helmuth, William T.
Hering, Constantine
Hinson, Eugene T.
Hodge, Hugh L.
Horner, William E.
Jackson, Algernon
Jackson, Chevalier
Jackson, Samuel
Jones, John
Kearsley, John
Keen, William W., Jr.
Kirkbride, Thomas S.
Kuhn, Adam
Leidy, Joseph
Leonard, Charles L.
Longshore, Hannah E. M.
McClellan, George
Macfarlane, Catharine
McKenzie, Robert T.
Marshall, Clara
Meigs, Arthur V.
Meigs, Charles D.

Meigs, John F.
Mills, Charles K.
Minton, Henry M.
Mitchell, John K.
Mitchell, S. Weir
Morgan, John
Morton, Samuel G.
Mossell, Nathan F.
Opie, Eugene L.
Orton, Samuel T.
Otto, John C.
Packard, Francis R.
Pancoast, Joseph
Parran, Thomas
Parrish, Isaac
Parrish, Joseph
Parvin, Theophilus
Passavant, William A.
Pattison, Granville S.
Pearce, Louise
Pennock, Caspar W.
Pepper, William
Physick, Philip S.
Potter, Ellen C.
Preston, Ann
Price, Joseph
Procter, William, Jr.
Redman, John
Richards, Alfred N.
Rodman, William L.
Rowntree, Leonard
Rubinow, Isaac M.
Rush, Benjamin
Schamberg, Jay F.
Shakespeare, Edward O.
Shippen, William
Shryock, Richard H.
Smith, Albert H.
Solis-Cohen, Jacob D.
Solis-Cohen, Solomon
Stille, Alfred
Stokes, Joseph, Jr.
Stubbs, Frederick D.
Tracy, Martha
Turner, John P.
Tyson, James
Wistar, Caspar
Wood, George B.
Wood, Horatio C.

Rhode Island

Bartlett, Elisha
Burgess, Alexander

Chapin, Charles V.
Hunter, William
Parsons, Usher
Ray, Isaac
Snow, Edwin M.

South Carolina

Babcock, James W.
Bull, William
Chisolm, Julian J.
Delany, Martin R.
Dickson, Samuel H.
Evans, Matilda A.
Fayssoux, Peter
Garden, Alexander
Geddings, Eli
Jervey, James W.
Lining, John
Lynch, Kenneth M.
McClennan, Alonzo C.
Moore, Samuel P.
Moultrie, John, Jr.
Olyphant, David
Porcher, Francis P.
Ramsay, David
Sims, J. Marion

South Dakota

Donahoe, William E.
Freeman, John W.
Hare, Lyle
Lommen, Christian P.
McGillycuddy, Valentine T.
Pettigrew, George A.
Phillips, Josiah L.
Spafford, Frederick A.

Tennessee

Blalock, Alfred
Bowling, William K.
Boyd, Robert F.
Briggs, William T.
Campbell, Willis C.
Clark, Sam L.
Ellett, Edward C.
Eve, Paul F.
Goodpasture, Ernest W.
Gunn, John C.
Haggard, William D., Jr.
Hale, John H.
Hubbard, George W.
Leathers, Waller
Lindsley, John B.

Lynk, Miles V.
Maury, Richard B.
Mitchell, Robert W.
Quinland, William S.
Robertson, Felix
Robinson, G. Canby
Rogers, William E.
Roman, Charles V.
Rose, Wickliffe
Shoulders, Harrison H.
Sutherland, Earl W., Jr.
West, Harold D.
Witherspoon, John A.
Yandell, Lunsford P.

Texas

Anderson, John W.
Bertner, Ernst W.
Carter, William S.
Cary, Edward H.
Covington, Benjamin J.
Cox, George W., Jr.
Gathings, Joseph G.
Moursund, Walter H.
Muller, Hermann J.
Nixon, Pat I.
Randall, Edward
Scott, Arthur C.
Smith, Ashbel
Wooten, Thomas D.

Utah

Beatty, Theodore
Behle, Augustus
Callister, Alfred C.
Marshall, Hyrum L.
Morrell, Joseph R.
Richards, George G.
Richards, Paul S.
Richards, Ralph T.
Shipp, Ellis R.
Viko, Louis E.

Vermont

Allen, Lyman
Beecher, Clarence H.
Brown, William E.
Carpenter, Walter
Caverly, Charles S.
Dodd, Walter J.
Gallup, Joseph A.
Gridley, Selah
Holton, Henry D.

Lincoln, Benjamin
Pomeroy, John
Raab, Wilhelm
Shew, Joel
Smith, Nathan R.
Thayer, Samuel W.
Tinkham, Henry C.
Wheeler, John B.
Witthaus, Rudolph
Woodward, Theodore

Virginia

Baynham, William
Blanton, Wyndham B.
Brown, William
Cabell, James
Craik, James
Curtis, Alva
Dunglison, Robley
Francis, Grossi H.
Hume, David M.
McCaw, James B.
McClurg, James
McGuire, Hunter H.
Maxcy, Kenneth F.
Moore, Samuel P.
Pott, John
Tennent, John

Washington

Eagleson, James B.
Harkins, Henry N.
Heg, Elmer E.
Lumsden, Leslie L.
Mason, James T.
Maynard, David S.
Smith, Clarence A.
Weed, Gideon A.
Whitman, Marcus

West Virginia

Evans, George
Frissell, John
Gage, E. Lyle

Gamble, Henry F.
Hullihen, Simon P.
Marshall, Hubert
Moore, Phoebia G.
Pride, Maynard P.
Simpson, John
Spray, Robb S.
Vest, Walter
Whittico, James M.

Wisconsin

Bardeen, Charles R.
Dearholt, Hoyt E.
Elvehjem, Conrad A.
Favill, Henry B.
Favill, John
Gundersen, Adolf
Harper, Cornelius
Jermain, Louis F.
Kempster, Walter
Kremers, Edward
McCollum, Elmer V.
Mendenhall, Dorothy R.
Middleton, William S.
Miller, William S.
Minoka-Hill, Lillie R.
Reeve, James T.
Senn, Nicholas
Sleyster, Rock
Steenbock, Harry
Wolcott, Erastus B.
Wolcott, Laura J. R.

Wyoming

Barber, Amos
Carter, C. Dana
Finfrock, John H.
Heath, Lillian
Hocker, William A.
Hoyt, John W.
Johnston, George P.
Maghee, Thomas G.
Osborne, John E.

Listing by Specialty or Occupation

In order to make the contents of the DAMB more generally available to readers, up to four areas of medical specialization have been entered for each subject. Every subject is included in at least one category. The subjects are categorized primarily on the basis of their contributions as opposed to their occupations or professions. Modern terminology is used. Hence, there are no categories for "botany," "materia medica," and "fevers," as appear in earlier medical reference works. Most of the physicians who practiced before the age of specialization have been included under either "surgery" or "internal medicine." Since many persons who are in the DAMB because of their scientific work were also leading figures in their medical schools, the education category is enlarged. Moreover, because half of the DAMB is devoted to state and local figures, inevitably certain fields of medical endeavor that are organized along state lines, notably medical education and public health, are over-represented. Finally, to increase the DAMB's usefulness, Appendix D contains many subspecialties of recent origin. These medical subspecialties have relatively few entries, as many of the founders and leaders were still alive on December 31, 1976, the cut-off date for inclusion in the DAMB. Categories with an asterisk (*) are so marked to indicate that they were intended to include a representative sample of leading figures, rather than any attempt to develop a complete listing which was impossible due to space limitations.

AEROSPACE MEDICINE

Bronk, Detlev W.
Crowe, Samuel J.
DuBois, Eugene F.
Glasser, Otto
Lovelace, William R., II
Warnshuis, Frederick C.

ALLERGY AND IMMUNOLOGY

Auer, John
Avery, Oswald T.
Blanton, Wyndham
Boylston, Zabdiel
Coca, Arthur F.
Cooke, Robert A.
Francis, Thomas, Jr.
Freedlander, Samuel O.
Gay, Frederick
Graham, Helen T.
Hall, James L.
Landsteiner, Karl
Longcope, Warfield T.
Macleod, Colin M.

Mather, Cotton
McMaster, Philip D.
Meltzer, Samuel J.
Meyer, Karl F.
Murphy, James B.
North, Elisha
Nuttall, George H.
Rivers, Thomas M.
Russell, Frederick
Salmon, Daniel E.
Schick, Bela
Schloss, Oscar M.
Sellards, Andrew W.
Sewall, Henry
Shope, Richard E.
Smith, Theobold
Stanley, Wendell M.
Stokes, Joseph, Jr.
Theiler, Max
Waterhouse, Benjamin
Wells, Harry G.
Wood, William B., Jr.
Wright, Louis T.
Wyman, Morrill
Zinsser, Hans

ANATOMY AND EMBRYOLOGY

Allen, Edgar
Bardeen, Charles R.
Bayless, George W.
Bayley, Richard
Baynham, William
Bodine, James M.
Brodel, Max
Clark, Sam L.
Godman, John D.
Harrison, Ross G.
Hoerr, Normand L.
Holmes, Oliver W.
Horner, William E.
Jackson, John B. S.
Leidy, Joseph
Mall, Franklin P.
March, Alden
Miller, William S.
Minot, Charles S.
Morgan, Thomas H.
Morton, Samuel G.
O'Leary, James L.
Pancoast, Joseph
Pattison, Granville S.
Post, Wright

Poynter, Charles W. M.
Ramsay, Alexander
Ranson, Stephen W.
Sabin, Florence R.
Scammon, Richard E.
Shippen, William
Smith, Philip E.
Streeter, George L.
Todd, Thomas W.
Warren, John
Weed, Lewis H.
Wistar, Caspar
Wyman, Jeffries

ANESTHESIOLOGY

Andrews, Edmund
Beecher, Henry K.
Bigelow, Henry J.
Blaney, James V.
Bowditch, Henry P.
Brainard, Daniel
Chisholm, Julian J.
Fisher, John D.
Guthrie, Samuel
Halsted, William S.
Henderson, Yandell
Hertzler, Arthur E.
Hirschfelder, Arthur D.
Jackson, Charles T.
Jarvis, William C.
Koller, Carl
Long, Crawford W.
Matas, Rudolph
Morton, William T. G.
Rovenstine, Emery A.
Van Hoosen, Bertha
Wells, Horace

BACTERIOLOGY. See MICROBIOLOGY

BIOCHEMISTRY

Abel, John J.
Avery, Oswald T.
Benedict, Francis G.
Benedict, Stanley R.
Chase, Will H.
Chittenden, Russell H.
Cohn, Edward J.
Cori, Gerty
Elvehjem, Conrad A.

Folin, Otto
Gamble, James L.
Gies, William J.
Hartmann, Alexis F.
Henderson, Lawrence
Herter, Christian
Hoerr, Normand L.
Kendall, Edward C.
Long, Cyril N.H.
McCollum, Elmer V.
Mendel, Lafayette B.
Osborne, Thomas B.
Shaffer, Philip A.
Stanley, Wendell M.
Steenbock, Harry
Sutherland, Earl W.
Takamine, Jokichi
Tatum, Edward L.
Van Slyke, Donald D.
Vaughan, Victor C.
Voegtlin, Carl
Waksman, Selman A.
Wells, Harry G.
West, Harold D.
Wilkerson, Vernon A.
Witthaus, Rudolph

BIOLOGY, GENETICS, AND PARASITOLOGY

Ashford, Bailey K.
Avery, Oswald T.
Barron, Moses
Barton, Benjamin
Bigelow, Jacob
Clapp, Ahasel
Colden, Cadwallader
Garden, Alexander
Godman, John D.
Harrison, Ross G.
Henderson, Lawrence
Hillebrand, Wilhelm
Hosack, David
Just, Ernest E.
Kuhn, Adam
Lam, Frederick K.
Leidy, Joseph
Lining, John
Loeb, Jacques
Lynch, Kenneth M.
MacLeod, Colin M.
Martin, Henry N.
Minot, Charles S.

Mitchill, Samuel L.
Morgan, Thomas H.
Morton, Samuel G.
Muller, Hermann J.
Nuttall, George H. F.
Pearl, Raymond
Pincus, Gregory G.
Pitcher, Zina
Smith, Theobold
Stiles, Charles W.
Storer, David H.
Tatum, Edward L.
Waterhouse, Benjamin
Wood, Horatio
Wyman, Jeffries

BOTANY (medical). See BIOLOGY and PHARMACOLOGY

CARDIAC SURGERY. See THORACIC SURGERY

CARDIOVASCULAR MEDICINE

Abbott, Maude
Abrams, Albert
Barker, Lewellys
Beck, Claude S.
Cohn, Alfred E.
Da Costa, Jacob M.
Erlanger, Joseph
Gibbon, John H., Jr.
Herrick, James B.
Hirschfelder, Arthur D.
Horine, Emmet F.
Howell, William H.
Johnson, John B.
Libman, Emanuel
Marshall F Kennerly, Jr.
Martin, Henry N.
Porter, William T.
Raab, Wilhelm
Reid, Mont R.
Richards, Dickinson W.
Robinson, G. Canby
Sewall, Henry
Smith, Fred M.
Thayer, William S.
Viko, Louis E.
Weiss, Soma
White, Paul D.

Wiggers, Carl J.
Wilson, Frank N.

COLON AND RECTAL SURGERY

Coller, Frederick
Lahey, Frank H.
Mathews, Joseph M.
Physick, Philip S.
Rousselot, Louis M.
Schwyzer, Arnold

DENTISTRY*

Black, Greene V.
Boyd, Robert F.
Brown, Solyman
Garretson, James E.
Gies, William J.
Greenwood, John
Harris, Chapin A.
Hayden, Horace H.
Howe, Percy R.
Hullihen, Simon P.
Morton, William T. G.
Parmly, Eleazar
Wells, Horace

DERMATOLOGY

Biddle, Andrew P.
Duhring, Louis A.
Dyer, Isadore
Fordyce, John A.
Gathings, Joseph G.
Henry, Morris H.
Keyes, Edward L.
Lawless, Theodore K.
Pusey, William A.
Schamberg, Jay F.
White, James C.

ECONOMICS (MEDICAL). See HEALTH CARE ORGANIZATION AND FINANCING

EDITING (MEDICAL). See LITERATURE

EDUCATION (MEDICAL SCHOOLS)

(Born prior to 1800)

Antony, Milton
Archer, John

Bache, Franklin
Bard, John
Bard, Samuel
Beck, T. Romeyn
Bigelow, Jacob
Brown, Samuel
Bull, William
Caldwell, Charles
Channing, Walter
Chapman, Nathaniel
Cooke, John E.
Davidge, John B.
Delameter, John
Dewees, William P.
Dickson, Samuel H.
Drake, Daniel
Dudley, Benjamin W.
Dunglison, Robley
Dunlap, Livingston
Eberle, John
Francis, John W.
Fussell, Bartholomew
Gallup, Joseph A.
Galt, William C.
Geddings, Eli
Gridley, Selah
Harrison, John P.
Horner, William E.
Hosack, David
Jackson, Samuel
Jones, John
Kuhn, Adam
March, Alden
McClellan, George
Middleton, Peter
Morgan, John
Paine, Martyn
Pattison, Granville S.
Pitcher, Zina
Pomeroy, John
Potter, Nathaniel
Redman, John
Ridgely, Frederick
Romayne, Nicholas
Shippen, William
Silliman, Benjamin
Smith, Nathan
Smith, Nathan R.
Spalding, Lyman
Woodward, Theodore

(Born 1800 to 1849)

Anderson, William H. (b. 1820)
Andrews, Edmund

Armsby, James H.
Arnold, Richard D.
Augusta, Alexander T.
Bancroft, Frederick J.
Bartlett, Elisha
Bayless, George W.
Bedford, Gunning
Bell, Simeon B.
Bentley, Edwin
Billings, John S.
Blackwell, Elizabeth
Blackwell, Emily
Blake, James
Bobbs, John S.
Bodine, James M.
Bosworth, Franke H.
Bowditch, Henry P.
Bowling, William K.
Bradford, Edward H.
Brainard, Daniel
Brinton, John H.
Broomall, Anna E.
Buckingham, Richard G.
Byford, William H.
Cabell, James L.
Calhoun, Abner W.
Campbell, Henry F.
Carmalt, William H.
Carpenter, Walter
Chaillé, Stanford
Cheever, David W.
Clarke, Edward H.
Cleveland, Emeline H.
Cole, Richard B.
Connor, Leartus
Cooper, Elias S.
Cordell, Eugene F.
Crosby, Alpheus B.
DaCosta, Jacob M.
Dalton, John C.
Davis, Nathan S.
Dibrell, James A., Jr.
Dugas, Louis A
Eliot, Charles W.
Evans, John
Eve, Paul F.
Fenner, Erasmus D.
Fitz, Reginald H.
Fitzbutler, (W.) Henry
Flint, Austin
Flint, Austin, Jr.
Ford, Lewis D.
Gerhard, William W.
Gilman, Daniel C.

Gregory, Samuel
Gross, Samuel D.
Gunn, Moses
Hall, G. Stanley
Hering, Constantine
Holmes, Oliver W.
Hooker, Worthington
Hooper, Philo O.
Hubbard, George W.
Hughes, John C.
Janeway, Edward G.
Jenks, Edward W.
Ketchum, George A.
Knapp, (J.) Herman
Lamb, Daniel S.
Lane, Levi C.
Lincoln, Benjamin
Lindsley, John B.
Loomis, Alfred L.
Lozier, Clemence S.
Lyster, Henry F. L.
Marshall, Clara
McCready, Benjamin W.
McDowell, Joseph N.
McGuire, Hunter H.
Mosher, Eliza M.
Osler, William
Palmer, Alonzo B.
Peck, Washington F.
Pepper, William
Peter, Robert
Phelps, Edward E.
Pope, Charles A.
Preston, Ann
Purvis, Charles B.
Rogers, William E.
Sanford, John F.
Sayre, Lewis A.
Shattuck, George C., Jr.
Shipp, Ellis R.
Skene, Alexander
Thayer, Samuel W.
Toland, Hugh H.
Tupper, Henry M.
Tyson, James
Westmoreland, John G.
White, James P.
Wooten, Thomas D.
Yandell, Lunsford P.
Zakrzewska, Marie E.

(Born after 1849)

Abell, Irvin
Adams, Numa P. G.

Allen, Lyman
Baird, David W. E.
Bardeen, Charles R.
Bayne-Jones, Stanhope
Beecher, Clarence H.
Beecher, Henry K.
Bertner, Ernst
Bevan, Arthur D.
Biddle, Andrew P.
Bierring, Walter L.
Bilderback, Joseph B.
Billings, Frank
Blackfan, Kenneth D.
Blake, Francis G.
Blumer, George
Boyd, Robert F.
Bronk, Detlev W.
Brown, William E.
Burgess, Alexander M.
Cabot, Richard C.
Callister, Alfred C.
Cannon, Walter B.
Carter, William S.
Cary, Edward H.
Chesney, Alan M.
Churchill, Edward D.
Clark, Sam L.
Coller, Frederick A.
Colwell, Nathan P.
Copeland, Royal S.
Cowie, David M.
Cullen, Thomas S.
Curtis, Austin M.
Cushing, Harvey W.
Davison, Wilburt C.
Dean, Lee W.
Dickinson, Robert L.
Dillehunt, Richard B.
Dock, George
Donahoe, William E.
Edsall, David Linn
Flexner, Abraham
Fordyce, John A.
Foster, Eugene
Frederick, Rivers
French, Harley E.
Fuller, Solomon C.
Greene, Clarence S.
Gundersen, Adolf
Haggard, William D., Jr.
Hale, John H.
Halsted, William S.
Harkins, Henry N.

Hatcher, Robert A.
Holmes, Christian
Howell, William H.
Howland, John
Hume, David M.
Hurty, John N.
Jackson, Edward
Jayne, Walter A.
Jermain, Louis F.
Johnson, John B.
Jones, Noble W.
Jordan, Edwin O.
Kelly, George L.
Keyes, Edward L.
Kober, George M.
Leathers, Waller
Lenow, James H.
Lommen, Christian
Long, Leroy
Lynk, Miles V.
Lyon, Elias P.
Mackenzie, Kenneth A. J.
MacNider, William
Manning, Isaac H.
Marriott, W. McKim
Mayo, William J.
Mayo, Charles H.
McNeill, William C.
Menninger, Charles F.
Menninger, William C.
Meserve, Charles F.
Meyer, Adolf
Middleton, William S.
Moursund, Walter H.
Opie, Eugene L.
Poynter, Charles W. M.
Randall, Edward
Rappleye, Willard C.
Richards, Alfred N.
Roberts, Carl G.
Robinson, G. Canby
Rosenau, Milton J.
Sedgwick, William T.
Shadd, Furman J.
Shaffer, Philip A.
Simpson, John
Smith, Morgan
Sollmann, Torald H.
Tait, F. Dudley
Tinkham, Henry C.
Tracy, Martha
Vaughan, Victor C.
Viko, Louis E.

Vinsonhaler, Frank
Wahl, Harry R.
Warfield, William A.
Weed, Lewis H.
Weiskotten, Herman G.
Welch, William H.
West, Harold D.
Whipple, George H.
Williams, Daniel H.
Williams, John W.
Wilson, Louis B.
Winternitz, Milton C.
Witherspoon, John A.
Wynn, Frank B.

EMBRYOLOGY. See ANATOMY AND EMBRYOLOGY

ENDOCRINOLOGY AND METABOLISM

Abel, John J.
Albright, Fuller
Allen, Edgar
Atwater, Wilbur O.
Barron, Moses
Battey, Robert
Benedict, Francis G.
Benedict, Stanley R.
Cannon, Walter B.
Cori, Gerty
Crowe, Samuel J.
Cushing, Harvey W.
DuBois, Eugene F.
Edsall, David L.
Elvehjem, Conrad A.
Gamble, James L.
Harris, Seale
Hartmann, Alexis F.
Hench, Philip S.
Howland, John
Hume, David M.
Kendall, Edward C.
Loeb, Leo
Loeb, Robert F.
Long, Cyril N. H.
Lusk, Graham
MacCallum, William G.
Moore, Carl V.
Pincus, Gregory G.
Plummer, Henry S.
Raab, Wilhelm
Rowntree, Leonard

Smith, Philip E.
Sutherland, Earl W., Jr.
Takamine, Jokichi
Timme, Walter
Voegtlin, Carl
Whipple, George H.
Wood, William B.

EPIDEMIOLOGY

Ashford, Bailey K.
Blake, Francis G.
Carter, Henry R.
Caverly, Charles S.
Chapin, Charles V.
Crawford, John
Emerson, Haven
Folks, Homer
Francis, Thomas, Jr.
Frost, Wade H.
Goldberger, Joseph
Greenberg, Morris
Hunt, Ezra M.
Kober, George M.
Lumsden, Leslie L.
Maxcy, Kenneth F.
Meyer, Karl F.
Mitchell, John K.
Paul, John R.
Potter, Nathaniel
Reed, Walter
Ricketts, Howard T.
Sedgwick, William T.
Shakespeare, Edward O.
Shope, Richard E.
Smillie, Wilson G.
Smith, Theobold
Sydenstricker, Edgar
Trask, James D.
Webster, Noah
Zinsser, Hans

ETHICS, LAW AND JURISPRUDENCE*

Alexander, Franz G.
Beck, T. Romeyn
Beecher, Henry K.
Cabot, Richard C.
Caldwell, Charles
Crosby, Dixi
Elwell, John
Fairchild, David S.
Harison, Beverly D.

Hooker, Worthington
MacCallum, William G.
Martland, Harrison S.
Ray, Isaac
Spitzka, Edward C.
Tibbals, Frank B.
Warnshuis, Frederick C.
Witthaus, Rudolph

EYE, EAR, NOSE AND THROAT

Barnes, William H.
Bosworth, Franke H.
Burch, Frank E.
Buxton, Lauren H.
Calhoun, Abner W.
Carmalt, William H.
Chisholm, Julian J.
Clarke, Edward H.
Coakley, Cornelius
Copeland, Royal S.
Crowe, Samuel J.
Dean, Lee W.
Delafield, Edward
de Schweinitz, George E.
Dickerson, Spencer C.
Ellett, Edward C.
Gifford, Harold
Gifford, Sanford R.
Green, Horace
Gruening, Emil
Hays, Isaac
Hill, Frederick
Holmes, Christian
Holt, Erastus E.
Howe, Lucien
Jackson, Chevalier
Jackson, Edward
Jarvis, William C.
Jervey, James W.
Knapp, (J.) Herman
Koller, Carl
Lefferts, George M.
McKay, Read J.
Morman, William D.
North, Elisha
Packard, Francis R.
Parrish, Isaac
Robinson, John L.
Roman, Charles V.
Shakespeare, Edward O.
Solis-Cohen, Jacob D.
Solly, S. Edwin

Spalding, James A.
Von Békésy, Georg
Weeks, John E.
Williams, Elkanah
Williams, Henry W.
Wood, Casey A.

FOLK MEDICINE. See POPULAR AND FOLK MEDICINE

GENETICS. See BIOLOGY, GENETICS, AND PARASITOLOGY

GYNECOLOGY. See OBSTETRICS AND GYNECOLOGY

HEALTH CARE ORGANIZATION AND FINANCING*

(Hospital founders and administrators, originators of group practice and health insurance plans)

Barlow, Walter T.
Becker, Harry F.
Bertner, Ernst W.
Billings, John S.
Blackwell, Emily
Bond, Thomas
Brown, Charlotte
Brunk, Andrew S.
Burrough, James W.
Burton, DeWitt
Busey, Samuel C.
Butler, Henry R.
Byford, William H.
Cabot, Hugh
Campbell, Willis C.
Carpenter, Walter
Carson, Simeon L.
Cheever, David W.
Chisolm, Julian J.
Clinton, Fred S.
Codman, Ernest A.
Coffey, Robert C.
Coit, Henry L.
Cole, Fern M.
Cole, Rufus
Coley, William B.
Covington, Benjamin J.

Cutler, Elliott C.
Dailey, Ulysses G.
Davis, Michael M.
Davison, Wilburt C.
De Lee, Joseph B.
Delafield, Edward
Dennis, Frederic S.
Dibble, Eugene H.
Donaldson, Mary E.
Dorsette, Cornelius N.
Dunlap, Livingston
Dyer, Isadore
Evans, Matilda A.
Finney, John M.
Fishbein, Morris
Flint, Austin
Folks, Homer
Goldwater, Sigismund S.
Greene, Cordelia
Gunderson, Adolf
Hale, John H.
Hall, G. Stanley
Hargrave, Frank S.
Hosack, David
Jackson, Algernon
Jackson, James
Jackson, James M., Jr.
Jones, John
Jones, Noble W.
Kenney, John A.
Kirkbride, Thomas S.
Lahey, Frank H.
Lambright, Middleton
Larsen, Nils P.
Larson, Leonard W.
Lovelace, William R. (b. 1883)
Manning, Isaac H.
Marshall, Hubert
Mason, James T.
Mayo, Charles H.
Mayo, William J.
Menninger, Charles F.
Menninger, William C.
Middleton, William S.
Minton, Henry M.
Moore, Aaron
Mossell, Nathan F.
Moten, Pierce S.
Northcross, David C.
Nott, Josiah C.
Perry, John E.
Porcher, Francis P.
Price, Joseph

Quain, Eric P.
Ramstad, Niles O.
Rappleye, Willard C.
Robinson, Paul T.
Rubinow, Isaac
Scott, Arthur C.
Smith, Stephen
Sprague, Edward W.
Sydenstricker, Edgar
Thompson, Solomon H.
Warfield, William A.
Warren, John C.
Weible, Ralph E.
White, William A.
Williams, Daniel H.,
Woodward, Samuel B.
Woodworth, John M.
Wyman, Morrill
Zakrzewska, Marie E.

**HEALTH INSURANCE. See HEALTH CARE
ORGANIZATION AND FINANCING**

HEMATOLOGY

Blackfan, Kenneth D.
Coca, Arthur F.
Cohn, Edwin J.
Cooley, Thomas B.
Dameshek, William
Downey, Hal
Drew, Charles R.
Ewing, James
Hektoen, Ludvig
Henderson, Lawrence
Herrick, James B.
Howell, William H.
Landsteiner, Karl
Libman, Emanuel
Minot, George R.
Moore, Carl V.
Nuttall, George H. F.
Osgood, Edwin E.
Otto, John C.
Rous, Peyton
Smith, Harry P.

HISTOLOGY

Delafield, Francis
Downey, Hal
Hoerr, Normand L.

Mallory, Frank B.
Prudden, T. M.
Wilson, Louis B.
Woodward, Joseph J.

HISTORY

Abbott, Maude
Allen, Lyman
Bayne-Jones, Stanhope
Beecher, Henry K.
Blanton, Wyndham
Chase, Will H.
Chesney, Alan M.
Chittenden, Russell H.
Clendening, Logan
Cordell, Eugene F.
Coxe, John R.
Crosby, Alpheus B.
Dock, Lavinia L.
Fairchild, David S.
Farber, Sidney
Findley, Palmer
Foster, Eugene
Fulton, John F.
Garrison, Fielding
Grassick, James
Harris, Seale
Hemmeter, John C.
Horine, Emmet F.
Hume, Edgar E.
Kremers, Edward
Lamb, Daniel S.
MacCallum, William G.
Major, Ralph H.
Mead, Kate C. H.
Merritt, John W.
Middleton, Peter
Middleton, William S.
Miller, William S.
Milroy, William F.
Mumford, James G.
Nixon, Pat I.
Nuttall, Mary A.
Packard, Francis R.
Pusey, William A.
Roman, Charles V.
Shryock, Richard H.
Sigerist, Henry E.
Smillie, Wilson G.
Toner, Joseph M.
Underwood, Felix J.
Van Ingen, Philip

Vinsonhaler, Frank
Walsh, James J.
Whipple, Allen O.
Wickes, Stephen
Winslow, Charles-Edward A.
Woodward, Julian J.
Zinsser, Hans

HOSPITAL ADMINISTRATION. See HEALTH CARE ORGANIZATION AND FINANCING

HOSPITAL FOUNDER. See HEALTH CARE ORGANIZATION AND FINANCING

IMMUNOLOGY. See ALLERGY AND IMMUNOLOGY

INTERNAL MEDICINE

(Born prior to 1800)

Appleton, Moses
Archer, John
Bard, John
Barker, Jeremiah
Bartlett, Josiah
Bates, James
Bond, Thomas
Boylston, Zabdiel
Brackett, Joshua
Brown, Samuel
Cadwalader, Thomas
Cartwright, Samuel A.
Chapman, Nathaniel
Church, Benjamin
Colden, Cadwallader
Cooke, John E.
Craik, James
Crawford, John
Cutter, Ammi R.
Darlington, William
Dexter, Aaron
Dickinson, Jonathan
Dickson, Samuel H.
Douglass, William
Drake, Daniel
Durham, James
Eberle, John
Elmer, Jonathan

Ewell, James
Farrar, Bernard G.
Fayssoux, Peter
Ferguson, Richard B.
Fisher, John D.
Francis, John W.
Galland, Isaac
Gallup, Joseph A.
Garden, Alexander
Geddings, Eli
Gridley, Selah
Harrison, John P.
Hersey, Ezekiel
Holyoke, Edward A.
Hopkins, Lemuel
Hosack, David
Hulse, Isaac
Jackson, Hall
Jackson, James
Kearsley, John
McClurg, James
Middleton, Peter
Moultrie, John, Jr.
Paine, Martyn
Pennock, Caspar W.
Pott, John
Ramsay, David
Ramsay, Alexander
Redman, John
Ridgely, Frederick
Robertson, Felix
Rush, Benjamin
Saugrain de Vigne, Antoine F.
Shattuck, George C.
Sibley, John
Thacher, James
Thornton, Matthew
Tufts, Cotton
Ware, John
Warren, Joseph
Wiesenthal, Charles F.

(Born 1800 to 1849)

Ah Fong, C. K.
Anderson, William H. (b. 1820)
Augusta, Alexander
Baldwin, Abel S.
Bartholow, Roberts
Bartlett, Elisha
Baruch, Simon
Benjamin, Dowling
Black, John J.
Blake, James

Blaney, James V.
Brown, William W.
Burrough, James W.
Bush, Lewis P.
Carpenter, Walter
Coffman, Victor H.
Cordell, Eugene F.
Da Costa, Jacob M.
Dana, Israel T.
Daniel, Richard P.
Delany, Martin R.
Dibrell, James A.
Dolley, Sarah R. A.
Fabrique, Andrew H.
Faget, Jean C.
Favill, John
Fitzbutler, (W.) Henry
Flint, Austin
Fortner, Benjamin F.
Garcelon, Alonzo
Gerhard, William W.
Gibbons, Henry
Gorrie, John
Handy, John C.
Hargis, Robert B.
Hillebrand, Wilhelm
Hocker, William A.
Hoyt, John W.
Hughes, Henry A.
Jacobi, Mary P.
Janeway, Edward G.
Jones, Joseph
Ketchum, George A.
Longshore, Hannah E. M.
Maynard, David S.
McGillycuddy, Valentine
McKinney-Steward, Susan M. S.
Monette, John W.
Morse, John F.
Noon, Adolphus H.
Osler, William
Palmer, Thomas M.
Parrish, Joseph
Pepper, William
Phares, David L.
Porcher, Francis P.
Remond, Sarah P.
Robertson, William S.
Rock, John S.
Rutherford, Frances A.
Sanford, John F.
Shattuck, George C.
Smith, Ashbel

Smith, James McC.
Smith, Thomas J.
Stevenson, Sarah A. H.
Still, James
Thomas, Mary F. M.
Walker, Delos
Wall, John P.
Whitehead, Peter F.
Wolcott, Laura J. R.
Young, John W.

(Born after 1849)

Abrams, Albert
Alexander, Walter G.
Anderson, John W.
Baird, David W. E.
Barber, Amos W.
Barker, Lewellys
Barlow, Walter J.
Barron, Moses
Beebe, James
Blanton, William P.
Blanton, Wyndham
Blumer, George
Boyd, Robert F.
Bradford, Claudius B.
Burgess, Alexander
Butler, Henry R.
Cannon, George E.
Carter, C. Dana
Cheatham, Anderson W.
Cole, Fern M.
Collister, George
Covington, Benjamin J.
Darrow, Edward M.
Davis, Abraham I.
Davis, George
Dibble, Eugene H.
Dock, George
Donnell, Clyde H.
Dorsette, Cornelius
Dyer, Isadore
Einhorn, Max
Espinosa, Tobias
Evans, George
Evans, Matilda A.
Frederick, Rivers
Freeman, John W.
Frisbie, Evelyn F.
Gamble, Henry F.
Gibson, Samuel C.
Hall, Josiah N.
Haralson, Hugh H.

Hare, Lyle
Harris, Seale
Harris, William H.
Heath, Lillian
Hemmeter, John C.
Jackson, Algernon
Jermain, Louis F.
Johnston, George P.
Jones, Noble W.
Lam, Frederick K.
Lattimore, John A.
Long, Francis A.
Mackenzie, Kenneth A. J.
Major, Ralph H.
McClennan, Alonzo C.
Milroy, William F.
Minoka-Hill, Lillie R.
Moeur, Benjamin B.
Montezuma, Carlos
Moore, Aaron
Moore, Phoebia G.
Parsons, Mary A.
Picotte, Susan LaF.
Pittenger, Fred A.
Plummer, Henry S.
Richards, George G.
Richardson, Rodney H.
Robins, Charles A.
Romig, Joseph H.
Smith, Fred M.
Smith, Warren G.
Solis-Cohen, Solomon
Spafford, Frederick
Stickney, Victor H.
Sullivan, John J.
Swift, Homer F.
Thayer, William S.
Tildon, Toussaint
Tillett, William S.
Vest, Walter
West, Archa K.
Whitehead, William M.
Whittico, James
Wylder, Meldrum K.

LARYNGOLOGY. See EYE, EAR, NOSE AND THROAT

LIBRARY SCIENCE (MEDICAL). See LITERATURE

LITERATURE*

(Editors, librarians, translators, collectors, illustrators, popular writers)

Abt, Isaac A.
Alexander, Walter G.
Anderson, William H. (b. 1886)
Antony, Milton
Bartholow, Roberts
Barton, Benjamin S.
Battey, Robert
Beck, T. Romeyn
Biddle, Andrew P.
Billings, John S.
Blaney, James V.
Blanton, Wyndham B.
Bowditch, Henry I.
Bowling, William K.
Brigham, Amariah
Brill, Abraham A.
Brödel, Max
Brown, Lawrason
Brown, Solyman
Campbell, Henry F.
Cartwright, Samuel A.
Chaillé, Stanford E.
Chapman, Nathaniel
Clark, Sam L.
Clendening, Logan
Coca, Arthur F.
Colden, Cadwallader
Cole, Richard B.
Connor, Leartus
Cooke, John E.
Cooper, Elias S.
Cordell, Eugene F.
Coxe, John R.
Curtis, Alva
Dailey, Ulysses G.
Dameshek, William
Davidson, Henry A.
Davis, Nathan S.
Dean, Lee W.
Dearholt, Hoyt E.
De Kruif, Paul H.
Dooley, Thomas A.
Drake, Daniel
Dugas, Louis A.
Dunglison, Robley
Dyer, Isadore
Eagleson, James B.
Eastman, Joseph

Eberle, John
Edsall, David L.
Einhorn, Max
Evans, George
Fenner, Erasmus D.
Fishbein, Morris
Flexner, Simon
Flint, Austin
Fordyce, John A.
Fulton, John F.
Fulton, Mary H.
Garland, Joseph
Garrison, Fielding
Garvin, Charles H.
Gibbons, Henry
Gies, William J.
Gifford, Harold
Godman, John D.
Gray, John P.
Gross, Samuel D.
Hamilton, Alice
Hamilton, John B.
Hammond, William A.
Haralson, Hugh H.
Harkins, Henry N.
Harris, Seale
Harrison, Ross G.
Hays, Isaac
Hektoen, Ludvig
Helmuth, William T.
Henry, Morris H.
Hertzler, Arthur E.
Hoerr, Normand L.
Holmes, Oliver W.
Holt, L. Emmett
Hopkins, Lemuel
Horsfall, Frank L., Jr.
Hurd, Henry M.
Hurty, John N.
Jackson, Edward
Jackson, James
Jacobi, Abraham
Jayne, Walter A.
Jelliffe, Smith Ely
Jordan, Edwin O.
Kelly, Howard A.
Kenney, John A.
Knapp, (J.) Herman
Long, Francis A.
Lynk, Miles V.
McCaw, James B.
McCormack, Arthur T.
Maddock, William O.

Martin, Franklin H.
Miller, William S.
Mitchell, S. Weir
Morse, John F.
Mumford, James G.
Newton, Robert S.
Osler, William
Patrick, Hugh T.
Pattison, Granville S.
Pilcher, Lewis P.
Potter, William W.
Purple, Samuel S.
Roman, Charles V.
Shrady, George F.
Simmons, George H.
Smith, Clarence A.
Smith, Nathan R.
Spivak, Charles D.
Thacher, James
Toner, Joseph M.
Westmoreland, John G.
Whipple, Allen O.
Williams, Stephen W.
Williams, William C.
Winslow, Charles-Edward A.
Wood, Casey A.
Wood, Thomas F.
Yandell, Lunsford P.

**MENTAL ILLNESS. See PSYCHIATRY/
MENTAL ILLNESS**

**METABOLISM. See ENDOCRINOLOGY
AND METABOLISM**

MICROBIOLOGY

Avery, Oswald T.
Bayne-Jones, Stanhope
Bierring, Walter L.
Biggs, Hermann M.
Blake, Francis G.
Blumer, George
Carrel, Alexis
Carroll, James
Carter, Henry R.
Cole, Rufus
Councilman, William T.
De Kruif, Paul H.
Dick, George F.
Dick, Gladys

Dochez, Alphonse
Flexner, Simon
Francis, Thomas, Jr.
Gay, Frederick
Goldberger, Joseph
Goodpasture, Ernest W.
Hektoen, Ludvig
Herter, Christian
Horsfall, Frank L., Jr.
Jones, Joseph
Jordan, Edwin O.
Just, Ernest E.
Keefer, Chester
Kinyoun, Joseph J.
Klebs, Theodore A.
Landsteiner, Karl
Lazear, Jesse W.
Libman, Emanuel
Loeb, Leo
Lynch, Kenneth M.
MacCallum, William G.
MacLeod, Colin M.
Meyer, Karl F.
Murphy, James B.
Noguchi, Hideya
North, Charles E.
Novy, Frederick G.
Nuttall, George H. F.
Opie, Eugene L.
Park, William H.
Paul, John R.
Pearce, Louise
Perkins, Roger G.
Prescott, Samuel C.
Prudden, T. Mitchell
Reed, Walter
Ricketts, Howard T.
Rivers, Thomas M.
Rosenau, Milton J.
Russell, Frederick
Salmon, Daniel E.
Sellards, Andrew W.
Shope, Richard E.
Smith, Margaret
Smith, Theobold
South, Lillian H.
Spray, Robb S.
Stanley, Wendell M.
Sternberg, George M.
Tatum, Edward L.
Theiler, Max
Tillett, William S.
Toomey. John A.

Trask, James D.
Tunnicliff, Ruth M.
Vaughan, Victor C.
Waksman, Selman A.
Welch, William H.
Wolbach, Simeon B.
Wollstein, Martha
Wood, William B., Jr.
Zinsser, Hans

MILITARY MEDICINE

Bartholow, Roberts
Barton, William P. C.
Bayne-Jones, Stanhope
Benites, Jose M.
Blake, Francis G.
Bowditch, Henry I.
Brinton, John H.
Brown, William
Carroll, James
Carter, C. Dana
Church, Benjamin
Churchill, Edward D.
Cochran, John
Craig, Winchell M.
Craik, James
Cutler, Elliott C.
Gihon, Albert L.
Gorgas, William C.
Hammond, William A.
Heermann, Lewis
Hulse, Isaac
Hume, Edgar E.
Letterman, Jonathan
McCaw, James B.
McCaw, Walter D.
McGee, Anita N.
McGuire, Hunter H.
Moore, Samuel P.
Morgan, John
Olyphant, David
Parsons, Usher
Porter, Henry R.
Reed, Walter
Rousselot, Louis M.
Russell, Frederick
Senn, Nicholas
Shippen, William
Sternberg, George M.
Tilton, James
Vedder, Edward B.

Walker, Mary E.
Woodward, Julian J.

MISSIONARY*

Carter, William S.
Dooley, Thomas A.
Eliot, Charles W.
Fulton, Mary H.
Judd, Gerrit P.
Kerr, John G.
McLean, Mary H.
Parker, Peter
Post, George E.
Swain, Clara
Whitman, Marcus
Wright, Eliphalet

NEPHROLOGY

Abel, John J.
Albright, Fuller
Delafield, Francis
Foley, Frederick E.B.
Hume, David M.
Kelly, Howard A.
Longcope, Warfield T.
Marshall, E. Kennerly, Jr.
Richards, Alfred N.
Rowntree, Leonard G.
Smith, Homer W.
Van Slyke, Donald D.

NEUROLOGY

Barker, Lewellys
Bartholow, Roberts
Beard, George M.
Bishop, George H.
Branche, George C.
Bronk, Detlev W.
Cannon, Walter B.
Clark, Sam L.
Dana, Charles L.
Donaldson, Henry H.
Erlanger, Joseph
Forbes, Alexander
Fuller, Solomon C.
Fulton, John F.
Gasser, Herbert S.
Graham, Helen T.
Hammond, William A.
Harrison, Ross G.

Herter, Christian
Huntington, George
Jelliffe, Smith Ely
Keen, William W., Jr.
Lennox, William G.
Meyer, Adolf
Mills, Charles K.
Mitchell, S. Weir
Neal, Josephine B.
O'Leary, James L.
Orton, Samuel T.
Patrick, Hugh T.
Putnam, James J.
Ranson, Stephen W.
Sachs, Bernard
Seguin, Edouard
Seguin, Edward C.
Southard, Elmer E.
Spitzka, Edward C.
Timme, Walter

NEUROSURGERY

Beck, Claude S.
Craig, Winchell
Cushing, Harvey W.
Dandy, Walter E.
Fenger, Christian
Gage, E. Lyle
Greene, Clarence S.
Keen, William W., Jr.
Murphy, John B.

NURSING*

Barton, Clara
Beard, Mary
Cannon, Ida M.
Delano, Jane A.
Dock, Lavinia L.
Goldmark, Josephine
Kenny, Elizabeth
Livermore, Mary A. R.
McGee, Anita N.
Nuttall, Mary A.
Passavant, William A.
Richards, Linda
Robb, Isabel A. H.
Thoms, Adah B.
Wald, Lillian D.
Winslow, Charles-Edward A.

NUTRITION AND DEFICIENCY DISEASES

Atwater, Wilbur O.
Babcock, James W.
Chase, Will H.
Chesney, Alan M.
Chittenden, Russell H.
Elvehjem, Conrad A.
Goldberger, Joseph
Graham, Sylvester
Hall, James L.
Hess, Alfred F.
Howland, John
Jackson, James C.
Kellogg, John H.
Ladd, Edwin F.
Lusk, Graham
Marine, David
McCollum, Elmer V.
Meigs, Arthur V.
Mendel, Lafayette B.
Minot, George R.
Osborne, Thomas B.
Steenbock, Harry
Vedder, Edward B.
Whipple, George H.
Wolbach, Simeon B.

OBSTETRICS AND GYNECOLOGY

Albright, Fuller
Atlee, John L.
Atlee, Washington
Bard, Samuel
Barker, B. Fordyce
Barringer, Emily D.
Battey, Robert
Bedford, Gunning
Bertner, Ernst W.
Bingham, Arthur W.
Blackwell, Emily
Bozeman, Nathan
Broomall, Anna E.
Brown, Charlotte
Byford, William H.
Channing, Walter
Cleveland, Emeline
Cole, Richard B.
Cullen, Thomas S.
De Lee, Joseph B.
Delameter, John
Dewees, William P.
Dickinson, Robert L.

Eastman, Joseph
Findley, Palmer
Frisbie, Evelyn F.
Gilliam, David T.
Hinson, Eugene T.
Hodge, Hugh L.
Holmes, Oliver W.
Howard, William T.
Hunter, William
Huson, Florence
Jenks, Edward W.
Jones, John
Kelly, Howard A.
Lambright, Middleton
Leighton, Adam P.
Lloyd, James
Lozier, Clemence S.
Macfarlane, Catharine
Martin, Franklin H.
Maury, Richard B.
May, Frederick
McLean, Mary H.
McNeill, William C.
Mead, Kate C. H.
Meigs, Charles D.
Meigs, John F.
Mendenhall, Dorothy R.
Mergler, Marie J.
Merrick, Myra K.
Miller, Henry, Jr.
Murray, Peter M.
Parvin, Theophilus
Potter, Ellen C.
Potter, William W.
Prevost, Francois M.
Price, Joseph
Ripley, Martha G.
Ross, Julian W.
Rubin, Isidore C.
Rutherford, Frances A.
Sanger, Margaret
Seaman, Valentine
Shipp, Ellis R.
Sims, J. Marion
Skene, Alexander
Smith, Albert H.
Stastny, Olga F.
Storer, David H.
Storer, Horatio R.
Taussig, Frederick
Taylor, Eugene T.
Thomas, T. Gaillard
Van Hoosen, Bertha

White, James P.
Williams, John W.
Yarros, Rachelle
Zakrzewska, Marie E.

OCCUPATIONAL MEDICINE

Davis, George G.
Edsall, David Linn
Gardner, Leroy U.
Hamilton, Alice
Jackson, James M., Jr.
Kelley, Florence
Kober, George M.
Larsen, Nils P.
Leavitt, Erasmus
Longcope, Warfield T.
Lynch, Kenneth M.
Martland, Harrison S.
McCready, Benjamin W.
McGee, Lemuel
Richards, Paul S.
Smith, Andrew H.
Thompson, William G.

ONCOLOGY

Bloodgood, Joseph C.
Coley, William B.
Ewing, James
Farber, Sidney
Graham, Evarts A.
Gross, Samuel W.
Hoffman, Frederick
Horsfall, Frank L., Jr.
Koch, William F.
Krebs, Ernest
Larson, Leonard W.
Loeb, Leo
Macfarlane, Catharine
Murphy, James B.
Osgood, Edwin E.
Papanicolaou, George N.
Rodman, William L.
Rous, Peyton
Taussig, Frederick
Tracy, Martha
Voegtlin, Carl
Woodward, Joseph

OPHTHALMOLOGY. See EYE, EAR, NOSE AND THROAT

ORTHOPEDIC SURGERY

Agnew, David H.
Bigelow, Henry J.
Bradford, Edward H.
Campbell, Willis C.
Codman, Ernest A.
Crosby, Dixi
Dandy, Walter E.
Davis, Henry G.
Dillehunt, Richard B.
Gillette, Arthur J.
Gunn, Moses
Murphy, John B.
Orr, Hiram W.
Physick, Philip S.
Sayre, Lewis A.
Steindler, Arthur
Taylor, Charles F.
Whitman, Royal
Wright, Louis T.

OTOLARYNGOLOGY. See EYE, EAR, NOSE AND THROAT

OTOLOGY. See EYE, EAR, NOSE AND THROAT

PARASITOLOGY. See BIOLOGY, GENETICS, AND PARASITOLOGY

PATENT MEDICINE*

Abrams, Albert
Ayer, James C.
Brandreth, Benjamin
Brinkley, John R.
Cramp, Arthur J.
Dyott, Thomas W.
Hartman, Samuel B.
Koch, William
Krebs, Ernest
Perkins, Elisha
Pinkham, Lydia
Reich, Wilhelm

Warner, Hulbert H.
Wiley, Harvey W.

PATHOLOGY

Abbott, Maude
Biggs, Hermann M.
Bloodgood, Joseph C.
Brinton, John H.
Cabot, Richard C.
Councilman, William T.
Cullen, Thomas S.
De Witt, Lydia M.
Delafield, Francis
Dickerson, Spencer C.
Ewing, James
Farber, Sidney
Fenger, Christian
Fitz, Reginald
Flexner, Simon
Fuller, Solomon C.
Gardner, Leroy U.
Gay, Frederick
Gerhard, William W.
Gilliam, David T.
Goodpasture, Ernest W.
Hektoen, Ludvig
Herter, Christian
Hertzler, Arthur E.
Horner, William E.
Jackson, John B. S.
Klebs, Theodore A.
Kline, Benjamin S.
Larson, Leonard W.
Libman, Emanuel
Loeb, Leo
Longcope, Warfield T.
Lynch, Kenneth M.
MacCallum, William G.
Mallory, Frank B.
Marine, David
Martland, Harrison S.
Mendenhall, Dorothy R.
Murphy, James B.
Opie, Eugene L.
Palmer, Alonzo B.
Pepper, William
Prudden, T. Mitchell
Quinland, William S.
Rous, Peyton
Shore, Clarence
Smith, Harry P.
Smith, Margaret

Stillé, Alfred
Welch, William H.
Wells, Harry G.
Whipple, George H.
Wilson, Louis B.
Winternitz, Milton C.
Wolbach, Simeon B.
Wollstein, Martha
Woodward, Joseph J.

PEDIATRICS

Abt, Isaac A.
Aldrich, Charles A.
Baker, S. Josephine
Becker, Harry F.
Bilderback, Joseph B.
Blackfan, Kenneth D.
Blalock, Alfred
Brown, Charlotte
Busey, Samuel C.
Butler, Henry R.
Coit, Henry L.
Cooley, Thomas B.
Cowie, David M.
Davison, Wilburt C.
Farber, Sidney
Gamble, James L.
Garland, Joseph
Gesell, Arnold L.
Greenberg, Morris
Hartmann, Alexis F.
Hess, Alfred F.
Holt, L. Emmett
Howland, John
Jacobi, Abraham
Knox, James H. M., Jr.
Koplik, Henry
Ladd, William E.
Levy, Julius
Marriott, W. McKim
McQuarrie, Irvine
Meigs, Arthur V.
Meigs, John F.
O'Dwyer, Joseph
Osgood, Edwin E.
Porter, William T.
Putnam, Charles P.
Ramsey, Walter R.
Ripley, Martha G.
Rotch, Thomas M.
Sachs, Bernard
Schick, Bela

Schloss, Oscar M.
Smith, Alonzo D.
Smith, Job L.
Stokes, Joseph, Jr.
Van Ingen, Philip
Veeder, Bordon S.
Wollstein, Martha

PERSONAL HYGIENE. See POPULAR AND FOLK MEDICINE

PHARMACOLOGY

Abel, John J.
Auer, John
Bache, Franklin
Barton, Benjamin
Bigelow, Jacob
Blake, James
Brown, William
Carrel, Alexis
Chase, Will H.
Chittenden, Russell H.
Coxe, John R.
Cushny, Arthur R.
De Witt, Lydia M.
Fearn, Thomas
Garden, Alexander
Graham, Helen T.
Hatcher, Robert A.
Henderson, Yandell
Hirschfelder, Arthur D.
Hunt, Reid
Jackson, Hall
Jackson, Samuel
King, John
Kremers, Edward
Lloyd, John U.
Loeb, Robert F.
Long, Perrin H.
MacLeod, Colin M.
MacNider, William
Maloney, Arnold H.
Marshall, E. Kennerly, Jr.
Meltzer, Samuel J.
Phares, David L.
Procter, William, Jr.
Richards, Alfred N.
Rowntree, Leonard G.
Schamberg, Jay F.
Sollmann, Torald H.
Spalding, Lyman

Squibb, Edward R.
Stillé, Alfred
Takamine, Jokichi
Voegtlin, Carl
Waksman, Selman A.
Weiss, Soma
Wood, George B.
Wood, Horatio C.
Wright, Louis T.

PHILANTHROPY*

(Primarily persons engaged in medical research and health care delivery)

Anderson, John W.
Bousfield, Midian O.
Gates, Frederick
Rose, Wickliffe
Schuyler, Louise L.
Stiles, Charles W.
Straus, Nathan

PHYSICAL MEDICINE AND REHABILITATION

Bradford, Edward H.
Dillehunt, Richard B.
Gillette, Arthur J.
Hench, Philip S.
Kenny, Elizabeth
Lothrup, Charles H.
McKenzie, Robert T.
Marshall, Hubert
Reid, William W.
Smith, Clarence A.
Steindler, Arthur
Taylor, Charles
Thompson, William G.
Toomey, John A.

PHYSIOLOGY

Allen, Edgar
Auer, John
Beaumont, William
Bishop, George H.
Blalock, Alfred
Bowditch, Henry P.
Bronk, Detlev W.
Campbell, Henry F.
Cannon, Walter B.
Carrel, Alexis

Carter, William S.
Crile, George W.
Cushny, Arthur R.
Dalton, John C.
Dragstedt, Lester
DuBois, Eugene F.
Dunglison, Robley
Erlanger, Joseph
Flint, Austin, Jr.
Forbes, Alexander
Fulton, John F.
Gasser, Herbert S.
Graham, Helen T.
Halsted, William S.
Hammond, William A.
Hemmeter, John C.
Henderson, Lawrence
Henderson, Yandell
Hirschfelder, Arthur D.
Howell, William H.
Kendall, Edward C.
Loeb, Jacques
Loeb, Robert F.
Long, Cyril N. H.
Mann, Frank C.
Marshall, E. Kennerly, Jr.
Martin, Henry N.
McMaster, Philip D.
Meltzer, Samuel J.
Oliver, Daniel
Papanicolaou, George N.
Porter, William T.
Richards, Dickinson W.
Sewall, Henry
Smith, Homer W.
Van Slyke, Donald D.
Von Békésy, Georg
Weiss, Soma
Wiggers, Carl J.

PLASTIC SURGERY

Blair, Vilray P.
Callister, Alfred C.
Davis, John S.
Kolle, Frederick S.
Ladd, William E.
Mott, Valentine
Padgett, Earl C.
Senn, Nicholas
Shrady, George F.
Whitehead, William R.

POPULAR AND FOLK MEDICINE*

(Personal hygiene reformers and writers of medical works for laymen)

Alcott, William A.
Aldrich, Charles A.
Baruch, Simon
Clendening, Logan
Evans, William A., Jr.
Ewell, James
Fishbein, Morris
Flower, Benjamin O.
Graham, Sylvester
Greene, Cordelia
Gregory, Samuel
Gunn, John C.
Hall, William W.
Hitchcock, Edward
Holt, L. Emmett
Hunt, Harriot K.
Hutchinson, Woods
Jackson, James C.
Jean, Sally L.
Kellogg, John H.
Knowlton, Charles
Lewis, Dio
Macfadden, Bernarr
Nichols, Mary S. N. G.
Sanger, Margaret
Shipp, Ellis R.
Smith, Peter
Stevenson, Sarah A. H.
Tennent, John
Thacher, Thomas
Trall, Russell T.
Walker, Mary E.
White, Ellen G.
Yarros, Rachelle

PROFESSIONAL ASSOCIATIONS*

Abell, Irvin
Alexander, Walter G.
Arnold, Richard D.
Atlee, John L.
Atlee, Washington
Awl, William M.
Baldwin, Abel S.
Baldwin, William O.
Barnes, William H.
Biddle, Andrew P.
Bierring, Walter L.

Bilderback, Joseph B.
Blanton, William P.
Blesh, Abraham L.
Bobbs, John S.
Bodine, James M.
Bosworth, Franke H.
Boyd, Robert F.
Bradford, Claudius
Bradford, Edward H.
Brainard, Daniel
Briggs, William T.
Brigham, Amariah
Brodie, William
Brown, Lawrason
Brown, Solyman
Busey, Samuel C.
Butler, Henry R.
Byford, William H.
Campbell, Willis C.
Chapman, Nathaniel
Cochran, Jerome
Coffey, Robert C.
Coffman, Victor H.
Colwell, Nathan P.
Connor, Leartus
Cooke, Robert A.
Cooley, Thomas B.
Cramp, Arthur J.
Daniel, Richard P.
Davis, Nathan S.
Dibble, Eugene H.
Dibrell, James A.
Dibrell, James A., Jr.
Dolley, Sarah R.
Donnell, Clyde H.
Dunlap, Livingston
Elmer, Jonathan
Engstad, John E.
Evans, John
Fairchild, David S.
Fishbein, Morris
Fortner, Benjamin
Francis, Grossi H.
Francis, John W.
Gamble, Henry F.
Gathings, Joseph G.
Giles, Roscoe C.
Gridley, Selah
Griscom, John H.
Gross, Samuel D.
Haggard, William D., Jr.
Hargrave, Frank S.
Harison, Beverly D.

Harris, William H.
Hays, Isaac
Haywood, Edmund B.
Holt, Erastus E.
Holyoke, Edward A.
Hooper, Philo
Hurd, Henry M.
Huson, Florence
Jackson, James M., Jr.
Johnson, Peter A.
Kenney, John A.
Ketchum, George A.
Knight, Jonathan
Larson, Leonard W.
Livingston, Robert R.
Main, John H. T.
Majors, Monroe A.
Martin, Franklin H.
McCormack, Joseph N.
McKean, Robert
McKee, William H.
Meltzer, Samuel J.
Millspaugh, Joseph G.
Munson, Eneas
Murray, Peter M.
Pittman, Newsome J.
Pride, Maynard P.
Rodman, William L.
Shoulders, Harrison
Simmons, George H.
Smith, Relliford S.
Van Hoosen, Bertha
Vinsonhaler, Frank
Von Mansfelde, Alexander S.
Warnshuis, Frederick C.
Warren, John
Watkins, William W.
Weatherly, Job S.
Weed, Gideon A.
Wilbur, Ray L.
Wynn, Frank B.

PSYCHIATRY/MENTAL ILLNESS

Alexander, Franz G.
Awl, William M.
Babcock, James W.
Bates, James
Beard, George M.
Beck, T. Romeyn
Beers, Clifford
Bell, Luther V.
Black, John J.

Bond, Thomas
Branche, George C.
Brigham, Amariah
Brill, Abraham A.
Bryce, Peter
Cogswell, Mason F.
Davidson, Henry A.
Dix, Dorothea
Earle, Pliny
Evans, John
Fuller, Solomon C.
Gesell, Arnold L.
Gray, John P.
Healy, William
Hocker, William A.
Hooper, Philo O.
Horney, Karen
Hurd, Henry M.
Jarvis, Edward
Jelliffe, Smith Ely
Kempster, Walter
Kirkbride, Thomas S.
Menninger, Charles F.
Menninger, William C.
Meyer, Adolf
Mitchell, S. Weir
Munsterberg, Hugo
Orton, Samuel T.
Prince, Morton
Putnam, James J.
Ray, Isaac
Rush, Benjamin
Seguin, Edouard
Sleyster, Rock
Smith, Lyndon A.
Smith, Stephen
Southard, Elmer E.
Spitzka, Edward C.
Steuart, Richard S.
Sullivan, Harry S.
Todd, Eli
White, William A.
Woodward, Samuel B.

PUBLIC HEALTH

(Primarily persons associated with government agencies or voluntary associations)

(Born prior to 1850)

Arnold, Richard D.
Baker, Henry B.
Baruch, Simon

Bayley, Richard
Blackwell, Elizabeth
Bowditch, Henry I.
Brackett, Cyrus F.
Brodie, William
Brown, Charlotte A.
Bush, Lewis P.
Cabell, James
Caldwell, Charles
Chaillé, Stanford
Chandler, Charles F.
Cochran, Jerome
Coffman, Victor H.
Daniel, Richard P.
Dibrell, James A., Jr.
Fenner, Erasmus D.
Garcelon, Alonzo
Gary, Thomas P.
Gerrish, Frederic H.
Gihon, Albert L.
Gorgas, William C.
Griscom, John H.
Hamilton, John B.
Handy, John C.
Hargis, Robert B. S.
Harris, Elisha
Hewitt, Charles N.
Hitchcock, Homer O.
Holt, Erastus E.
Holton, Henry D.
Howe, Lucien
Hunt, Ezra M.
Jackson, Samuel
Jacobi, Abraham
Janeway, Edward G.
Jarvis, Edward
Jones, Joseph
Kane, John K.
Kempster, Walter
Lam, Frederick K.
Lamb, Daniel S.
Leavitt, Erasmus
Lindsley, John B.
Livermore, Mary A.
Lyster, Henry F. L.
Magruder, George L.
McCormack, Joseph N.
Miller, Thomas
Mitchell, Robert W.
Moore, Edward M.
North, Elisha
Ohage, Justus
Owens-Adair, Bethenia A.

Parker, Willard
Porter, Joseph Y.
Prudden, T. Mitchell
Putnam, Charles P.
Rauch, John H.
Reeve, James T.
Robertson, William S.
Schuyler, Louise L.
Shattuck, Lemuel
Smith, Stephen
Snow, Edwin M.
Souchon, Edmund
Steele, Henry K.
Steele, William L.
Straus, Nathan
Towne, Solon R.
Waring, George E.
Weatherly, Job S.
Wiley, Harvey W.
Wood, Thomas F.
Woodworth, John M.

(Born after 1849)

Ashford, Bailey K.
Baker, S. Josephine
Barker, Lewellys F.
Beard, Mary
Beatty, Theodore
Beers, Clifford
Bierring, Walter L.
Biggs, Hermann M.
Bingham, Arthur W.
Brown, William E.
Campbell, Elizabeth
Carter, Henry R.
Caverly, Charles S.
Chapin, Charles V.
Cogswell, William F.
Coit, Henry L.
Copeland, Royal S.
Council, Walter
Cowie, David M.
Cox, George W., Jr.
Crumbine, Samuel J.
Darrow, Edward M.
Dearholt, Hoyt E.
Donahoe, William E.
Emerson, Haven
Evans, Matilda A.
Evans, William A., Jr.
Favill, Henry B.
Flick, Lawrence F.
Folks, Homer

Foster, Eugene
Francis, Grossi H.
French, Harley E.
Frost, Wade H.
Gant, Harris A.
Garrison, Charles W.
Gibson, Samuel C.
Goldberger, Joseph
Goldmark, Josephine
Goldwater, Sigismund S.
Goodfellow, George E.
Grassick, James
Greenberg, Morris
Hargrave, Frank S.
Harper, Cornelius
Healy, Henry H.
Heg, Elmer E.
Hess, Alfred F.
Hoffman, Frederick
Holt, L. Emmett
Hood, William H.
Hume, Edgar E.
Hunter, John F.
Hurty, John N.
Jackson, James M., Jr.
Jean, Sally L.
Johnson, Peter A.
Johnston, George P.
Jordan, Edwin O.
Kelley, Florence
Kiefer, Guy L.
Kinyoun, Joseph J.
Knox, James H. M., Jr.
Kober, George M.
Koplik, Henry
Ladd, Edwin F.
Lam, Frederick
Larsen, Nils P.
Lathrop, Julia C.
Leathers, Waller
Levy, Julius
Livermore, Mary A. R.
Lovejoy, Esther P.
Lumsden, Leslie L.
Mahoney, John F.
Marshall, Hyrum
McCormack, Arthur T.
McLean, Mary H.
Mead, Kate C. H.
Mendenhall, Dorothy R.
Meyer, Karl F.
Morrell, Joseph R.
Mouritz, Arthur A.

North, Charles E.
Park, William H.
Parran, Thomas
Payne, Howard M.
Perkins, Roger G.
Picotte, Susan LaF.
Potter, Ellen C.
Quain, Fannie A.
Riis, Jacob A.
Rose, Wickliffe
Rosenau, Milton J.
Sabin, Florence R.
Salmon, Daniel E.
Schick, Bela
Scott, James R.
Sedgwick, William T.
Smillie, Wilson G.
Smith, Andrew C.
Smith, Morgan
Snow, William F.
South, Lillian H.
Southard, Elmer E.
Squibb, Edward R.
Stastny, Olga F.
Stiles, Charles W.
Sydenstricker, Edgar
Taussig, Frederick
Underwood, Felix J.
Van Ingen, Philip
Vaughan, Victor C.
Viko, Louis E.
Wald, Lillian D.
Washburn, Victor D.
Weedon, Leslie W.
Welch, William H.
Wende, Ernest
Winslow, Charles-Edward A.
Wylder, Meldrum K.
Yount, Clarence E.

PULMONARY MEDICINE

Boswell, Henry
Bowditch, Henry I.
Brown, Lawrason
Cole, Rufus
Dearholt, Hoyt E.
Denison, Charles
Dochez, Alphonse
Flick, Lawrence F.
Gardiner, Charles F.
Gardner, Leroy U.
Grassick, James

Hargrave, Frank S.
Heg, Elmer E.
Hopkins, Lemuel
Jackson, Chevalier
Jackson, James, Jr.
Laurey, James R.
Loomis, Alfred L.
Matson, Ralph C.
Matson, Ray W.
Meriwether, Clinton P.
Moorman, Lewis J.
O'Dwyer, Joseph
Opie, Eugene L.
Payne, Howard M.
Pennock, Caspar W.
Sabin, Florence R.
Sewall, Henry
Solly, S. Edwin
Trudeau, Edward L.
Werner, Walter I.

RADIOLOGY

Brown, Percy
Caldwell, Eugene W.
Dandy, Walter E.
Dodd, Walter J.
Glasser, Otto
Graham, Evarts A.
Kolle, Frederick S.
Leonard, Charles L.
Martland, Harrison S.
Minot, George R.
Moore, Carl V.
Muller, Hermann J.
Pusey, William A.
Williams, Francis H.
Wolbach, Simeon B.

RHINOLOGY. See EYE, EAR, NOSE AND THROAT

SANITARY ENGINEERING*

Eddy, Harrison P.
Gorgas, William C.
Hazen, Allen
Kirkwood, James P.
Mills, Hiram F.
Sedgwick, William T.
Waring, George E.

SOCIAL WORK* (MEDICAL)

Cabot, Richard C.
Cannon, Ida M.
Folks, Homer
Hamilton, Alice
Holt, Winifred
Jean, Sally L.
Lathrop, Julia C.
Meyer, Adolf
Potter, Ellen C.
Putnam, Charles P.
Ripley, Martha G.
Rubinow, Isaac
Southard, Elmer E.
Wald, Lillian D.

SPECIAL EDUCATION*
(*For physically and mentally handicapped*)

Buckingham, Richard G.
Cogswell, Mason
Dunglison, Robley
Fisher, John Dix
Gallaudet, Thomas
Gesell, Arnold L.
Holt, Winifred
Howe, Samuel G.
Orton, Samuel T.
Seguin, Edouard
Wilbur, Hervey B.

STATISTICS

Baker, Henry B.
Billings, John S.
Blaney, James V.
Boylston, Zabdiel
Chapin, Charles V.
Earle, Pliny
Emerson, Haven
Frost, Wade H.
Gihon, Albert L.
Harris, Elisha
Hitchcock, Edward
Hoffman, Frederick
Hunt, Ezra M.
Jarvis, Edward
Mather, Cotton
Miller, Thomas
Pearl, Raymond
Rubinow, Isaac
Shattuck, Lemuel

Snow, Edwin M.
Spalding, Lyman
Sutton, William L.
Sydenstricker, Edgar

SURGERY. See also under various Subspecialties

(Born prior to 1800)

Antony, Milton
Bates, James
Bayley, Richard
Baynham, William
Beaumont, William
Belisle, Henri
Benites, Jose M.
Coffin, Nathaniel
Cogswell, Mason
Davidge, John B.
Delameter, John
Dorsey, John S.
Dudley, Benjamin W.
Hunter, William
Jackson, Hall
Jones, John
Knight, Jonathan
Lloyd, James
March, Alden
McClellan, George
McDowell, Ephraim
Mott, Valentine
Mussey, Reuben D.
Parsons, Usher
Pell, Thomas
Physick, Philip S.
Post, Wright
Prevost, Francois M.
Seaman, Valentine
Smith, Alban G.
Smith, Nathan
Smith, Nathan R.
Twitchell, Amos
Warren, John
Warren, John C.

(Born 1800 to 1849)

Abbott, Anderson
Agnew, David H.
Andrews, Edmund
Bancroft, Frederick
Battey, Robert
Bayless, George W.

Bigelow, Henry J.
Blackwell, Emily
Bobbs, John S.
Brainard, Daniel
Briggs, William I.
Brinton, John H.
Brodie, William
Campbell, Henry F.
Carmalt, William H.
Cheever, David W.
Chisholm, Julian J.
Cleveland, Emeline
Coffman, Victor H.
Cooper, Elias S.
Crosby, Alpheus B.
Crosby, Dixi
Den, Richard S.
Dibrell, James A., Jr.
Dimock, Susan
Dugas, Louis A.
Eastman, Joseph
Eve, Paul F.
Fairchild, David S.
Fenger, Christian
Finfrock, John H.
Fitz, Reginald
Fowler, George R.
Frissell, John
Garcelon, Alonzo
Gary, Thomas P.
Gerrish, Frederic
Gilliam, David T.
Griffin, John S.
Gross, Samuel D.
Gross, Samuel W.
Gunn, Moses
Hall, G. Stanley
Hamilton, John B.
Haywood, Edmund B.
Helmuth, William T.
Henry, Morris H.
Hodgen, John T.
Hughes, John C.
Hullihen, Simon P.
Keen, William W., Jr.
Krackowizer, Ernst
Lane, Levi C.
Livingston, Robert R.
Lothrop, Charles H.
Lozier, Clemence M.
Maghee, Thomas G.
Maury, Richard B.
Mayo, William W.

McBurney, Charles
McDowell, Joseph N.
McGraw, Theodore A.
McGuire, Hunter H.
Moore, Edward M.
Nott, Josiah C.
Ohage, Justus
Pancoast, Joseph
Parker, Willard
Parrish, Isaac
Peck, Washington F.
Phillips, Josiah L.
Pilcher, Lewis
Pope, Charles A.
Purvis, Charles B.
Reyburn, Robert
Rogers, William E.
Senn, Nicholas
Sims, J. Marion
Smith, Stephen
Souchon, Edmund
Steele, William L.
Stone, Warren
Thayer, Samuel W.
Thompson, Mary H.
Toland, Hugh H.
Warren, Edward
Warren, J. Collins
Watson, Beriah A.
Whitehead, William R.
Wolcott, Erastus B.
Wood, James R.
Wyman, Morrill

(Born after 1849)

Abell, Irvin
Allen, Lyman
Anderson, William H. (b. 1886)
Andrews, Edward W.
Barber, Amos
Barringer, Emily D.
Beck, Claude S.
Behle, Augustus
Bevan, Arthur D.
Blakemore, Arthur H.
Blalock, Alfred
Blanton, William P.
Blesh, Abraham L.
Bloodgood, Joseph C.
Brödel, Max
Cabot, Hugh
Carrel, Alexis
Carson, Simeon L.

Carter, C. Dana
Churchill, Edward D.
Clement, Kenneth W.
Coffey, Robert C.
Coley, William B.
Coller, Frederick
Council, Walter W.
Crile, George W.
Crowe, Samuel J.
Cullen, Thomas S.
Curtis, Austin M.
Cushing, Harvey W.
Cutler, Elliott C.
Dailey, Ulysses G.
Dandy, Walter E.
Darrow, Edward M.
Davis, George G.
Davis, John S.
Deaver, John B.
Dennis, Frederic S.
Dragstedt, Lester
Drew, Charles R.
Eagleson, James B.
Engstad, John E.
Finney, John M.
Fite, Francis B.
Frederick, Rivers
Freedlander, Samuel O.
Freeman, John W.
Gamble, Henry F.
Giles, Roscoe C.
Goodfellow, George E.
Graham, Evarts A.
Gundersen, Adolf
Haggard, William D.
Haight, Cameron
Hale, John H.
Hall, George C.
Halsted, William S.
Harkins, Henry N.
Heg, Elmer E.
Hertzler, Arthur E.
Hill, Luther L.
Howard, William F.
Hume, David M.
Huson, Florence
Jackson, Algernon
Jayne, Walter A.
Johnson, Peter A.
Johnson, A. Holmes
Johnston, George P.
Kelly, Howard A.
Ladd, William E.

Lahey, Frank H.
Laurey, James R.
Lilienthal, Howard
Lovelace, William R.
Lovelace, William R., II
Mann, Frank C.
Martin, Franklin H.
Mason, James T.
Matas, Rudolph
Matson, Ralph C.
Matson, Ray W.
Mayo, Charles H.
Mayo, William J.
McCaw, Walter D.
McClennan, Alonzo C.
Mergler, Marie J.
Meyer, Willy
Mumford, James G.
Murphy, John B.
Orr, Thomas G.
Palmer, Erroll P.
Park, Roswell
Pettigrew, George A.
Price, Joseph
Quain, Eric P.
Ramstad, Niles O.
Reid, Mont R.
Richards, Paul S.
Richards, Ralph T.
Richardson, Maurice H.
Roberts, Carl G.
Robinson, Paul T.
Rodman, William L.
Rousselot, Louis M.
Schwyzer, Arnold
Scott, Arthur C.
Shoulders, Harrison
Smith, Andrew C.
Sprague, Edward W.
Stubbs, Frederick D.
Summers, John E., Jr.
Tait, F. Dudley
Thomas, William M.
Turner, Delos A.
Turner, John P.
Tuthill, Alexander
Van Hoosen, Bertha
Vaughan, George T.
Warfield, William A.
Warnshuis, Frederick C.
Weible, Ralph E.
Wheeler, John B.
Whipple, Allen O.

Whitehead, William M.
Williams, Daniel H.
Wishard, William N.
Wright, Louis T.

THORACIC SURGERY

Auer, John
Beck, Claude S.
Blakemore, Arthur H.
Blalock, Alfred
Churchill, Edward D.
Cutler, Elliott C.
Freedlander, Samuel O.
Gibbon, John H., Jr.
Graham, Evarts A.
Haight, Cameron
Hill, Luther L.
Laurey, James R.
Lilienthal, Howard
Matas, Rudolph
Matson, Ralph C.
Meyer, Willy
Mott, Valentine
Murphy, John B.
Reid, Mont R.
Schwyzer, Arnold
Stubbs, Frederick D.
Vaughan, George T.

UNORTHODOX MEDICINE*

(Sectarian practitioners)

Beach, Wooster
Brandreth, Benjamin
Brinkley, John R.
Curtis, Alva
Eddy, Mary Baker
Flower, Benjamin O.
Graham, Sylvester
Helmuth, William T.
Hering, Constantine
Jackson, James C.
King, John
Lloyd, John U.
Merrick, Myra K.
Newton, Robert S.
Nichols, Mary S. N. G.
Palmer, Bartlett J.
Palmer, Daniel D.
Ruggles, David
Scudder, John M.

Shew, Joel
Still, Andrew T.
Thomson, Samuel
Trall, Russell T.
Wesselhoeft, Conrad

UROLOGY

Alcock, Nathaniel
Bigelow, Henry J.
Blanton, William P.
Boylston, Zabdiel
Briggs, William T.
Cabot, Hugh
Dudley, Benjamin W.
Eve, Paul F.
Flocks, Rubin H.
Foley, Frederick
Garvin, Charles H.
Gross, Samuel W.
Keyes, Edward L.
Lilienthal, Howard
Martin, Franklin H.
McGuire, Hunter H.
Meyer, Willy
Physick, Philip S.
Timberlake, Gideon
Vincent, Hubert C.
Wishard, William N.
Young, Hugh H.

VENEREAL DISEASES

Barringer, Emily D.
Branche, George C.
Chesney, Alan M.
Fordyce, John A.
Garrison, Charles W.
Gathings, Joseph G.
Henry, Morris H.
Hinton, William A.
Keyes, Edward L.
Kline, Benjamin S.
Landsteiner, Karl
Lawless, Theodore K.
Mahoney, John F.
Noguchi, Hideya
Parran, Thomas
Pusey, William A.
Schamberg, Jay F.
Snow, William F.
Swift, Homer F.
Young, Hugh H.
Yarros, Rachelle

WRITING (MEDICAL). See LITERATURE

WRITING (POPULAR). See LITERATURE and POPULAR AND FOLK MEDICINE

Listing by Medical College or Graduate Level College

Graduates of a medical college or graduate-level college are listed in Appendix E. Foreign graduates are listed by country where their institutions are located and not by the individual colleges. The American colleges that are represented here are those that had four or more graduates among the individuals selected for inclusion.

ALBANY MEDICAL COLLEGE (N.Y.)

Blackfan, Kenneth D.
Fairchild, David S.
Hewitt, Charles N.
Smith, Theobold
Wright, Eliphalet N.

AUSTRIA AND HUNGARY

Alexander, Franz G.
Koller, Carl
Krackowizer, Ernst
Landsteiner, Karl
Raab, Wilhelm
Reich, Wilhelm
Schick, Bela
Steindler, Arthur
Von Békésy, Georg

BELLEVUE HOSPITAL MEDICAL COLLEGE: See NEW YORK UNIVERSITY SCHOOL OF MEDICINE

BERKSHIRE MEDICAL COLLEGE (Mass.)

Buckingham, Richard G.
Frissell, John
Parker, Willard

Stone, Warren
Wilbur, Hervey B.

BOWDOIN MEDICAL SCHOOL (MEDICAL SCHOOL OF MAINE)

Barker, B. Fordyce
Brackett, Cyrus F.
Gerrish, Frederic
Holt, Erastus E.
Leighton, Adam P.
Lincoln, Benjamin
Ray, Isaac

BRITISH ISLES

Bard, Samuel
Blake, James
Brown, Samuel
Brown, William
Cushny, Arthur R.
Davidge, John B.
Den, Richard S.
Douglass, William
Fayssoux, Peter
Fulton, John F.
Garden, Alexander
Kuhn, Adam
Long, Cyril N. H.
McClurg, James
McDowell, Ephraim

Martin, Henry N.
Middleton, Peter
Mitchill, Samuel L.
Morgan, John
Morton, Samuel G.
Moultrie, John, Jr.
Mouritz, Arthur A.
Olyphant, David
Physick, Philip S.
Redman, John
Romayne, Nicholas
Rush, Benjamin
Shippen, William
Smith, James McC.
Theiler, Max
Todd, Thomas W.
Warren, John C.
Wistar, Caspar

UNIVERSITY OF BUFFALO SCHOOL OF MEDICINE

Bancroft, Frederick J.
Dorsette, Cornelius N.
Flint, Austin, Jr.
Wende, Ernest

UNIVERSITY OF CALIFORNIA

McQuarrie, Irvine
Nuttall, George H. F.
Smith, Harry P.
Waksman, Selman A.

CANADA

Abbott, Anderson
Abbott, Maude
Augusta, Alexander
Barker, Lewellys
Cogswell, William F.
Cullen, Thomas S.
Drew, Charles R.
Evans, George
Harison, Beverly D.
Horsfall, Frank L., Jr.
Livingston, Robert R.
Long, Cyril N. H.
McKenzie, Robert T.
Mackenzie, Kenneth A. J.
MacLeod, Colin M.
Osler, William
Rowntree, Leonard G.
Wood, Casey A.

CASE WESTERN RESERVE UNIVERSITY: See WESTERN RESERVE UNIVERSITY SCHOOL OF MEDICINE

CASTLETON MEDICAL COLLEGE (Vt.) (Includes Middlebury College)

Armsby, James H.
Green, Horace
Jenks, Edward W.
Maynard, David S.
Reeve, James T.
Wood, James R.

CHICAGO MEDICAL COLLEGE: See NORTHWESTERN UNIVERSITY

UNIVERSITY OF CHICAGO (Includes Rush Medical College graduates through 1940)

Adams, Numa P. G.
Beatty, Theodore
Behle, Augustus
Bevan, Arthur D.
Cohn, Edwin J.
Colwell, Nathan P.
Darrow, Edward M.
Davis, George G.
Dearholt, Hoyt E.
Dick, George F.
Dickerson, Spencer C.
Dillehunt, Richard B.
Dragstedt, Lester
Engstad, John E.
Favill, Henry B.
Fishbein, Morris
Folin, Otto
Graham, Evarts A.
Graham, Helen T.
Grassick, James
Hall, James L.
Hamilton, John B.
Harkins, Henry N.
Healy, Henry H.
Healy, William
Herrick, James B.
Hoerr, Normand L.
Hume, David M.
Jones, Noble W.
Just, Ernest E.
Lyon, Elias P.
McGee, Lemuel

Morrell, Joseph R.
Murphy, John B.
O'Leary, James L.
Phillips, Josiah L.
Ranson, Stephen W.
Robins, Charles A.
Simmons, George H.
Smith, Fred M.
Spray, Robb S.
Tunnicliff, Ruth M.
Von Mansfelde, Alexander S.
Weed, Gideon A.
Weible, Ralph E.
Wells, Harry G.

CINCINNATI MEDICAL COLLEGE: See UNIVERSITY OF CINCINNATI COLLEGE OF MEDICINE

UNIVERSITY OF CINCINNATI COLLEGE OF MEDICINE (Includes Medical College of Ohio and Cincinnati Medical College)

Billings, John S.
Bowling, William K.
Byford, William H.
Evans, John
Finfrock, John W.
Garcelon, Alonzo
Gilliam, David T.
Johnston, George P.
Wynn, Frank B.

MEDICAL COLLEGE OF THE CITY OF NEW YORK: See NEW YORK UNIVERSITY SCHOOL OF MEDICINE

UNIVERSITY OF THE CITY OF NEW YORK MEDICAL DEPARTMENT: See NEW YORK UNIVERSITY SCHOOL OF MEDICINE

CLEVELAND MEDICAL COLLEGE: See WESTERN RESERVE UNIVERSITY SCHOOL OF MEDICINE

COLLEGE OF PHYSICIANS AND SURGEONS OF CHICAGO: See UNIVERSITY OF ILLINOIS

COLLEGE OF PHYSICIANS AND SURGEONS OF THE WESTERN DISTRICT OF NEW YORK: See FAIRFIELD MEDICAL SCHOOL

COLUMBIA UNIVERSITY

Avery, Oswald T.
Barlow, Walter J.

Beard, George M.
Beck, T. Romeyn
Bingham, Arthur W.
Blanton, Wyndham
Brill, Abraham A.
Brodie, William
Carmalt, William H.
Cohn, Alfred E.
Coit, Henry L.
Connor, Leartus
Cooke, Robert A.
Dana, Charles L.
Dana, Israel T.
Davis, Michael M.
Delafield, Edward
Delafield, Francis
Drew, Charles R.
Du Bois, Eugene F.
Emerson, Haven
Ewing, James
Ford, Lewis D.
Francis, John W.
Greenberg, Morris
Gruening, Emil
Halsted, William S.
Harris, Elisha
Herter, Christian
Hess, Alfred F.
Hitchcock, Homer O.
Holt, Erastus E.
Holt, L. Emmett
Hunt, Ezra M.
Huntington, George
Janeway, Edward G.
Jayne, Walter A.
Jelliffe, Smith Ely
Kendall, Edward C.
Koplik, Henry
Lazear, Jesse W.
Lefferts, George M.
Levy, Julius
Libman, Emanuel
Loomis, Alfred L.
McBurney, Charles
McCaw, Walter D.
McCormack, Arthur T.
McCready, Benjamin W.
McGraw, Theodore A.
Marshall, Hyrum L.
Martland, Harrison S.
Milroy, William F.
Mott, Valentine
Muller, Hermann J.

North, Charles E.
O'Dwyer, Joseph
Park, William H.
Richards, Alfred N.
Richards, Dickinson W.
Rousselot, Louis M.
Rubin, Isidore C.
Rubinow, Isaac M.
Russell, Frederick
Sayre, Lewis A.
Seguin, Edward C.
Shrady, George F.
Smith, Andrew H.
Smith, Clarence A.
Smith, Job L.
Smith, Stephen
Snow, Edwin M.
Sternberg, George M.
Streeter, George L.
Sullivan, John J.
Summers, John E., Jr.
Thompson, William G.
Timme, Walter
Trudeau, Edward L.
Van Ingen, Philip
Vinsonhaler, Frank
Welch, William H.
Whipple, Allen O.
Zinsser, Hans

COLUMBIAN COLLEGE MEDICAL DEPARTMENT: See GEORGE WASHINGTON UNIVERSITY

COOPER MEDICAL COLLEGE (Now STANFORD UNIVERSITY SCHOOL OF MEDICINE)
(Includes Medical College of the Pacific)

Blumer, George
Handy, John C.
Scott, James R.
Smith, Andrew C.
Snow, William F.
Wilbur, Ray L.

CORNELL UNIVERSITY

Barringer, Emily D.
Giles, Roscoe C.
Howland, John
Larsen, Nils P.
Marriott, W. McKim
Menninger, William C.
Neal, Josephine B.

Salmon, Daniel E.
Smith, Philip E.
Smith, Warren G.
Trask, James D.
Weiss, Soma

DARTMOUTH MEDICAL SCHOOL

Bell, Luther V.
Carpenter, Walter
Crosby, Alpheus B.
Crosby, Dixi
Gallup, Joseph A.
Mussey, Reuben D.
Pettigrew, George A.
Shattuck, George C.
Smith, Lyndon A.
Spafford, Frederick A.
Stickney, Victor H.
Towne, Solon R.
Twitchell, Amos

DETROIT COLLEGE OF MEDICINE (Now WAYNE STATE UNIVERSITY COLLEGE OF MEDICINE)

Biddle, Andrew P.
Koch, William F.
Laurey, James R.
McGillycuddy, Valentine T.

FAIRFIELD MEDICAL SCHOOL (COLLEGE OF PHYSICIANS AND SURGEONS OF THE WESTERN DISTRICT OF NEW YORK)

Davis, Nathan S.
Gorrie, John
Judd, Gerrit P.
Palmer, Alonzo B.
Whitman, Marcus
Wolcott, Erastus B.

FRANCE

Abel, John J.
Carrel, Alexis
Faget, Jean C.
Jacobi, Mary C. P.
Jones, John
Loeb, Jacques
Prevost, Francois
Sachs, Bernard
Tait, F. Dudley

GENEVA MEDICAL COLLEGE (NY): See SYRACUSE UNIVERSITY COLLEGE OF MEDICINE

GEORGETOWN UNIVERSITY

Ashford, Bailey K.
Eastman, Joseph
Garrison, Fielding
Kinyoun, Joseph J.
Kober, George M.
Lamb, Daniel S.
Magruder, George L.
Parran, Thomas
Porter, Henry R.
Yount, Clarence E.

GEORGE WASHINGTON UNIVERSITY (Includes Columbian College Medical Department and National Medical College)

Dana, Charles L.
Harper, Cornelius A.
McGee, Anita N.
Scott, James R.

MEDICAL COLLEGE OF GEORGIA (Includes University of Georgia Medical Department)

Campbell, Henry F.
Foster, Eugene
Kelly, George L.
Westmoreland, John G.

GERMANY

Abrams, Albert
Barton, Benjamin
Benedict, Francis G.
Chandler, Charles F.
Dunglison, Robley
Einhorn, Max
Fordyce, John A.
Glasser, Otto
Harrison, Ross G.
Heermann, Lewis
Hering, Constantine
Hillebrand, Wilhelm
Horney, Karen
Jacobi, Abraham
Klebs, Theodore A.
Knapp, (J.) Hermann
Kremers, Edward
Lane, Levi C.
Lusk, Graham

Meltzer, Samuel J.
Meyer, Willy
Munsterberg, Hugo
Nuttall, George H. F.
Papanicolaou, George N.
Senn, Nicholas
Stiles, Charles W.
Voegtlin, Carl

HARVARD UNIVERSITY

Albright, Fuller
Appleton, Moses
Babcock, James W.
Beecher, Henry K.
Bigelow, Henry J.
Blake, Francis G.
Bowditch, Henry I.
Bowditch, Henry P.
Bradford, Edward H.
Brown, Percy
Brown, William E.
Burgess, Alexander
Cabot, Hugh
Cabot, Richard C.
Callister, Alfred C.
Cannon, Walter B.
Channing, Walter
Cheever, David W.
Churchill, Edward D.
Codman, Ernest A.
Coley, William B.
Coller, Frederick
Cushing, Harvey W.
Cutler, Elliott C.
Dalton, John Call
Dameshek, William
Dana, Israel T.
Donnell, Clyde H.
Farber, Sidney
Favill, John
Finney, John M. T.
Fisher, John Dix
Fitz, Reginald H.
Flint, Austin
Forbes, Alexander
Fulton, John F.
Gamble, James L.
Garland, Joseph
Haight, Cameron
Hall, G. Stanley
Hall, Josiah N.
Henderson, Lawrence J.
Hill, Frederick T.

Hinton, William A.
Hitchcock, Edward
Holmes, Oliver W.
Hooker, Worthington
Howe, Samuel G.
Hume, Edgar E.
Jackson, Charles T.
Jackson, James
Jackson, James, Jr.
Jackson, John B. S.
Jarvis, Edward
Ladd, William E.
Lahey, Frank H.
Leavitt, Erasmus
Lennox, William G.
Lilienthal, Howard
Loeb, Robert F.
Lovelace, William R., II
Mallory, Frank B.
May, Frederick
Minot, Charles S.
Minot, George R.
Mumford, James G.
Paine, Martyn
Parker, Willard
Parsons, Usher
Pincus, Gregory G.
Prince, Morton
Putman, Charles P.
Putnam, James J.
Rappleye, Willard C.
Richards, Paul S.
Richardson, Maurice H.
Rotch, Thomas M.
Shaffer, Philip A.
Shattuck, George C., Jr.
Smillie, Wilson G.
Smith, Nathan
Southard, Elmer E.
Spalding, James A.
Spalding, Lyman
Storer, David H.
Storer, Horatio R.
Stubbs, Frederick D.
Thayer, William S.
Tildon, Toussaint T.
Viko, Louis E.
Ware, John
Warren, J. Collins
Wesselhoeft, Conrad
Wheeler, John B.
White, James C.
White, Paul D.

Whitman, Royal
Williams, Francis H.
Williams, Henry W.
Wolbach, Simeon B.
Wright, Louis T.
Wyman, Jeffries
Wyman, Morrill

HOLLAND: See NETHERLANDS

HOWARD UNIVERSITY COLLEGE OF MEDICINE

Clement, Kenneth W.
Dibble, Eugene H.
Garvin, Charles H.
Gathings, Joseph G.
Greene, Clarence S.
McClennan, Alonzo C.
McNeill, William C.
Morman, William D.
Murray, Peter M.
Parsons, Mary A.
Payne, Howard M.
Ross, Julian W.
Shadd, Furman J.
Thompson, Solomon H.
Warfeld, William A.

UNIVERSITY OF ILLINOIS (Includes College of Physicians and Surgeons of Chicago)

Donahoe, William E.
Eagleson, James B.
Evans, William A., Jr.
Frederick, Rivers
Frisbie, Evelyn F.
Hare, Lyle
Hektoen, Ludvig
Northcross, David C.
Roberts, Carl G.
Sleyster, Rock
Stanley, Wendell M.
Turner, Delos A.
West, Harold D.

INDIANA UNIVERSITY SCHOOL OF MEDICINE (Includes Medical College of Indiana)

Hurty, John N.
Maloney, Arnold H.
Mann, Frank C.
Rovenstine, Emery A.

Wiley, Harvey W.
Wishard, William N.

STATE UNIVERSITY OF IOWA

Bierring, Walter L.
Dean, Lee W.
Long, Francis A.
Shope, Richard E.
Wilkerson, Vernon A.

JEFFERSON MEDICAL COLLEGE OF PHILADELPHIA

Atlee, Washington
Battey, Robert
Beebe, James
Bobbs, John S.
Brainard, Daniel
Brinton, John H.
Calhoun, Abner W.
Coffman, Victor H.
Cole, Richard B.
Da Costa, Jacob M.
Davidson, Henry A.
Flick, Lawrence F.
Flint, Austin, Jr.
Gibbon, John H., Jr.
Gross, Samuel D.
Gross, Samuel W.
Hartman, Samuel B.
Hill, Luther L.
Hooper, Philo O.
Howard, William T.
Jackson, Algernon
Jackson, Chevalier
Kane, John K.
Keen, William W., Jr.
Kerr, John G.
Lane, Levi C.
Lenow, James H.
Letterman, Jonathan
Minton, Henry M.
Mitchell, S. Weir
Pattison, Granville S.
Porter, Joseph Y.
Reeve, James T.
Robertson, William S.
Rodman, William L.
Rogers, William E.
Sims, J. Marion
Solis-Cohen, Solomon
Spivak, Charles D.
Squibb, Edward R.
Toner, Joseph M.

Warren, Edward
White, James P.
Whitehead, Peter F.

JOHNS HOPKINS UNIVERSITY

Auer, John
Bardeen, Charles R.
Bayne-Jones, Stanhope
Beck, Claude S.
Blakemore, Arthur H.
Blalock, Alfred
Brown, Lawrason
Chesney, Alan M.
Cole, Rufus
Craig, Winchell
Crowe, Samuel J.
Dandy, Walter E.
Davis, John S.
Davison, Wilburt C.
Dick, Gladys
Dochez, Alphonse
Donaldson, Henry H.
Erlanger, Joseph
Flocks, Rubin H.
Foley, Frederick
Gasser, Herbert S.
Gay, Frederick
Goodpasture, Ernest W.
Harrison, Ross G.
Hemmeter, John C.
Hirschfelder, Arthur D.
Howell, William H.
Hume, Edgar E.
Hunt, Reid
Keefer, Chester S.
Kline, Benjamin S.
Knox, James H. M., Jr.
Longcope, Warfield T.
MacCallum, William G.
McQuarrie, Irvine
Major, Ralph H.
Marine, David
Marshall, E. K., Jr.
Maxcy, Kenneth F.
Mendenhall, Dorothy R.
Merritt, John W.
Morgan, Thomas H.
Murphy, James B.
Nixon, Pat I.
Opie, Eugene L.
Orr, Thomas G.
Paul, John R.
Pearce, Louise

Perkins, Roger G.
Reid, Mont R.
Rivers, Thomas M.
Robinson, G. Canby
Rous, Peyton
Sabin, Florence R.
Schloss, Oscar M.
Sedgwick, William T.
Sellards, Andrew W.
Sewall, Henry
Shore, Clarence A.
Simpson, John
Smith, Homer W.
Smith, Margaret G.
Tillett, William S.
Wahl, Harry R.
Weed, Lewis H.
Whipple, George H.
Winternitz, Milton C.
Wood, William B., Jr.

UNIVERSITY OF KANSAS SCHOOL OF MEDICINE (Includes Kansas City [Mo.] Medical College)

Bradford, Claudius B.
Clendening, Logan
Clinton, Fred S.
Howard, William F.
Menninger, Charles F.
Scammon, Richard E.

KENTUCKY SCHOOL OF MEDICINE (Includes Transylvania University Medical Department)

Baldwin, William O.
Bodine, James M.
Briggs, William T.
Coffey, Robert C.
Farrar, Bernard G.
Fenner, Erasmus D.
Hall, William W.
Horine, Emmet F.
McDowell, Joseph N.
Miller, Henry, Jr.
Monette, John W.
Peter, Robert
Sutton, William L.
Toland, Hugh H.

LEONARD MEDICAL SCHOOL (SHAW UNIVERSITY MEDICAL DEPARTMENT) (N.C.)

Hargrave, Frank S.
Kenney, John A.

Moore, Aaron M.
Turner, John P.

LONG ISLAND COLLEGE HOSPITAL (Now STATE UNIVERSITY OF NEW YORK, DOWNSTATE MEDICAL CENTER COLLEGE OF MEDICINE)

Dickinson, Robert L.
Howe, Lucien
Johnson, Peter A.
Kempster, Walter
Kolle, Frederick S.
Manning, Isaac H.
Skene, Alexander J. C.
Smith, Alonzo de G.
White, William A.

UNIVERSITY OF LOUISIANA MEDICAL DEPARTMENT: See TULANE UNIVERSITY SCHOOL OF MEDICINE

UNIVERSITY OF LOUISVILLE SCHOOL OF MEDICINE (Includes Louisville Medical Institute and Louisville Medical College)

Abell, Irvin
Bozeman, Nathan
Flexner, Simon
Hughes, Henry A.
Long, Leroy
Marshall, Hubert
Mathews, Joseph M.
Moorman, Lewis J.
Newton, Robert S.
Williams, Elkanah
Wooten, Thomas D.

MEDICAL SCHOOL OF MAINE: See BOWDOIN MEDICAL SCHOOL

UNIVERSITY OF MARYLAND SCHOOL OF MEDICINE

Bartholow, Roberts
Cabell, James
Carroll, James
Carter, Henry R.
Cordell, Eugene F.
Councilman, William T.
Dugas, Louis A.
Fussell, Bartholomew
Godman, John D.
Hemmeter, John C.
Hughes, John C.

Hulse, Isaac
Jarvis, William C.
Palmer, Thomas M.
Steuart, Richard S.
Sutton, William L.
Werner, Walter I.
Williams, John W.
Yandell, Lunsford P.

MEHARRY MEDICAL COLLEGE (Tenn.)

Anderson, John W.
Boyd, Robert F.
Burton, De Witt
Butler, Henry R.
Covington, Benjamin J.
Davis, Abraham I.
Francis, Grossi H.
Hale, John H.
Harris, William H.
Lambright, Middleton
Lattimore, John A.
Lynk, Miles V.
Majors, Monroe A.
Moten, Pierce S.
Perry, John E.
Quinland, William S.
Robinson, Paul T.
Roman, Charles V.
Smith, Relliford S.
Taylor, Eugene T.
Thomas, William M.
Whittico, James M.

UNIVERSITY OF MICHIGAN

Andrews, Edmund
Becker, Harry F.
Bronk, Detlev W.
Carson, Simeon L.
Cooley, Thomas B.
Copeland, Royal S.
Cowie, David M.
De Kruif, Paul H.
De Witt, Lydia M.
Fitzbutler, (W.) Henry
Gifford, Harold
Hamilton, Alice
Hood, William H.
Hurd, Henry M.
Huson, Florence
Hutchinson, Woods
Kiefer, Guy L.
Koch, William
Long, Perrin H.

Lyster, Henry F. L.
McLean, Mary H.
Mall, Franklin P.
Mayo, William J.
Millspaugh, Joseph G.
Mosher, Eliza M.
Novy, Frederick G.
Orr, Hiram W.
Owens-Adair, Bethenia A.
Pearl, Raymond
Pilcher, Lewis S.
Quain, Fannie A.
Tibbals, Frank B.
Van Hoosen, Bertha
Van Slyke, Donald D.
Vaughan, Victor C.
Walker, Delos
Weeks, John E.
Wiggers, Carl J.
Wilson, Frank N.

MIDDLEBURY COLLEGE (Vt.): See CASTLETON MEDICAL COLLEGE

UNIVERSITY OF MINNESOTA (Includes St. Paul Medical College)

Barron, Moses
Burch, Frank E.
Downey, Hal
Foley, Frederick
Gillette, Arthur J.
Larson, Leonard W.
Quain, Eric P.
Ramsey, Walter R.
Ramstad, Niles O.
Wilkerson, Vernon A.
Wilson, Louis B.

MISSOURI MEDICAL COLLEGE: See WASHINGTON UNIVERSITY SCHOOL OF MEDICINE

UNIVERSITY OF NASHVILLE MEDICAL DEPARTMENT

Boswell, Henry
Cochran, Jerome
Fortner, Benjamin F.
Hubbard, George W.
Shoulders, Harrison H.

**NATIONAL MEDICAL COLLEGE: See
GEORGE WASHINGTON UNIVERSITY**

NETHERLANDS (HOLLAND)

Bull, William
Crawford, John
Douglass, William
Waterhouse, Benjamin

**NEW YORK UNIVERSITY SCHOOL OF
MEDICINE (Includes Medical College of
the City of New York, University of the
City of New York, and Bellevue Hospital
Medical College)**

Baker, Henry B.
Baker, S. Josephine
Bentley, Edwin
Biggs, Hermann M.
Bosworth, Franke H.
Bryce, Peter
Caldwell, Eugene W.
Cary, Edward H.
Chapin, Charles V.
Coakley, Cornelius G.
Dennis, Frederic S.
Eastman, Joseph
Fowler, George R.
Freeman, John W.
Gardiner, Charles F.
Goldberger, Joseph
Goldwater, Sigismund S.
Gorgas, William C.
Hammond, William A.
Heg, Elmer E.
Hill, Luther L.
Hocker, William A.
Holton, Henry D.
Howe, Lucien
Howland, John
Jackson, James M., Jr.
Jenks, Edward W.
Kellogg, John H.
Keyes, Edward L.
Kinyoun, Joseph J.
Lothrop, Charles H.
McCaw, James B.
McKay, Read J.
Maghee, Thomas G.
Maury, Richard B.
Morse, John F.
Patrick, Hugh T.

Peck, Washington F.
Post, George E.
Purple, Samuel S.
Pusey, William A.
Reed, Walter
Richards, George G.
Richards, Ralph T.
Rubinow, Isaac M.
Scott, Arthur C.
Seguin, Edouard
Spitzka, Edward C.
Steele, Henry K.
Swift, Homer F.
Tait, F. Dudley
Vaughan, George T.
Watson, Beriah A.
Weatherly, Job S.
Weedon, Leslie W.
Witthaus, Rudolph A.

**NORTHWESTERN UNIVERSITY
(Includes Chicago Medical College)**

Abt, Isaac A.
Alcock, Nathaniel
Aldrich, Charles A.
Andrews, Edward W.
Billings, Frank
Black, Greene V.
Blesh, Abraham L.
Bousfield, Midian O.
Cheatham, Anderson
Cole, Fern M.
Curtis, Austin M.
Dailey, Ulysses G.
De Lee, Joseph B.
Findley, Palmer
Fordyce, John A.
French, Harley E.
Hertzler, Arthur E.
Jermain, Louis F.
Johnson, Arthur H.
Lawless, Theodore K.
Martin, Franklin H.
Mayo, Charles H.
Montezuma, Carlos
Park, Roswell
Pittenger, Fred A.
Plummer, Henry S.
Ricketts, Howard T.
Senn, Nicholas
Thompson, Mary H.
Williams, Daniel H.
Woodworth, John M.

MEDICAL COLLEGE OF OHIO: See UNIVERSITY OF CINCINNATI COLLEGE OF MEDICINE

UNIVERSITY OF OREGON MEDICAL SCHOOL

Baird, David W. E.
Bilderback, Joseph B.
Lovejoy, Esther P.
Maddock, William O.
Matson, Ralph C.
Matson, Ray W.
Osgood, Edwin E.

MEDICAL COLLEGE OF THE PACIFIC: See COOPER MEDICAL COLLEGE

UNIVERSITY OF PENNSYLVANIA (Includes College of Philadelphia Department of Medicine)

Agnew, David H.
Archer, John
Arnold, Richard D.
Atlee, John L.
Bache, Franklin
Barber, Amos
Barnes, William H.
Barton, William P. C.
Bayless, George W.
Benjamin, Dowling
Bigelow, Jacob
Black, John J.
Blaney, James Van Z.
Bloodgood, Joseph C.
Busey, Samuel C.
Bush, Lewis P.
Caldwell, Charles
Carter, William S.
Channing, Walter
Chapman, Nathaniel
Clarke, Edward H.
Coca, Arthur F.
Cooke, John E.
Coxe, John R.
Daniel, Richard P.
Darlington, William
de Schweinitz, George E.
Deaver, John B.
Dewees, William P.
Dibrell, James A.
Dibrell, James A., Jr.
Dickson, Samuel H.

Dock, George
Dorsey, John S.
Drake, Daniel
Dudley, Benjamin W.
Duhring, Louis A.
Earle, Pliny
Eberle, John
Edsall, David Linn
Ellett, Edward C.
Elmer, Jonathan
Eve, Paul F.
Fearn, Thomas
Gage, E. Lyle
Gant, Harris A.
Garretson, James E.
Gerhard, William W.
Gibbons, Henry
Gray, John P.
Griffin, John S.
Griscom, John H.
Harrison, John P.
Hays, Isaac
Haywood, Edmund B.
Hinson, Eugene T.
Hodge, Hugh L.
Horner, William E.
Hosack, David
Jackson, Edward
Jackson, Samuel
Jones, Joseph
Kelly, Howard A.
Ketchum, George A.
Kirkbride, Thomas S.
Leidy, Joseph
Leonard, Charles L.
Lindsley, John B.
Long, Crawford W.
McClellan, George
McKee, William H.
McMaster, Philip D.
Meigs, Arthur V.
Meigs, Charles D.
Meigs, John F.
Middleton, William S.
Miller, Thomas
Mills, Charles K.
Mitchell, John K.
Moore, Edward M.
Morton, Samuel G.
Mossell, Nathan F.
Mussey, Reuben D.
Nott, Josiah C.
Oliver, Daniel

Orton, Samuel T.
Otto, John C.
Packard, Francis R.
Pancoast, Joseph
Parrish, Isaac
Parrish, Joseph
Parvin, Theophilus
Pennock, Caspar W.
Pepper, William
Pittman, Newsome J.
Pope, Charles A.
Potter, Nathaniel
Price, Joseph
Ramsay, David
Randall, Edward
Rauch, John H.
Richardson, Rodney H.
Robertson, Felix
Rosenau, Milton J.
Schamberg, Jay F.
Seaman, Valentine
Shakespeare, Edward O.
Shattuck, George C.
Shryock, Richard H.
Silliman, Benjamin
Smith, Albert H.
Smith, Thomas J.
Solis-Cohen, Jacob D.
Stillé, Alfred
Stokes, Joseph, Jr.
Tilton, James
Tracy, Martha
Tyson, James
Vedder, Edward B.
Veeder, Bordon S.
Vincent, Ubert C.
Walsh, James J.
Wende, Ernest
Whitehead, William R.
Wickes, Stephen
Williams, William C.
Wistar, Caspar
Witherspoon, John A.
Wood, George B.
Wood, Horatio C.
Woodward, Joseph J.

RUSH MEDICAL COLLEGE: See UNI-VERSITY OF CHICAGO

ST. LOUIS MEDICAL COLLEGE: See WASHINGTON UNIVERSITY

SHAW UNIVERSITY MEDICAL DEPARTMENT: See LEONARD MEDICAL SCHOOL

MEDICAL COLLEGE OF SOUTH CAROLINA (Includes Medical College of the State of South Carolina)

Chisolm, Julian J.
Gary, Thomas P.
Geddings, Eli
Jervey, James W.
Moore, Samuel P.
Porcher, Francis P.
Steele, William L.
Thomas, T. Gaillard
Wall, John P.

STANFORD UNIVERSITY: See COOPER MEDICAL COLLEGE

STATE UNIVERSITY OF NEW YORK, DOWNSTATE MEDICAL CENTER COLLEGE OF MEDICINE: See LONG ISLAND COLLEGE HOSPITAL

STATE UNIVERSITY OF NEW YORK, UPSTATE MEDICAL CENTER COLLEGE OF MEDICINE: See SYRACUSE UNIVERSITY COLLEGE OF MEDICINE

SWITZERLAND

Dimock, Susan
Loeb, Leo
Meyer, Adolf
Meyer, Karl F.
Schwyzer, Arnold
Sigerist, Henry E.

SYRACUSE UNIVERSITY COLLEGE OF MEDICINE (Includes Geneva Medical College)

Baldwin, Abel S.
Blackwell, Elizabeth
Gunn, Moses
Weiskotten, Herman G.

TRANSYLVANIA UNIVERSITY MEDICAL DEPARTMENT: See KENTUCKY SCHOOL OF MEDICINE

TULANE UNIVERSITY SCHOOL OF MEDICINE (Includes University of Louisiana Medical Department)

Anderson, William H. (b. 1886)
Chaillé, Stanford
Cox, George W., Jr.
Dyer, Isadore
Evans, William A., Jr.
Haralson, Hugh H.
Hargis, Robert B.
Hatcher, Robert A.
Hunter, John F.
Matas, Rudolph
Mitchell, Robert W.
Phares, David L.
Souchon, Edmund
Young, John W.

UNIVERSITY OF VERMONT COLLEGE OF MEDICINE

Allen, Lyman
Beecher, Clarence H.
Buxton, Lauren H.
Caverly, Charles S.
Denison, Charles
Dodd, Walter J.
Henry, Morris H.
Osborne, John E.
Taylor, Charles F.
Tinkham, Henry C.

MEDICAL COLLEGE OF VIRGINIA

Baruch, Simon
McCaw, Walter D.
McGuire, Hunter H.
Vest, Walter

UNIVERSITY OF VIRGINIA

Anderson, William H. (b. 1820)
Campbell, Willis C.
Council, Walter W.
Frost, Wade H.
Harris, Seale
Leathers, Waller
Lumsden, Leslie L.
Mason, James T.
Maury, Richard B.
Reed, Walter

Timberlake, Gideon
Vaughan, George T.
Warrren, Edward
Whitehead, William M.
Young, Hugh H.

WASHINGTON UNIVERSITY (Includes Missouri Medical College and St. Louis Medical College)

Blair, Vilray P.
Carter, C. Dana
Clark, Sam L.
Cooper, Elias S.
Gibson, Samuel C.
Hartmann, Alexis F.
Hodgen, John T.
Lam, Frederick K.
Lovelace, William R.
Mayo, William W.
Meriwether, Clinton P.
Moore, Carl V.
Ohage, Justus
Padgett, Earl C.
Porter, William T.
Sutherland, Earl W., Jr.
Taussig, Frederick J.
Watkins, William W.
Wylder, Meldrum K.

WAYNE STATE UNIVERSITY COLLEGE OF MEDICINE: See DETROIT COLLEGE OF MEDICINE

WESTERN RESERVE UNIVERSITY SCHOOL OF MEDICINE (Includes Cleveland Medical College and University of Wooster Medical Department)

Blackwell, Emily
Crile, George W.
Donaldson, Mary E.
Elwell, John J.
Freedlander, Samuel O.
Goodfellow, George E.
Greene, Cordelia
Johnson, John B.
Pride, Maynard P.
Purvis, Charles B.
Sollmann, Torald H.
Toomey, John A.
Zakrzewska, Marie E.

UNIVERSITY OF WISCONSIN

Bishop, George H.
Elvehjem, Conrad A.

Maloney, Arnold H.
Senn, Nicholas
Steenbock, Harry
Tatum, Edward L.

WOMAN'S MEDICAL COLLEGE OF PENNSYLVANIA

Broomall, Anna E.
Brown, Charlotte
Cleveland, Emeline H.
Evans, Matilda A.
Fulton, Mary H.
Jacobi, Mary P.
Longshore, Hannah E. M.
Macfarlane, Catharine
Marshall, Clara
Mead, Kate C. H.
Minoka-Hill, Lillie R.
Picotte, Susan La F.
Potter, Ellen C.
Preston, Ann
Rutherford, Frances A.
Shipp, Ellis R.
South, Lillian H.
Swain, Clara
Thomas, Mary F. M.
Tracy, Martha
Wolcott, Laura J. R.
Yarros, Rachelle S.

UNIVERSITY OF WOOSTER MEDICAL DEPARTMENT: See WESTERN RESERVE UNIVERSITY SCHOOL OF MEDICINE

YALE UNIVERSITY

Alcott, William A.
Atwater, Wilbur O.
Benedict, Stanley R.
Chittenden, Russell H.
Davis, Henry G.
Francis, Thomas, Jr.
Gamble, Henry F.
Gardner, Leroy U.
Gesell, Arnold L.
Gies, William J.
Henderson, Yandell
Knox, James H. M., Jr.
McCollum, Elmer V.
Mendel, Lafayette B.
Miller, William S.
Osborne, Thomas B.
Parker, Peter
Phelps, Edward E.
Prudden, T. M.
Smith, Ashbel
Smith, Nathan R.

Listing of Females

Abbott, Maude	1869	Kelley, Florence	1859
Baker, S. Josephine	1873	Kenny, Elizabeth	1886
Barringer, Emily D.	1876	Lathrop, Julia C.	1858
Barton, Clara	1821	Livermore, Mary A.	1821
Beard, Mary	1876	Longshore, Hannah E.	1819
Blackwell, Elizabeth	1821	Lovejoy, Esther P.	1870
Blackwell, Emily	1826	Lozier, Clemence S.	1813
Broomall, Anna E.	1847	Macfarlane, Catharine	1877
Brown, Charlotte	1846	McGee, Anita N.	1864
Campbell, Elizabeth	1862	McKinney-Steward, Susan M. S.	1847
Cannon, Ida M.	1877	McLean, Mary H.	1861
Cleveland, Emeline H.	1829	Marshall, Clara	1847
Cori, Gerty	1896	Mead, Kate C. H.	1867
De Witt, Lydia M.	1859	Mendenhall, Dorothy R.	1874
Delano, Jane A.	1862	Mergler, Marie J.	1851
Dick, Gladys	1881	Merrick, Myra K.	1825
Dimock, Susan	1847	Minoka-Hill, Lillie R.	1876
Dix, Dorothea	1802	Moore, Phoebia G.	1872
Dock, Lavinia L.	1858	Mosher, Eliza M.	1846
Dolley, Sarah R. A.	1829	Neal, Josephine B.	1880
Donaldson, Mary E.	1851	Nichols, Mary S. N. G.	1810
Eddy, Mary Baker	1821	Nutting, Mary A.	1858
Evans, Matilda A.	1872	Owens-Adair, Bethenia A.	1840
Frisbie, Evelyn F.	1873	Parsons, Mary A.	1850
Fulton, Mary H.	1854	Pearce, Louise	1885
Goldmark, Josephine	1877	Picotte, Susan La F.	1865
Graham, Helen T.	1890	Pinkham, Lydia E.	1819
Greene, Cordelia	1831	Potter, Ellen C.	1871
Hamilton, Alice	1869	Preston, Ann	1813
Heath, Lillian	1865	Quain, Fannie A.	1874
Holt, Winifred	1870	Remond, Sarah P.	1826
Horney, Karen	1885	Richards, Linda	1841
Hunt, Harriot K.	1805	Ripley, Martha G.	1843
Huson, Florence	1857	Robb, Isabel A. H.	1860
Jacobi, Mary P.	1842	Rutherford, Frances A.	1842
Jean, Sally L.	1878	Sabin, Florence R.	1871

Sanger, Margaret H.	1879	Tracy, Martha	1876
Schuyler, Louise L.	1837	Tunnicliff, Ruth M.	1876
Shipp, Ellis R.	1847	Van Hoosen, Bertha	1863
Smith, Margaret G.	1896	Wald, Lillian D.	1867
South, Lillian H.	1879	Walker, Mary E.	1832
Stastny, Olga F.	1878	White, Ellen G. H.	1827
Stevenson, Sarah A. H.	1841	Wolcott, Laura J. R.	1826
Swain, Clara	1834	Wollstein, Martha	1868
Thomas, Mary F. M.	1816	Yarros, Rachelle S.	1869
Thompson, Mary H.	1829	Zakrzewska, Marie E.	1829
Thoms, Adah B. S.	1863		

Index

705, 707, 712, 717-18, 721, 726, 728, 737, 739, 748, 755, 762, 776-77, 782, 787, 799, 815, 819-20, 823, 830; anti-trust case of, 112; black delegates in, 548; black physicians in Directory of, 292; Bureau of Investigation, 165; Council on Health and Public Instruction, 242; Council on Medical Education, 61, 696, 746, 787, 805, 815; reorganization of, 475

American Medical Association, Journal of the, 187, 248, 322, 663, 683, 773

American Medical College (Philadelphia), 645

American Medical College Association, 155. *See also* Medical Colleges, Association of American

American Medical Digest, 685

American Medical Directory, 683

American Medical Editors' Association, 155

American Medical Education Society, 307

American Medical Journal, 304

American Medical Library and Intelligencer, 585

American Medical Missionary College of Chicago, 408

American Medical Recorder, 225, 585

American Medical Review, 697

American Medical Times, 680-81, 699-700

American Medical Women's Association, 478, 510, 759

American Medico-Legal Association, 776

American Medico-Psychological Association, 104, 380, 707

American Men of Science, women scientists in, 301

American Museum of Natural History, 531, 692

American Neurological Association, 36, 178, 322, 524, 562, 566, 584, 610, 614, 660, 671, 710

American Nurses Association, 193, 741

American Nursing Association, 640

American Opthalmological and Otological Association, 158

American Ophthalmological Society, 120, 191, 197, 229, 310, 357, 385, 786, 807-8

American Orthopedic Association, 90, 117, 565, 716, 801

American Orthopsychiatric Association, 338

American Otological Society, 188, 310, 357, 571

American Pediatric Society, 7, 11, 71, 108, 157, 274, 359, 389, 421, 424, 694, 721, 760, 764, 818

American Pharmaceutical Association, 451, 712

American Pharmacological Association, 611

American Philosophical Society, 28, 41, 81, 407, 451, 510-11, 536, 657, 681, 683, 814, 820

American Physicians and Surgeons, Congress of, 250

American Physiological Society, 85, 119, 135, 302, 370, 494, 500

American Practitioner, 583

American Proctological Society, 504

American Psychiatric Association, 94, 515, 566, 798. *See also* Insane, Association of Medical Superintendents of American Institutions for the

American Psychiatric Association, Journal of the, 184

American Psychoanalytical Association, 519

American Pyschoanalytic Association, 798

American Psychological Association, 317

American Psychopathological Association, 337, 798

American Public Health Association, 29, 67, 111, 147, 231, 261, 291, 327, 329, 377, 393, 422, 439, 474, 578, 626, 649, 656-60, 669, 700, 702-3, 717, 748, 757, 812, 822, 825

American Red Cross. *See* Red Cross

American Revolution. *See* Revolutionary War

American Rheumatism Association, 341

American Roentgen Ray Society, 100

American Sanatorium Association, 82, 99

American School of Osteopathy (Kirksville, Missouri), 720

American Social Hygiene Association, 38, 804, 832

American Social Science Association, 29

American Statistical Association, 677

American Surgeon, 566

American Surgical Association, 61, 93, 120, 132, 136, 153, 173, 185, 196, 248, 287, 312, 374, 407, 480-81, 502, 508, 535, 566, 588, 637, 779-80, 794

American Surgical Society, 262, 309

American Therapeutic Society, 319, 526, 632

American Trudeau Society, 82, 536

American University (Washington, District of Columbia), 692

American University of Beirut (Lebanon), 136, 603, 794-95

American Urological Association, 5, 814, 833

American Urology Association, 255

American Vegetarian Society, 677
American Veterinary Medical Association, 660
American Woman's War Hospital, 153
American Women's Hospital (France), 713
American Women's Hospitals, 461
Amherst College, 215, 236, 253, 302, 352, 544, 579, 753, 783, 804
Amidon, E. L., 53
Amory, Robert, 138
Amoss, Harold, 818
Amputation, American method of, 183
Anaerobic bacteria, 711; cultivation of, 557
Anatomical Record, 34, 355, 492
Anatomists, American Association of, 12, 527, 625, 659, 698, 724
Anatomists, Association of American, 441, 492
Anatomy, 890
Anatomy, Hamann Museum of Comparative, 747
Anatomy, Philadelphia School of, 8, 278, 295, 575
Anatomy, American Journal of, 36, 137, 492
Anatomy Act (New York), 572
Anatomy and Surgery, Annals of, 262, 596
Ancker Hospital (St. Paul), 257, 293, 623
Ancon Hospital (Canal Zone), 474, 795
Anderson, Donald G., 406
Anderson, Dr. (Canada), 561
Anderson, J. F., 296
Anderson, John F., 649
Anderson, John Wesley, *13-14*
Anderson, William Henry, *14-15*
Anderson Hospital for Cancer Research (Texas), 61
Andersonian Institution (Glasgow), 584
Anderson's Clinic (Mississippi), 14
Anderson's College (Glasgow), 731
Andrew Clinical Society (Tuskegee, Alabama), 176, 199, 412
Andrew Memorial Hospital (Tuskegee, Alabama), 199, 273, 411
Andrews, Edmund, *15-16*
Andrews, Edward Wyllys, *15-16*
Anemia: cause of tropical, 20; hookworm as a cause of, 441; pernicious, 528; treatment of, 795
Anesthesia, 512, 759; cocaine as local, 424; conduction, 85; discovery of, 384, 455, 540, 790; first public demonstration of, 64; introduction of to West Virginia, 267; laboratory for research in, 54; local, 347; opera-

tions using, 88; spinal, 727; in thoracic surgery, 22; use of in childbirth, 129
Anesthesia, American Society of Regional, 653
Anesthesiology, 890
Anesthesiology, American Board of, 653
Anthon, George Christian, 56
Anthony, William A., 89
Antibiotics, 770
Antioch College, 317, 372, 398
Antirabies station, first, 558
Antiseptic surgery, 286, 310
Antiseptic techniques, 779; introduction of, 15, 241
Antivivisection, 85, 133
Antony, Milton, *16-17*, 455
Apothecaries, Society of, 219, 705
Appendicitis, 469; diagnosis and treatment of, 250; operation for, 548, 579; surgery for, 189
Appendix, diagnosis of perforated, 43
Appleton, Moses, *17*
Appleton, Nathaniel W., 361
Archer, John, *17-18*
Archiv for Soziale Gesetzgeburg, 407
Archiv für Verdauungs-Krankheiten (Berlin), 227
Argentina, 857
Arizona, 859, 873
Arizona, University of, 323
Arizona Board of Medical Examiners, 373
Arizona Medical Society, 373
Arizona State University, 532
Arizona Territorial Asylum, 373
Arkansas, 859, 873; medical education in, 443; medical licensing in, 199-200; medical societies in, 490
Arkansas, State Medical Society of, 362, 490
Arkansas, University of, 60, 279, 443, 516, 695, 766
Arkansas Association for the Relief and Control of Tuberculosis, 516
Arkansas Industrial University, 60, 200, 362, 443, 532, 516
Arkansas Medical Society, 60, 199-200, 443, 516, 695, 766
Arkansas Medical Society, Journal of the, 60
Arkansas State Board of Health, 279, 695
Arkansas State Lunatic Asylum, 362
Arkansas State Medical Association, 199-200, 362
Arkansas State Pediatric Society, 696
Arkansas Tubercular Sanitarium, 516

Brown, Dr. (Tacoma, Washington), 123
Brown, James B., 73
Brown, Lawrason, *99-100*
Brown, Percy, *100*
Brown, Samuel, *100-101*, 242, 638
Brown, Solyman, *101-2*, 580
Brown, Wade Hampton, 132, 587
Brown, William, *102*
Brown, William Eustis, *102-3*
Brown, William Wells, *103*
Brown University, 12, 40, 106, 129, 249, 369, 406, 461, 495, 582, 702, 781
Bruce, David, 519
Bruce, Roscoe C., 541
Brucellosis, 519
Brunk, Andrew S., *103-4*
Brunswick, D., 259
Bryant, Henry, 63
Bryant, Ira, 800
Bryce, Peter, *104*
Bryce Hospital (Alabama), 104
Bryn Mawr College, 296, 301, 331, 452, 537, 750
Bubonic plague, 252, 416; commission to study existence of in San Francisco, 36
Buchholtz, M., 490
Buckingham, Richard Green, *104-5*
Bucknell, Martha E., 99
Bucknell University, 406
Budapest, University of, 11, 767
Buffalo (New York), public health in, 790
Buffalo, University of, 32, 177, 193, 211, 241, 254, 262, 368, 382, 534-35, 577, 606, 790, 797, 815
Buffalo Eye and Ear Infirmary, 368
Buffalo General Hospital, 368, 577, 606, 790
Buffalo Medical College, 699
Buffalo Medical Journal, 254-55, 606, 790
Buffalo Women's Hospital, 606
Buford, C. G., 245
Bull, William, *105*
Bullitt, H. M., 80
Bunch, C. C., 168
Bunnell, W. W., 585-86
Burch, Frank Earl, *105-6*
Burchell, Albert R., 652
Burgess, Alexander Manlius, *106-7*
Burnham, C. F., 168
Burnham, F. R., 410
Burns, Allan, 584-85
Burns, Robert Bruce, 422
Burrage, Walter L., 410, 735
Burrough, James William, *107*

Burton, De Witt T., *107*
Burton Mercy Hospital (Detroit), 107
Busey, Samuel Clagett, *107-8*, 422
Bush, J. M., 217
Bush, Lewis Potter, *108-9*
Bush Hill Hospital (Philadelphia), 595
Butler, A. M., 274
Butler, Henry Rutherford, *109*
Butler Hospital (Providence, Rhode Island), 56, 627
Butler University, 804
Buxton, Lauren Haynes, *109-10*
Byars, L., 73
Byford, William Heath, *110*, 515

Cabell, George, 111
Cabell, James Lawrence, *111*
Cabot, Hugh, *111-12*, 208
Cabot, Richard Clarke, *112-13*, 118, 210
Cadwalader, Thomas, *113*, 398, 405
Caesarean section, 194, 609
Caglieri, G., 731
Cain, D.J.C., 133
Caisson Disease, 689
Calanthe, Courts of, of Alabama, 542
Caldwell, Charles, *113-14*, 831
Caldwell, Eugene Wilson, *114-15*, 613
Caldwell Memorial Hospital (Idaho), 151
Calhoun, Abner Wellborn, *115*
Calhoun, Andrew B., 115
Calhoun, F. Phinizy, 115
Calhoun, F. Phinizy, Jr., 115
Calhoun, S., 606
California, 859, 873; health conditions in early, 59; medical care in early, 107
California, University of, 37, 79, 151, 232, 284, 298, 316, 342, 352, 444, 452, 487, 496, 519, 558, 625, 667, 691, 698, 713, 731, 748, 769, 795
California Academy of Medicine, 804
California Academy of Sciences, 74
California Board of Medical Examiners, 731
California Department of Public Health, 519
California Institute of Technology, 537
California Medical Association, 776
California State Board of Health, 288, 703
California State Medical Journal, 539
California State Medical Society, 99, 157, 288, 434
California State Normal School (Pennsylvania), 811
Calkins, L. A., 664
Callister, Alfred Cyril, *115-16*

Harvard University, 9, 17, 22, 27, 44, 50, 54, 57, 64, 71, 73, 84, 87-90, 100, 102, 106, 109, 112, 115, 119, 127-29, 132, 136, 138, 148, 152-53, 161, 171, 173-74, 177, 179, 193, 198, 207, 210, 216, 226, 228, 231, 241, 243, 247, 249-51, 253-54, 257-58, 268, 274, 277-78, 283-84, 287, 298, 305, 316-17, 319, 321, 334, 337, 342, 345, 347, 349, 351-52, 357, 360, 362, 365, 368-70, 375, 377-78, 384-86, 388, 392, 406, 430, 439, 442-43, 445, 447, 450, 453, 462, 469, 479, 483, 486, 493, 503, 507, 527, 540, 545-46, 549, 555, 563, 566, 572, 579, 582, 591, 597, 603, 607, 610, 613-14, 618, 621, 623, 625, 635-36, 644, 649-50, 658, 660, 664, 666, 671, 674, 676, 686, 692, 696, 700, 707-9, 722-24, 733, 735-37, 739, 743, 752, 765, 767, 773-74, 778-81, 787, 790-91, 794, 796-97, 801, 805, 807-8, 816, 820, 822, 825, 827-29, 836

Harvey Society, 216, 366, 454, 465, 643, 651, 698, 729

Hashinger, E. H., 140

Haskins, H. H., 568

Hassall, Albert, 719

Hatch Act (1887), 21

Hatcher, Robert Anthony, *334*, 705

Havana, eradication of yellow fever in, 628

Havana Yellow Fever Commission, 127, 716

Haverford College, 142, 721, 756

Hawaii, 860, 875; public health in, 434

Hawaii, University of, 767

Hawaii Academy of Family Physicians, 431

Hawaiian Medical Society, 350

Hawaii Board of Health, 543

Hawaii Bureau of Communicable Diseases, 431

Hawaii Insane Asylum, 350

Hawaii Medical Association, 402, 431

Hawaii Territorial Board of Health, 431

Hawkes, E. Zeh, 711

Hay, Thomas H., 188

Hayden, Horace H., 328, *334-35*

Hay fever, 829; treatment of, 156

Hayhurst, Emery R., 422

Haymarket Square Relief Station (Boston), 430

Hays, Isaac, *335*

Hays, Joseph, 641

Haywood, Edmund Burke, *335-36*

Haywood, Egbert, 646

Haywood, Fabius J., 335

Hazen, Allen, *336-37*

Health, child, 30

Health Authorities, Conference of State and Provincial, 474, 757

Health care organizations, 896-97

Health education, 393; municipal bureau of, 297

Health insurance, 112; AMA opposition to, 776

Health Insurance Plan of Greater New York, 626

Health Journal and Advocate of Physiological Reform, 552

Health Journal and Independent Magazine, 552

Health Officers, Association of State and Territorial, 148

Health officers, certification of, 89

Health Officers of North America, State and Provincial, 148, 327

Health Reformer, 408

Healy, Henry Herbert, *337*

Healy, W., 11

Healy, William, *337-38*

Heard, F. F., 723

Hearing: mechanism of, 767; physiology and pathology of, 168

Heart: irritable, 175; suture of the, 350

Heart Disease, Association for Prevention of, 148

Heart-lung machine, 288

Heath, Clark W., 528

Heath, Lillian, *338*

Hebra, Ferdinand (Von), 218, 796

Hebrew Hospital (Baltimore), 368

Hebrew University, 447

Heerman, Lewis, *338-39*

Heg, Elmer Ellsworth, *339-40*

Heidelberg, University of, 6, 57, 134, 142, 241, 294, 352, 419, 546, 707

Heidelberger, Michael, 485-86

Heinbecker, Peter, 69, 562

Hektoen, Ludvig, 245, *339-40*

Hektoen Institute for Medical Research, 340

Helmholtz, Hermann von, 808

Helmuth, William S., 340

Helmuth, William Tod, *340*

Hematology, 528, 691, 897; father of, 178

Hematology, American Society of, 178

Hemmeter, John Conrad, *340-41*

Hemophilia: clinical diagnosis of, 570; treatment of, 528

Hench, Philip Showalter, *341-42*, 411

Henderson, Lawrence Joseph, *342-43*

Henderson, Yandell, *343*

Viral growth, chick-embryo inoculation for, 298
Virchow, Hans, 347
Virchow, Rudolph, 250, 391, 418, 773
Virginia, 870, 887
Virginia, Medical College of, 43, 77, 183, 375, 471, 481, 764, 822
Virginia, Medical Society of, 111, 471, 473, 481
Virginia, University of, 14, 76, 111, 117, 124, 160, 219, 267, 330, 438, 464, 474, 502, 505-6, 628, 692, 745, 761, 777, 799, 833
Virginia Clinical Record, 471
Virginia Commonwealth University, 375-76
Virginia Mason Hospital (Seattle), 502, 799
Virginia Medical and Surgical Journal, 471
Virginia Medical Journal, 471
Virginia Medical Monthly, 77
Virginia Military Institute, 159, 799
Virology, development of as a specialty, 639
Virus laboratory, diagnostic, 721
Visiting Nurse Association (Cincinnati), 116
Vital statistics, 677, 775; registration of, 76
Vitamins, 513, 715, 763; discovery of, 473
Vocational Education, Federal Board for, 725
Voegtlin, Carl, 470, 766-67
Voit, Carl, 343, 465
Von Békésy, Georg, 767-68
Von Eiselberg, Toldt, 607
Von Hebra, Ferdinand, 218, 796
Von Hess, C. L., 625
Von Mansfelde, Alexander Siedschlag, 768
Von Muller, Friedrich, 643
Von Neusser, Edmund, 634
Von Pirquet, Clemens, 665
Von Winckel, Franz, 72
Voorhees, Arthur B., Jr., 75
Vosburgh, Dr. (Syracuse), 211

Wabash College (Indiana), 653, 813
Waddell, J., 230
Wagner Free Institute of Science, 441
Wahl, Harry Roswell, 769
Wahl, Henry S., 769
Waisman, Harry A., 230
Wake Forest College, 754
Waksman, Selman Abraham, 769–70
Wald, Lillian D., 770-71
Walden University (Nashville), 316, 466, 541, 801
Waldeyer, Wilhelm, 120, 347
Walker, Alvah, 771

Walker, Delos, 771
Walker, Dr. (Virginia), 47
Walker, E. L. 671
Walker, Mary Edwards, 771-72
Wall, John Perry, 181, 281, 772-73
Wallach, Otto, 426
Wally-Sternburg, Freida, 791
Walsh, James Joseph, 773
Walter Reed Hospital, 745
Walzer, Matthew, 142
Ward, Elizabeth J., 438
War Disease Control Station, 679
Ware, John, 773-74
Warfield, William Alonza, 774
Waring, C. H., 296
Waring, George Edwin, 774-75
Waring, W. R., 19
War Medicine, 330
Warner, A. R., 186
Warner, E. D., 692
Warner, Hulbert Harrington, 775-76
Warner's Safe Kidney and Liver Cure, 775
Warnshuis, Frederick Cook, 776-77
War of 1812, 28, 42-43, 50, 225, 244, 313, 364, 388, 582, 744, 781
Warren, Edward, 777-78
Warren, J. H., 360
Warren, John, 198, 572, 778-79, 780
Warren, John C., 64, 167, 253, 540, 572, 828
Warren, John Collins, 722, 779
Warren, J[ohn] Collins, 779-80
Warren, Joseph, 778
Warren, Joseph, III, 780
Warren, William Christian, 777
Warren Anatomical Museum (Harvard University), 388
Warrington, Joseph, 71
Washburn, Victor Duke, 780
Washburn College (Kansas), 514, 727
Washburne, A. W., 529
Washington, District of Columbia, 860, 874-75. *See also* District of Columbia
Washington (state of), 870, 887
Washington, Pathological Society of, 507
Washington, University of, 326, 810
Washington Academy of Sciences (District of Columbia), 108
Washington and Lee University, 624, 730
Washington College (Virginia), 244
Washington Infirmary (District of Columbia), 523
Washington Life Insurance Company, 475

About the Contributors

Paul Addis is completing a Ph.D. in history from the University of Maryland. He holds an M.A. in history from Maryland and an M.S. in public health from the University of Minnesota. Addis has taught at Maryland and has worked as a senior research associate on environmental issues for the AFL-CIO in Washington, D.C. He is the author of several articles about occupational health and is completing a history of dentistry in Va.

Virginia Allen is a specialist in the history of medicine of Okla. She received a doctorate from the University of Oklahoma, where she studied under Dr. Palmer Howard. Allen has taught medical history at the University of Oklahoma and has served as historian of the University of Texas Cancer Center in Houston. She is author of articles about the history of medicine and public health, focusing on medicine and health of the Plains Indians.

Rima D. Apple is project coordinator of the Center for Photographic Images of Medicine and Health Care, the State University of New York at Stony Brook. She received a Ph.D. in the history of medicine and history of science from the University of Wisconsin-Madison in 1981. Apple has lectured on a wide range of topics in the history of women and medicine and has published articles in the *Bulletin of the History of Medicine, Women and Health, Notable American Women*, and *Wisconsin Women, Graduate School and the Professions*.

William Barlow is professor of history at Seton Hall University. He received a Ph.D. from Ohio State University and has published articles on the history of medicine in various state and national professional journals.

Ronald Elmer Batt graduated from the University of Buffalo Medical School in 1958 and holds the position of clinical associate professor of gynecology-obstetrics at the State University of New York at Buffalo. He is a microsurgeon who specializes in reproductive surgery and is co-author, with Dr. John Naples, of the monograph *Conservative Surgery for Endometriosis in the Infertile Couple* (1982). Batt is also a specialist in the history of medicine of western N.Y. and is co-author, with Glenn Atwell, of a book on local history, *The Chapel* (1979).

Harold Bauman is associate professor of history at the University of Utah, teaching courses in the history of science and medicine. He received a Ph.D. from the University of Iowa in 1964 and taught at the College of Idaho, Cornell College, University of Illinois at Normal, and University of Oregon before assuming his position in Salt Lake City, Utah, in 1965.

William K. Beatty is professor of medical bibliography at Northwestern University, teaching courses in medical writing and the history of medicine. He received an M.S. from Columbia University in 1952 and was at the College of Physicians of Philadelphia and the University of Missouri before assuming his position in Chicago in 1962. Beatty is co-author of five popular works in the history of medicine, most recently *Epidemics* (1976), and has written historical articles for publications such as *JAMA, Practitioner,* and *Bulletin of the New York Academy of Medicine.*

Irving A. Beck is an internist in Providence, R.I. whose avocations are medical history and book collecting. He received an M.D. from Harvard University in 1936. Beck holds an appointment as lecturer in medical science at Brown University and contributes to the teaching of clinical subjects and the history of medicine.

Leland V. Bell is professor of history at Central State University in Ohio. He received a Ph.D. degree from West Virginia University in 1968 and has had extensive experience as both a college teacher and researcher. Bell is author of *In Hitler's Shadow: The Anatomy of American Nazism* (1973), *Treating the Mentally Ill: From Colonial Times to the Present* (1980), and several journal articles.

Whitfield J. Bell, Jr., received a Ph.D. from the University of Pennsylvania, where he studied under Dr. Richard H. Shryock. He also studied medical history at the Welch Library and the Johns Hopkins Institute for the History of Medicine, where he worked with Dr. Henry Sigerist and Dr. Owsei Temkin. Bell published a full-length biography of John Morgan (1965) and has written numerous articles about the history of American medicine. A sampling of his writings was published in 1975 (*The Colonial Physician and Other Essays*). He has taught history, worked on the papers of Benjamin Franklin, and served as librarian of the American Philosophical Society.

David W. Boilard is director of libraries for the School of Medicine, University of North Dakota. He received a masters of library science degree from the University of Michigan in 1975 and was associate director of the medical library of the University of South Dakota before moving to Grand Forks, N.Dak. Boilard has published and presented national and international papers in librarianship.

Charles Bonsett is a specialist in neurology and in the history of medicine and medical education of Ind. He received a medical degree from Indiana University in 1952 and was board certified in neurology in 1959. Bonsett is clinical professor of neurology at Indiana University Medical Center and director of its Muscular Dystrophy Clinic. He is also director of the Indiana Medical History Museum, editor of the *Indiana Medical History Quarterly,* and author of *Pseudohypertrophic Muscular Dystrophy* (1969) and numerous articles about neurology and Ind. medical history.

Charlotte Borst is a doctoral student at the University of Wisconsin in the Department of the History of Medicine. She is writing her dissertation on the change from midwife to physician-assisted childbirth in the late nineteenth and early twentieth centuries, focusing on Wisconsin. She received an M.A. in History from Tufts University in 1977 and an M.A. in the History of Science from the University of Wisconsin in 1980.

John A. Breinich is director of the Hawaii Medical Library. He received a B.A. in psychology from the University of Iowa, and in 1966 he received an M.S. in library science from the University of Illinois.

Patrick W. Brennen is director of the Lommen Health Sciences Library at the University of South Dakota School of Medicine. He received an M.L.S. in 1971 from the University of Illinois. In addition to being an author of several articles in library science, and an international library consultant, he is also in charge of the archives and history of medicine collection in the Lommen Library.

Gert H. Brieger is director, Institute of the History of Medicine, Johns Hopkins University. He studied the history of medicine at Johns Hopkins University and taught there, at Duke, and at the University of California, San Francisco. Brieger has written extensively about medicine in America and the history of public health and surgery.

Simon Rulin Bruesch specializes in neuroscience and the history of medicine. He received a Ph.D. (anatomy) in 1940 and an M.D. in 1941, both from Northwestern University. He has served for 41 years on the faculty of the University of Tennessee and is presently Goodman Professor of Anatomy at the University of Tennessee Health Sciences Center, Memphis. In June 1982 it was announced that his former students had subscribed $1.2 million to establish the S. R. Bruesch Alumni Professorship in Anatomy. Bruesch is author of articles about neuroscience and the history of medicine.

Chester Burns is the James Wade Rockwell Professor of Medical History at the University of Texas Medical Branch at Galveston. He received an M.D. from Vanderbilt University School of Medicine and a Ph.D. in the history of medicine from the Johns Hopkins University School of Medicine. Burns has published 30 essays on various aspects of medical history, especially the history of medical ethics. He is the editor of *Legacies in Law and Medicine* (1977) and *Legacies in Ethics and Medicine* (1977).

Philip Cash is professor of history at Emmanuel College, Boston, Mass., where he teaches courses on the political and social aspects of American history and on American medical history. He received a Ph.D. from Boston College in 1968. Cash is author of *Medical Men at the Siege of Boston* (1973) and senior editor of *Medicine in Massachusetts, 1620-1820* (1980) and has contributed articles about medical history to the *Bulletin of the History of Medicine, Harvard Medical Alumni Bulletin, Journal of the American Medical Association,* and *New England Journal of Medicine.*

James H. Cassedy is an historian at the History of Medicine Division, National Library of Medicine (NLM), and former president (1982-84) of the American Association for the History of Medicine. He received a Ph.D. in American Civilization from Brown University in 1959. Before joining the NLM in 1968, Cassedy directed U.S. cultural centers in Haiti, Burma, and Pakistan and was executive secretary of NIH's History of the Life Sciences Study Section. He is author of *Charles V. Chapin and the Public Health Movement* (1962), *Demography in Early America* (1969), the forthcoming *American Medicine in a Numerical Age,* and numerous articles.

Sandra L. Chaff is director of the Archives and Special Collections on Women in Medicine and research instructor in the history of medicine at the Medical College of Pennsylvania. She received an M.S. in library science from Case Western Reserve University and is one of the editors of *Women in Medicine: A Bibliography of the Literature on Women Physicians.*

Betty Clements is librarian and editor in the Department of Family Practice at the University of Iowa College of Medicine. She received a master's degree in English literature from Duke University in 1968 and a master's degree in library science from the University of California, Los Angeles, in 1971. She has worked in the rare book room of the University of Alabama and in the Missionary Research Library at Union Theological Seminary (New York City). Clements has been reference librarian at Scripps College and archivist and acting head of the special collection at Samford University (Birmingham, Ala.). Since going to the University of Iowa in 1975, she has contributed research and editorial skills to book and journal publications of faculty, residents, and staff in the Department of Family Practice.

Thomas E. Cone, Jr., is professor of clinical pediatrics, emeritus, at Harvard Medical School and senior associate in clinical genetics and medicine at the Children's Hospital Medical Center, Boston. He received a medical degree from the Columbia University College of Physicians and Surgeons in 1939 and is author of *200 Years of Feeding Infants in America* (1976) and *History of American Pediatrics* (1979).

Eugene H. Conner, a specialist in anesthesiology, is in private practice. His avocation is the history of medicine. Conner received a medical degree from the University of Maryland College of Medicine in 1945, with postgraduate studies at the University of Pennsylvania School of Medicine. He has taught at Maryland, Pennsylvania, and Louisville and, while chairman of anesthesiology at the University of Louisville, 1957-71, conducted lecture courses in medical history. He is the historian of the Kentucky Medical Association and has contributed articles to the *Bulletin of the History of Medicine, Journal of the History of Medicine and Allied Sciences,* and other journals.

David L. Cowen is professor emeritus of history at Rutgers University. Trained in American history at Rutgers and Columbia, he was on the Rutgers faculty from 1933 until his retirement in 1974. From 1945 to 1974 he was chairman of the Department of History of University College, Rutgers, and from 1952 he was lecturer in the history of pharmacy at the Rutgers College of Pharmacy. Cowen has long been a contributor to the fields of the history of pharmacy and the history of medicine. Among his books are *Medicine and Health in New Jersey: A History* (1964), *The New Jersey Pharmaceutical Association, 1870-1970* (1970), and *The Spread and Influence of British Pharmacopoeial and Related Literature* (1974).

Charlotte Lazear Cutter is a freelance historian and writer. She holds an M.A. in history from the University of New Mexico, Albuquerque. Her writing and research interests are in the history of medicine, science, and social welfare.

Marc H. Dawson is instructor of the history of medicine and African history at Union College, Schenectady, N.Y., and is completing his dissertation at the University of Wisconsin. He has been a research associate at the University of Nairobi, Kenya, and has published an article about smallpox in Kenya, which appeared in *Social Science and Medicine*.

Gordon B. Dodds is professor of history at Portland State University, teaching courses on the history of the Pacific Northwest and Oreg. He received a Ph.D. from the University of Wisconsin in 1959. Dodds is author of several books and articles about the history of the West, including *Oregon: A Bicentennial History* (1977).

John P. Dolan served as professor of the history of public health at the University of South Carolina, Columbia, before his untimely death. He published several books and articles about the history of American medicine and public health.

Craig Donegan is an instructor in history at Southwest Texas State University in San Marcos. His current work is in labor and medical history under the directorship of John Duffy at the University of Maryland, and he is completing his dissertation on attitudes toward industrial workers' health in the northern United States from 1830 to 1870.

Virginia Drachman is professor of history at Tufts University, teaching courses on the history of medicine and the history of women. She received a Ph.D. from SUNY, Buffalo, in 1976 and a Rockefeller Foundation Humanities Fellowship in 1977. She was also a fellow of the Bunting Institute of Radcliffe College in 1978 and a Radcliffe Research Scholar in 1982. Drachman is author of articles about the history of medicine and the history of women, most recently "Female Solidarity and Professional Success: The Dilemma of Women Doctors in Late Nineteenth Century America," in the *Journal of Social History*.

John Duffy, who received a Ph.D. from the University of California, Los Angeles, in 1946, recently retired from the Priscilla Alden Burke Chair of American History at the University of Maryland. He specializes in the history of American medicine and public health and has written or edited ten books, including a two-volume history of medicine in La., a two-volume history of public health in New York City, a study of epidemics in colonial America, and a thematic text, *The Healers*. Duffy also has published some 70 articles, has served as the editor of the *American Historical Review*, and has held offices in various historical associations.

Jerome Edwards is professor of history at the University of Nevada, Reno. He contributed the biographical sketches of Nev. physicians to this dictionary.

Ralph Edwards is dean of administration and planning and professor of health science at Kingsborough Community College of the City University of New York. He received a doctorate from Columbia University in 1959. Edwards helped found Kingsborough Community College and served in several deanships at that college. Before going to Kingsborough, he was in charge of the health education department and was chief premedical-predental advisor at Columbia College, N.Y. (1957-64). He has taught health education at Queens College, University of Illinois, Teachers College of Columbia University, and New York University, and his recent articles have been about the history of medicine and health care.

Samuel Eichold is a specialist in internal medicine, with a special interest in diabetes, which led to the founding and operation of Camp Seale Harris for Children with Diabetes, the first such camp east of the Mississippi and south of the Mason-Dixon line. His undergraduate and graduate training was at Tulane University. With the establishment of the University of South Alabama College of Medicine in Mobile, Eichold entered the academic world and now is professor in the Department of Medicine and preceptor for the senior elective in the history of medicine. He was founder of and is curator of the Heustis Medical Museum at the college, is author of numerous papers in his specialty, and serves on the editorial board of the *Alabama Journal of the Medical Sciences*.

G. E. Erikson is professor of medical science and chairman of the section of morphology at Brown University. He teaches courses in human, comparative, and surgical anatomy and in the history of biology and medicine. He received a Ph.D. from Harvard University in 1948 and taught there until 1965. Erikson is archivist and historian for the American Association of Anatomists and archivist and co-historian for the American Association of Physical Anthropologists. He is currently working on a history of anatomy in America from 1888 to 1937.

J. Worth Estes is professor of pharmacology, also specializing in the history of pharmacology, at the Boston University School of Medicine. He received an M.A. in pharmacology (1963) and a medical degree (1964) from Boston University. Estes is author of *Hall Jackson and the Purple Foxglove* (1979) and co-author of *Medicine In Massachusetts, 1620-1820* (1980) and has contributed articles to journals of medicine and medical history.

Leslie A. Falk received an M.D. in 1942 at the Johns Hopkins School of Medicine, where he studied medical history under Dr. Henry Sigerist, and received a doctorate of philosophy in medical sciences from Oxford University. He taught at the University of Pittsburgh from 1953 to 1963 and then moved to Meharry Medical College, where he specializes in black medical history. Falk is author of many articles about the history of blacks in medicine and the health of blacks and has worked on a history of Meharry Medical College.

Daniel M. Fox is professor of humanities in medicine at the State University of New York at Stony Brook. He received a Ph.D. in history from Harvard University, where he was assistant professor of history and public administration. Fox is author of *Engines of Culture* (1963), *The Discovery of Abundance* (1967), *Economists and Health Care* (1979), and articles in journals in the fields of history and health services research.

Norman Gevitz is assistant professor of the social sciences at the Illinois Institute of Technology. He received a Ph.D. in sociology from the University of Chicago in 1980. Gevitz is author of *The D.O.'s: Osteopathic Medicine in America* (1982).

John S. Goff is professor of social science at Phoenix College, and he has been interested in Ariz. history since he arrived there in 1960. He received a Ph.D. in history from the University of Southern California in 1960 and a J.D. from Arizona State University in 1974. A member of the Ariz. bar, Goff is author of several books and monographs.

Gerald N. Grob is professor of history and chairperson of the Department of History at Rutgers University. He received a Ph.D. from Northwestern University in 1958 and taught at Clark University in Worcester, Mass., before moving to N.J. He has taught courses on American social history and the history of medicine and disease in America. Grob's books include *The State and the Mentally Ill* (1966), *Mental Institutions in America: Social Policy to 1875* (1973), *Edward Jarvis and the Medical World of Nineteenth Century America* (1978), and a forthcoming book tentatively entitled *Institutional Care in Modern America*.

E. Ashby Hammond is professor of history, emeritus, at the University of Florida, Gainsville. In 1941 he received a Ph.D. from the University of North Carolina, Chapel Hill, where his major interest was the history of medieval England. Hammond is co-author of *The Medical Practitioners of Medieval England* (1965) and has published articles in the *Bulletin of the History of Medicine*, *Journal of the History of Medicine and Allied Sciences*, and *Medical History*. In recent years, his interest in medical practice in nine-teenth-century Fla. has resulted in numerous articles in the *Journal of the Florida Medical Association* and *Florida Historical Quarterly*.

Arthur A. Hart is director of the Idaho State Historical Society. During the past 12 years, he has published 4 books and more than 700 articles about western history. After receiving a master of fine arts degree from the University of Washington in 1948, he taught at colleges in Idaho, N.H., and Mass. before assuming his present position in 1969.

Andrea Rose Carroll Helms is associate professor of political science at the University of Alaska-Fairbanks. She received a Ph.D. from the University of Connecticut in 1968 and taught at Moorhead State University (Minn.) and Central Michigan University before going to the University of Alaska in 1973. Her specialties include Alaskan politics and history.

Bernice M. Hetzner is emeritus professor and librarian for Nebr. medical history at the University of Nebraska Medical Center, Omaha. Before her retirement, she was director (1948-73) of both the University of Nebraska Medical Center Library of Medicine and the Midcontinental Regional Medical Library Program. She received a library science degree from the University of Denver and an M.A. from the University of Northern Colorado. Hetzner has done extensive research in Nebr. medical history and has published and edited in that field, including a revision with index of Albert F. Tyler and Ella F. Auerbach, *History of Medicine in Nebraska* (1977).

Robert Hudson is trained in internal medicine and the history of medicine. He received a medical degree from the University of Kansas in 1952 and an M.A. in the history of medicine from Johns Hopkins in 1966. Hudson is chairman of the Department of the History and Philosophy of Medicine at the University of Kansas Medical Center and serves as president (1984-86) of the American Association for the History of Medicine.

Marion Hunt is a doctoral candidate in the history of social welfare at Washington University, St. Louis, where she held an Olin Fellowship from 1976 to 1980. Her dissertation is a study of women's role in the development of pediatrics. She has published articles on women and nineteenth-century medicine in the *Bulletin of the Missouri Historical Society*.

John W. Ifkovic is associate professor of history at Westfield State College, teaching courses in early American history and Mass. history. He received a Ph.D. in history from the University of Virginia in 1974, after having received an M.A.T. from Yale. Ifkovic has done extensive research in the history of Conn. and the New England region and is author of *Connecticut's Nationalist Revolutionary: Jonathan Trumbull, Junior* (1977).

Glen Pierce Jenkins, a graduate of Scripps College in Calif., received a master's degree in library science from Case Western Reserve University in 1972. Currently she is rare book librarian and archivist for the historical division of the Cleveland Health Sciences Library and lectures on rare book librarianship and medical history at the university.

Mary Van Hulle Jones is a registered nurse and historian of nursing. She received a B.S.N. in 1952 and an M.A. in the history of science in 1981 from the University of Wisconsin-Madison, where she is presently a doctoral candidate in the history of medicine. Jones is author of an article on Wis. hospitals, in Ronald Numbers and Judith Leavitt, eds., *Wisconsin Medicine-Historical Perspectives* (1981).

Robert J. T. Joy is professor and chairman of the section of medical history at the Uniformed Services University of the Health Sciences in Bethesda, Md. He is an internist who received a medical degree from Yale and just retired as a colonel in the Army Medical Corps. Joy is the editor of the *Journal of the History of Medicine and Allied Sciences*.

Charles S. Judd, Jr., is professor of surgery and executive of the Division of Medical History at the University of Hawaii School of Medicine. He received an M.D. from Yale University and has written several articles on the history of medicine.

Elizabeth Barnaby Keeney is a graduate student in the history of science at the University of Wisconsin-Madison, with an interest in science, medicine, and popular culture in America.

Ramunas A. Kondratas is a curator in the Division of Medical Sciences of the Smithsonian Institution's National Museum of American History. He received a Ph.D. from Harvard University in 1977 and is author of articles on the history of health sciences in the United States and Eastern and Western Europe. At the museum, Kondratas collects, interprets, and exhibits artifacts that document the history of public health and pharmacy in America.

Donald Konold is professor of history at Arkansas State University, where he has been teaching since receiving the Ph.D. from the University of Missouri in 1954. He is author of *A History of American Medical Ethics* (1962) and "Codes of Medical Ethics, I. History," in the *Encyclopedia of Bioethics* (1978).

Dorothy I. Lansing is a specialist in gynecology and the history of medicine. She received a medical degree from Indiana University in 1947 and obtained subsequent training at Philadelphia General Hospital. Married to W. Robert Penman, who also specializes in the history of medicine along with obstetrics and gynecology, Lansing is the editor of *Medicine and Science in Early America* (1982) and the *Serum Cestricum* series of her local medical society. She is historian to the Obstetrical Society of Philadelphia, having also been clerk of the Section on Medical History, College of Physicians of Philadelphia.

Judith Walzer Leavitt is associate professor of the history of medicine, the history of science, and women's studies at the University of Wisconsin-Madison, where she also serves as chair of the Department of the History of Medicine. Leavitt received an M.A. (1966) and a Ph.D. (1975) from the University of Chicago, where she specialized in American urban and public health history. She is the co-editor of three books about American medical history and the author of *The Healthiest City: Milwaukee and the Politics of Health Reform* (1982). Her current research focuses on the history of childbirth in America.

Susan Eyrich Lederer is a doctoral candidate in the Department of the History of Science at the University of Wisconsin-Madison. Her dissertation is about the history of human experimentation in America in the Progressive era.

Marshall Scott Legan is associate professor of history and head of the Department of History and Government at Northeast Louisiana University. He received a Ph.D. from the University of Mississippi in 1968 and is author of articles about medical history and public health in the South that have appeared in the *Bulletin of the History of Medicine, Journal of the History of Medicine and Allied Sciences*, and *Journal of Mississippi History*.

Brian C. Lister is professor of history at the University of Maine at Farmington. He received a Ph.D. from the University of Maine at Orono in 1975 and has done postdoctoral work at the University of Arizona, Tucson, funded by the National Endowment for the Humanities. His Ph.D. dissertation was a study of Dr. Alonzo Garcelon, one of Maine's foremost early physicians.

Lawrence D. Longo is professor of physiology and obstetrics and gynecology at the School of Medicine, Loma Linda University. He received a medical degree from that institution in 1954, after which he taught at the University of Southern California, University of California, Los Angeles, and University of Pennsylvania. Longo edited *Respiratory Gas Exchange and Blood Flow in the Placenta* (1973) and *Fetal and Newborn Cardiovascular Physiology* (2 vols., 1978) and has written numerous scientific and historical papers. Currently he edits the section "Classic Pages in Obstetrics and Gynecology" in the *American Journal of Obstetrics and Gynecology*.

Berit Midelfort is a physician who was trained in medical history at the University of Wisconsin-Madison, studying under Gunter Risse, Ronald Numbers, and Judith Leavitt.

Genevieve Miller is the retired director of the Howard Dittrick Museum of Historical Medicine, Cleveland, Ohio, and associate professor emeritus of Case Western Reserve University School of Medicine. She is currently research associate at the Johns Hopkins Institute of the History of Medicine, where, as the first graduate of the Institute, she received an M.A. in 1939. Miller obtained a Ph.D. in the history of science from Cornell University in 1955. Her publications include *The Adoption of Inoculation for Smallpox in England and France* (1957), *Bibliography of the History of Medicine in the U.S. and Canada, 1939-1960* (1964), and articles about smallpox inoculation, American medical history, medical education, and medical historiography. She is a past president of the American Association for the History of Medicine.

Regina Morantz received a Ph.D. in American history from Columbia University in

1971. She now teaches women's history, history of the family, and the social history of medicine at the University of Kansas and, for several years, has been working on a historical study of women physicians in America. From 1976 to 1978 she served as academic consultant and principal interviewer for the Oral History Project on Women in Medicine sponsored by the Medical College of Pennsylvania. Morantz is editor of *In Her Own Words, Oral Histories of Women Physicians* (1982) and has published numerous articles about the history of women and health in the *American Quarterly, Journal of Social History, Reviews in American History, Journal of American History, Sickness and Health in America, Clio's Consciousness Raised,* and *Medicine Without Doctors.*

James Polk Morris III is a postdoctoral fellow at the School of Public Health, University of Texas Health Science Center, Houston, Tex., and historian of the Methodist Hospital (since 1980). He received a master's degree in American history from the University of New Orleans (1969) and a Ph.D. in American social history from Tulane University (1973), where he studied under John Duffy. He received an M.P.H. in community health from the University of Texas in 1983. Morris has taught medical history at Tulane University School of Medicine (1972-74), University of Texas Medical Branch at Galveston (1974-76), and Texas A & M University (1976-79).

Pierce C. Mullen is professor of history at Montana State University, teaching courses in the history of science and medicine. He received a Ph.D. from the University of California, Berkeley, in 1964. Mullen has published articles about nineteenth-century German medical and biological science and about the history of medicine in Mont.

Robert L. Murphy is director of learning resources (medical library, photography, television, and illustrations) at the West Virginia University Medical Center. He received an undergraduate degree from George Washington University and an M.L.S. from the Catholic University of America (1970). Murphy was previously a technical information specialist with the Library of Congress, National Science Foundation, and National Aeronautics and Space Administration.

Kenneth R. Nodyne is professor of history at West Liberty State College, in W. Va. He received a master's degree from the University of Pennsylvania (1962) and a Ph.D. from New York University (1969). Nodyne recently completed *History of Dentistry in West Virginia,* sponsored by the state dental association. He is co-author of *Wheeling: An Annotated Bibliography*; has written articles in various historical journals; is editor of the *Upper Ohio Valley Historical Review*; and is a member of the editorial board of *West Virginia History.*

Ynez Violé O'Neill is associate professor of medical history at the University of California, Los Angeles. A fourth-generation Californian, she received a Ph.D. from the University of California, Los Angeles, in 1964. A trustee of the California Historical Society, O'Neill has written articles for the *California Historical Quarterly* and *California History* as well as for the *Journal of the American Medical Association, Bulletin of the History of Medicine,* and *Journal of the History of Medicine.* She is author of *Speech and Speech Disorders in Western Thought before 1600* (1980).

William J. Orr is curator of manuscripts of the Center for Western Studies of the Joslyn Art Museum in Omaha, Nebr. He received a Ph.D. in modern European history from the University of Wisconsin-Madison in 1971, after which he taught at Beloit College and Carroll College. He also served as a research associate in the Department of the History of Medicine of the University of Wisconsin. Orr is author of various articles including "William Beaumont's Reception at Home and Abroad," in *Isis* (1982), co-authored with Ronald L. Numbers.

Anthony Palmieri III is associate professor of pharmaceutics at the University of Wyoming. He received a master's degree from the University of Rhode Island (1973) and a Ph.D. in pharmaceutics from the University of Georgia (1976). Palmieri has published numerous scientific, educational, and historical articles in journals such as the *Journal of Pharmaceutical Sciences, American Journal of Pharmaceutical Education, Pharmacy in History,* and *Annals of Wyoming.* He is also the editor of *The Mask of Kappa Psi.*

Steven J. Peitzman is associate professor of medicine at the Medical College of Pennsylvania. He received a medical degree from Temple University in 1971 and then did postgraduate clinical training in internal medicine and nephrology at the Medical College of Pennsylvania, where he now practices and teaches these disciplines. His historical investigations of various subjects in American and English medicine have appeared in the *Bulletin of the History of Medicine* and other journals.

Martin S. Pernick is assistant professor of history at the University of Michigan, where he teaches in both the history department and the Inteflex Medical Program. He received a Ph.D. from Columbia University in 1979 and has taught at the Hershey Medical Center of Pennsylvania State University and Harvard University. Pernick is author of *A Calculus of Suffering: Pain, Professionalism, and Anesthesia in Nineteenth Century American Medicine* (1983) and articles in the *William and Mary Quarterly, Hastings Center Report, Encyclopedia of Bioethics,* and several anthologies.

Charles V. Pollack, Jr., is currently a student at Tulane University School of Medicine. He received a masters degree in history from Emory University (1980), where he studied under James Harvey Young, and is continuing research in the history of medicine.

David O. Powell is professor of history at the C. W. Post Center of Long Island University. He received a Ph.D. from the Ohio State University and is author of articles in the *Bulletin of the History of Medicine* and *Journal of the History of Medicine and Allied Sciences.*

Robert E. Rakel is professor and head of the department of family practice at the University of Iowa College of Medicine, where he established the History of Medicine Society. He received a medical degree from the University of Cincinnati in 1958 and, after four years of postgraduate study, was a practicing family physician in Newport Beach, Calif., until joining the faculty of the College of Medicine at the University of California, Irvine. He went to Iowa in 1971 to join the faculty of the College of Medicine. Rakel is editor of the textbook *Family Practice* (1973) and the *Yearbook of Family Practice* (1980), author of *Principles of Family Medicine* (1977), and co-editor of the journal *The Female Patient.* He serves on the editorial boards of several journals, including the *Journal of the American Medical Association* and *Archives of Internal Medicine.*

Larry Remele is historian-editor and acting director of the Education and Interpretation Division of the State Historical Society of North Dakota at Bismarck. Author of both scholarly and informal works about state and local history, he edits *North Dakota History: Journal of the Northern Plains.* Remele holds a master's degree from the University of North Dakota.

Frank Bradway Rogers is professor of surgery, emeritus, at the University of Colorado. He was educated at Yale (B.A.), Ohio State (M.D.), and Columbia (M.L.S.). He served as first director of the National Library of Medicine (1949-63) and was president of the Medical Library Association (1962-63) and American Association for the History of Medicine (1966-68). Rogers is the compiler of *Selected Papers of John Shaw Billings* (1965). His most recent contributions are in *Centenary of Index Medicus* (1980) and *A Celebration of Medical History* (1982).

Barbara Gutmann Rosenkrantz is professor of the history of science at Harvard University. She received a Ph.D. in history from Clark University in 1970 and teaches courses in the history of public health and medicine in both the Faculty of Arts and Sciences and the Faculty of Public Health. Rosenkrantz is author of *Public Health and the State* (1972) and articles about disease and its consequence in the nineteenth century and is editor of "Public Health Then and Now" in the *American Journal of Public Health*.

Robert Rosenthal retired after 57 years of pediatric practice. He graduated from the medical school of Vienna (Austria) University in 1922 and is assistant professor of pediatrics emeritus of the University of Minnesota and historian emeritus of the Ramsay County Medical Society. Rosenthal has published a number of articles dealing mainly with medico-historical subjects.

David Rosner is associate professor of health administration at Baruch College and Mt. Sinai School of Medicine and teaches courses in health administration and the history of health care. He received a Ph.D. in the history of science from Harvard University in 1978, where he was a Macy Fellow in the History of Medicine and Biology. Presently he is a National Endowment for the Humanities Fellow at the Hastings Center. Rosner is author of *A Once Charitable Enterprise: Hospitals and Health Care in Brooklyn and New York, 1885-1915* (1982) and is an editor of *Health Care in America: Essays in Social History* (1979). He has also published articles in *Health and Society, American Quarterly, American Journal of Public Health,* and other journals.

Lewis P. Rubin is a resident in pediatrics at the Children's Hospital Medical Center in Boston. He received an M.D. in 1982 and is completing a Ph.D. in the history of science and medicine from Yale University. Rubin has taught at Yale and the University of Hartford and is author of several articles about science, medicine, and public health during the seventeenth to twentieth centuries.

Guillermo C. Sanchez received a medical degree from Harvard University and is a practicing internist at the Massachusetts General Hospital. He also is a member of the faculty of the Harvard Medical School. Sanchez has a special interest in the history of anesthesia and the history of medicine in Boston, especially during the nineteenth century.

Rennie B. Schoepflin is a doctoral candidate in the History of Science and Medicine Department at the University of Wisconsin-Madison, where he received an M.A. in 1980. He is completing a dissertation in "Christian Science Healing in American Society: Theory and Practice from 1865 to 1910."

Edward Shoemaker is a graduate student in the history department of Emory University, where he studies under the direction of James Harvey Young. Shoemaker specializes in the social history of the United States in the nineteenth century and is completing a dissertation on the Irish of Savannah, 1840-80.

Dale C. Smith teaches the history of preventive medicine and medical history at the Uniformed Services University of the Health Sciences. In 1979 he received a Ph.D. in history of medicine from the University of Minnesota, where he studied with Leonard Wilson. He taught at Minnesota before assuming his position in Bethesda, Md. Smith is author of several articles about the history of infectious diseases and the history of medical education.

Duane R. Sneddeker is completing a Ph.D. dissertation in history at Washington University of St. Louis. His dissertation is about the development of the Washington University Medical Center, 1910-41. Sneddeker has assisted in the chancellor's Oral History Project at Washington University and also did work in local history for the Landmarks Association of St. Louis, Mo.

Michael M. Sokal is professor of history at the Worcester Polytechnic Institute in Mass. A historian of science and technology with a Ph.D. from Case Western Reserve University (1972), he has written extensively on the history of psychology, particularly in the United States. His articles and reviews have appeared in numerous journals, including *Isis, American Psychologist, Journal of the History of Behavioral Sciences,* and *Annals of Science, 1880-1888* (1981), and he compiled (with Patrice A. Rafail) *A Guide to Manuscript Collections in the History of Psychology and Related Areas* (1982).

Phinizy Spalding is associate professor of history at the University of Georgia. Spalding received a Ph.D. from the University of North Carolina (Chapel Hill, N.C.) in 1963 and taught at the College of Charleston before going to the University of Georgia in 1966. He is author of *Oglethorpe in America* (1977), which was nominated by the University of Chicago Press for a Pulitzer Prize in two categories. He also is co-author of *A History of Georgia* (1977), recently published *The Book of Accessions, Georgia Depositories* (1981), and was editor of the *Georgia Historical Quarterly* (1973-80). Spalding's history of the Medical College of Georgia is soon to be published.

Elizabeth H. Thomson is a research associate in the section of the history of medicine at the Yale University School of Medicine. Educated at Simmons College and Mount Holyoke, she served as an editor of the *Yale Journal of Biology and Medicine* (1950-60) and *Journal of the History and Science of Medicine* (1948-72). Thomson also is author (with John F. Fulton) of a biography of Benjamin Silliman (1948), a life of Harvey Cushing (1950, reissued in 1980), and a number of articles in various medical and historical journals.

Lester J. Wallman is a neurosurgeon who received a medical degree from Yale in 1938 and his specialty training in Stockholm, Sweden, and New Haven and Hartford, Conn. Since 1946 he has been on the faculty of the University of Vermont College of Medicine, where he is now emeritus professor. Wallman has taught and written about Vt. medical history.

John Harley Warner received an M.A. in the history of science from the University of Wisconsin in 1977 and an A.M. from Harvard University in 1978. He is completing his dissertation on medical therapeutics in nineteenth-century America, to fulfill requirements for the Ph.D. in the history of science from Harvard University. Warner has published essays on the history of medicine in *Perspectives in American History, Bulletin of the History of Medicine, Medical History,* and *Journal of the History of Medicine and Allied Sciences,* as well as in Ronald L. Numbers, ed., *The Education of American Physicians* (1980).

Margaret Humphreys Warner received an A.M. in the history of science from Harvard University, where she is currently a Ph.D. medical student. She is author of articles in the *Journal of the History of Medicine and Allied Sciences* and *Journal of Southern History*.

James Clifton Whorton is associate professor of biomedical history at the University of Washington, teaching courses in the history of medicine and public health. He received a Ph.D. in history of science from the University of Wisconsin in 1969 and has taught in Seattle since that time. Whorton has authored *Before Silent Spring* (1975), *Crusaders for Fitness* (1982), and articles in the *Bulletin of the History of Medicine* and *Journal of Sport History*.

William H. Williams is an associate professor of history, University of Delaware Parallel Program, Georgetown, Del. He received a Ph.D. from the University of Delaware in 1971 and has taught history for that institution since 1967. Williams is author of *Anglo-*

America's First Hospital: The Pennsylvania Hospital (1976) and articles in the *Journal of the American Medical Association, Pennsylvania Magazine of History and Biography, American Journal of Hospital Pharmacy,* and *Dictionary of American Biography.*

James Harvey Young is Charles Howard Candler Professor of American Social History at Emory University, where he has taught since receiving a Ph.D. from the University of Illinois in 1941. His research field has been the history of quackery and of food and drug regulation in America. Young is author of *The Toadstool Millionaires* (1961), *The Medical Messiahs* (1967), and *American Self-Dosage Medicine* (1974).

About the Editors

Martin Kaufman received a doctorate from Tulane University in 1969, where he was a Josiah Macy, Jr., Fellow in the History of Medicine. He developed an interest in the history of medicine as a student of John Duffy, both at the University of Pittsburgh and at Tulane University. Kaufman is author of *Homeopathy in America* (1971), *American Medical Education: Formative Years* (1976), *The University of Vermont College of Medicine* (1979), and articles, essays, and reviews in a large number of journals. He is editorial director of the *Historical Journal of Massachusetts*, director of the Institute for Massachusetts Studies of Westfield State College, and professor of history at Westfield State College in Mass.

Stuart Galishoff is associate professor of history at Georgia State University, teaching courses in American urban history and the history of American public health and social welfare. He received a doctorate in urban history from New York University, where he studied under Bayrd Still. Galishoff is author of *Safeguarding the Public Health: Newark, 1895-1918* (1975) and articles in the *Bulletin of the History of Medicine* and *Journal of the History of Medicine and Allied Sciences*.

Todd L. Savitt is associate professor of medical humanities at the East Carolina University School of Medicine, Greenville, N.C., where he holds an affiliate appointment in the history department. He attended the University of Rochester School of Medicine (1965-68) before entering the University of Virginia, where he received a Ph.D. in history in 1975. Savitt studied the history of medicine and the history of science at Duke University and then taught medical humanities and history for six years (1976-82) at the University of Florida. He is author of *Medicine and Slavery* (1978) and several articles on black health in the United States.

Joseph Carvalho III is the supervisor of the genealogy and local history department at the Springfield (Mass.) City Library. He received an M.A. from the College of William and Mary in 1977. Carvalho has served on the editorial board of the *Historical Journal of Massachusetts* since its inception in 1972 and has been associate editor since 1978. A certified genealogical records searcher, he is also president of the local history section of the Massachusetts Library Association and is an M.L.S. candidate at the University of Rhode Island.